MANAGEMENT GUIDELINES FOR NURSE PRACTITIONERS WORKING WITH ADULTS

D1516859

New Editions of F. A. Davis's
Management Guidelines for Nurse Practitioners Serie

Unique clinical references created to help nurse practitioners manage problems the encounter with clients throughout the life span

❖ *Management Guidelines for Nurse Practitioners*
Working with Adults, 2nd Edition
By Lynne M. Hektor Dunphy
ISBN 0-8036-1117-X

> ❖ *Management Guidelines for Nurse Practitioners*
> *Working with Children and Adolescents, 2nd Edition*
> By Nancy L. Herban Hill and Linda M. Sullivan
> ISBN 0-8036-1102-1

❖ *Management Guidelines for Nurse Practitioners*
Working with Women, 2nd Edition
By Kathleen M. Pelletier Brown
ISBN 0-8036-1116-1

PDA versions of these books, including a free trial available at www.fadavis.com

> ❖ *Management Guidelines for Nurse Practitioners*
> *Working with Older Adults, 2nd Edition*
> By Laurie Kennedy-Malone, Kathleen Ryan Fletcher,
> and Lori Martin Plank
> ISBN 0-8036-1120-X

Each book:
- Is pocket-sized for on-the-spot consultation,
- Focuses on health promotions, anticipatory guidance, and disorder guideli
- Focuses on recommendations and guidelines, not theory,
- Includes ICD-9 codes for all the disorders,
- Includes diagnostic test information tables with test name, results indicatin disorder, and CPT codes,
- Lists one or two "Signal Symptoms" for each disorder that helps nurse practitioners quickly target potential differential diagnoses.

Recently Published:

> ❖ *Management Guidelines for Nurse Practitioners*
> *Working in Family Practice*
> By Alice F. Running and Amy E. Berndt
> ISBN 0-8036-0810-1
> - Organized by anatomical areas, it covers 310 disorders and conditions, with rationales and causes provided for abnormal test values.

Purchase copies of one or all of the books in F. A. Davis's
Management Guidelines Series
as well as **related PDA software**
from your local health science bookstore or directly from F. A. Davis
by shopping online at www.fadavis.com
or calling 800-323-3555 (US), 800-665-1148 (CAN).

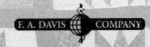

F. A. DAVIS COMPANY

MANAGEMENT GUIDELINES FOR NURSE PRACTITIONERS WORKING WITH ADULTS

Second Edition

Lynne M. Hektor Dunphy, PhD, APRN-BC

Professor and Assistant Dean for the Graduate Program
Christine E. Lynn College of Nursing
Florida Atlantic University
Boca Raton, FL
and
Family Nurse Practitioner
Palmetto Park Medical Associates
Boca Raton, FL

F. A. DAVIS COMPANY | Philadelphia

10/07

F. A. Davis Company
1915 Arch Street
Philadelphia, PA 19103

Printed in Canada

Last digit indicates print number: 10 9 8 7 6 5 4 3 2 1

Acquisitions Editor: Joanne Patzek DaCunha, RN, MSN
Developmental Editor: Diane Blodgett
Cover Designer: Louis J. Forgione

As new scientific information becomes available through basic and clinical research, recommended treatments and drug therapies undergo changes. The authors and publisher have done everything possible to make this book accurate, up to date, and in accord with accepted standards at the time of publication. The authors, editors, and publisher are not responsible for errors or omissions or for consequences from application of the book, and make no warranty, expressed or implied, with regard to the contents of the book. Any practice described in this book should be applied by the reader in accordance with professional standards of care used with regard to the unique circumstances that may apply in each situation. The reader is advised always to check product information (package inserts) for changes and new information regarding dose and contraindications before administering any drug. Caution is especially urged when using new or infrequently ordered drugs.

Library of Congress Cataloging-in-Publication Data

Management guidelines for nurse practitioners working with adults/ [edited by] Lynne M. Hektor Dunphy.—2nd ed.
    p. ; cm.
Includes index.
Prev. ed. published as: Management guidelines for adult nurse practitioners, c1999.
ISBN 0-8036-1117-X
  1. Primary care (Medicine) 2. Nurse practitioners. 3. Medical Protocols. I. Dunphy, Lynne M. Hektor. Management guidelines for adult nurse practitioners.
  [DNLM: 1. Primary Nursing Care. 2. Nursing Assessment. WY 101 M266 2003]
RT82.8.M33 2003
610.73—dc21

                                                                        2003053077

To the Memory of my Mother
My Biggest Cheerleader and Strongest Supporter
For all of her love, which is much missed

PREFACE

Management Guidelines for Nurse Practitioners Working with Adults,
2E, is designed for advanced practice nurses and students who are providing primary care to adults. These guidelines were developed by clinical experts to provide fast and easy access to information needed to
provide comprehensive care to adult patients in the primary care setting.
This information will also be of use to physicians and physician assistants
in primary care, clinical nurse specialists, case managers, community
health nurses, school nurses, and RNs providing ambulatory care and
home health care. This book, owing to its size and portability, would also
be of use to undergraduate students who are new to disease process in a
variety of settings that they enter for the first time. Bringing the *Guidelines* book with them will enable them to access information easily about
diseases that they are encountering, as well as what to do about them.

Unit I, "The Healthy Adult," reviews information to provide holistic
care. Chapter One, entitled "Health Promotion," provides information on
planning health promotion and health promotion activities, as well as
identifying barriers to preventive care and health promotion. Additionally,
important information regarding nutrition and approaches to nutrition
counseling are included, important to integrate in all phases of practice
caring for adults.

Unit II, "Managing Illness," is the heart of the book. Twelve chapters
provide a condensed approach to disease management. This handy
reference allows you to quickly locate the important information you
need to diagnose and treat your patients effectively. Chapter Two,
"Common Presenting Symptoms and Problems" presents the symptom-
based problems that adults frequently bring to their primary care
provider. An overview of the differential diagnoses and diagnostically
oriented algorithms guide you to an appropriate diagnosis and management plan. Subsequent chapters contain common disorders for each

respective body system organized in a head-to-toe approach. The final chapter, Chapter 13, covers very important psychosocial problems and issues that advanced practice nurses know can significantly affect one's health.

The discussion of each problem and disorder follows a consistent, easy-to-follow monograph format:

- Definition, including ICD-9-CMs
- Etiology
- Occurrence
- Age
- Ethnicity
- Gender
- Contributing Factors
- Signs and Symptoms
- Diagnostic Tests, including CPT Codes
- Differential Diagnosis
- Treatment, including pharmacologic, physical, surgical and complementary therapies
- Follow-up
- Sequelae
- Prevention/Prophylaxis
- Referral
- Education, including Web sites

This book is written by—and for—advanced practice nurses involved in the day-to-day primary health care of adult patients. It provides you with essentials of medical management required for safe and effective practice. However, it is your unique nursing-based perspective that differentiates and strengthens your application of these generic guidelines. Use this book and make it your own by jotting down experiences from your own individual practice as well as new and updated medical treatment approaches. This will enable you to bring skill and knowledge to today's health-care arena things that we know our patients, today's health care consumers, are calling out for: astute, individualized, current, state-of-the-art compassionate management of symptoms; an increased focus on quality-of-life, prevention and health promotion. Perhaps most importantly, and simply, someone who listens to them, someone who cares for them, someone who hears them. This is what we, as advanced practice nurses, do best.

Lynne M. Hektor Dunphy

ACKNOWLEDGMENTS

Special thanks and acknowledgment go to Bruce Wishnov, D.O., Family Practice—a wonderful colleague, a great mentor, and most of all, a truly great doctor, who truly cares about his patients.

Additionally, many thanks to Joanne P. DaCunha, my publisher and longtime friend and nursing colleague from FA Davis; and special thanks to Diane Blodgett, Developmental Editor, for all her great work and support during a difficult year.

With thanks to all at FA Davis, from Production to the wonderful sales department, for all support and hard work to make our books successful.

CONTRIBUTORS

Terry J. Apt, MSN, APRN-BC
VA Primary Care Clinic
Sterling Medical
Leesburg, FL

Naomi Breiner, MSN, APRN-BC
Adult Nurse Practitioner
Neurology Associates
Miami, FL

Phillip Britton, MSN, APRN-BC
Family Nurse Practitioner
Dermatology
Boca Raton, FL

Kathleen Jett, PhD, GNP-BC
Assistant Professor
Florida Atlantic University
Christine E. Lynn College of Nursing
Boca Raton, FL

Barbara Lamb, MSN, APRN-BC
Emergency Services
Jackson Memorial Hospital
Miami, FL

Pamela Brinker Lester, APRN-BC, MSN
Visiting Assistant Professor
Florida Atlantic University
Christine E. Lynn College of Nursing
Boca Raton, FL
and
Family Nurse Practitioner
Western Communities Family Practice
Wellington, FL

Ruth McCaffrey, ND, APRN-BC
Assistant Professor
Florida Atlantic University
Christine E. Lynn College of Nursing
Boca Raton, FL
and
Family Nurse Practitioner
Palm Beach Family Physicians
West Palm Beach, FL

Janice M. Muzic, MSN, APRN-BC
Cardiology Nurse Practitioner
Cardiology Partners of the Palm Beaches
Loxahatchee, FL

Patricia M. Siccardi, EdD, APRN-BC
Psychiatric Clinical Practice
Boca Raton, FL
and
Adjunct Faculty
Florida Atlantic University
Christine E. Lynn College of Nursing
Boca Raton, FL

Linda D. Scott, DNS, APRN-BC
Family Nurse Practitioner
Spectrum Healthcare Resources
Fort Bragg, NC

Ann Marie Szoke-Halal, RN, MSN, CRNP, ONC
Trauma Nurse Practitioner
St. Luke's Hospital
Bethlehem, PA

Mary Beth Thompson, MSN, APRN-BC
Family Nurse Practitioner
Hahn and Adler
Internal Medicine and Gastroenterology
Plantation, FL

Sharon A. Thrush, MSN, APRN-BC
Family Nurse Practitioner
Palm Beach Family Physicians
West Palm Beach, FL
and
Adjunct Faculty
Florida Atlantic University
Christine E. Lynn College of Nursing
Boca Raton, FL

CONSULTANTS

Ellen M. Chiocca, RNC, MSN, CPNP
Assistant Professor
Loyola University Chicago
Marcella Niehoff School of Nursing
Chicago, IL

Gretchen Hope Miller Heery, APRN, BC
Occupational Health Nurse Practitioner
WorkForce Wellness Program
Family Nurse Practitioner
Gnaden Huetten Memorial Hospital
Lehighton, PA

Anita Hunter, RN, PhD, PNP
Assistant Professor
Clemson University School of Nursing
Clemson, SC

Marjorie Thomas-Lawson, PhD, RN-CS, FNP
Associate Professor
University of Southern Maine
Portland, ME

Donna G. Nativio, PhD, CRNP, FAAN
Associate Professor
Director of the Family Nurse Practitioner Program
University of Pittsburgh School of Nursing
Pittsburgh, PA

Kristy Kiel Martyn, PhD, RN
Assistant Professor
University of Michigan School of Nursing
Ann Arbor, MI

CONTENTS

Unit **1**

Chapter 1

HEALTH PROMOTION

Health Promotion: ICD-9-CM: V70.0

Promoting health and preventing illness are constants of clinical practice and of increased importance as limited resources and cost restraints continue to constrain the treatment of disease. The focus of *Healthy People 2010,* health goals for the United States from the surgeon general, is to change risky behaviors into healthy behaviors to maintain health, prevent or control health problems, preserve functional independence, reduce the likelihood of disability, and preserve quality of life. Many of the serious clinical problems encountered in daily clinical practice are preventable or postponed by primary prevention (healthier lifestyles, immunizations, and chemoprophylaxis) or by secondary prevention (screening and early treatment). Confusion exists as to what constitutes proper screening and prevention programs. Research constantly produces new findings, and government agencies, professional organizations, voluntary associations, and academic experts recommend an array of preventive services.

In 1984, the U.S. Department of Health and Human Services commissioned the U.S. Preventive Service Task Force to study health promotion activities. The task force issued a guide for preventive services. The principal findings of the task force include the following: (1) Counseling and patient education are more effective than traditional clinical activities, such as diagnostic testing; (2) patients are assuming increased responsibility for their own health; (3) individual risk profiles are needed to individualize preventive services; and (4) more effective interventions address the personal health practices of patients. All health care providers should assess health risk factors routinely and encourage modified behaviors related to smoking, alcohol, seat-belt use, diet, exercise, stress, and safe sex. The guidelines and recommendations presented here are based on areas of agreement among authorities in the *Clinician's Handbook of Preventive Services* and current literature (Table 1–1).

TABLE 1–1 Adult Preventive Care Timeline Recommendations of Major Authorities

Diagnostic Tests	
Blood pressure	Yearly
Height and weight	Yearly
Total blood cholesterol Fasting lipoprotein profile (total cholesterol, LDL cholesterol, HDL cholesterol, triglycerides)	Complete risk factor assessment Adults age ⩾20: every 5 years
Hearing	Periodically (age ⩾65)
Mammography	Baseline at age 35 Age 40–50 years: every 2 years Age ⩾50: every 1–2 years with or without clinical breast examination
Pap smear	Sexually active and have cervix: every 1–3 years Age ⩾65: based on indication
Prostate-specific antigen	Age ⩾50: yearly
Sigmoidoscopy	Age ⩾50: every 3–5 years
Stool for occult blood	Age ⩾50: yearly
Digital rectal examination	Begin at age 40: yearly
Urinalysis	Age ⩾60: periodically
Examinations	
Dental	Yearly
Vision and glaucoma	Age 40–60: every 2–4 years Age ⩾60: every 2 years
Breast	Age 18–40: every 1–2 years (by some authorities) Age ⩾40: yearly
Cancer screening Thyroid, mouth, skin, ovaries, testicles, lymph nodes, rectum Prostate Colon	Age 18–40: every 3 years (by some authorities) Age ⩾40: yearly Men age ⩾50: with PSA yearly Age ⩾50: annual fecal occult; flexible sigmoidoscopy (nonspecified)
Immunizations	
Tetanus/diphtheria	Every 10 years
Pneumococcal	Once at age 65 (by some authorities)
Influenza	Yearly (age ⩾65)
Health Promotion Counseling	
Smoking	Ask and document every visit
Alcohol and drugs	Periodically
Sexual behavior	Periodically
AIDS	Periodically
Nutrition	Periodically
Physical activity	Periodically
Violence and firearm use and storage	Periodically

(continued)

TABLE 1–1   Adult Preventive Care Timeline Recommendations of Major Authorities *(continued)*

Health Promotion Counseling	
Motor vehicle safety	Periodically
Smoke detector	Periodically
Injury prevention	Periodically
Occupational health	Periodically
Dental health	Periodically
Aspirin	Men age $\geqslant$40
Family planning	Periodically
Folate	Women age 12–45 0.4 mg daily
Estrogen	Women age $\geqslant$45
Calcium intake	Men and women age 25–50 1000 mg daily Postmenopausal women age 50–65, 1500 mg daily (1000 mg if on estrogen) Men and women $\geqslant$65 1500 mg daily
Estrogen	Women age $\geqslant$45

Sources:
Expert Panel on Detection, Evaluation, and Treatment of High Blood Cholesterol in Adults: Executive Summary of the third report of the National Cholesterol Education Program (NCEP) (Adult Treatment Panel III). JAMA, *285:* 2486, 2001.
Shapiro, JA, et al: Colorectal cancers screening test and associated health behaviors. Am J Prev Med *21:* 132, 2001.
US Public Health Service: Put Prevention into Practice: Clinician's Handbook of Preventive Services, ed 2. International Medical Publishers,McLean, Va., 1997.
US Public Health Service: Quick Reference Guide for Clinicians: Treating Tobacco Use and Dependence. 2001. Contact: http://www.surgeongeneral.gov/tobacco/tobaqrg.htm. Retrieved December 22, 2001.
US Preventive Services Task Force: Guide to Clinical Preventive Services, ed 2. 1996. Contact: http://odphp.osophs.dhhs.gov/pubs/guidecps. Retrieved December 22, 2001.

PLANNING HEALTH PROMOTION

The nursing process effectively guides the planning, implementation, and evaluation of health promotion activities.

Assess

The first priority is to complete an assessment or risk factor profile of your clinical patient base. Local or state health departments provide relevant data on specific populations to identify the types of health promotion activities and preventive care important to a patient population. Evaluation of the feasibility of providing these services is essential on a routine basis. Individualization of these activities is crucial for each patient. A useful strategy is to supply the waiting area with short, risk factor–oriented patient questionnaires for patients to complete while they are waiting to be seen.

Plan

Determine a specific strategy, such as a systematic approach to provide the basic set of health promotion activities and preventive services for patients on a regular basis that yields significant results. A basic tool for tracking and prompting health promotion activities and preventive care is a flow sheet in each patient's medical record.

Implement

Seeking active patient involvement in health care insures successful attainment of health promotion activities and preventive care. Self-care and education are essential components to empower patients in making collaborative health care decisions. Research shows that most patients are interested in preventive care. Provide patients with a variety of educational materials to enhance their interest and knowledge. The U.S. Public Health Service (202-653-5075) provides a "Put Prevention into Practice Education and Action Kit" that contains a variety of patient educational materials, risk-assessment forms, reminder postcards for preventive services, and other materials. Studies have shown that patient-held records, such as childhood immunizations, are useful in tracking and prompting child and adult preventive care services. It is important to use every opportunity to model and teach preventive health care. Every staff member needs to be committed to practice health promotion activities and disease prevention.

Evaluate

An ongoing evaluation plan is essential to monitor the success and effectiveness of health promotion activities and preventive care plans. Research has shown that most practitioners overestimate the amount of time they spend in preventive care. Objective evaluations, such as random audits of patient records or computer-based tracking systems, are essential to modify and enhance prevention activities of patients. Compiling preventive care databases over time is useful to show the cost-effectiveness of preventive health care in a persuasive way for third-party payers to reimburse the health promotion role of the advanced practice nurse.

HEALTH PROMOTION ACTIVITIES

The two major health promotion activities of the advanced practice nurse are promoting immunizations and providing patient education and counseling. Education enables individuals to make informed decisions and adopt behaviors that promote health.

Immunizations

Immunization requirements vary by state; however, the Centers for Disease Control and Prevention makes specific recommendations for adult immunizations (Table 1–2). Immunization guidelines change frequently, and current ones are issued annually, usually in January. Numerous government websites, such as the Center for Disease Control and Health Promotion, National Immunization Program (http://www.cdc.gov/nip), are easily accessible.

Patient Education and Counseling

Positive and effective health promotion strategies require personal involvement. Individuals, families, and communities make choices that optimize their health potential. A therapeutic nurse-patient relationship reflects the application of scientifically based knowledge of human behavior and communication, an attitude of caring and commitment for the patient's well-being, and knowledge of effective approaches for patient education and counseling. Strategies for effective counseling and education include the following:

Seek the patient's attention and interest in the topic.

Be specific. For example, write a prescription for the patient to walk 1 mile in 45 minutes 4 times weekly.

Be direct. Make direct, simple, and specific statements, such as "I want you to stop smoking."

Provide a clear rationale for suggested changes with expected outcomes.

Obtain a specific commitment from the patient. For example, ask "When will you begin?"

Use the contract process, informally or formally, to describe specifically the patient's plans for achievement that includes measurable goals with time frames, such as "We agree that you will lose 5 lb by the next office visit."

Develop a realistic time frame for changes to occur so that the patient knows when to expect an effect or change.

Encourage small steps to build the patient's confidence in his or her ability to change. Large steps are overwhelming and hasten failure.

Individualize the counseling. Plan teaching strategies for the individual patient and in accordance to his or her health, cultural, and spiritual beliefs.

Use written literature for more complex information that is appropriate for the patient's reading, language, and educational level.

Use a combination of strategies. Integrate individual counseling efforts with classes and audiovisual and written educational materials.

Encourage the patient's social support system to participate actively in the plan for greater adherence of changes.

Provide positive feedback and praise for positive outcomes. Avoid negative comments.

TABLE 1–2   Adult Immunization Schedule Recommendations

Vaccine	Dosage and Administration	Comments
Hepatitis A (Hep A)	Dosage: 1.0 mL IM Administer: First dose, then second dose 6–12 months later	Two doses are recommended for persons requiring long-term protection Travelers to countries where the disease is common should get the first dose at least 4 weeks before departure *Contraindicated* in persons with allergy to alum or preservative 2-phenoxyethanol
Hepatitis B (Hep B)	Dosage: 1.0 mL IM (deltoid) Administration: First dose, then second dose 1 month later, then third dose 5 months after second dose	If the vaccination doses are interrupted after the first dose, the second dose should be administered as soon as possible and the third dose at least 2 months after the second May be given with other vaccines, but at a different site *Contraindicated* in persons with allergy to yeast
Influenza (Flu)	Dosage: 0.5 mL IM Administration: One dose every fall	For persons age ≥50 Residents of nursing homes or other facilities for patients with chronic medical conditions For persons <50 years old; who have chronic medical problems, such as heart disease, lung disease, diabetes, renal dysfunction, hemoglobinopathies, immunosuppressive disorders, or immunodeficiency disorders Others persons who work or live with high-risk individuals Consult your physician to determine your level of risk *Contraindicated* in persons with acute febrile illness and anaphylactic allergy to eggs
Measles, mumps, rubella (MMR)	Dosage: 0.5 mL SC (deltoid) Administration: One dose	Two doses 1 month apart are recommended for adults born in 1957 or later if immunity cannot be proved Not to be given to pregnant women or women considering pregnancy within 3 months of vaccination *Contraindicated* in persons on immunosuppressive therapy or with immunodeficiency; untreated, active tuberculosis; anaphylactic allergy to neomycin; pregnancy; immune globulin preparation
Pneumococcal	Dosage: 0.5 mL IM or SC Administration: One dose any time during the year	Usually given once at age ≥65 For people <65 who have chronic illnesses, such as those listed for influenza and with kidney disorders and sickle cell anemia For Alaskan Natives and certain Native American populations

(continued)

TABLE 1–2 Adult Immunization Schedule Recommendations *(continued)*

Vaccine	Dosage and Administration	Comments
Pneumococcal	Dosage: 0.5 mL IM or SC Administration: One dose any time during the year	A repeat dose 5 years after initial dose may be given to those at highest risk or if vaccinated before age 65 Consult your physician to determine your level of risk May be given simultaneously with influenza, but at a different site
Tetanus, diphtheria (Td)	Dosage: 0.5 mL IM Administration: *If initial series not given during childhood* First dose, then second dose 4–6 weeks later, then third dose 6–12 months after second dose; booster shot every 10 years	Needs booster as part of severe wound management
Chickenpox (varicella)	Dosage: 0.5 mL SC (deltoid) Administration: First dose, then second dose 1–2 months later	Persons age ≥13 who have not had chickenpox Not to be given to pregnant women or women considering pregnancy within 1 month of vaccination Contraindicated in persons with anaphylactic allergy to gelatin or neomycin; untreated, active tuberculosis; immunosuppressive therapy or immunodeficiency; pregnancy; immune globulin preparation or blood product received in last 5 months

Source: National Immunization Program: Adult immunization recommendations. 2002. Contact: http://www.cdc.gov/nip. Retrieved January 2, 2002.

Refer for needed resources from major referral sources, such as community agencies, national voluntary health organizations, instructional references, other patients, and other professionals (Table 1–3).

Develop an interdisciplinary team for community education and counseling to maximize expert community resources for target groups.

SPECIFIC AREAS

Changes in patient behaviors are more valuable for health than the many screening tests and immunizations available. Patients value the advice of their health care providers. Brief, simple advice is beneficial even if

Table 1–3 Websites

Agency, Organization, Association	Website
Agency for Healthcare Research and Quality	http:www.ahrq.gov/clinic
American Heart Association	http://americanheart.org
American Whole Health, Integrative Medicine	http://wholehealthmd.com
Centers for Disease Control and Prevention	http://www.cdc.gov
Guide to Clinical Preventive Services, ed 2.	http:odphp.osophs.dhhs.gov/pubs/guideceps/
Health Finder	http://healthfinder.gov
National Immunization Program	http://www.cdc.gov/nip
National Health Information Center	http://health.gov/NHIC
National Heart, Lung, and Blood Institute	http://nhlbi.nih.gov/health
National Institutes of Health	http://www.nih.gov/ninr
US Preventive Services Task Force Screening	http://www.ahrq.gov/clinic/uspstfix.html
US Department of Health and Human Resources	http://www.usdhhs.gov

results are not immediately apparent. Specific areas of health promotion, preventive care, patient education, and counseling should be included in patient care.

Exercise

Planned, regular exercise is an important health promotion activity. Established exercise programs have shown that exercise reduces the risk of developing cancer, cardiovascular disease, depression, and other diseases, while improving one's general sense of well-being. Recommend 30 minutes of exercise activity every day that an individual identifies as being positive, available, convenient, and enjoyable activity, such as brisk mall walking, bicycling, or water-based activity. Evaluation of the patient's health history, physical examination, exercise level, activity tolerance, exercise pattern, functional capabilities, changes in patterns of activity, and potential barriers is important before beginning an exercise program. Moderation and safety, including proper clothing and equipment, are key because overexertion often leads to abandonment of the prescribed activity.

Rest and Sleep

The need for rest and relaxation varies among individuals. The number of hours of sleep needed to maintain positive health and functioning decreases as one grows older. Problems with sleep are associated with physiologic problems, mental health issues, activity tolerance, diet, lifestyle changes, medication changes, and personal relationships. A sleep diary is a valuable tool to assess if a patient is receiving adequate rest and sleep and is waking rested. Asking a patient about issues such as insomnia, difficulty awakening, and nightmares assesses the patient's need for rest. Continued periods of sleeping for more than 9 continuous hours in a 24-hour period may require a more detailed workup.

Nutrition

Four of the leading 10 causes of death, including heart disease, stroke, diabetes, and certain cancers, are linked to diet. Diet-related health conditions cost an estimated $250 billion annually in medical costs and lost productivity. Overconsumption of calories, specifically fat, and declining levels of physical activity make overweight or obesity a public health problem. Approximately 33% of Americans are overweight, and the numbers continue to increase. Underconsumption of nutrients, such as calcium, iron, and folate, causes health problems for individuals, particularly women.

Good nutrition is essential to health throughout life, and dietary intervention is an important component of health promotion, prevention, and treatment of disease. Health care providers need to counsel and educate patients about their dietary habits and consumption of dietary supplements. Basic patient dietary education includes the following:

Eat a variety of foods.

Balance the food you eat with physical activity to maintain or improve your weight to decrease low-density lipoprotein (LDL) levels and increase high-density lipoprotein (HDL) levels.

Eat foods high in soluble fiber (20–30 g daily), such as cereal grains, beans, peas, legumes, and many vegetables and fruits.

Choose a diet low in fat (25–35% of total calories), saturated fat (<7% of total calories), cholesterol (<200 mg daily), and carbohydrates (50–60% of total calories).

Use plant stanols and sterols (2 g daily) (found in certain margarine and salad dressings) and soluble fiber (10–25 g daily) to boost LDL-lowering power.

Eat a diet moderate in sugars.

Consume moderate amounts of salt and sodium (<2400 mg daily).

Drink alcohol in moderation (no more than 1 drink daily for women and 2 drinks daily for men). One drink is 12 oz. of beer, 5 oz. of wine, or 1.5 oz. of 80-proof distilled spirits.

Recommend a diet with fewer total calories of fat and a modest increase in physical activity for patents who are overweight.

The weight loss goal should be 0.5 to 1 lb weekly.

The National Cholesterol Education Program's Adult Treatment Panel III (ATP III) Guidelines recommend a stepped approach with aggressive cholesterol-lowering treatment for Americans. The stepped approach focuses on therapeutic lifestyle changes to lower LDL levels by completing a risk assessment, emphasizing reduction in saturated fat and cholesterol, encouraging physical activity, evaluating LDL levels, and beginning LDL-lowering therapy. The risk assessment tool translates clinical conditions and lifestyle factors into a single, easy-to-read risk category of a patient's chance of a heart attack within 10 years. The risk factors are calculated separately for men and women and are based on age, total cholesterol, HDL, systolic blood pressure, treatment for hypertension, and cigarette smoking. A fasting lipoprotein profile measures the level of total cholesterol, total HDL, total LDL, and tryglycerides in adults ≥20 years old every 5 years. The blood levels are as follows:

Total cholesterol	Desirable: ≤200 mg/dL Borderline high: 200–239 mg/dL High: ≥240 mg/dL
Total HDL	Low: ≤40 mg/dL High: ≥60 mg/dL (protective against heart disease and desirable)
Total LDL	Optimal LDL: ≤100 mg/dL Borderline high: 130–159 mg/dL High: 160–189 mg/dL Very high: ≥190 mg/dL
Triglyceride levels	Desirable: ≤150 mg/dL Borderline high:150–199 mg/dL High: 200–499 mg/dL Very high : ≥500 mg/dL

The *metabolic syndrome* identifies risk factors linked to insulin resistance that dramatically increase the risk of coronary events. This syndrome is a strong contributor to early heart disease and an underlying etiology of type 2 diabetes; it is important to recognize risk factors and defining levels and treat the metabolic syndrome. Risk factors include the following:

Abdominal obesity (waist circumference)
    Men
    Women
	
	>102 cm(>40 inches)
	>88 cm(>35 inches)

Triglyceride levels	≥150 mg/dL

HDL cholesterol
    Men
    Women
	
	<40 mg/dL
	<50 mg/dL

Blood pressure	≥130/≥85 mm Hg
Fasting glucose	≥110 mg/dL

The implementation of the ATP III Guidelines into practice and patient education is crucial to improve nutrition and decrease heart disease. For risk calculators, patient information sheets, guidelines, and other data, refer to the National Institutes of Health at http://www.nhlbi.nih.gov/guideines/cholesterol/index.html.   Patients need ongoing support and reinforcement to undertake significant dietary changes, especially through plateaus and regression periods. Recommend small, achievable steps over time to promote continuation of the diet. Plan frequent follow-up times to provide support and monitor the patient's efforts. Refer patients with multiple or severe nutritional problems for counseling with a professional dietitian.

Stress Management

The ability to control stress is paramount for positive health. Evidence suggests that 75% of hospitalizations and visits to acute care practitioners are related directly or indirectly to the inability to cope with stressful situations. It is important to recognize the interrelationships between work, family, environmental stressors, coping abilities, and the degree an individual controls actual and perceived stress. Many questionnaires, such as the Social Readjustment Rating Scale, are useful in evaluating the patient. A stress awareness diary requires a patient to record stressful events when they occur, record the appearance of any physical or emotional symptoms, and rate the effectiveness of coping techniques used. Patient education is the key to decrease stress and includes a variety of stress reduction techniques, such as meditation, visualization, music, art, and biofeedback.

Self-Examination

The monthly self-examination of breasts or testicles and the reporting of findings are an important health promotion activity. Both genders need to be educated about the importance of a breast examination and provide a return demonstration. Men and some clinicians believe that men are excluded from breast self-examinations; however, approximately 1% of all breast cancers are documented in men. Women need a baseline mammogram at age 35, follow-up tests every other year beginning at age 40, then annually beginning at age 50. Early detection of testicular cancer is accomplished best by monthly self-palpation of the testes during a hot shower beginning at age 14 years. Skin self-examination is important because the patient is usually the best person to recognize changes in his or her skin, especially changes in moles beginning in adolescent years.

Avoidance of Tobacco, Alcohol, and Drugs

Tobacco dependence is the most damaging substance to an individual's health, the leading cause of preventable death, and a chronic condition requiring repeated intervention. The current clinical guidelines from the Public Health Service for *Treating Tobacco Use and Dependence* employ the *5As* (ask, advise, assess, assist, and arrange) approach. The most important assessment for smoking cessation is to ask about and document tobacco use of every patient on every visit. Research shows that more patients effectively stopped smoking because of a health care provider's questions, concern, and support. In a clear, strong, and personalized message, urge every tobacco user to quit and assist in setting a quit date. Acknowledging and discussing the obstacles that the patient faces, such as fear of failing; weight gain; stress; withdrawal symptoms; and spouse, friends, and coworkers who smoke, are helpful.

The epidemic of alcoholism in the United States suggests that health care providers need to be assertive and assess the alcohol intake of patients. Some studies cited primary care providers' detection rates of alcohol and drug problems are only 30%. A health-risk appraisal, such as CAGE or TACE questionnaires, determines the risk of alcohol abuse. Responses regarding alcohol consumption, health patterns, and life satisfaction provide clues to alcohol dependence.

Substance abuse of prescription and nonprescription medications is of epidemic proportions. During each visit, ascertain a thorough medication history that includes over-the-counter (OTC) medications and whether or not the patient is receiving medication from another health care provider. Drug interactions need to be reviewed closely. Treatment for substance abuse is difficult, and relapse is common. The first step begins with a trusting therapeutic relationship with the patient.

Support Groups

A referral to supportive services is effective therapy. Support groups comprise individuals who have common links and assist one another in providing emotional support for the individual and the family. Networking between groups facilitates the availability of resources and educational and prevention programs.

SCREENING

A major component of disease prevention is screening for diseases before they occur. Screenings are popular because they decrease costs of health care, screening tests are available over-the-counter, and public education stresses the importance of screenings. Authorities vary in screening recommendations; however, most practitioners and researchers agree that the general criteria for screenings include the following: (1) The condition must have a significant effect on the quality and quantity of life; (2) acceptable methods of treatment must be available; (3) the condition must have an asymptomatic period during which detection and treatment significantly reduce mortality and morbidity rates; (4) tests that are acceptable to patients must be available, at a reasonable cost, to detect the condition in the asymptomatic period; and (5) the incidence of the condition must be sufficient to justify the cost of the screening. Close tracking of results and appropriate follow-up enhance the value of performing screening tests. Adherence to the concepts of test sensitivity (the proportion of people with a condition who correctly test positive when screened), specificity (the proportion of people without the disease who correctly test negative when screened), and positive predictive value (the proportion of people with a positive test who actually have the condition; most screening tests have positive predictive values of 10–30%) is essential when evaluating and selecting screening tests.

BARRIERS TO HEALTH PROMOTION AND PREVENTIVE CARE

Health promotion and disease prevention are practiced through many channels and include modifying personal risk factors to prevent disease, controlling communicable diseases, protecting the environment, and preventing or reducing the severity of chronic diseases. There are notable decreases in morbidity and mortality rates; however, significant numbers of people, specifically minority and lower socioeconomic groups, do not receive appropriate health promotion and preventive care services. Existing barriers or limitations include the following: (1) Preventive services are limited by logistic, political, religious, and financial barriers; (2) environment-specific preventive measures often face vigorous political opposition; (3) vaccine and screening services are costly and often unavailable to individuals who cannot pay or have limited access to health care; (4) unhealthy behaviors are often enjoyable or deeply ingrained in culture and lifestyles; (5) behavior changes forced on society, such as legislating the use of seat belts or motorcycle helmets, often conflict with values of individual rights; (6) health care practitioners lack the time to implement services; (7) it is unclear to health care practitioners how to obtain reimbursement for health promotion and preventive care services; (8) personal or financial incentives to health care providers to institute the care and activities are lacking; (9) confusion and skepticism exist about which prevention guidelines are effective; and (10) knowledge is lacking about patients' perceptions about the importance of health promotion activities and preventive health services. It is imperative for the advanced practice nurse to increase personal awareness of these barriers so that he or she can determine strategies to overcome them.

REFERENCES

Agency for Healthcare Research and Quality: What's new in preventive services. 2002. Contact: http:www.ahrq.gov/clinic/prevnew.htm. Retrieved January 2, 2002.

American Heart Association: Comprehensive risk reduction for patients with coronary and other vascular diseases. 2001. Contact: http://americanheart.org/ presenter.jhtml?identifer=1316. Retrieved December 21, 2001.

American Heart Association: Managing your lifestyle. 2001. Contact: http://americanheart.org/presenter.jhtml?identifer=1200014. Retrieved December 21, 2001.

American Heart Association: My heart watch. 2001. Contact: http://www.myheartwatch.org/myheartwatch/inc/public.asp?&REVISITED=1007070199406. Retrieved December 21, 2001.

American Heart Association: Older Americans and physical activity. 2001. Contact: http://americanheart.org/presenter.jhtml?identifer=811. Retrieved December 21, 2001.

American Heart Association: Physical activity and cardiovascular health: Questions and answers. 2001. Contact: http://americanheart.org/presenter.jhtml?identifer=830. Retrieved December 21, 2001.

American Heart Association: Physical activity and cardiovascular health fact sheet. 2001. Contact: http://americanheart.org/presenter.jhtml?identifer=820. Retrieved December 21, 2001.

American Heart Association: Tips for exercise success. 2001. Contact: http://americanheart.org/presenter.jhtml?identifer=801. Retrieved December 21, 2001.

Anonymous: AHA dietary guidelines revised for the new millennium. Clin Rev 11:58, 2001.

Anonymous: Cholesterol testing and management: Updated guidelines. Consultant 1399, 2001.

Antai-Otong, D: Proactive response to workplace violence: Nurses' role in health promotion. Texas Nursing 72:4, 1998.

Balducci, L, and Kennedy, BJ: Cancer screening in older patients. Patient Care for the Nurse Practitioner 4:41, 2001.

Blackie, C, et al: Promoting health in young people. Nursing Standard 12:39, 1998.

Callaghan, P: Social support and locus of control as correlates of UK nurses' health-related behaviours. J Adv Nurs 28:1127, 1998.

Clarke, A: Changing attitudes through persuasive communication. Nursing Standard 13:45, 1999.

Coffield, AB, et al: Priorities among recommended clinical preventive services. Am J Prev Med 21:1, 2001.

Cook, R: Promoting women's health. Nursing Standard 14:38, 2000.

Cotter, VT, and Strumpf, NE (eds): Advanced Practice Nursing with Older Adults. McGraw-Hill, New York, 2002.

Diebold, CM, et al: A health promotion practicum targeting the college-age population. Nurse Educator 25:48, 2000.

Dunphy, LM, and Winland-Brown, JE: Primary Care: The Art and Science of Advanced Practice Nursing. FA Davis, Philadelphia, 2001.

Eldeman, CL, and Mandle, CL: Health Promotion Throughout the Lifespan, ed 4. Mosby, St. Louis, 1998.

Expert Panel on Detection, Evaluation, and Treatment of High Blood Cholesterol in Adults: Executive Summary of the third report of the National Cholesterol Education Program (NCEP) (Adult Treatment Panel III). JAMA 285:2486, 2001.

Feingold, C, and Perlich, L: Teaching critical thinking through a health-promotion contract. Nurse Educator 24:42, 1999.

Green, PM, and Adderley-Kelly, B: Partnership for health promotion in an urban community. Nursing and Health Care Perspectives 20:76, 1999.

Kashyap, M: Clinical aspects of dyslipidemia. Managed Care 10:4, 2001.

Lai, SC, and Cohen, MN: Promoting lifestyle changes. Am J Nurs 99:63, 1999.

Maciosek, MV, et al: Methods for priority setting among clinical preventive services. Am J Prev Med 21:10, 2001.

National Immunization Program: Adult immunization schedule. 2002. Contact: http://www.cdc.gov/nip/recs/adult-schedule.html. Retrieved January 2, 2002.

Nawaz, H, and Katz, DL: American College of Preventive Medicine Practice policy statement: Weight management counseling of overweight adults. Am J Prev Med 21:73, 2001.

Norton, L: Health promotion and health education: What role should the nurse adopt in practice? Issues and innovations in nursing practice. J Adv Nurs 28:1269, 1998.

Piper, SM, and Brown, PA: The theory and practice of health education applied to nursing: A bi-polar approach. J Adv Nurs 27:383, 1998.

Redman, BK: The Practice of Patient Education, ed 8. Mosby, St. Louis, 1997.

Risi, GF, and Tomascak, V: Prevention of infection in the immunocompromised host. Am J Infect Control 26:594, 1998.

Rush, KL: Health promotion ideology and nursing education. J Adv Nurs 25:1292, 1997.

Schauffler, HH, et al: Adoption of the AHCPR clinical practice guideline for smoking cessation: A survey of California's HMOs. Am J Prev Med 21:153, 2001.

Shapiro, JA, et al: Colorectal cancers screening test and associated health behaviors. Am J Prev Med 21:132, 2001.

Sheahan, SL: Documentation of health risks and health promotion counseling by emergency department nurse practitioners and physicians. Journal of Nursing Scholarship 23:2445, 2000.

Sinclair, BP: Advanced practice nurses in integrated health care systems. J Obstet Gynecol Neonatal Nurs 26:217, 1997.

Sortet, JP, and Banks, SR: Health beliefs of rural Appalachian women and the practice of breast self-examination. Cancer Nurs 20:231, 1997.

Stanley, M, and Beare, PG (eds): Gerontological Nursing: A Health Promotion/Protection Approach, ed 2. FA Davis, Philadelphia, 1999.

Stevenson, A: Immunizations for women and infants. J Obstet Gynecol Neonatal Nurs 28:534, 1999.

Stuifgergen, AK, et al: An explanatory model of health promotion and quality of life in chronic disabling conditions. Nurs Res 49:122, 2000.

Sword, W: A socio-ecological approach to understanding barriers to prenatal care for women of low income. J Adv Nurs 29:1170, 1999.

Thomson, P, and Kohli, H: Health promotion training needs analysis: An integral role for clinical nurses in Lanarkshire, Scotland. J Adv Nurs 26:507, 1997.

US Department of Health and Human Services: Healthy people 2010: Understanding and improving health. 2000. Contact: http://www.health.gov/healthypeople. Retrieved December 22, 2001.

US Preventive Services Task Force: Guide to Clinical Preventive Services, ed 2. 1996. Contact: http://odphp.osophs.dhhs.gov/pubs/guidecps. Retrieved December 22, 2001

US Preventive Services Task Force: Screening for asymptomatic coronary artery disease. In: Guide to Clinical Preventive Services, ed 2. 1996. Contact: http://hstat.nlm.nih.gov/ftrs/pick?collect=cps&dbName=0&cc=1&t=1009200137. Retrieved December 22, 2001

US Public Health Service: Put prevention into Practice: Clinician's Handbook of Preventive Services, ed 2. International Medical Publishers, McLean, Va., 1997.

US Public Health Service: Quick reference guide for clinicians: Treating tobacco use and dependence. 2001. Contact: http://www.surgeongeneral.gov/tobacco/tobaqrg.htm. Retrieved December 22, 2001.

Whitehead, D: Applying collaborative practice to health promotion. Nursing Standard 15:33, 2001.

Winslow, EH: Patient education materials: Can patients read them or are they ending up in the trash? Am J Nurs 101:33, 2001.

Young, LE, and Hayes, V: Transforming Health Promotion Practice: Concepts, Issues, and Applications. FA Davis, Philadelphia, 2002.

Unit *II*

Chapter 2
SYMPTOM-BASED PROBLEMS

BACK PAIN

Intervertebral disk disorder	ICD-9-CM: 722.9
Back pain, low	ICD-9-CM: 724.2
Backache, unspecified	ICD-9-CM: 724.5

Description: Low back pain, sometimes called *sciatica,* is defined as activity intolerance produced by lower back or back-related leg symptoms of <3 months' duration. It may or may not involve the rupture of an intervertebral disk with herniation (nucleus pulposus) into the spinal canal. Back pain without sciatica is rarely due to disk herniation. About 90% of acute low back pain episodes in adults are related to mechanical causes that resolve within 4 weeks without serious sequelae.

Etiology: Caused by muscle or ligament strain (or both), degenerative joint disease, spinal stenosis, or a combination of these as well as potentially serious conditions, such as spinal fracture, tumor, or infection. A herniated disk often is preceded by years of intermittent episodes of localized back pain corresponding to repeated damage to the annular fibers of the disk. Herniation occurs when the nucleus pulposus protrudes through tears in the annular fibers resulting in nerve root compression.

Occurrence: One of the most frequent complaints for which adults seek medical attention; second to the common cold for time missed from work. Lifetime prevalence is 60% to 90%; 1 out of 20 patients has nerve root involvement; 95% of diseased disks are localized to L4-5 and L5-S1; <2% of patients have infection, neoplasms, or inflammatory spondyloarthropathies.

Age: Occurs most commonly between ages 24 and 45. The intervertebral disks begin to degenerate in the 20s. As they grow thinner, they are more likely to herniate out of the central cavity. After age 50, there is a lower incidence of disk herniation because the nucleus pulposus becomes more fibrotic and dehydrated.

Ethnicity: No significant ethnic predisposition.

Gender: Occurs about equally in men and in women.

Contributing factors: Obesity; sedentary lifestyle; trauma; lifting of heavy object; use of poor body mechanics; vibration, such as driving motor vehicles with a standard shift; aging process; osteoporosis; stress; tension; cigarette smoking.

Signs and symptoms:

History

The patient usually complains of an inability to move related to low back pain. Ascertain limitations to activities of daily living and the length of time for the limitations.

Associated Signs and Symptoms

The patient may complain of a sharp, shooting, or "electric" type of pain in the buttock or posterior thigh that radiates along the lateral thigh, leg, and foot. This is radicular pain, which commonly is referred to as sciatica and usually is increased with walking and relieved by sitting. Paresthesia or numbness may occur in the sensory distribution of the nerve root.

Physical Examination

Deep tendon reflexes are absent or depressed in the distribution of the nerve root. Muscular weakness and atrophy also may result. Only true sciatica from nerve compression radiates below the knee to the foot. The straight-leg raise test can assess tension in the L5 or S1 nerve root. In the supine position, elevation of the affected leg produces pain at 15° to 30° in severe cases and 30° to 60° in milder cases. Crossover pain occurs when straight-leg raise of the patient's well limb elicits pain in the leg with sciatica. A herniated disk is suggested when <70° of leg elevation produces pain below the knee; pain is aggravated by ankle dorsiflexion or hip rotation.

Diagnostic tests:

Tests	Results Indicating Disorder	CPT Code
Lumbosacral x-rays*	Determine structural abnormalities, such as fracture, tumor, osteophytes (bone spurs), or vertebral infection	72100

*Lumbosacral x-rays are not indicated in the first 4 weeks of acute-onset low back pain without neurologic signs.

Differential diagnosis:

- Acute spinal: spinal fracture, infection, cauda equina syndrome, tumor, sciatica, musculoskeletal strain
- Chronic spinal: lumbosacral strain, spondylolisthesis, ankylosing spondylitis, spinal stenosis, osteoporosis

- Nonspinal: dissecting aortic aneurysm, gallstones, pyelonephritis, pleuritis, pelvic inflammatory disease

Treatment: Treat cause or refer as appropriate.

Red Flag: Cauda equina syndrome (compression of the lower portion of the nerve root) is a medical emergency and requires immediate referral. Symptoms include loss of sphincter control or disturbance in bowel and bladder function (especially of rapid onset); severe or rapidly progressive neurologic deficit in the lower extremities, such as perianal or perineal sensory loss; and major muscle weakness.

Symptomatic Treatment

Conservative management is effective for most episodes of acute low back pain, including radiculopathy, and includes bed rest in the acute phase with a gradual return to activity as tolerated after pain is controlled. A midline support (back brace) may be helpful. Occasionally, pelvic traction is needed. Other conservative management therapies include heat or cold therapies, physical therapy, a progressive walking program (short walks four times a day, lengthened as tolerated), application of transcutaneous electrical nerve stimulation, the use of shoe insole inserts, manipulation, biofeedback, and acupuncture.

Pharmacologic therapies include nonsteroidal anti-inflammatory drugs (NSAIDs) for 10 days then as needed, narcotic analgesia (opioids), and mild sedation as indicated. Muscle relaxants are controversial for herniation but may be helpful in lumbosacral strain. Epidural, trigger point, ligamentous, and facet joint injections also may be performed. Diskectomy is recommended only with cauda equina or in cases of intolerable pain, multiple recurrent episodes of severe pain, or severe postural tilt.

Follow-up: See the patient as indicated by cause of symptom. See the patient in 1 week and monitor every 2 weeks until the patient has full return of function. Monitor physical therapy, activity, and exercise program.

Sequelae: Possible complications depend on cause of symptom. General complications may include footdrop, limitation of movement and activity, depression, and addiction to pain medication.

Prevention/prophylaxis: Prevention strategies depend on cause of symptom. General prevention strategies include advising the patient to use proper body mechanics, to maintain a regular exercise program (walking and abdominal exercises are recommended) to help stretch and strengthen the back muscles, to lose weight if overweight, to wear a back brace or modify job habits (including prolonged sitting or standing) as indicated, to stop smoking, and to practice stress management.

Referral: Refer to or consult with appropriate specialist as indicated by cause of symptom. Referral to a physical therapist or pain management specialist may be indicated.

Education: Explain cause of symptoms, tests or procedures used to determine the cause, and symptomatic treatment, if any. Advise the patient when to seek medical care. Discuss prevention strategies.

CHEST PAIN

Chest pain, central	ICD9-CM: 786.5
Chest pain, musculoskeletal	ICD9-CM: 786.5
Chest pain, noncardiac	ICD9-CM: 786.59
Chest pain, respiratory	ICD9-CM: 786.52
Chest pain, abdominal nonspecified	ICD9-CM: 789.0
Chest pain, psychogenic	ICD9-CM: 307.88

Description: Chest pain is an unpleasant sensation in the chest area. The first task is to identify if the pain is cardiac or noncardiac in nature and to identify life-threatening conditions.

Etiology: Caused by many disorders involving the cardiovascular, pulmonary, gastrointestinal (GI), musculoskeletal, and neurologic systems or may be psychological or idiopathic in nature. Pain that arises from the cardiopulmonary, GI, or musculoskeletal systems is transmitted through the T1-5 spinal cord segments, making it difficult to differentiate a specific location of the pain.

Occurrence: Common in adults.

Age: Occurs at any age. If associated with coronary artery disease (CAD), incidence increases in men >35 years old and in postmenopausal women.

Ethnicity: If associated with CAD, incidence is higher in blacks.

Gender: If associated with CAD, occurs more in men up to age 50, then occurs equally in men and women.

Contributing factors:
- Cardiac etiology: hyperlipidemia, hypertension, cigarette smoking, diabetes mellitus, genetic predisposition, obesity, sedentary lifestyle, hormonal changes, congenital anomalies, and aging (CAD); alcohol use; viral, idiopathic, infectious, and infiltrative disease such as hemochromatosis (congestive heart failure [CHF]); rheumatic fever; valvular disease; drug toxicity; cocaine abuse (in younger patients)
- Pulmonary etiology: immobility, pregnancy, CHF, sickle cell anemia, surgery, use of oral contraceptives (pulmonary emboli), trauma, genetics, invasive procedures (pneumothorax), infection, malignancy
- GI etiology: genetics, ingestion of certain types and amount of foods, obesity, use of nicotine or alcohol, postprandial positioning
- Musculoskeletal etiology: trauma (usually rib fractures); unusual physical activity; excessive coughing; degenerative or inflammatory joint disease of shoulders, thorax, or cervical spine
- Neurologic etiology: immunosuppressed states, trauma, herpes zoster
- Psychological etiology: anxiety/panic disorder

Signs and symptoms: It is important first to exclude cardiac etiology as the primary cause of chest pain because the patient may have a life-threatening emergency. Refer chest pain of cardiac origin to a clinical emergency department for evaluation and treatment.

Cardiac Etiology

The patient with chest pain related to cardiac etiology may have a history of CAD risk factors, such as smoking, sedentary lifestyle, hyperlipidemia, hypertension, diabetes mellitus, and obesity or a past medical history or family history of cardiovascular disease. Cardiac chest pain usually cannot be reproduced on palpation, although 15% of cardiac chest pain may be reproduced. There are no swollen areas on palpation; pulses may be bounding, weak, or absent; abnormal heart sounds, including extra heart sounds, murmurs, and clicks, may be present. The classic chest pain of cardiac etiology is usually a dull, substernal pain that may radiate to the left shoulder and arm or to the neck or lower jaw. These symptoms are found more frequently in men. Women present with more atypical symptoms, such as shortness of breath, fatigue, abdominal or jaw pain, and nausea. These symptoms are present for hours rather than minutes. The elderly and diabetic patients also present with more atypical symptoms. Suspect angina if a patient appears anxious; has midsternal chest pain lasting <10 minutes that is aggravated by exertion, stress, anxiety, anger, or physical activity; complains of dyspnea; and has the pain relieved by rest or nitroglycerin. If the patient has sudden, crushing, substernal chest pain lasting ≥30 minutes with pallor, cyanosis, diaphoresis, dyspnea, anxiety, nausea, or vomiting, suspect an acute myocardial infarction. The pain may or may not be relieved by nitroglycerin. A dissecting thoracic or aortic aneurysm should be suspected if a patient presents with onset of sudden, severe anterior chest pain or abdominal or back pain that has lasted for hours. The patient also may appear anxious and seemingly in distress and complain of limb ischemia. The patient may have a widened pulse pressure, pulse asymmetry, and abnormal vital signs with an elevated or decreased blood pressure. Nitroglycerin does not improve the pain. Pericarditis should be suspected if there is a pericardial friction rub. A mitral valve prolapse should be suspected if there is variable chest pain, palpitations or dysrhythmias, a midsystolic click, and patient anxiety. Suspect mitral regurgitation if there is a holosystolic murmur, heard best at the apex in the left lateral position that may radiate to the axilla or back, which is associated with exertional chest pain, fatigue, dyspnea on exertion, palpitations, and dizziness or syncope. Aortic stenosis should be suspected with a systolic murmur heard best at the second right intercostals space when the patient leans forward with associated symptoms of exertional chest pain, fatigue, dyspnea on exertion, palpitations, and dizziness or syncope.

Pulmonary Etiology

Respiratory inflammation should be suspected if the patient has a past medical history or family history of respiratory diseases or exposure to environmental allergens, such as cigarette smoke. Sudden, severe pain (often described as a stabbing pain) over the lung area or the lateral thorax that occurs on normal inspiration or expiration with cyanosis, dyspnea, cough (productive or nonproductive), hemoptysis, tachycardia, tachypnea, deviated trachea, fever, diminished or absent lung sounds, friction rub, wheezes, rhonchi, or crackles also may indicate respiratory inflammation. If the patient has pain and a history of recent trauma to the thorax, suspect rib fractures. Suspect a pneumothorax with sharp, tearing chest pain radiating to the ipsilateral shoulder, which is associated with dyspnea, asymmetric chest expansion, diminished or absent breath sounds or bronchial breath sounds on the affected side, and decreased tactile fremitus. A tension pneumothorax should be suspected if there is marked tachycardia, hypotension, tracheal shift, subcutaneous crepitus, and hyperresonance on percussion. Suspect a pulmonary embolus if there is an acute onset of shortness of breath, associated with pleuritic pain; restlessness and anxiety; cough; hemoptysis; and decreased breath sounds, crackles, or wheezes.

Gastrointestinal Etiology

The chest pain may be gradual or a sudden, sharp pain that is usually midsternal and may be described as a dull, pressure-like, gripping, or burning sensation. Suspect esophageal spasm if the patient complains of chest pain aggravated by food, cold liquids, and exercise. The pain may be alleviated by nitroglycerin or calcium channel blockers but not as quickly. If the pain is aggravated after eating a heavy meal or lying down and is relieved by walking, by being in an upright position, or by taking antacids, suspect a hiatal hernia or esophageal reflux disease. A peptic ulcer should be suspected if acidic food or a lack of food aggravates the pain or if the pain is alleviated by food or antacids. The patient may have a history of smoking or alcohol abuse and may experience hematemesis or tarry stools. If the patient has pain aggravated by fatty foods or by lying down and complains of nausea or vomiting, suspect cholecystitis. Pancreatitis should be suspected with severe left upper quadrant pain radiating to the chest or with epigastric pain radiating to the back that is worse in a supine position and is associated with nausea and vomiting, mild abdominal distention, diminished bowel sounds, and fever.

Musculoskeletal Etiology

The chest pain is variable and may be sudden or gradual, lasting a few seconds to several days. Suspect costochondritis if the patient has a history of a recent respiratory infection with possible excessive cough and a complaint of sharp pain, which is usually anterior at the costochondral junction and worsens on deep inspiration. If the patient complains of pain that increases on movement or has been involved recently in excessive physical activity and the pain can be reproduced, suspect musculoskeletal pain. Suspect nerve root compression if the patient has pain and motor weakness.

Neurologic Etiology

If the patient has a history of a previous exposure to a viral process or is immunocompromised and complains of a persistent burning sensation with a vesicular rash and pain that follows a dermatome pattern, suspect herpes zoster. The patient also may complain of irritation from clothing near the rash, pain on palpation of the rash, diminished sensation caused from nerve root compression, and swelling of regional lymph nodes.

Psychological Etiology

If the patient describes a generalized, unrelenting quality of chest pain that is aggravated by any effort and signs and symptoms such as dyspnea, anxiety, fatigue, palpitations, headache, insomnia, nausea, vomiting, diarrhea, and tremors, suspect a psychological etiology for the chest pain. With anxiety, pain is often atypical and prolonged.

Diagnostic tests: Specific tests performed are based on the patient's history, risk factors, physical examination, and suspected cause.

Cardiac Etiology

Tests	Results Indicating Disorder	CPT Code
ECG	Depression in the ST segment or T wave inversion suggests myocardial ischemia; elevation of the ST segment suggests myocardial injury	93000
Cardiac enzymes (CK-MB, troponin T or I)	Elevation suggests acute myocardial infarction; CK-MB elevates within 6 hours and peaks in 24 hours; troponin T or I are more specific and remain elevated 7–10 days post infarction	82553, 84512
CBC with differential	Elevation of WBC count may be seen from day 2–7	85004
Echocardiography	Determines left ventricular function by looking at position, size, and movement of heart valves and chambers	93320
Exercise stress testing or radionuclide testing	Indicated with anginal chest pain to determine myocardial ischemic areas	93015, 89.44
Chest x-ray	Determine cardiac size and pulmonary infiltration of edema	71020
Thoracic CT scan	Determine aortic dissection	71250

ECG, electrocardiogram; CBC, complete blood count; WBC, white blood cell; CT, computed tomography.

Pulmonary Etiology

Tests	Results Indicating Disorder	CPT Code
Pulse oximetry	Oxygen saturation should be >90%	94760
Arterial blood gases	Determine oxygenation of blood, acidosis, alkalosis	82803
Chest x-ray	Determine pulmonary infiltration, masses	71020
Lung scan or ventilation-perfusion scan	Determine pulmonary embolism by diminished blood supply to affected area or lack of air movement in the lung	78588

Gastrointestinal Etiology

Tests	Results Indicating Disorder	CPT Code
CBC with differential	Elevation of WBC count with left shift suggests bacterial infection	85004
Serum amylase, lipase	Elevation of amylase suggests pancreatic inflammation; elevation of lipase suggests pancreatic damage	82150, 83690
Abdominal ultrasound	Determines masses, fluid collection, and infection; useful to determine pancreatitis and gallbladder disease	76700
Stool for occult blood	Positive test suggests GI bleeding	82270
Endoscopy	Determine gastroesophogeal reflux or problems with upper GI system	43200

Musculoskeletal Etiology

Tests	Results Indicating Disorder	CPT Code
Chest x-ray	Determine cardiac size and pulmonary masses, rib fractures	71020
CT scan	Determine pulmonary etiology	71250

Differential diagnosis:

Cardiac Etiology
- Acute myocardial infarction: history of CAD risk factors. Classic symptoms of substernal chest pressure that may radiate to the shoulder, neck, or jaw for >30 minutes, dyspnea, diaphoresis, nausea or vomiting. Women present with more atypical symptoms of chest pain, such as dyspnea, fatigue, nausea, and abdominal or jaw pain occurring over hours rather than minutes. The elderly and diabetics also present with more atypical symptoms.
- Aortic aneurysm dissection: sudden tearing anterior chest or back pain radiating to arms, abdomen, and legs; pulse deficit; hypertension or hypotension; possible neurologic changes in lower extremities

- Angina pectoris: substernal chest pressure during or after exercise or stress that is relieved by rest or nitroglycerin, nausea, dyspnea, diaphoresis
- Pericarditis: sharp, stabbing chest pain with radiation to left shoulder increased with coughing or deep breathing; fever; tachycardia; pericardial friction rub
- Mitral valve prolapse: variable chest pain, palpitations, anxiety, dysrhythmias, midsystolic click
- Mitral regurgitation: chest pain with exercise, fatigue, dyspnea on exertion, palpitations, dizziness or syncope, holosystolic murmur heard best at apex in left lateral position and may radiate to axilla or back
- Aortic stenosis: chest pain with exercise, fatigue, dyspnea on exertion, palpitations, dizziness or syncope, systolic murmur heard best at second right intercostal space with patient leaning forward

Pulmonary Etiology

- Pulmonary embolus: acute onset of dyspnea, pleuritic pain, hemoptysis, restlessness and anxiety, cough, tachycardia, tachypnea, decreased breath sounds, crackles or wheezes
- Pneumothorax: sharp, tearing pain radiating to ipsilateral shoulder, dyspnea, tachycardia, decreased breath sounds and tactile fremitus; with tension pneumothorax, hyperresonance and tracheal shift are present
- Pneumonia: pleuritic chest pain; dyspnea; productive cough of green, yellow, or rust-colored sputum; fever; tachycardia, tachypnea, inspiratory crackles, dull percussion sounds, bronchophony or egophony over area of consolidation
- Pleuritis: mild, localized chest pain worse with deep breath and recent history of upper respiratory infection, shallow respirations, local tenderness, pleural friction rub

Gastrointestinal Etiology

- Esophageal spasm: pain similar to angina pectoris and may be relieved by nitroglycerin but not as quickly
- Gastroesophageal reflux disease (GERD): burning lower chest and upper abdominal pain that occurs 30 to 60 minutes after eating, is worse lying down or bending over, and is relieved by antacids; sour taste in mouth; chronic cough; chronic laryngitis; sore throat; asthma
- Peptic ulcer disease: epigastric pain 1 to 2 hours after eating that may be relieved by antacids, epigastric tenderness to palpation; may have history of smoking and alcohol abuse
- Pancreatitis: severe left upper quadrant abdominal pain radiating to chest or epigastric pain radiating to back, pain worse in supine position, nausea and vomiting, mild abdominal distention, fever, diminished bowel sounds

- Cholecystitis: epigastric or right upper quadrant colicky abdominal pain radiating to ipsilateral shoulder or back, nausea and vomiting, positive Murphy's sign; may be precipitated by high-fat or spicy meal

Musculoskeletal Etiology

- Chostochondritis (Tietze's syndrome): pain along sternal border that increases with deep breath, pain on palpation over costochondral joints; may have history of upper respiratory infection or exercise
- Trauma (rib fracture): history of trauma, chest pain with deep breath, splinting of breathing with shallow respirations, pain on palpation
- Cervical or thoracic disk disease: chest pain associated with movement of the arm or shoulder, paresthesia

Neurologic Etiology

- Herpes zoster: unilateral chest pain with vesicular rash following dermatome

Psychological Etiology

- Anxiety/panic disorder: precordial chest pain with history of stressful situation or anxiety

Treatment: Treat cause or refer as appropriate.

 Red Flag: Exclude life-threatening causes of chest pain, such as myocardial infarction, aortic dissection, pulmonary embolus, and pneumothorax. If these are suspected, refer to an emergency department for evaluation and treatment.

Follow-up: See patient as indicated by cause of symptom.

Sequelae: Possible complications depend on cause of symptom.

Prevention/prophylaxis: Prevention strategies depend on cause of symptom.

Referral: Refer to or consult with appropriate specialist as indicated by cause of symptom.

Education: Explain cause of symptoms, tests or procedures used to determine the cause, and symptomatic treatment, if any. Advise patient when to seek medical care.

CONSTIPATION

Constipation	ICD-9-CM: 564.0

Description: Constipation is a highly subjective symptom often used by patients to refer to stools that are too hard, difficulty in defecating with infrequent bowel movements, excessive straining to expel stool, abdominal pain, and a feeling of incomplete evacuation. There is a lack of general agreement on normal stool. Constipation should be considered when there are two or fewer bowel movements per week or excessive straining at defecation.

Etiology: The most common cause is poor dietary or behavior (bowel) habits. Other causes include metabolic disorders, such as hypothyroidism, hyperparathyroidism, diabetes mellitus, hypokalemia, hypercalcemia, and uremia; neurologic problems, such as paralysis, Parkinson's disease, multiple sclerosis, depression, and surgery involving the pelvic nerves; perianal disease; colonic mass or lesion (adenocarcinoma) or stricture (diverticulosis); pregnancy; and painful anal conditions, such as hemorrhoids and fissures.

Occurrence: Common; affects almost everyone at some time.

Age: Occurs in all ages; highest incidence in the elderly.

Ethnicity: No significant ethnic predisposition.

Gender: Occurs more in women than in men.

Contributing factors: Lack of dietary fiber; inadequate intake of fluids; aging; suppression of the urge to defecate; uncomfortable bathrooms and surroundings; travel; side effect of medications such as opiate analgesics, diuretics, calcium channel blockers, anticholinergics, aluminum-based antacids, antihistamines, iron supplements, antiparkinson and antipsychotic agents; and laxative abuse over time.

Signs and symptoms:

History

Obtain history and pattern regarding the patient's normal bowel habits, including laxative use, suppositories, and enemas; diet including fluid intake; activity level; and medications.

Presenting Symptoms

Symptoms vary and may include abdominal pain, cramping or fullness, blood or mucus in stool, weight loss, fever, diarrhea alternating with constipation, and decreased defecation.

Physical Examination

The physical examination may reveal abdominal tenderness, distention, masses, and diminished bowel sounds. During the perianal examination, observe for fissures, strictures, tears, hemorrhoids, and rectal prolapse. A digital rectal examination may reveal a dilated rectum with stool, rectocele, or masses.

Diagnostic tests: Diagnosis usually is based on history, signs, and symptoms.

Tests	Results Indicating Disorder	CPT Code
CBC	Decreased RBCs, hemoglobin, and hematocrit suggest bleeding; decreased hemoglobin with changes in MCV, MCH, and MCHC suggests anemia (macrocytic, microcytic, thalassemia)	85004
Serum electrolytes	Hypokalemia or hypercalcemia can cause constipation	80051
TSH	Increased levels suggest hypothyroidism	84443
Fecal occult blood test	Positive result may suggest ulcerative or malignant GI lesion	82270
Abdominal x-ray	Determine pathology for intestinal obstruction, masses	74000
Sigmoidoscopy/ colonoscopy	Determine cause of bowel pathology; recommended after failure of conservative treatment or if positive occult blood or anemia present	45330, 45378
Barium enema	Determine masses, polyps, diverticula	74270

RBCs, red blood cells; MCV, mean corpuscular volume; MCH, mean corpuscular hemoglobin; MCHC, mean corpuscular hemoglobin concentration; TSH, thyroid-stimulating hormone.

Differential diagnosis:
- Simple constipation: history of decreased bulk and fiber in diet, fluid intake, activity level; pain with bowel movement
- Irritable bowel sydrome: onset in young adults; alternating constipation and diarrhea, mucus in stool
- Anorectal lesions (fissures, hemorrhoids): pain on defecation, blood on toilet tissue or in toilet
- Systemic diseases: such as diabetes mellitus, hypothyroidism, electrolyte imbalance
- Intestinal obstruction (masses, feces): hypoactive or absent bowel sounds, abdominal pain
- Medication induced: such as laxative abuse, calcium channel blockers, narcotic use

Treatment: Treat cause or refer as appropriate.

Physical
Dietary modifications include increasing fiber to 15–30 g/day and increasing fluid intake to 1.5 to 2 L/day. Lifestyle changes include increasing physical exercise and activities; developing bowel training routines; considering alternative medications if patient currently is taking medications that cause constipation; and advising against the long-term use of laxatives, suppositories, and enemas.

Pharmacologic
Add the following to the treatment regimen if dietary modifications and lifestyle changes fail. Hydrophilic colloids or bulk-forming agents are available over-the-counter in many forms and are not considered

laxatives. Use psyllium fiber in powder form or as chewable tablets or wafers taken as directed one to three times daily; methylcellulose powder, 1 tablespoon taken one to three times daily; or polycarbophil, 2 tablets taken one to four times daily. Surfactants or stool softeners, such as docusate sodium, 100 to 300 mg, or docusate calcium, 240 mg, may be given daily and can be given in addition to bulk-forming laxatives for short periods. The emollient action of these drugs should produce soft stools in 1 to 3 days. Osmotic laxatives are used for acute constipation but are not intended for long-term use. These drugs include magnesium hydroxide suspension, 30 to 60 mL in one dose; magnesium citrate, 240 mL in one dose; or sodium phosphate, 20 to 30 mL in one dose. The desired effect usually is produced within 0.5 to 3 hours.

Follow-up: See patient as indicated by cause of symptom.

Sequelae: Possible complications depend on cause of symptom; may include chronic constipation, fecal impaction, and bowel obstruction.

Prevention/prophylaxis: Prevention strategies depend on the cause but include advising the patient on the importance of maintaining healthy dietary, bowel, and lifestyle patterns. These include daily exercise; increase fluid intake to 1.5 to 2 L/day; and increase daily dietary fiber, including whole-grain breads and cereals, bran powder, green leafy vegetables, and fruit. Encourage the patient not to ignore the urge to defecate and to establish a set routine allowing enough time to defecate.

Referral: Refer to or consult with appropriate specialist as indicated by cause of symptom. Refer to physician if patient fails to respond to conventional treatment, if patient is >50 years old and has a sudden unexplainable change in bowel pattern, if patient has stools that test positive for blood, or if patient has weight loss.

Education: Explain cause of symptoms, tests or procedures used to determine the cause, and symptomatic treatment if any. Advise patient when to seek medical care. Discuss prevention strategies. Advise patient to take other medications 1 to 2 hours before the laxative because laxatives may alter the rate of medication absorption. Also strongly advise patient not to take any laxative for a prolonged period without medical supervision.

COUGH

Cough	ICD9-CM: 786.2

Description: Cough is a forceful, sometimes violent expiratory effort preceded by a preliminary inspiration. Coughing promotes airway clearance of secretions and foreign bodies. An acute cough most often is caused by a bacterial or viral respiratory infection. A chronic cough is a cough that lasts >3 weeks and most likely is caused by chronic lung or heart disease.

Etiology: Coughing is a reflex initiated by the stimulation of sensory nerve endings found in the trachea and tracheobronchial tree. Receptor sites in the periphery respond to irritation from inflammation, mechanical or chemical irritation, or extremes of temperature causing the cough reflex center located in the medulla oblongata of the brainstem to be stimulated. Efferent nerve fibers carry impulses back to the periphery causing contraction of effector muscles and cough.

Occurrence: One of the most common symptoms for which patients seek medical attention in an ambulatory setting.

Age: Occurs in all ages; increases with aging.

Ethnicity: No significant ethnic predisposition.

Gender: Occurs slightly more in men than in women.

Contributing factors: Smoking, exposure to secondhand smoke or other environmental irritants, postnasal drip, asthma, GERD, chronic sinusitis, chronic bronchitis, transient airway hyperresponsiveness, bronchiectasis, lung cancer, tuberculosis, interstitial lung disease, aspirated foreign body, CHF, cystic fibrosis, psychogenic cough, pneumonia, and pulmonary embolism.

Signs and symptoms:

History

Obtain information on the duration and character of the cough; precipitating, aggravating, and relieving factors; presence and character of sputum; and associated symptoms. Determine if the patient has been exposed recently to someone with an illness, such as an upper respiratory infection. Ascertain the patient's history of smoking or exposure to secondhand smoke or environmental stimuli (occupational and leisure) and family history of asthma, allergies, and tuberculosis exposure. Obtain information on the patient's current medication use, including over-the-counter (OTC) medications; especially be alert to the use of angiotensin-converting enzyme inhibitors and β-blockers. Determine if there are any associated constitutional symptoms, such as fever or weight loss.

Associated Signs and Symptoms

Signs and symptoms may include wheezing, postnasal drip, chest pain, frequent throat clearing, shortness of breath, heartburn or other reflux symptoms, fever, chills, and night sweats. The patient with a chronic cough related to postnasal drip also may have a history of seasonal allergies, atopy, or sinus infections and may complain of a sensation of having something drip into the throat or having the need to clear the throat frequently. The physical examination may reveal mucopurulent secretions or a cobblestone appearance of the nasopharyngeal mucosa. If there is hemoptysis with the cough and recent unexplained weight loss, suspect lung cancer. Suspect asthma if the patient has cough with episodic wheezing or shortness of breath, although cough can be the sole presenting symptom of asthma. If the patient has a history of cough with sputum production on most days for at least 3 months of the year for at least 2 years, suspect chronic bronchitis, especially if the patient has a history of smoking or exposure to environmental irritants. Suspect bronchiectasis if the patient complains of the production of large amounts of sputum, weight loss, fever, and malaise. The chest x-ray usually shows findings consistent with bronchiectasis. Suspect tuberculosis if there is a cough associated with weight loss, fatigue, and possible night sweats. If the patient has cough with heartburn and a sour taste in the mouth, suspect GERD. There also may be evidence of reflux on upper GI studies, evidence of esophagitis on esophagogastroduodenoscopy, or episodic evidence of acid reflux on esophageal pH monitoring. Pulmonary embolism may be suggested by cough; tachypnea; tachycardia; diminished breath sounds; and adventitious sounds such as wheezes, crackles, or pleural friction. A chronic, dry, nonproductive cough that begins after the initiation of angiotensin-converting enzyme inhibitors may indicate a side effect to the medication.

Physical Examination

Assess vital signs; an elevated temperature and pulse may indicate an acute bacterial or viral infection. Assess the ears for occlusion of the tympanic membrane and the nose and throat for mucus discharge, cobblestone pharynx, or postnasal drip. Evaluate the lymphatic system for enlarged nodes; if the supraclavicular nodes are enlarged, suspect lung cancer. Auscultate lung sounds; bibasilar crackles may suggest interstitial lung disease or CHF; general wheezing, especially expiratory, suggests asthma; localized wheezing may suggest partial bronchial obstruction; and stridor may indicate foreign body obstruction. Evaluate the cardiovascular system for valvular disease or CHF and the extremities for clubbing and edema. Assess mental status to determine level of consciousness, confusion, or restlessness, which may indicate hypoxemia.

Diagnostic tests:

Tests	Results Indicating Disorder	CPT Code
Chest x-ray	Determine infectious or noninfectious disease process or malignancy	71020
CBC with differential	Increase in WBC count with left shift suggests bacterial infection; increase in lymphocytes suggests viral infection; increase in eosinophils suggests allergy	85004
Sinus x-ray	Determine inflammation, masses of sinuses	70220
Bronchoscopy	Determine cause of cough if hemoptysis, significant cough, smoker, or age >50 years	31622
Spirometry	Assess for asthma; perform before and after use of bronchodilator or methacholine challenge test	94060

(Continued)

Tests	Results Indicating Disorder	CPT Code
Sputum for culture, Gram stain, or cytology	Determine cause of infectious process or cancer	87070
Tuberculosis skin testing	Positive test suggests tuberculosis	86580
Upper GI series	Determine acid reflux (GERD)	74240
Upper GI endoscopy	Determine acid reflux (GERD)	43200

Differential diagnosis:

Acute Cough

- Upper respiratory infection: cough, nasal congestion, pharyngitis, myalgia, fever, chills
- Lower respiratory infection (pneumonia): cough, dyspnea, pleurisy, sputum, fever, tachycardia, inspiratory crackles
- Asthma: cough, dyspnea, wheezing or diminished breath sounds, tachypnea, use of accessory muscles of respiration
- Pulmonary embolus: sudden onset of cough, dyspnea, chest pain, tachycardia, tachypnea, decreased breath sounds, crackles, wheezes or pleural friction rub; history of deep venous thrombosis risk factors
- CHF (pulmonary edema): cough, dyspnea, fatigue, tachycardia, tachypnea, use of accessory muscles of respiration, frothy sputum that may be blood tinged, wheezes or crackles; may have weight gain and lower extremity edema

Chronic Cough

- Asthma: dry hacking cough worse at night, prolonged expiratory respiratory phase with wheezing
- GERD: cough worse at night, foul taste in mouth, heartburn, may have epigastric pain on palpation; may have history of smoking or alcohol use
- Angiotensin-converting enzyme inhibitor–induced: nonproductive, dry cough beginning hours to months after initiation of angiotensin-converting enzyme inhibitor.
- Bronchogenic cancer: cough with hemoptysis, dyspnea, enlarged supraclavicular lymph nodes; history of smoking and weight loss
- Chronic sinusitis: mucopurulent rhinorrhea for at least 7 days
- Tuberculosis: cough, weight loss, fatigue, may have fever and night sweats

Treatment: Treat cause or refer as appropriate.

Red Flag: If patient is coughing and has signs and symptoms or history indicating a partially obstructed airway, such as stridor, retractions, and use of accessory muscles of respiration, maintain a patent airway and monitor patient for complete obstruction. Notify emergency medical services and transport to the emergency department.

Symptomatic Treatment

General measures include smoking cessation, avoiding secondhand smoke and other environmental irritants, and maintaining adequate hydration. Suppression of a productive cough is not recommended because coughing serves the protective function of ridding the airways of secretions and debris. A cough suppressant (prescription or OTC) may be indicated if the cough is persistent or severe or if cough-related complications develop. Central cough suppressors, such as codeine and dextromethorphan, affect the medullary cough center. Peripheral cough suppressors are thought to affect the cough receptors in the pharynx, larynx, and upper airway. Cough medications (prescription and OTC) are found in a variety of forms, including syrups and lozenges. Expectorants, such as guaifenesin, also may be used. If the patient has cough from postnasal drip, treatment commonly includes oral decongestants or a combination decongestant/antihistamine, such as pseudoephedrine sulfate, twice daily for several weeks. Nasal corticosteroids, such as fluticasone propionate (Flonase) or flunisolide (Nasalide), also may be used twice daily.

Follow-up: See patient as indicated by cause of symptom.

Sequelae: Possible complications depend on the cause of the symptom and may include strain on the intercostal muscles, sleep disturbance, irritation of the larynx and trachea, retching, and vomiting. Occasionally, rib fracture or tear of the rectus abdominis muscle and stress incontinence may occur. Pneumothorax, rupture of the subconjunctival or nasal veins, bradycardia, wound dehiscence after surgery, and cough syncope may be seen infrequently.

Prevention/prophylaxis: Prevention strategies depend on cause of symptom. Advise the patient to stop smoking at each session and to avoid secondhand smoke and other environmental irritants.

Referral: Refer to or consult with appropriate specialist as indicated by cause of symptom.

Education: Explain cause of symptoms, tests or procedures used to determine the cause, and symptomatic treatment, if any. Advise patient when to seek medical care. Discuss prevention strategies.

DIARRHEA

Diarrhea, acute   ICD-9-CM: 787.91

Description: Diarrhea is an increase in the frequency, volume, or fluid content of stools. In the United States, where dietary fiber is low and the daily stool usually weighs <200 g, diarrhea is defined as a stool volume >200 g/day or a frequency of three or more bowel movements a day. Chronic diarrhea is the passage of loose stools >200 g/day for >3 weeks.

Etiology: Acute diarrhea lasts 1 to 3 days. The most common cause of acute diarrhea is a self-limiting viral infection caused by rotavirus or Norwalk virus. Other causes include bacterial (specifically *Escherichia coli, Salmonella,* or *Shigella*) or protozoal infections (e.g., *Giardia lamblia, Cryptosporidium,* or *Entamoeba histolytica*) and travel to foreign countries (traveler's diarrhea). Sudden onset of diarrhea within hours after a meal may suggest diarrhea secondary to toxins such as *Staphylococcus* and *E. coli.* Chronic diarrhea, lasting >3 weeks, is probably not bacterial. Causes of chronic diarrhea include drug ingestion, inflammatory bowel disease, malabsorption syndromes, lactose intolerance, altered intestinal motility, and parasites.

Occurrence: Common.

Age: Occurs in all ages; most seriously affects the elderly.

Ethnicity: No significant ethnic predisposition.

Gender: Occurs equally in men and in women.

Contributing factors: Foreign travel; infected food or water sources; immunosuppression; abdominal surgery; laxative abuse; effects or side effects of certain medications (often from a cholinergic agent, such as a magnesium-containing antacid or antibiotics); and underlying medical conditions, such as hyperthyroidism, liver or gallbladder disease, certain neoplasias, and diabetes mellitus. Ingestion of certain foods containing sorbitol or mannitol may cause osmotic diarrhea; lactose intolerance is a type of osmotic diarrhea.

Signs and symptoms:

History

Obtain detailed information about the volume, frequency, and character of the stools; the presence of blood and mucus; and exposure to others with illnesses. A dietary history assists in the diagnosis of lactose intolerance. Inquire about recent travel because traveler's diarrhea typically begins 3 to 7 days after arrival in a foreign country and is usually quite acute. Assess for contributing stress-related symptoms and anxiety.

Associated Signs and Symptoms

Signs and symptoms may include nausea and vomiting, fever, and malaise. Suspect acute diarrhea if the patient has an abrupt onset of loose, liquid stools (with or without blood and mucus), fever, myalgia, headache, and anorexia. Chronic diarrhea often is accompanied by weight loss, steatorrhea, azotorrhea, and large volumes of stool. If the patient has chronic diarrhea characterized by pale greasy stools, abdominal cramping, and weight loss, suspect infection with *Giardia.* A secretory syndrome, such as carcinoid or Zollinger-Ellison syndrome, should be suspected if the patient has diarrhea alternating with constipation that is not improved by fasting. If the patient has a systemic illness or extraintestinal manifestations, such as arthritis, uveitis, or vasculitis, with the diarrhea or alternating diarrhea and constipation, suspect underlying inflammatory bowel disease, such as colon cancer, irritable bowel disease, and diverticulitis.

Physical Examination

Obtain vital signs, including weight. Inspect the skin and sclera for jaundice; the thyroid gland for signs of tenderness, nodules, or increased size; and the abdomen for evidence of surgical scars, localized swelling, or ascites. Auscultation may reveal hyperactive bowel sounds. Palpate lymph nodes. Patients with lymphadenopathy and chronic diarrhea may have human immunodeficiency virus/acquired immunodeficiency syndrome (HIV/AIDS) or lymphoma. Palpate and percuss the liver, spleen, and kidneys to assess size and locate areas of tenderness. Perform a rectal examination to assess for evidence of masses or polyps and to obtain stool to test for occult blood.

Diagnostic tests: Diagnosis usually is based on history, signs, and symptoms; however, certain clinical features, such as bloody stool, high fever, evidence of dehydration, recent antibiotic usage, and foreign travel, should trigger a stool examination.

Tests	Results Indicating Disorder	CPT Code
Fecal leukocytes	Positive result suggests inflammatory diarrheal disease and bacterial infections that invade intestinal wall (e.g., *E. coli, shigella, Salmonella, Campylobacter*)	85032
Fecal occult blood	Positive result suggests enteropathic bacteria or protozoa	82270
Stool for ova and parasites	Determine presence of parasites, such as hookworm, tapeworm, and *Giardia* (protozoan)	87177
Stool for *C. difficile* toxin assay	Positive result suggests malabsorption syndrome	87324
Fecal fat	Positive result suggests malabsorption syndrome	82710
D-xylose absorption test	Abnormal result in blood or urine suggests malabsorption syndrome	84620
CBC with differential	Increased leukocytes suggests infection; microcytic, hypochromic anemia may suggest chronic disease	83004
Serum electrolytes	Increased K^+ may suggest severe or persistent diarrhea or laxative abuse; increased Na^+, BUN, and creatinine and decreased pH may suggest dehydration	80051
Abdominal x-ray	Indicated if bowel obstruction or ischemia suspected	74000
Sigmoidoscopy	indicated if bloody diarrhea or if pseudomembranous or ulcerative colitis suspected	45330
Colonoscopy	Indicated if biopsy needed	45380

Differential diagnosis:

Acute Diarrhea

- Viral gastroenteritis (Norwalk, rotavirus): abrupt onset (6–12 hours postexposure), watery diarrhea without blood lasting <1 week, nausea, vomiting, fever, abdominal pain, tenesmus, hyperactive bowel sounds
- Bacterial gastroenteritis: acute onset within hours of exposure; symptoms dependent on specific bacteria (e.g., *Shigella, S. aureus, E. coli, Salmonella, Clostridium perfringens, Campylobacter jejuni, Vibrio choleraa, Entamoeba histolytica*)
- Protozoan gastroenteritis (*G. lamblia*): foul, watery diarrhea, low-grade fever
- Antibiotic induced: mild, watery diarrhea begins after taking antibiotics, abdominal cramping

Chronic Diarrhea

- Irritable bowel syndrome: diarrhea alternating with constipation, rectal urgency, stool with mucus, abdominal distention
- Ulcerative colitis: severe bloody diarrhea, initially without fever, weight loss, or abdominal pain; this occurs with moderate colitis
- Crohn's disease: chronic bloody diarrhea, abdominal cramping, tenderness, weight loss, rectal bleeding with fistulas
- Malabsorption (lactose): diarrhea caused by ingestion of lactose, flatus, bloating, abdominal pain
- Adenocarcinoma (with obstruction): pseudodiarrhea, fever, abdominal pain, hematochezia

Treatment: Treat cause or refer as appropriate.

Red Flag: Severe diarrhea can cause dehydration, especially in the elderly. Transport the patient to the emergency department for evaluation and possible hospitalization if signs and symptoms of acute dehydration are present.

Physical

General measures include placing the patient on a clear liquid diet to replace fluids and electrolytes and rest the bowel. Examples of recommended liquids include Gatorade or other sports or electrolyte-replacement drinks, tea, clear broth, and clear caffeine-free carbonated beverages such as ginger ale. Discontinue possible causative agents, such as antibiotics and antacids. After the diarrhea has decreased for 12 hours, advise the patient to try salted crackers or dry toast, then gradually add rice, baked potato, and chicken soup with noodles. As stools begin to gain shape, add applesauce, ripe bananas, baked fish, and poultry as tolerated until the patient has resumed a full diet. Have the patient avoid caffeine-containing foods and fluids, alcohol, dairy products, most fruits and vegetables, red meats, and spicy or heavily seasoned foods. Encourage rest and activity as tolerated. Provide reassurance.

Pharmacologic

Mild diarrhea: loperamide, 4 mg followed by 2-mg capsules; bismuth subsalicylate, 30 mL every half hour up to eight doses; or kaolin-pectin, 2 to 16 teaspoons daily, after each unformed stool

Infectious diarrhea: Use antiperistaltic agents with caution in patients with infectious diarrhea or antibiotic-associated colitis. Advise patients taking metronidazole to avoid alcoholic beverages.

  Giardia: metronidazole, 250 mg three times daily for 14 to 20 days

  E. histolytica: metronidazole, 750 mg three times daily for 10 days.

  C. difficile: metronidazole, 250 mg four times daily for 10 to 14 days

  Shigella: trimethoprim-sulfamethoxazole, 160 mg (trimethoprim) and 800 mg (sulfamethoxazole) twice daily for 5 days, or ciprofloxacin, 500 mg twice daily for 7 days

  Campylobacter: erythromycin, 250 mg four times daily, or ciprofloxacin, 500 mg orally twice daily for 3 days

  Cyclospora: trimethoprim-sulfamethoxazole, one double-strength tablet twice daily for 7 days

Traveler's diarrhea: trimethoprim-sulfamethoxazole, one double-strength tablet twice daily for 3 days, or ciprofloxacin, 500 mg twice daily for 3 days

Chronic diarrhea: psyllium or another hydrophilic agent to increase stool consistency; decrease caffeine, chocolate, and alcohol intake and stress

Secretory diarrhea: opiates, diphenoxylate-atropine, 5 to 20 mg daily, or loperamide, 4 to 16 mg daily, may be helpful

Lactose intolerance–related diarrhea: lactase

Follow-up: See patient as indicated by cause of symptom. Closely follow the patient. If diarrhea continues for 3 to 5 days, reassess the patient for hydration and reevaluate or modify the treatment plan.

Sequelae: Possible complications depend on cause of symptom. Complications may include dehydration, shock, sepsis, anemia, fluid and electrolyte abnormalities, malnutrition, anal excoriation, anal fissure, and hemorrhoids.

Prevention/prophylaxis: Prevention strategies depend on cause of symptom. To prevent traveler's diarrhea, avoid tap water or ice made from tap water; unpasteurized milk or dairy products; raw fruits or vegetables; lettuce and other leafy vegetables; cut-up fruit salad; raw or rare meat and fish; cold meat or shellfish; food from street vendors; and food from meals, such as buffets, that are left out for several hours. Safe foods include carbonated soft drinks, carbonated or bottled water if the patient is the one breaking the seal, and hot drinks if the water was boiled in preparing the drink. Use bottled water for brushing teeth and making ice cubes. Consider a prophylactic antibiotic.

Referral: Refer to or consult with appropriate specialist as indicated by cause of symptom.

Education: Explain cause of symptoms, tests or procedures used to determine the cause, and symptomatic treatment, if any. Advise patient when to seek medical care. Discuss prevention strategies.

DIZZINESS

| Dizziness | ICD-9-CM: 780.4 |

Description: Dizziness or vertigo is a sensation of abnormal movement of the body or surroundings. The sensation of moving around in space is called *subjective vertigo*; the sensation of having objects move around the person is called *objective* or *true vertigo*.

Etiology: Normal balance is a result of proper brainstem and cerebellar integration of three sensory systems: the vestibular apparatus located within the inner ear, the proprioceptive tracts of the central nervous system (CNS), and the visual pathways. An alteration in any of these three areas may result in dizziness. Other causes of dizziness include cerebrovascular ischemia from vertebrobasilar disease or transient ischemic attack or cardiovascular problems such as arrhythmias or orthostasis. Objective vertigo is usually a result of a disturbance of the equilibrium. Psychiatric problems are the second most common cause of dizziness after peripheral nervous system disorders.

Occurrence: Dizziness is a common presenting symptom in primary care; <2% of young adults and >30% of older adults seek medical attention for dizziness.

Age: Occurrence tends to increase with age.

Ethnicity: No significant ethnic predisposition.

Gender: No significant gender differentiation.

Contributing factors: Systemic disease; altered homeostasis; multisensory deficits; certain medications, either directly or as a side effect; head injuries; middle or inner ear infection; Ménière's disease; acoustic neuroma; cerebrovascular ischemia; multiple sclerosis; subclavian steal syndrome; hypoventilation; and psychological disorders such as anxiety, depression, and panic attacks.

Signs and symptoms:

History

During the history, it is important to establish what type of dizziness or vertigo the patient has and if the patient has dizziness, syncope, or dysequilibrium. Questions should be directed toward the quality and duration of the dizziness, precipitating factors, associated signs and symptoms or triggering factors, and medications.

Associated Signs and Symptoms

Dizziness may be classified into peripheral vestibular, central vestibular, presyncopal, psychiatric, and dysequilibrium etiologies. Peripheral vestibular dizziness includes benign positional vertigo, which is the most common cause of dizziness and may occur after trauma or viral infections or may be idiopathic in origin. It is characterized by brief episodes of intense vertigo that is associated with changes in head position but no change in hearing. Ménière's disease is an abnormal collection of endolymphatic fluid in the inner ear. It presents as episodic attacks of whirling vertigo that lasts for hours and is associated with nausea and vomiting, a neurosensory hearing loss, tinnitus, and ear fullness. Peripheral vestibulopathy is associated with a history of recent upper respiratory infection or GI infection and features severe vertigo associated with position changes but no change in hearing. Central vestibular dizziness is associated with CNS problems, including acoustic neuroma and vertebrobasilar disease. Acoustic neuroma is a tumor involving cranial nerve VIII. Clinically the patient presents with a gradual loss of hearing and tinnitus that is associated with dizziness/vertigo. Facial numbness and weakness may be seen as the condition progresses. Vertebrobasilar disease involves ischemic attacks of the brainstem areas. It is manifested by dizziness that is associated with signs of brainstem involvement, such as ataxia; visual disturbances; dysarthria; and weakness or sensory complaints on one, both, or alternating sides of the body. Presyncopal dizziness is a feeling of impending loss of consciousness and is associated with cardiovascular disease, postural hypotension, and metabolic disorders. Cardiovascular causes should be suspected if the patient presents with dizziness associated with syncope. Dizziness related to psychiatric etiologies, such as depression, anxiety, or panic attacks, may be manifested as lightheadedness. Dysequilibrium is seen more commonly in the elderly and results from a combination of sensory deficits. It is manifested as unsteadiness while walking but no dizziness when sitting or lying down.

Physical Examination

The physical examination and tests performed are based on the patient's history and the possible cause of the vertigo. Assess sensory functions. If a hearing problem is suspected, perform the whisper test to assess for hearing acuity. Perform the Weber test to determine lateralization of hearing using a 512-Hz tuning fork. Also check the external auditory canal, and perform the fistula test by occluding the external auditory canal with your finger. Vertigo occurs if a middle ear fistula is present. If a visual or nervous system problem is suspected, assess vision for nystagmus and visual acuity. Perform extraocular eye muscles (EOMs) to evaluate cranial nerves III, IV, and VI looking for weakness that could cause diplopia. Check for cataracts and perform a funduscopic examination of the lens. To evaluate neurologic function further, test cranial nerves V, VI, VII, VIII, IX, and X. Check for the presence of Horner's sign, which indicates brainstem dysfunction. Assess coordination and gait by performing tandem walking and the Romberg test, which evaluates brainstem and cerebellum function and assesses the vestibulospinal system. Evaluate proprioception by testing vibratory sensation in the feet using a 128-Hz tuning fork on the bony prominence or the toe or ankle malleoli and position sensation by testing the patient's perception of passive movement of the toes. If proprioception is impaired, there also may be an abnormal Romberg test and difficulty tandem walking. Test the vestibulo-ocular system by asking the patient to read newsprint while walking about or while the head is moving or perform the Hallpike maneuver. Have the patient sit on the examining table with the head turned to the side and eyes open. Grasp the patient's head and briskly bring the patient into a supine position with the head hanging below the head of the table. After 30 seconds, bring the patient back to the original sitting position. Repeat the maneuver with the head turned to the opposite side. Normally the patient experiences no vertigo. If the patient has a moderate sensation of vertigo with lateral and rotary nystagmus lasting about 1 minute, suspect a peripheral cause of positional vertigo. If the patient has a central cause of vertigo, repeated Hallpike maneuvers usually do not fatigue the nystagmus and the vertigo sensation.

If a cardiovascular cause is suspected, assess orthostatic vital signs, checking the blood pressure and pulse while lying and standing. A decrease in the systolic blood pressure of 20 mm Hg or in the diastolic blood pressure of 10 mm Hg and an increase in the pulse by 10 beats/min is a positive sign. Also auscultate the neck for carotid bruits.
Diagnostic tests:

Tests	Results Indicating Disorder	CPT Code
Audiometry	Low-frequency loss with Ménière's disease and acoustic neuroma	92557
Electronystagmography	Detects nystagmus that is spontaneous or induced by lateral gaze, positional change, or caloric testing	92543
MRI	Determine pathology involving brainstem or cerebellum	70551
Cerebral angiography (vertebral)	Determine pathology involving brainstem or cerebellum	75685

MRI, magnetic resonance imaging.

Differential diagnosis:
- Peripheral vestibulopathy: benign positional vertigo occurs with change in position, recurs, lasts a few minutes; no hearing loss or tinnitus. Ménière's syndrome has sudden onset, has fullness in ears, is recurrent, lasts hours, and has nystagmus.
- Central vestibulopathy (acoustic neuroma, vertebrobasilar disease): has gradual onset, mild dizziness, and tinnitus; may have facial numbness or weakness (or both). Cerebellar origin has acute onset, lack of coordination, ataxia, and nystagmus.
- Presyncopal (associated with cardiovascular disease, postural hypotension, metabolic disorder): orthostatic blood pressure, may have history of cardiovascular disease or antihypertensive medications
- Psychiatric (depression, anxiety, panic attacks): vague symptoms that recur; may indicate anxiety
- Dysequilibrium: combination of sensory deficits
- Peripheral nervous system disorder (e.g., multiple sclerosis): No specific findings; may have neurologic symptoms
- Trauma: symptoms depend on type and location of injury

Treatment: Treat cause or refer as appropriate.

Symptomatic Treatment

For benign paroxysmal positional vertigo, prescribe meclizine, 12.5 to 25 mg orally three or four times daily with dosage tapered as symptoms resolve, or dimenhydrinate, 50 mg orally three or four times daily. Prescribe prochlorperazine, 5 to 10 mg orally every 4 hours as needed for nausea. Bed rest may be necessary depending on the severity of the symptoms. To promote vestibular compensation, an exercise program may be helpful, although it may take several weeks to be effective. Exercises include having the patient repeat the head or body movements that cause the dizziness about five times every 8 hours until symptoms abate or having the patient move from a sitting to side-lying position, then repeating the maneuver on the opposite side. Peripheral vestibulopathy (acute labyrinthitis, vestibular neuronitis) usually resolves spontaneously within 3 to 6 weeks; the above-mentioned medications may be used for symptomatic relief if necessary.

Follow-up: See patient as indicated by cause of symptom. If the patient has a benign vestibular disorder, see immediately if the symptoms continue to worsen; see the patient in 3 to 6 weeks if the symptoms continue to resolve.

Sequelae: Possible complications depend on the cause of the symptom. Most benign vestibular disorders resolve without incident. There is always the danger of falls and motor vehicle accidents, however, during the acute phase of the disease. Without proper treatment, these disorders can lead to self-imposed isolation and a decrease in social contacts and activities because of the fear of falling and discomfort from the dizziness.

Prevention/prophylaxis: Prevention strategies depend on the cause of the symptom. Advise patient on safety methods to prevent falls, and caution against using machinery or driving motor vehicles.

Referral: Refer to, or consult with, appropriate specialist as indicated by cause of symptom.

Education: Explain cause of symptoms, tests or procedures used to determine the cause, and symptomatic treatment, if any. Educate the patient on safety precautions to take during attacks. Advise patient when to seek medical care. Reassure the patient with a benign vestibular disorder that it is usually self-limiting and resolves spontaneously.

FATIGUE

Fatigue	ICD-9-CM: 780.79

Description: Fatigue is a feeling of excessive tiredness, lethargy, lassitude, or exhaustion. It is a normal response to overexertion, lack of sleep, and stress.

Etiology: Fatigue may be a presenting symptom to many diseases, including endocrine disorders, such as hypothyroidism, hyperthyroidism, diabetes mellitus, and Addison's disease; cardiac disease; anemia; infections; respiratory disorders, such as sleep apnea and chronic obstructive pulmonary disease; systemic disorders, such as rheumatoid arthritis and systemic lupus erythematosus; cancer; obesity; and alcohol and other substance abuse. It also may be a side effect of medications and a symptom of a psychological disorder, especially depression.

Occurrence: One of the most common presenting symptoms in primary care.

Age: Occurs in all age groups.

Ethnicity: No significant ethnic predisposition.

Gender: No significant gender differentiation.

Contributing factors: Mental and physical overexertion, inadequate rest, poor nutritional intake, poor physical conditioning and stamina, prolonged emotional stress, drug use or abuse.

Signs and symptoms:

History

A detailed history is important to help determine the cause. Obtain information about the onset of the fatigue, its relationship to exertion, and any other accompanying signs and symptoms. Fatigue that is not present in the morning, becomes worse with exertion, and improves with rest usually is related to a physical problem. If the fatigue progressively increases over time, suspect anemia or cancer. Fatigue that is worse in the morning and improves as the day progresses may be related to a psychological problem or sleep disturbance. Fatigue, daytime somnolence, excessive snoring, obesity, and apneic periods during sleep may suggest a sleep disorder. If the patient has a flat affect, appetite or weight changes, feelings of guilt, or sexual dysfunction and fatigue, suspect depression. Review the social and family history and include the use of illicit drugs, alcohol dependency or abuse, and medications used by the patient. Anticholinergic agents, antidepressants, antihistamines, β-blockers, and centrally acting α-blockers have the potential to cause fatigue.

Associated Signs and Symptoms

Suspect an underlying infection if the patient has fever, lymphadenopathy, and cough. Fatigue accompanied by weight loss is seen with malignancies, endocrine disorders, poor nutrition, malabsorption syndromes, and chronic infectious diseases. If the patient has conjunctival or skin pallor with fatigue, suspect anemia. Joint abnormalities, muscle weakness, and fatigue may indicate a connective tissue disorder. Polydipsia, polyuria, polypepsia, heat or cold intolerance, weight changes, and fatigue can be seen with an endocrine disorder. Depression may be manifested by fatigue, sadness, indecisiveness, and sleep disturbances. Increased irritability or symptoms of autonomic hyperactivity, such as palpitations, sweating, dry mouth, or GI distress, with fatigue may suggest anxiety.

Diagnostic tests: Primarily diagnosed (85%) by history and physical examination. When diagnosis is not apparent, the following tests may be performed.

Tests	Results Indicating Disorder	CPT Code
CBC with differential	Increase in lymphocytes suggests viral infection; increase in WBC count with left shift suggests bacterial infection; increase in monocytes may suggest tuberculosis, CMV, lymphoma, metastatic cancer; increased eosinophils associated with drug reaction, allergy, lymphoma, vasculitis; decreased hematocrit suggests loss or diminished production of RBCs; decreased hemoglobin with changes in MCH, MCHC, and MCV suggests anemia (macrocytic, microcytic, thalassemia)	85004
Serum electrolytes, glucose, BUN/ creatinine ratio	Determine electrolyte balance, renal function, glucose; elevation in glucose may suggest diabetes mellitus; elevation in BUN/creatinine ratio suggests renal insufficiency or failure	80051, 82947, 82565, 84520
TSH	Increased level suggests hypothyroidism; decreased level suggests hyperthyroidism	84443
ESR	Increased level suggests infection, inflammation, neoplasm	85652
Monospot	Increased level suggest infectious mononucleosis	86308
Stools for occult blood	Positive results suggest GI bleeding, neoplasm	82270
Tuberculin skin test	Positive result suggests tuberculosis exposure	86580
Enzyme-linked immunosorbent assay	Positive results need to be confirmed by Western blot test to determine HIV status	87390– 87391

Differential diagnosis:

- Psychiatric problem (depression or anxiety): vague symptoms; may indicate anxiety
- Chronic fatigue syndrome: requires a 6-month history of new onset of fatigue accompanied by infectious, rheumatologic, and neuropsychiatric symptoms that cannot be explained by other medical diagnosis
- Organic disease: use laboratory tests to rule out organic problems, such as infection, anemia, malignancies, endocrine disorders, poor nutrition, and malabsorption syndromes
- Immune suppression: use HIV testing to rule out HIV/AIDS; other laboratory tests to rule out cancer or other immunosuppressive problems

Treatment: Treat cause or refer as appropriate.

Follow-up: See patient as indicated by cause of symptom.

Sequelae: Possible complications depend on cause of symptom and may include chronic fatigue syndrome.

Prevention/prophylaxis: Prevention strategies depend on cause of symptom. Advise the patient to maintain a healthy lifestyle, including regular exercise, balanced diet, and adequate sleep and relaxation, and to use healthy stress management techniques.

Referral: Refer to or consult with appropriate specialist as indicated by cause of symptom. Patients with psychological causes may need to be referred for counseling.

Education: Explain cause of symptoms, tests or procedures used to determine the cause, and symptomatic treatment, if any. Instruct the patient to get adequate rest and to plan and prioritize activities to optimize energy. Strenuous activities may require assistance. Medical care should be sought if symptoms do not improve.

FEVER

| Fever of unknown origin | ICD-9-CM: 780.6 |

Description: Fever is the abnormal elevation of body temperature >38°C (100.4°F) when taken orally.

Etiology: Fever is a sign that can reflect a disorder in any body system. There are three physiologic reasons for fever. The first involves the raising of the hypothalamic set-point, which results in a higher core body temperature and an elevation of helper T-cell production. Common causes of this type of fever include infection, collagen disease, vascular disease, and malignancy. The second type of fever is the consequence of heat production exceeding loss. This occurs when the environmental heat exceeds the normal heat loss mechanisms. It also can occur when the metabolic heat production of the body is increased. Causes of this second type of fever include malignant hypertension, hyperthyroidism, hypernatremia, and aspirin overdose. The third type of fever occurs when the body cannot contend with a normal heat load because of a defect in the heat loss mechanism. Heatstroke and burns can cause this type of fever.

Occurrence: Common.

Age: Occurs at any age.

Ethnicity: No significant ethnic predisposition.

Gender: No significant gender differentiation.

Contributing factors: Dehydration, heatstroke, thyroid storm, malignant hyperthermia, CNS lesions.

Signs and symptoms:

History

Note the onset, duration, and pattern of fever. Associated complaints, such as stiff neck, rash, wounds, injuries, earache, sore throat, cold symptoms, cough, nausea, vomiting, diarrhea, abdominal pain, night sweats, and urinary symptoms, can assist in determining the cause. A history of recent travel may provide clues to infectious diseases endemic in that region. Exposures to communicable disease, exposure to animals, tick bites, drug use, work environment, and HIV risk should be sought. A complete history of medications taken by the patient can provide clues to the possible cause. Also note patient's response to self-medication with antipyretics.

Accompanying Signs and Symptoms

Signs and symptoms may include warm, flushed skin; shivering or chills; sweating; night sweats; tachycardia; tachypnea; malaise; fatigue; headache; myalgia; and enlarged lymph nodes. The patient also presents with local or systemic manifestations of the underlying cause.

Diagnostic tests:

Tests	Results Indicating Disorder	CPT Code
CBC with differential and platelets	Increase in lymphocytes suggests viral infection; increase in WBC count with left shift suggests bacterial infection; increase in monocytes suggests tuberculosis, CMV, lymphoma, or metastatic cancer; increased eosinophils associated with drug reaction, allergy, lymphoma, and vasculitis; increased hemoglobin and decreased hematocrit associated with dehydration; increased platelets and anemia associated with acute and chronic infections, neoplasms, and inflammatory diseases; decreased platelets occasionally associated with acute infection, immune-mediated disorder, and leukemia	85025
ESR	Increased level suggests inflammation, infection, or neoplasm	85652
Serum electrolytes	Determine electrolyte balance and renal function	80051
Culture and sensitivity	Identify causative infectious agent and appropriate antibiotic therapy	87077–87084
Urinalysis	Urinary tract infection associated with increased WBC count, nitrates, and bacteria in urine	81001

Differential diagnosis:
- Respiratory (including tonsillitis, sinusitis, pneumonia): fever usually <38.7°C (101.5°F). Systemic symptoms are common along with cough and nonpurulent sputum. Pharyngeal erythema may be present with pharyngitis.
- GI: bacterial or viral gastroenteritis, acute abdomen
- Urinary: upper urinary tract infections commonly produce systemic symptoms with flank pain and fever
- Pelvic inflammatory disease: associated with lower abdominal tenderness, suprapubic tenderness, cervical motion tenderness, vaginal discharge, and fever
- Drug reaction or alcohol withdrawal
- Fever of unknown origin: if fever persists for at least 14 days with undetermined cause, consider fever of unknown origin. The etiology of 20% of fevers remains unknown despite an extensive medical workup.

Treatment: Treat cause or refer as appropriate.

 Red Flag: Fever >41°C (106°F) requires emergency treatment and continuous monitoring because it can cause CNS dysfunction. Administer antipyretics and cool the body rapidly with tepid sponges or hypothermia blanket.

Symptomatic Treatment

Antipyretic therapy is effective with the first type of fever. Acetaminophen, aspirin, or ibuprofen given every 4 hours can help decrease symptoms associated with fever and decrease the incidence of chills and diaphoresis. Fever <40°C (104°F) is usually tolerated well; however, symptomatic treatment, such as cool sponge baths, antipyretic therapy, and replacement of fluids lost through insensible perspiration and diaphoresis, may be required. Appropriate antibiotic therapy should be given to a patient with an identified source of infection. If the patient is immunocompromised or has suspected sepsis, empirical use of broad-spectrum antibiotics before confirmation of an infection is indicated.

Follow-up: See patient as indicated by cause of symptom. Telephone the patient in 24 to 48 hours. If the fever persists for >3 days, see patient for additional evaluation.

Sequelae: Possible complications depend on cause of symptom.

Prevention/prophylaxis: Prevention strategies depend on cause of symptom. Advise the patient to avoid contact with sources of communicable diseases. A healthy lifestyle promotes an overall physical well-being, which is the most important factor in maintaining an intact immune system.

Referral: Refer to or consult with appropriate specialist as indicated by cause of symptom. Immediately refer to clinical emergency department if the patient has a fever >41°C (106°F), changes in level of consciousness, or neurologic symptoms. Refer to a physician if the patient has marked dehydration, appears septic, or has a fever for 7 to 10 days despite antibiotic therapy.

Education: Explain cause of symptoms, tests or procedures used to determine the cause, and symptomatic treatment, if any. Explain to the patient how to take a temperature properly. Advise patient when to seek medical care.

HEADACHE

Headache	ICD-9-CM: 784.0
Headache, cluster	ICD-9-CM: 346.2
Headache, tension	ICD-9-CM: 307.81
Migraine, unspecified	ICD-9-CM: 346.9
Classic, migraine	ICD-9-CM: 346.0

Description: A headache is a diffuse pain in the head. Headaches are categorized into primary and secondary. Primary headaches are headaches without structural pathology or systemic disease; they account for >90% of all headaches and include migraine, tension, and cluster headaches. Secondary headaches are headaches caused by identifiable organic pathology of the meninges or cerebral parenchyma. Headaches also may be categorized as acute, recurrent, or chronic.

Etiology: Causes of headaches include traction on pain-sensitive structures, inflammation of vessels and meninges, vascular dilation, excessive muscle contraction, and dysregulation of the ascending brainstem serotoninergic systems.

Occurrence: Most individuals experience some form of headache at some time in their lives; 50% of individuals have severe headaches, and 10% to 20% consult a health care provider.

Age: Occurs in all ages. Migraine headaches often begin in childhood. Cluster headaches often begin in the 30s.

Ethnicity: No significant ethnic predisposition.

Gender: Tension headaches and migraine headaches are more common in women, and cluster headaches occur predominantly in men.

Contributing factors:

- General headache: food intolerance (e.g., chocolate, red wine, foods that contain nitrates or monosodium glutamate), alcohol ingestion, caffeine withdrawal, certain medications (e.g., reserpine, vasodilators, birth control pills), stress, and hunger
- Migraine headache: specified foods, alcohol, caffeine, skipped meals, hormonal changes, stress, birth control pills, hormone replacement therapy, changes in weather or barometric pressure, female gender, genetic predisposition
- Tension headache: depression, anxiety, and chronic headaches may coexist with combination migraine and tension headaches; dental

malocclusion; stress; abnormal positions of neck; excessive caffeine; obstructive sleep apnea

- Cluster headache: short naps, small amounts of vasodilators such as alcohol or nitroglycerin, tyramine, emotional stress

Signs and symptoms: Symptoms suggesting a tension headache include a slowly progressing, bilateral, nonthrobbing or bandlike sensation around the head that is a mild-to-moderate dull pressure usually located in the occipital and suboccipital areas. The physical examination is normal, but the neck muscles might be tight.

A migraine headache may present as a common migraine (without aura) or classic migraine (with aura). Common migraine presents as a unilateral, throbbing headache that is usually in the frontotemporal or supraorbital region. Nausea, vomiting, photophobia, and phonophobia may be present. Classic migraine has a prodrome that is abrupt in onset, lasts 15 minutes, is contralateral to the headache, and occurs 15 to 30 minutes before the headache. Visual auras include scotomata, transient blindness, blurred vision, and hemianopsia. Nonvisual auras include weakness, aphasia, and photophobia. The headache is severe and is accompanied by nausea, vomiting, photophobia, and phonophobia.

Symptoms that suggest a cluster headache include a sudden, severe, unilateral, burning or stabbing pain behind the eye that usually begins at night. Ipsilateral rhinorrhea, nasal stuffiness, conjunctival injection, and ptosis also may be seen.

Diagnostic tests: Headache is usually diagnosed by history, signs, and symptoms.

Tests	Results Indicating Disorder	CPT Code
CBC with differential	Increased WBC count with left shift suggests bacterial infection	85004
Cervical x-ray	Detect cervical radiculopathy	72040
CT scan	Detect cerebral pathology	72125
MRI	Detect cerebral pathology	72141
Lumbar puncture	Viral infection suggested with normal or slightly increased protein, 10–500 lymphocytes (PMVs); bacterial infection suggested with protein 50–1500 mg/100 mL, decreased glucose usually <20 mg/dL, 25–10,000 polymorphonuclear neutrophils	62270

Differential diagnosis:

Primary Headache

- Migraine without aura (common migraine): Diagnosis cannot be made unless there are five attacks that fulfill the following criteria: (1) headache lasts 4 to 72 hours; (2) headache has at least two of the following characteristics—unilateral, pulsating, moderate-to-severe, aggravated by walking stairs or similar activity; and (3) during the headache, at least one of the following occurs—nausea or vomiting, photophobia, or phonophobia.

- Migraine with aura (classic migraine): Diagnosis cannot be made unless there are two attacks with at least three of the following features: (1) fully reversible aura symptoms indicating focal brain dysfunction, (2) at least one aura symptom that develops gradually over >4 minutes or two or more symptoms that occur in succession, (3) no single aura symptom lasting >60 minutes, and (4) headache usually follows aura within 1 hour.
- Tension: bilateral pain banding head, history of stress, anxiety, tight neck muscles
- Cluster: severe, nighttime, unilateral headache, periorbital pain, ptosis, ipsilateral nasal stuffiness or rhinorrhea

Secondary Headache

 Red Flag: Red flags include papilledema, abnormal visual fields, abnormal gait, change in headache pattern, new-onset headache in a person >50 years old, abrupt onset of headache, or unusual neurologic symptoms.

- Intracerebral hemorrhage: sudden onset of severe headache with or without history of trauma, neurologic findings associated with site of bleeding
- Meningitis: severe headache, chills, myalgia, stiff neck, positive Kernig's and Brudzinski's signs, fever, photophobia, mental status change, petechial rash
- Intracranial tumor: headache that is progressive, exacerbated by coughing or exercise, worse in the morning, papilledema, vomiting, neurologic findings associated with location of tumor
- Dental disease: localized pain in jaw and top of head, malocclusion, caries, abscess, or tooth or gum disease
- Temporomandibular joint disorder: pain in temporomandibular joint or ear, temporoparietal headache, bruxism
- Sinusitis: frontal, upper molar, or periorbital pain or pressure; cough; rhinorrhea; may have low-grade fever, pain on palpation of sinuses, purulent nasal or postnasal discharge
- Other medical disorder: including hypoglycemia, hypertension, temporal arteritis, drug withdrawal

Treatment: Treat cause or refer as appropriate.

Symptomatic Treatment

Pharmacologic therapy usually is initiated with the least-addictive medications, such as acetaminophen, aspirin, and NSAIDs. Therapy for migraines is divided into abortive or prophylactic. Abortive therapy should begin as soon as symptoms occur. The medication is more effective the sooner it is taken. Waiting too long to begin abortive therapy is a primary reason for failure of the medication. In some cases, Excedrin, an

OTC drug, has proved to be effective. Other abortive drugs include ergotamines, which cause vasoconstriction. Ergotamines are contraindicated in patients with cerebrovascular or cardiovascular disease and must not be used within 24 hours of a triptan medication. Triptan medications are serotonin agents that inhibit 5-hydroxytryptamine 1B/1D receptors located in the intracranial blood vessels to prevent vasodilation. These agents are used exclusively for the treatment of migraine headache and include sumatriptan (Imitrex), zolmitriptan (Zomig), and naratriptan (Amerge), which may be administered in a variety of methods. Nonpharmacologic approaches, such as biofeedback, stress management, relaxation, and exercise, also may be of benefit. For a tension headache, amitriptyline, 50 to 100 mg at bedtime; psychotherapy; or behavior modification aided by biofeedback or social counseling may help severe chronic muscle-contraction headaches. Massage, exercise, and a healthy diet may help to decrease headaches.

Follow-up: See patient as indicated by cause of symptom. See patient if headache is unrelieved or if it increases in severity, duration, or frequency from the usual pattern.

Sequelae: Possible complications depend on cause of symptom. A cycle of drug-dependency headache and caffeine-withdrawal headache or drug addiction and drug-seeking behavior may occur with a patient with a tension headache.

Prevention/prophylaxis: Prevention strategies depend on cause of symptom. Migraine prophylactic therapy includes medications used to prevent the headache, including β-blockers, calcium channel blockers, antiseizure drugs, and tricyclic and selective serotonin reuptake inhibitor antidepressants.

Referral: Refer to or consult with appropriate specialist as indicated by cause of symptom. Refer to or consult with a physician if the patient has any of the following signs: abnormal physical signs; new-onset, unilateral headache, particularly in patients >35 years old; severe headache or headache different from previous ones; headaches becoming more continuous and intense; or headaches accompanied by vomiting but not nausea.

Education: Explain cause of symptoms, tests or procedures used to determine the cause, and symptomatic treatment, if any. Advise patient when to seek medical care.

HEARING LOSS

Hearing loss, sensorineural	ICD-9-CM: 389.10
Hearing loss, conductive	ICD-9-CM: 389.0

Description: Hearing loss is the decreased ability or complete inability to hear. Conductive hearing loss is usually reversible and may involve the external or middle ear, which indicates a mechanical or conductive problem. Sensorineural hearing loss is usually irreversible and involves the inner ear, which indicates a nerve or sensorineural problem causing distortion of sound and misinterpretation of speech. Hearing loss may have conductive and sensorineural components and may be unilateral or bilateral.

Etiology:

Sensorineural

Sensorineural hearing loss is caused by a lesion in the organ of Corti or in the central pathways, including the eighth cranial nerve and auditory cortex. Age-related hearing loss (presbycusis) is a form of sensorineural hearing loss. Sensorineural hearing loss also may be caused by Ménière's disease, tumor, noise damage, genetics, ototoxicity from a variety of medications, syphilis, metabolic disorder such as hypothyroidism, an inner ear fistula, and viral syndromes such as mumps.

Conductive

Conductive hearing loss is caused by a lesion involving the outer and middle ear to the level of the oval window. This hearing loss may result from a variety of structural abnormalities, cerumen impaction, perforation of the tympanic membrane, middle ear fluid, damage to the ossicles from trauma or infection, otosclerosis, tympanosclerosis, cholesteatoma, middle ear tumors, temporal bone fractures, injuries related to trauma, and congenital problems.

Occurrence: Increased prevalence after age 40; affects 30% of all adults age 65 to 74 and 50% of all adults >85 years old.

Age: Sensorineural hearing loss increases with age; degenerative decline starts at age 20.

Ethnicity: No significant ethnic predisposition.

Gender: Occurs equally in men and women.

Contributing factors: Exposure to loud noises; heredity; ototoxic drugs such as aminoglycoside antibiotics, acetylsalicylic acid, furosemide, and quinine; eustachian tube obstruction; chronic middle ear infections; chronic cerumen impaction; trauma.

Signs and symptoms:

History

Obtain a complete history of current and past prescription and OTC medications. The social and occupational history should include specific questions regarding noise or toxin exposure and any blast injuries. The review of systems should focus on the neurologic system, including cranial nerve function, such as facial weakness or tingling, loss of taste, or dysphagia.

Associated Signs and Symptoms

The patient may complain of difficulty hearing associated with pain, pressure, discharge, nausea, vomiting, discomfort, vertigo, or loss of balance.

Other associated symptoms include tinnitus, dizziness, blockage, popping, crackling, distant sounds, stiffness, fever, or upper respiratory infection.

Physical Examination

The whisper test is abnormal if much more than a 40-db loss is present. In unilateral disease, the Rinne test shows air conduction less than bone conduction, and the Weber test lateralizes to the involved ear. The physical examination includes inspection of the external auditory canal. During the otoscopic examination, note redness, foreign objects, discharge, scaling, lesions, and cerumen. Expect to see minimal cerumen, a pink color, and hairs in the outer third of the ear. The tympanic membrane should be a translucent pearly gray without perforations. Note if the tympanic membrane moves from the pressure of the pneumatic otoscope. Changes in the tympanic membrane may be consistent with conductive hearing loss.

Diagnostic tests:

Tests	Results Indicating Disorder	CPT Code
Audiometry	Include pure tone and speech testing and impedance testing to determine type and degree of loss	92557
MRI	Determine cause, such as acoustic neuroma, cholesteatoma	70480, 70551

Differential diagnosis:

Conductive Hearing loss

- Cerumen impaction
- Otosclerosis
- Middle ear effusion: usually unilateral hearing loss; tympanic membrane is dull, is hypomobile, and may have air bubbles in the middle ear

Sensorineural Hearing Loss

- Ototoxicity: causative drugs include salicylates, aminoglycosides, and loop diuretics
- Trauma: may have perforated tympanic membrane or hemotympanum
- Presbycusis: progressive high-frequency symmetric hearing loss associated with aging
- Ménière's disease: hearing loss associated with tinnitus and vertigo
- Acoustic neuroma: unilateral hearing loss associated with tinnitus

Treatment: Treat cause or refer as appropriate. Encouragement, follow-up, and support are important for the patient with hearing loss.

Conductive Hearing Loss

If hearing loss is caused by cerumen buildup, disimpaction is performed using a 1:1 mixture of hydrogren peroxide and mineral oil. Place three drops in the external ear and wait 1 hour, then lavage with warm saline.

If hearing loss is caused by infection, treat as appropriate. Refer if a tympanic perforation is present or if there is damage to ossicles, tympanosclerosis, otosclerosis, tumor, or temporal bone injury.

Sensorineural Hearing Loss

Refer patient. Stop medications if indicated. Treat the underlying cause. If the patient has sudden sensorineural hearing loss with no apparent cause, high doses of steroids (80 mg/day of prednisone or equivalent) sometimes are used. No specific treatment reverses the process of presbycusis. Treatment involves hearing aids. It is important to educate and support the patient so that no further damage occurs. Suggest that the patient reduce noise exposure and avoid ototoxic medications. Refer to a speech therapist to learn lip-reading when appropriate and instruct the family to speak clearly. Complete a home assessment for the need of assistive devices, such as a special telephone or closed-captioned television.

Follow-up: See patient as indicated by cause of symptom.

Sequelae: Possible complications depend on cause of symptom but may include permanent hearing loss. The patient may need a hearing aid. Cerumen removal may cause damage to the external auditory meatus or perforation of the tympanic membrane or otitis media if not done properly. Middle ear problems may progress to chronic ear problems, such as perforations or cholesteatoma. Severe nerve deafness, particularly associated with tinnitus, may produce severe depression and social isolation.

Prevention/prophylaxis: Prevention strategies depend on cause of symptom. Advise the patient to use devices to protect against occupational or recreational hearing loss, to equalize ear pressure when diving, to chew gum in airplanes or use decongestants, to avoid flying or diving if an upper respiratory infection is present, and to avoid ototoxic medications. Teach the patient proper techniques for cerumen removal. Advise the patient not to use Q-tips.

Referral: Refer to or consult with appropriate specialist as indicated by cause of symptom. Referral to audiometry may be indicated.

Education: Explain cause of symptoms, tests or procedures used to determine the cause, and symptomatic treatment, if any. Advise patient when to seek medical care. Discuss prevention strategies. Teach the importance of the use of hearing aids if indicated because this can make a significant difference in quality of the patient's life. Advise the patient to contact rehabilitation centers to learn lip-reading skills, sign language, or both. Provide support and help the patient resist the temptation to withdraw socially. Educational resource materials are available from the Better Hearing Institute, PO Box 1840, Washington, DC 20013 (800-424-8576) and the National Hearing Aid Helpline, 20361 Middlebelt Road, Livonia, MD 48152 (800-521-5247).

HOARSENESS

| Voice loss (aphonia) | ICD-9-CM: 784.41 |

Description: Hoarseness describes a voice with a harsh quality and low pitch. It also may include weakness, raspiness, or simply a change from the usual voice quality.

Etiology: Hoarseness is caused by an abnormality somewhere along the vocal tract that causes an abnormal flow of air past the vocal cords. An abnormal harsh quality in the voice is caused by turbulence created by irregularity in the vocal cords. Hoarseness can be acute or chronic. Acute hoarseness is the result of an infectious or inflammatory process in the larynx. Hoarseness lasting >3 weeks is termed *persistent (chronic)* and may indicate structural changes to the vocal cords from polyps, nodules, or malignant or benign tumors and from vocal cord paralysis. Hoarseness also may be a symptom of a systemic disease, such as hypothyroidism or rheumatoid arthritis, and laryngeal muscle atrophy seen with aging. Gastroesophageal reflux also can cause laryngeal irritation resulting in hoarseness.

Occurrence: Common.

Age: Occurs at any age.

Ethnicity: No significant ethnic predisposition.

Gender: Occurs equally in men and in women.

Contributing factors: Laryngeal trauma caused by excessive alcohol intake, inhalation of noxious fumes and cigarette smoke, allergies, and excessive talking and shouting.

Signs and symptoms:

History

Note the duration of symptoms and lifestyle. Acute onset (<3 weeks' duration) is more likely to be from upper respiratory infection or overuse of the voice. Chronic symptoms or a complaint of progressively increasing hoarseness is more likely to be from structural change in the larynx or a systemic disease process. If the hoarseness becomes progressively worse during the day, suspect myasthenia gravis. A professional singer or weekend football fan can suffer voice overuse and abuse. A cigarette smoker of two packs per day for 45 years may have irritation or malignancy. A scratchy throat the morning after eating spicy foods late in the evening suggests gastroesophageal reflux. Recurrent episodes of hoarseness may indicate allergies or sinusitis.

Associated Signs and Symptoms

Hoarseness accompanied by a sore throat and otalgia is seen frequently in malignant tumors of the larynx or pharynx. Dysphagia or odynophagia with hoarseness may indicate a disease affecting the pharynx or esophagus. Cough and hoarseness suggest irritation of the endolarynx or pulmonary disease. Hemoptysis and hoarseness may indicate a malignant process of the pharyngeal, laryngeal, or pulmonary areas. Fever; oral, nasal, or otalgic discharge; and hoarseness suggest an infectious process. Progressive dysarthria and dysphagia may indicate Parkinson's disease, myasthenia gravis, or amyotrophic lateral sclerosis.

Physical Examination

The physical examination may reveal infection, masses, or neurologic disorders.

Diagnostic tests:

Tests	Results Indicating Disorder	CPT Code
CBC with differential	Increase in lymphocytes may suggest viral infection; increase in WBC count with left shift suggests bacterial infection; increased monocytes suggest tuberculosis, CMV, lymphoma, metastatic cancer; increased eosinophils may suggest drug reaction, allergy, lymphoma, vasculitis	85004
Culture and sensitivity of discharge	Determine causative infectious agent and appropriate antibiotic therapy	87070
Laryngoscopy with or without biopsy	If hoarseness persisted >2 weeks, determine structural problems of larynx	31505, 31510
CT scan	Determine structural problems of larynx, vagus, or laryngeal nerves	70490

Differential diagnosis:

- Acute laryngitis: voice overuse; exposure to environmental irritants; recent upper respiratory infection as shown by aphonia, cervical lymphadenopathy, pharyngitis, edema of vocal cords
- Chronic laryngitis: hoarseness >3 weeks' duration with history of chronic smoking or alcohol use; exposure to environmental irritants with edema or nodules of vocal cords
- Vocal cord paralysis: chronic cough; stridor with exertion; weak, soft voice
- Polyps: hoarseness >3 weeks' duration or progressive hoarseness worse at the end of the day but almost normal in the morning; history of allergy, voice abuse, GERD, smoking
- Hypothyroidism: systemic symptoms of cold intolerance, fatigue, weight gain, dry skin and hair, prolonged deep tendon reflexes
- GERD: history of upper GI burning and cough, chronic use of alcohol, NSAIDs, aspirin, smoking
- Psychogenic: breathy, low voice with normal examination

Treatment: Treat cause or refer as appropriate. Referral for laryngoscopy with or without biopsy is indicated if hoarseness has persisted >3 weeks. Laryngeal papillomatosis, vocal polyps, and tumors require surgical removal.

Symptomatic Treatment

Smoking cessation, voice rest, and humidification may relieve irritation.

Follow-up: See patient as indicated by cause of symptom. See patient until problem resolves.

Sequelae: Possible complications depend on cause of symptom. Airway obstruction may occur if patient has inflammation or lesions. Refer immediately for emergency treatment if symptoms of airway obstruction are present.

Prevention/prophylaxis: Prevention strategies depend on cause of symptom. Advise patient to maintain a healthy lifestyle and avoid noxious inhalants, alcohol, and overuse of the voice.

Referral: Refer to or consult with appropriate specialist as indicated by cause of symptom. Referral to a speech therapist may be indicated.

Education: Explain cause of symptoms, tests or procedures used to determine the cause, and symptomatic treatment, if any. Advise patient when to seek medical care.

INSOMNIA

Sleep disturbance, unspecified	ICD-9-CM: 780.50
Insomnia with sleep apnea	ICD-9-CM: 780.51
Other insomnia	ICD-9-CM: 780.52

Description: Insomnia is a sleep disorder in which there is an abnormality in the amount, quality, or timing of sleep. It may be experienced as a difficulty in falling asleep (sleep-onset insomnia), frequent or prolonged awakenings from sleep (sleep-maintenance insomnia), early morning awakening, or a combination of these. Insomnia can be categorized as transient, short-term, or long-term (chronic). Transient insomnia usually lasts a few days; is often the result of jet lag, anticipation of an important event, or sleeping in a strange place; and usually is caused by situation anxiety. Short-term insomnia usually lasts a few weeks and often is associated with the loss of a job, death in the family, or divorce. Chronic insomnia usually lasts months to years and can be the result of physical or emotional illnesses. Insomnia may cause significant distress in social, occupational, or other areas of functioning.

Etiology: Caused by psychological factors (psychological insomnia), such as situational anxiety or stress, or physiologic factors (physiologic insomnia), such as abnormalities or disruption of the body's circadian rhythm, especially body temperature. Patients with insomnia often have higher core body temperatures than good sleepers and less variation in their temperature curve throughout the 24-hour period.

Occurrence: Occurs in about 30% of adults; one of the most common complaints seen in primary care. Frequently these cases are undiagnosed and untreated.

Age: Prevalence rises with age. Average age of onset is in the mid-30s for sleep-onset difficulties and mid-50s for sleep-maintenance problems.

Ethnicity: No significant ethnic predisposition.

Gender: Occurs equally in men and in women. Sleep apnea is more common in men.

Contributing factors: Chronic illnesses, such as arthritis, fibromyalgia, chronic fatigue disorders, hyperthyroidism, GERD, Alzheimer's disease, sleep apnea, restless leg syndrome, respiratory disorders, and painful conditions; psychiatric illnesses, such as depression, anxiety, alcohol or substance abuse, and schizophrenia; pregnancy; age; obesity; polypharmacy (multiple drug intake); medications, such as β-blockers, corticosteroids, bronchodilators, respiratory stimulants, stimulating antidepressants, methyldopa, thyroid supplements, CNS stimulants, decongestants, and phenytoin; circadian rhythm disturbances, such as work shift changes, time zone changes, irregular sleep-wake pattern, and daytime napping, which may be due to sleep apnea or narcolepsy; excessive use of caffeine, alcohol, or nicotine; vigorous exercise or mental activity near bedtime; inadequate maintenance of a comfortable sleep environment, such as excessive room temperature, light, or noise.

Signs and symptoms:

History

Obtain information on the patient's past and present sleep and activity patterns, current medications, daily habits, diet, exercise pattern, occupation, work schedule, social routines, and other psychosocial factors. Determine the severity and duration of the problem. Is it a chronic problem, or is it transient (<4 weeks)? Assess for depression and chronic pain. If possible, assess the patient's sleeping partner for additional observations.

Associated Signs and Symptoms

Along with the complaint of insomnia, the patient may appear fatigued, haggard, and irritable. The patient may complain of impaired daytime functioning, including poor concentration, reduced work performance, and daytime sleepiness, and have an increased incidence of stress-related psychophysiologic problems, such as tension headache, increased muscle tension, or GI distress. There may be excessive worry about not sleeping or about falling asleep at the wheel while driving.

Diagnostic tests: Insomnia usually is diagnosed by history.

Test	Results Indicating Disorder	CPT Code
Polysomnography	Records sleep, heart rate, respiratory movement, and oxygen saturation; determines sleep continuity	95808

Differential diagnosis:

- Sleep apnea: sleepiness during the day, snoring, restless sleep, and periods of apnea at night
- Medication effects or side effects: caffeine, nicotine, β-blockers, corticosteroids, bronchodilators, respiratory stimulants, thyroid supplements, CNS stimulants, decongestants, phenytoin
- Alcohol or substance abuse
- Chronic medical or psychiatric conditions: hyperthyroidism, GERD, Alzheimer's disease, arthritis, fibromyalgia, depression, manic disorders, schizophrenia

Treatment: Treat cause or refer as appropriate.

General Treatment Measures

Plan for activities during the daytime to stimulate wakefulness, and use measures to promote sleep at night. Discuss with the patient and family comfort measures, sleep-promoting techniques, or lifestyle changes to promote sleep. General treatment measures include advising the patient to do the following:

Establish and maintain a regular bedtime and bedtime rituals conducive to sleep, such as reducing stimuli in the environment at bedtime, relaxing in a warm bath, drinking a glass of warm milk, creating a comfortable sleep setting, using eyeshades, using earplugs, and playing soft music or relaxation tapes.

Avoid daytime napping.

Avoid caffeine, nicotine, and alcohol (especially within 6 hours of bedtime) as well as heavy meals before bedtime. A daily exercise routine promotes sleep, but physical activities close to bedtime disturb sleep.

If unable to sleep after 30 minutes, get out of bed and participate in a quiet activity, such as reading. Use the bed and bedroom only for sleeping.

Transient Insomnia

Provide appropriate counseling, reassurance, and general treatment measures to reduce anxiety.

Chronic Insomnia

Treat the underlying cause. Provide appropriate counseling, reassurance, and general treatment measures. Evaluate for depression. If these measures do not result in adequate sleep, pharmacologic therapy may be used. If the patient is to receive sleep medications, plan a program for withdrawal from the medication to prevent addiction; do not give the patient a standing prescription for the medication. Pharmacologic therapy includes use of analgesics if indicated for pain and hypnotic agents, such as the benzodiazepines (flurazepam, 15–30 mg at bedtime; temazepam, 15 mg 1–2 hours before bed; triazolam, 0.125–0.25 mg at bedtime [useful for jet lag]); tricyclic antidepressants, which are usually

prescribed for insomnia associated with depression (amitriptyline, 50–100 mg at bedtime); and nonbenzodiazepines (zolpidem, 5–10 mg orally at bedtime). Other medications include OTC medications such as diphenhydramine (Benadryl), 25 to 50 mg at bedtime. By some reports, the dietary supplement melatonin (a pineal hormone) may be useful for jet lag, but this use is not approved by the Food and Drug Administration.
Follow-up: See patient as indicated by cause of symptom.
Sequelae: Possible complications depend on cause of symptom. General complications include transient insomnia becoming chronic, increase in daytime sleepiness, and falling asleep while performing activities of daily living such as driving a motor vehicle. Initiate medications over the weekend to evaluate for any side effects.
Prevention/prophylaxis: Prevention strategies depend on cause of symptom. To promote continuous and effective sleep, advise the patient to maintain sleep hygiene conditions and practices such as maintaining a regular bedtime; avoiding caffeine, nicotine, alcohol, and heavy meals before bedtime; timing exercise and physical activities so that they enhance rather than disturb sleep; and reducing stimuli in the environment at bedtime.
Referral: Refer to or consult with appropriate specialist as indicated by cause of symptom. Refer for a more complete workup if the patient requires benzodiazepine hypnotic medication for more than a few weeks.
Education: Explain cause of symptoms, tests or procedures used to determine the cause, and symptomatic treatment, if any. Advise patient when to seek medical care. Discuss prevention strategies.

JAUNDICE

Jaundice	ICD-9-CM: 782.4

Description: Jaundice or icterus is the yellowish discoloration of the skin, sclera, and mucous membranes from the breakdown of the heme in bilirubin. It is the hallmark sign of underlying hepatobiliary disease. Clinically, jaundice may be divided into two types. Jaundice with few symptoms is called *unconjugated hyperbilirubinemia (indirect jaundice)*, and jaundice with multiple symptoms is called *conjugated hyperbilirubinemia (direct jaundice)*.
Etiology: Unconjugated hyperbilirubinemia is the result of bilirubin overproduction that may be due to hemolysis, ineffective erythropoiesis, or impaired conjugation such as from Gilbert's syndrome. Conjugated hyperbilirubinemia is caused by an impaired excretion of bilirubin that may be the result of obstructive hepatocellular disease, intrahepatic biliary obstruction (cholestasis), or extrahepatic biliary obstruction.
Age: Highest rate is in young adults and is the result of hepatitis. Of patients age 30 to 60, 33% of patients with jaundice have cirrhosis.

Ethnicity: No significant ethnic predisposition.

Gender: No significant gender differentiation.

Contributing factors: Contact with another person with jaundice. Use of hepatotoxic substances, such as intravenous drugs, alcohol, chemical solvents, exposure to blood or blood transfusion in past 6 months; hepatotoxic drugs, such as isoniazid (INH); phenothiazines (e.g., chlorpromazine [Thorazine, prochlorperazine [Compazine]); oral contraceptives; halothane anesthesia; methyldopa. History of alcoholism, gallstones, liver disease, drug addiction, malignancy, mononucleosis. Foreign travel in the past 6 months.

Signs and symptoms:

History

If the patient has a history of weight loss and depression with the jaundice, this may suggest a malignancy. Suspect hepatocellular dysfunction if the patient has a history of travel to areas of high risk for hepatitis, raw shellfish consumption, excessive alcohol intake, or intravenous drug use.

Associated Signs and Symptoms

A common generalized associated symptom is pruritus. Suspect obstructive jaundice if the patient complains of abdominal pain or has a history of gallstones or biliary surgery. If the patient complains of lethargy, fatigue, anorexia, nausea, vomiting, or right upper quadrant pain, suspect hepatitis.

Physical Examination

Observation may reveal excoriations, a yellowish to greenish hue in the skin or sclera, testicular atrophy, gynecomastia, petechiae, spider angiomas, palmer erythema, wasting, and dark urine. Palpation may reveal epigastric or right upper quadrant tenderness, enlarged liver, splenomegaly, palpable gallbladder, or lymphadenopathy. Percussion may reveal an increased area of dullness over the left upper abdominal quadrant or the right upper abdominal quadrant. See Figure 2–1 for steps in the differential diagnosis of jaundice.

Diagnostic tests:

Tests	Results Indicating Disorder	CPT Code
CBC with differential	Decreased hematocrit suggests loss or diminished production of RBCs; decreased hemoglobin with changes in MCH, MCHC, and MCV suggests anemia (macrocytic, microcytic, thalassemia)	85004
AST, ALT	Increased levels suggest hepatocellular damage or inflammation; ALT more specific for liver disease; ALT levels more elevated than AST levels suggests viral hepatitis; AST levels at least twice ALT levels suggest liver injury from alcoholism	80053

(Continued)

Tests	Results Indicating Disorder	CPT Code
Alkaline phosphatase	Increased levels suggest cholestasis or infiltrative liver disease; may be elevated with bone and intestinal problems	80053
Bilirubin, total	Increased levels suggest liver injury, biliary obstruction, hemolysis	80053
Bilirubin, direct	Increased levels suggest biliary obstruction/cholestasis (≥50% conjugated bilirubin)	82248
Bilirubin, indirect	Increased levels suggest hemolysis of RBCs (>80% of total bilirubin level)	82247
Serum albumin/ total protein	Decreased levels suggest liver disease	82053, 84155
Prothrombin time	Increased levels suggest liver disease, vitamin K deficiency	85610
Drug screen	Determine specific drugs such as alcohol that can cause liver damage	80100
Hepatitis screening: AbsAg, anti-AbcIgM, Anti-HAV IgM	Determine acute/chronic hepatitis	86706, 86705, 86708, 86709, 86803
Abdominal ultrasound	Determine cause of hepatic lesions, biliary disease	76705
CT scan	Determine cause of hepatic lesions, biliary disease	74150
Endoscopic retrograde cholangiopan- creatography	Determine location and extent of biliary obstruction	74328

AST, aspartate aminotransferase; ALT, alanine aminotransferase.

Differential diagnosis:

- Hepatitis: malaise, anorexia, low-grade fever, enlarged and tender liver, greenish hue, dark urine; splenomegaly with chronic disease
- Cirrhosis: fatigue, anorexia, weight loss, abdominal pain, enlarged liver, spider angioma, palmar erythema, gynecomastia, testicular atrophy, amenorrhea, hematemesis
- Biliary obstruction: colicky right upper quadrant pain, greenish hue, light-colored stools, dark urine; fever and chills with cholangitis
- Primary or metastatic liver cancer: cachexia, weakness, weight loss, ascites, enlarged and tender liver; may have palpable mass, bruit, or friction rub; generally associated with cirrhosis
- Hemochromatosis: autosomal recessive disease causing increased accumulation of iron in the liver, pancreas, heart, adrenals, testes, pituitary, and kidneys causing multisystem failure
- Hemolytic diseases: diminished RBC survival owing to short RBC survival or inability of the bone marrow to produce RBCs

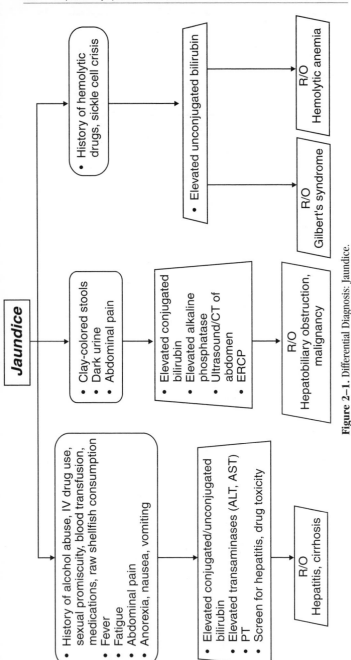

Figure 2–1. Differential Diagnosis: Jaundice.

- Drug/toxin-induced liver disease: drugs such as acetominophen, alcohol, heavy metals, valproic acid, niacin, and vitamin A may cause inflammatory or noninflammatory liver disease

Treatment: Treat cause or refer as appropriate. Surgery usually is indicated for obstructive jaundice and medical therapy for nonobstructive jaundice. Instruct patient to avoid contributing factors, such as alcohol and liver-impairing medications. The patient may require treatment for itching secondary to hyperbilirubinemia.

Follow-up: See patient as indicated by cause of symptom.

Sequelae: Possible complications depend on cause of symptom.

Prevention/prophylaxis: Prevention strategies depend on cause of symptom. Advise patient at risk for hepatitis A or B to receive immunization. Postexposure prophylaxis with immune globulin or hepatitis B immune globulin is recommended. Advise the patient to follow proper hand-washing techniques, standard precautions, and safe sex practices. Teach patient about disease transmission and factors that may exacerbate the condition.

Referral: Refer to or consult with appropriate specialist as indicated by cause of symptom. Referral for alcohol and drug counseling also may be indicated.

Education: Explain cause of symptoms, tests or procedures used to determine the cause, and symptomatic treatment, if any. Advise patient when to seek medical care. Discuss prevention strategies.

NAUSEA AND VOMITING

Vomiting	ICD-9-CM: 787.03
Vomiting and nausea	ICD-9-CM: 787.01
Psychogenic	ICD-9-CM: 306.4

Description: Nausea is a subjective, unpleasant sensation usually preceding vomiting. Vomiting is the forceful ejection of gastric contents as opposed to passive reflux. Nausea and vomiting often occur together.

Etiology: Nausea is caused by alterations in the motility of the stomach and small intestine. Parasympathetic activity, such as pallor, diaphoresis, salivation, and other vasovagal signs such as hypotension and bradycardia, often accompanies nausea. Vomiting is a reflex involving visceral and somatic components that are integrated in the vomiting center and the chemoreceptor trigger zone of the medulla oblongata. The vomiting reflex begins with the stimulation of receptor sites in the mucosa of the upper GI tract, the labyrinthine apparatus (inner ear), higher cortical centers (e.g., emotional stimuli), or the chemoreceptor trigger zone (dopamine receptors) by specific mediators in the blood. The afferent nerves carry the impulses to the vomiting center, then the efferent pathways (including the phrenic nerves to the diaphragm, spinal nerves to the abdominal musculature, and visceral nerves to the stomach and esophagus) carry the impulses to the effector muscles, causing relaxation of the gastric fundus and gastroesophageal sphincter, contraction of the gastric pylorus, and reverse peristalsis in the esophagus. The glottis closes, increasing intrathoracic pressure and preventing aspiration. Intra-abdominal pressure is increased when the abdominal wall muscles and the diaphragm contract, resulting in the forcing of the stomach contents through the mouth.

Occurrence: Common.

Age: Occurs in all ages.

Ethnicity: No significant ethnic predisposition.

Gender: Occurs more in women than in men, primarily because of pregnancy and hormonal fluctuations in general.

Contributing factors: Numerous. Structural malformations, such as hiatal hernia; GI disorders, such as gastroenteritis or obstruction; abdominal surgery; CNS disorders and dysfunction, such as migraine headache or tumor; pancreatic and biliary disturbances; underlying chronic conditions, such as diabetes, heart disease, or renal insufficiency; vestibular disturbances; psychological disorders; pregnancy; sight or odor of noxious or emotionally upsetting stimuli; motion sickness; toxins; drug ingestion; fever; and infection.

Signs and symptoms:

History

Obtain information about the timing, frequency, and duration of the nausea/vomiting. A 1- to 2-day history of nausea/vomiting in an otherwise healthy patient suggests an acute gastroenteritis that is usually self-limiting. Nausea/vomiting in the morning often is associated with early pregnancy, uremia, and alcoholic gastritis. If it occurs shortly after eating, suspect pylorospasm, gastritis, or a psychogenic cause. Vomiting 4 to 6 hours after eating with the vomitus composed of undigested food suggests gastric distention.

Associated Signs and Symptoms

Symptoms of dehydration include dry mucous membranes, orthostatic hypotension, weight loss, excessive thirst, and decreased urination. The presence of jaundice suggests hepatitis or cholestasis. If the patient complains of vomiting without nausea and muscular contraction of the diaphragm or abdominal wall, suspect hiatal hernia or GERD. Projectile vomiting without nausea is an ominous symptom suggesting a CNS disturbance, such as a lesion. Blood in the vomitus warrants further assessment because the cause may be minor, such as swallowed blood from a nosebleed, or major, such as GI bleeding. A putrid odor (feculent vomitus) is associated with lower intestinal obstruction or gastrocolic fistula. Bile-colored vomitus suggests upper gastrointestinal contents, but bile is present with prolonged vomiting of any cause. Vomiting that is clear suggests gastric fluid.

Physical Examination

Abdominal distention suggests ileus, obstruction, or ascites. The absence of bowel sounds suggests ileus; high-pitched, tinkling sounds suggest intestinal obstruction; hyperactive bowel sounds may indicate acute gastroenteritis. If the patient has tenderness with guarding (muscular rigidity) or rebound tenderness, suspect peritoneal or visceral inflammation. The location of these signs may help pinpoint the underlying cause. A neurologic, cardiovascular, or pelvic examination also may be indicated by patient history and complaint.

Diagnostic tests:

Tests	Results Indicating Disorder	CPT Code
Pregnancy test urine	Positive results suggest pregnancy	81025
Urine specific gravity	Increased level suggests volume depletion	81001
CBC with differential	Increase in lymphocytes suggests viral infection; increase in WBC count with left shift suggests bacterial infection	85004
Serum electrolytes, glucose, BUN/creatinine ratio	Evaluate renal function, electrolyte and acid-base balance, dehydration. Increased glucose may suggest diabetes mellitus; decreased level may suggest pancreatic disorders. Increased BUN/creatinine ratio suggests renal insufficiency or failure	80053
AST, ALT	Increased levels suggest hepatocellular damage or inflammation; ALT more specific for liver disease; ALT levels more elevated than AST levels suggests viral hepatitis; AST levels at least twice ALT levels suggest liver injury from alcoholism	80053
Alkaline phosphatase	Increased levels suggest cholestasis or infiltrative liver disease; may also be elevated with bone and intestinal problems	80053
Serum amylase, lipase	Increased levels >3 times upper limit suggests pancreatic disease, obstruction	82150, 83690
Bilirubin, total	Increased levels suggest liver injury, biliary obstruction, hemolysis	80053
Bilirubin, direct	Increased levels suggest biliary obstruction/cholestasis ($\geq$50% conjugated bilirubin)	82247
Bilirubin, indirect	Increased levels suggest hemolysis of RBCs (>80% of total bilirubin level)	82247
Drug screen	Determine specific drugs that can cause liver toxicity	80100
Hepatitis screening: AbsAg, anti-, AbcIgM, anti-HAV IgM, anti-HepC	Determine acute/chronic hepatitis	86706, 86705, 86708, 86709, 86803
Abdominal x-ray	Determine pathology of obstruction or ileus	74000

(Continued)

Tests	Results Indicating Disorder	CPT Code
Abdominal ultrasound	Determine cause of hepatic lesions, biliary disease, pancreatitic problems	76705
Upper GI endoscopy	Determine GERD	43200
ECG	Depression in the ST segment or T wave inversion suggests myocardial ischemia; elevation of the ST segment suggests myocardial injury	93000

Differential diagnosis: Self-limiting versus acute (serious) nausea/vomiting.

- Acute myocardial infarction: history of CAD risk factors; atypical symptom of myocardial infarction
- Gastroenteritis (viral or bacterial): crampy, diffuse abdominal pain, nausea/vomiting, hyperactive bowel sounds
- Pancreatitis: left upper quadrant pain radiating to back, nausea/vomiting, diarrhea, fever, abdominal distention, decreased bowel sounds, diffuse rebound tenderness
- Cholecystitis/lithiasis: right upper quadrant pain may radiate to right subscapular area, nausea/vomiting, tenderness to palpation, positive Murphy's sign
- Bowel obstruction: crampy abdominal pain, nausea/vomiting, abdominal distention, hyperactive, high-pitched bowel sounds

Treatment:

 Red Flag: Projectile vomiting may indicate a CNS problem. Immediate evaluation or referral may be indicated.

Symptomatic Treatment
Treat cause or refer as appropriate.

Physical
General measures include placing the patient on a clear liquid diet to replace fluids and electrolytes and prevent dehydration when the acute episode has subsided. During the acute episode, recommend small sips of clear fluids or ice chips. Examples of recommended liquids include Gatorade or other sports or electrolyte-replacement drinks, tea, clear broth, and clear caffeine-free carbonated beverages, such as ginger ale. After the nausea/vomiting has decreased for 12 hours, advise the patient to try salted crackers or dry toast and gradually add rice, baked potato, and chicken soup with noodles, then eat foods as tolerated, returning gradually to a full diet. Have the patient avoid caffeine-containing foods and fluids, alcohol, dairy products, most fruits and vegetables, red meats, and spicy or heavily seasoned foods until fully recovered. If the patient is pregnant, suggest dietary changes such as eating small frequent meals, separating wet and dry food, avoiding foods with strong odors, and eating dry salted crackers first thing on awaken-

ing. For all patients, provide reassurance and encourage resting as much as possible.

Pharmacologic

Adjusting the timing, dosage, or preparation of medications may help relieve nausea/vomiting associated with medication use. Antiemetic medications may provide symptomatic relief. Many medications have combined anticholinergic, antihistamine, and CNS depressant activity: Use prochlorperazine, 5 to 10 mg orally every 4 to 6 hours as needed or 25 mg in prolonged-release form every 6 hours as needed; metoclopramide (for diabetic gastroparesis or postoperatively), 10 mg orally three or four times daily; or antihistamines, such as dimenhydrinate or hydroxyzine (for motion sickness, postoperative nausea, or drug-induced nausea).

Follow-up: See patient as indicated by cause of symptom. See patient in 3 days to assess whether or not nausea/vomiting has stopped or for reevaluation.

Sequelae: Possible complications depend on cause of symptom. Complications may include dehydration, metabolic acidosis, electrolyte imbalances, and aspiration pneumonia.

Prevention/prophylaxis: Prevention strategies depend on cause of symptom. Monitor and prevent dehydration during acute episode. Advise patient of dietary precautions, such as avoiding fatty or spicy foods, if appropriate; the proper handling of food; proper hand-washing techniques; and, if appropriate, precautions to take when traveling outside of the United States.

Referral: Refer to or consult with appropriate specialist as indicated by cause of symptom.

Education: Explain cause of symptoms, tests or procedures used to determine the cause, and symptomatic treatment, if any. Advise patient when to seek medical care.

PALPITATIONS

| Palpitations | ICD-9-CM: 785.1 |
| Palpitations, psychogenic | ICD-9-CM: 306.2 |

Description: Palpitations are a conscious awareness of one's own heartbeat. They may be described as pounding, fluttering, skipping, or thumping sensations felt over the precordium or in the throat or neck. Palpitations may indicate rapid or slow rates and regular or irregular rhythms.

Etiology: The most common causes are anxiety; exercise; fever; stimulants, such as caffeine and alcohol; drugs, such as amphetamines, cocaine, and thyroid hormone medications; and cardiac disease. As people age, there is often a decreasing tolerance to caffeine, alcohol, and

medications, which then results in palpitations. Other causes include anemia, hypoglycemia, thyrotoxicosis, conduction disturbances, and hypoxia.
Occurrence: Common.
Age: Occurs in all ages; more common in adults.
Ethnicity: No significant ethnic predisposition.
Gender: Occurs in both genders. Palpitations associated with mitral valve prolapse are more common in women.
Contributing factors: Ingestion of food and beverages containing caffeine; use of alcohol, nicotine, recreational drugs, and OTC weight-reducing agents; use of decongestants that contain ephedrine; exercise; stressful events; thyroid replacement therapy; history of cardiac disease; discontinuation of medications; use of certain medications such as clonidine, phenytoin, β-blockers, and antiarrhythmics; pregnancy; menopause.
Signs and symptoms:

History
Refer immediately if the patient has a history of cardiac problems or presents with palpitations and accompanying dizziness; confusion; chest pain; syncope; pale, cool, clammy skin; and abnormal vital signs. Suspect an underlying medical problem if the patient's palpitations are not related to exercise, anxiety, fever, or drugs. If palpitations occur in the late afternoon and early evening several hours after eating, suspect reactive hypoglycemia. Ask the patient to describe or tap out the rhythm of the palpitation, then check the patient's pulse rate and rhythm. Fluttery feelings in the sternum or throat and rates >160 beats/min are associated with supraventricular tachycardia. Rates <150 beats/min and regular are more likely to be related to sinus tachycardia, exercise, fever, drugs, or thyrotoxicosis. Rapid irregular tachycardia with a pulse deficit suggests atrial fibrillation.

Associated Signs and Symptoms
Suspect an acute anxiety attack if the patient has flushing of the face, diaphoresis, hyperventilation, trembling, tachycardia, and a sense of doom. If the patient has pallor, fatigue, and dyspnea on exertion, suspect anemia. Suspect hypertension if the patient has headache, dizziness, nausea, vomiting, and a change in level of consciousness. If the patient has weakness, fatigue, paresthesia, muscle twitching, and hyperreflexia, suspect hypocalcemia. Hypoglycemia should be suspected if the palpitations occur late in the afternoon or are associated with meals. Suspect hyperthyroidism or thyrotoxicosis if the patient has sustained palpitations, nervousness, tremors, diarrhea, heat intolerance, weight loss, and possibly exophthalmus and an enlarged thyroid. Mitral valve prolapse should be suspected if the patient has paroxysmal palpitations accompanied by a sharp, aching precordial pain, dyspnea, fatigue, anxiety, and a midsystolic click followed by a late systolic murmur.

Diagnostic tests:

Tests	Results Indicating Disorder	CPT Code
CBC with differential	Decreased hematocrit suggests loss or diminished production of RBCs; decreased hemoglobin with changes in MCH, MCHC, or MCV suggests anemia (macrocytic, microcytic, thalassemia)	85004
Serum electrolytes, calcium, magnesium	Electrolyte, calcium, and magnesium imbalance can cause arrhythmias	80051, 82330, 83735
Glucose	Hypoglycemia can cause cardiac abnormalities	82947
TSH	Decreased level with hyperthyroidism	84443
ECG	Determine arrhythmias, cardiac abnormalities	93000
Halter monitor	Determine cardiac arrhythmias over time (necessary if history of syncope, dizziness, chest pain, or arrhythmia on ECG)	93224
Echocardiogram	Determine left ventricular function by looking at size, position, and movement of heart valves and chambers	93307
Hyperventilation	3-4 minutes of hyperventilation may reproduce arrhythmia in patient with anxiety; record on ECG	93000

Differential diagnosis:
- Acute myocardial infarction: history of CAD risk factors. Classic symptoms of substernal chest pressure that may radiate to the shoulder, neck, or jaw for >30 minutes; dyspnea; nausea and vomiting. Decreased cardiac output causes tachycardia.
- Arrhythmia (atrial, ventricular, Wolff-Parkinson-White syndrome): may be precipitated by hypokalemia, hypomagnesemia, hypoglycemia, thyrotoxicosis. Drug withdrawal/reactions can cause arrhythmias (including digitalis, phenytoin, β-blockers, calcium channel blockers, caffeine, alcohol, nicotine).
- Mitral valve prolapse: associated with a midsystolic click followed by a late systolic murmur, dyspnea, fatigue, and anxiety
- Anxiety: associated with stress, panic attack
- Fever: elevation of temperature associated with inflammation or infection
- Hormonal change: associated with pregnancy or menopause
- Anemia: associated with decreased hemoglobin, hematocrit

Treatment: Treat cause or refer as appropriate.

Red Flag: Patients with cardiac complaints of chest pain, shortness of breath, diaphoresis, or palpitations associated with dizziness, syncope, confusion, and abnormal vital signs must be transported to the hospital for emergency evaluation and management.

Symptomatic Treatment

Measures include avoiding food and beverages containing caffeine and alcohol and causative medications, stopping smoking, and using relaxation techniques to decrease anxiety. Treat fever with antipyretics and antibiotics as indicated. Readjust, eliminate, or resume medications as needed to stop palpitations. Prescribe iron supplements to correct anemia.

Follow-up: See patient as indicated by cause of symptom. Usually the healthy patient requires no follow-up or can be seen in several weeks; if the patient is receiving antiarrhythmic therapy, see weekly for the first several weeks of therapy, then monthly.

Sequelae: Possible complications depend on cause of symptom; usually none in the healthy patient.

Prevention/prophylaxis: Prevention strategies depend on cause of symptom. Advise patient to limit use of stimulants, alcohol, and caffeine; to stop smoking; and to use relaxation techniques to reduce stress.

Referral: Refer to or consult with appropriate specialist as indicated by cause of symptom.

Education: Explain cause of symptoms, tests or procedures used to determine the cause, and symptomatic treatment, if any. Advise the patient to seek medical care if heart rate is extremely rapid or there is lower extremity edema or weight gain, increasing dyspnea on exertion, or chest pain. Teach methods of breaking the arrhythmia to patients with occasional symptoms, including vagal maneuvers such as Valsalva maneuver (straining against a closed glottis), gagging by sticking a finger down the throat, or immersing the face in cold water (diving reflex).

PERIPHERAL EDEMA

Edema, legs	ICD-9-CM: 782.3

Description: Peripheral edema is the accumulation of fluid within the interstitial spaces of the extremities. Edema of the lower extremities is a symptom of an underlying process, not the primary disorder.

Etiology: Caused by a disturbance in hydrostatic pressure, such as from thrombophlebitis, hepatic obstruction, chronic venous insufficiency, heart failure, and sodium and water retention. Disturbance in the colloid oncotic pressure, such as from renal and hepatic disease, hemorrhage, burns, protein malnutrition, or conditions resulting in a serum albumin level <2.5 g/100 mL, can cause peripheral edema. Obstruction in the lymphatic flow caused by tumors, inflammation, or after surgical removal of lymph nodes or an increase in capillary permeability, such as from trauma, allergy, infection, and neoplasms, also can result in peripheral edema.

Occurrence: Common.

Age: Occurs in all ages; higher incidence in older adults.

Ethnicity: No significant ethnic predisposition.

Gender: No significant gender differentiation.

Contributing factors: Prolonged sitting, standing, immobility, constrictive clothing, excessive dietary sodium intake, certain medications such as NSAIDs and estrogen, pregnancy (especially third trimester), and large pelvic masses.

Signs and symptoms:

History

Obtain information about the onset, duration, and location of the edema and any associated symptoms including pain. If the patient complains of numbness and tingling and presents with diminished or absent pulses, pallor or mottling, and coolness in the extremity, steps to preserve the limb become imperative. Refer the patient immediately for evaluation of arterial insufficiency or occlusion to the affected extremity.

Associated Signs and Symptoms

Acute onset of edema over hours or days that is primarily unilateral and accompanied by pain indicates an acute process, such as deep vein thrombosis (DVT), cellulitis, abscess, compartment syndrome, a rupture of a Baker's cyst, or strained gastrocnemius muscle. Fever, chills, and erythema accompanying the edema suggest an infectious process, such as cellulitis, lymphangitis, osteomyelitis, and venous thrombosis. Leg trauma and fracture cause rapidly developing leg edema and possibly associated ecchymotic areas.

Painless swelling of a lower extremity involving the dorsum of the toes and feet could be either the earliest symptom of lymphedema or obstruction of lymphatic drainage. The edema starts in the foot and ankle and progresses proximally, usually subsiding in the morning and progressing with activity. It may become permanent secondary to fibrosis and thickening of the skin and subcutaneous tissue and diminished fatty tissue. Chronic edema is usually a symptom of a systemic disease process, such as heart failure, hepatic or renal disease, endocrine dysfunction (Cushing's disease or thyroid dysfunction), and metabolic dysfunction (protein deficiency). The patient presents with edema and the signs and symptoms of the disease process. Chronic edema of the lower legs accompanied by hyperpigmentation, pruritus, excoriation, weeping, and crusting may suggest chronic venous insufficiency secondary to varicose veins or DVT. Edema accompanied by skin that has a thick, dimpled (orange peel) appearance and that may be hyperpigmented or pruritic on the dorsum of the feet (pretibial myxedema) as well as signs and symptoms of hyperthyroidism may indicate Graves' disease. Peripheral edema also may occur in the later stages of hypothyroidism. Painless, bilateral edema may be seen as a side effect of sodium-retaining medications and with prolonged immobility and dependent position. Cyclic or idiopathic bilateral edema occurs frequently in obese women. Assess the lower extremities carefully. In the obese patient, fat accumulation in the lower extremities may be mistaken for edema. Usually fat stops accumulating, so the ankle and the dorsum of the foot are spared.

Diagnostic tests: Usually diagnosed by history and physical examination.

Tests	Results Indicating Disorder	CPT Code
CBC with differential	Increase in lymphocytes associated with viral infection; increase in WBC count with left shift associated with bacterial infections; decreased hematocrit suggests loss or diminished production of RBCs; decreased hemoglobin with changes in MCH, MCHC, or MCV suggests anemia (macrocytic, microcytic, thalassemia)	85004
Electrolytes, BUN/creatinine ratio	Determine electrolyte, acid-base balance; increased BUN/creatinine ratio suggests renal failure, prerenal azotemia, postrenal obstruction; decreased ratio suggests starvation, liver failure	80051, 84520, 82565
AST, ALT	Increased levels suggest hepatocellular damage or inflammation; ALT more specific for liver disease; ALT levels more elevated than AST levels suggest viral hepatitis; AST levels at least twice ALT levels suggest liver injury from alcoholism	84450, 84460
Serum albumin/total protein	Decreased levels suggest liver disease	82040, 84155
Prothrombin time	Increased levels suggest liver disease, vitamin K deficiency	85610
TSH	Increased level with hypothyroidism; decreased level with hyperthyroidism	84443
Thyroxine	Increased level with hyperthyroidism; decreased level with hypothyroidism	84439
Chest x-ray	Determine cardiac size and pulmonary infiltrates of edema	71020
ECG	Determine cardiac abnormalities, arrhythmias	93000
Doppler ultrasound	Determine venous obstruction (DVT)	76880
Pelvic ultrasound	Determine obstruction of lymph flow, masses	76856

Differential diagnosis:

Unilateral Edema

- DVT: edema of extremity associated with pain in calf of leg; positive Homan's sign; may have history of CHF, recent surgery, oral contraceptive use, prolonged inactivity

- Chronic venous insufficiency: progressive edema of lower extremity and secondary changes in the skin and subcutaneous tissue, brownish discoloration, itching, dull pain worse on standing
- Trauma (strain, sprain, fracture): edema accompanied by pain after extremity injury
- Cellulitis: edema, erythema, pain in affected area

Bilateral Edema

- CHF: edema of lower extremities without pain, which decreases with elevation; symptoms of cardiac disease
- Renal disease: edema of lower extremities without pain; symptoms of renal disease
- Cirrhosis: edema of lower extremities without pain; symptoms of hepatic disease
- Nutritional disorders: decreased albumin level causing edema of lower extremities.
- Pelvic obstruction (lymphedema): edema particularly on dorsum of feet and toes, thickening of subcutaneous tissue that does not respond to elevation
- Medication side effect: calcium channel blockers, NSAIDs, and estrogen can cause lower extremity edema

Treatment: Treat cause or refer as appropriate.

Red Flag: Transport the patient to the hospital for emergency evaluation and management if the patient presents with acute CHF, pulmonary edema, or acute arterial occlusion (patient complains of paresthesia and extremity pallor or mottling, pain, poikilothermia [coolness], pulses diminished or absent, and paralysis).

Symptomatic Treatment

Fluid restriction, dietary changes, correction of electrolytes, drug therapy including use of diuretics, or change in medication may be required. Compression leg pumps or compression stockings and exercise help increase venous return. Weight reduction also may be indicated if the patient is overweight.

Follow-up: See patient as indicated by cause of symptom. See patient until problem resolves or is controlled.

Sequelae: Possible complications depend on cause of symptom. Peripheral edema can cause tissue ischemia resulting from compressed and diminished arterial circulation.

Prevention/prophylaxis: Prevention strategies depend on cause of symptom. Advise patient to maintain a healthy lifestyle.

Referral: Refer to or consult with appropriate specialist as indicated by cause of symptom.

Education: Explain cause of symptoms, tests or procedures used to determine the cause, and symptomatic treatment, if any. Advise patient when to seek medical care.

PRURITUS

Pruritus	ICD9-CM: 698.9

Description: Pruritus (itching) is an unpleasant sensation that affects the skin, certain mucous membranes, and the eyes and provokes a desire to scratch. It may be localized or general.

Etiology: Caused most commonly by dermatologic disorders and allergic reactions. Other causes include systemic disorders such as renal failure, hepatobiliary disease, thyroid dysfunction, malignant disorders, iron deficiency anemia, neurologic disorders, and psychiatric disorders. Pruritus also can be a side effect of certain medications.

Occurrence: Common.

Age: Occurs at any age.

Ethnicity: No significant ethnic predisposition.

Gender: No significant gender differentiation.

Contributing factors: Climatic conditions, such as cold dry air or extreme heat and cold; dry skin; contact of skin with irritants; pregnancy; pain; poor hygiene; and nutritional state.

Signs and symptoms:

History

Obtain a family history. If multiple family members are experiencing pruritus, consider parasitic infestations, such as scabies or pediculosis, as the cause.

Associated Signs and Symptoms

Pruritus with skin lesions or eruptions suggests a dermatologic cause. Generalized pruritus without visible skin eruptions may indicate a systemic problem. Increased pruritus after bathing may be caused by dry skin or pityriasis rosea. Pruritus that is worse at night may indicate scabies. Hepatobiliary disorders commonly associated with jaundice are accompanied by pruritus. Pruritis associated with medications may indicate an allergic response to the medication. Assess skin excoriation from trauma caused by scratching for infection and scarring.

Diagnostic tests: Usually diagnosed by history and physical examination.

Tests	Results Indicating Disorder	CPT Code
Skin biopsy	Determine diagnosis	11100

If the patient has persistent pruritus with no visible skin pathology, diagnostic tests may help determine a systemic cause.

Tests	Results Indicating Disorder	CPT Code
CBC with differential	Decreased hematocrit suggests loss or diminished production of RBCs; decreased hemoglobin with changes in MCH, MCHC, or MCV suggests anemia (macrocytic, microcytic, thalessemia); elevation in eosinophils suggests drug reaction, allergy; increased reticulocyte count suggests polycythemia; abnormalities in the WBC count may suggest leukemia	85004
Serum glucose	Increased level may suggest diabetes mellitus	82947
BUN/creatinine ratio	Increased levels suggest renal insufficiency or renal failure	84520, 82565
TSH	Decreased levels suggest hyperthyroidism; elevated levels suggest hypothyroidism	84443
AST, ALT	Increased levels suggest hepatocellular damage or inflammation; ALT more specific for liver disease; ALT levels more elevated than AST levels suggest viral hepatitis; AST levels at least twice ALT levels suggest liver injury from alcoholism	84450, 84460
Bilirubin, total	Increased levels suggest liver injury, biliary obstruction, hemolysis	82247
Bilirubin, direct	Increased levels suggest biliary obstruction/cholestasis ($\geq$50% conjugated bilirubin)	82248
Bilirubin, indirect	Increased levels suggest hemolysis of RBCs (>80% of total bilirubin level)	82247

Differential diagnosis:
- Skin disorders: dermatitis, insect bites, parasitic infestations, urticaria, allergic reactions, folliculitis, sunburn, herpes simplex and zoster, pityriasis rosea, psoriasis, and fungal infections
- Allergic reaction: associated with medications, cosmetics, fabrics, and laundry detergent
- Systemic disorders: renal disease, hepatobiliary disease, anemia, lymphoma, leukemia, multiple myeloma, polycythemia vera, and thyroid dysfunction
- Psychological: emotional disorders, anxiety

Treatment: Treat cause and refer as appropriate.

Symptomatic Treatment
Antihistamines, minor tranquilizers, and topical steroids may provide symptomatic relief from itching. Emollients and increased humidity may provide relief for dry skin. Sitz baths, Burrow's compresses, or UVB phototherapy may reduce symptoms. Help patient identify stress factors and alternative approaches to dealing with stress.

Follow-up: See patient as indicated by cause of symptom. See patient until problem resolves.

Sequelae: Possible complications depend on cause of symptom. Skin infections and permanent scarring from scratching may occur.

Prevention/prophylaxis: Prevention strategies depend on cause of symptom. Advise the patient to maintain a healthy lifestyle with good nutrition, hygiene, and skin care, including protection from sunburn and the avoidance of extreme temperatures.

Referral: Refer to or consult with an appropriate specialist as indicated by cause of symptom.

Education: Explain cause of symptoms, tests or procedures used to determine the cause, and symptomatic treatment, if any. Advise patient when to seek medical care.

SYNCOPE

| Syncope, near, presyncope | ICD-9-CM: 780.2 |

Description: Syncope is a sudden, transient loss of consciousness and postural tone as a result of inadequate cerebral blood flow. Recovery to full consciousness is usually spontaneous.

Etiology: Caused by a transient reduction of blood to the brain, usually from vasomotor instability, severe reduction of cardiac output secondary to obstruction in the flow of cardiac and pulmonary circulation, cardiac arrhythmias that cause transient decrease in cardiac output, or cerebrovascular disease causing decreased cerebral perfusion.

Occurrence: Common; 3% of all emergency department visits and 1% to 6% of all medical admissions annually are attributed to syncope; 5% to 20% of the population experience a syncopal episode by age 75. Most likely to occur in patients with known heart disease.

Age: Occurs at any age; most common in older men and younger women.

Ethnicity: No significant ethnic predisposition.

Gender: More common in older men and younger women.

Contributing factors: Vasovagal instability caused by certain situations, such as coughing, swallowing, micturition, defecation, orthostatic hypotension, and after a large meal or ingestion of alcohol; emotional response such as stress; pain; unpleasant sight, smell, or sound; psychiatric disorders; use of cocaine, marijuana, and alcohol; medications such as vasodilators, antiarrhythmics, diuretics, psychoactive drugs, β-blockers, digitalis, and insulin.

Signs and symptoms: Prodromal symptoms, such as confusion, light-headedness, weakness, tinnitus, visual disturbances, nausea, diaphoresis, and pallor, are seen commonly if the patient has vasovagal syncope. Have the patient lie flat to avert loss of consciousness if these prodromal symptoms are present. Syncope caused by cardiac arrhythmias occurs even if the patient is supine. After the syncopal episode, the patient usually regains consciousness spontaneously and is oriented, although there may

be some residual weakness. Suspect orthostatic hypotension if there is a decline of 20 mm Hg from supine to standing in the blood pressure. If there is a difference of 20 mm Hg in each arm, suspect aortic dissection. Syncope that is sudden in onset with no prodromal symptoms or a brief prodrome and occurring during or after exertion usually suggests a cardiac problem. Syncope with diplopia or other visual disturbances, auditory disturbances, dysarthria, vertigo, and other motor and sensory symptoms suggests a cerebrovascular etiology. If the patient has syncope while wearing a tight shirt collar, shaving, or turning the head, carotid sinus syncope may be the cause. Auscultate the carotid arteries for bruits.
Diagnostic tests: Diagnosed primarily by history and physical examination.

Tests	Results Indicating Disorder	CPT Code
CBC with differential	Decreased hematocrit suggests loss or diminished production of RBCs; decreased hemoglobin with changes in MCH, MCHC, or MCV suggests anemia (macrocytic, microcytic, thalassemia)	85004
Serum electrolytes, glucose, calcium	Hypocalcemia, hyponatremia, or hypoglycemia may precipitate syncope	80051, 82947, 82330
ECG	Determine cardiac arrhythmias, abnormalities	93000
Halter monitor	Determine cardiac arrhythmias over time with recurrent syncopal episodes	93224
Tilt-table testing	Determine cause of postural hypotension	93660

Differential diagnosis:
- Cardiovascular: Syncope may be caused by mechanical problems, such as aortic stenosis or arrhythmias. Episodes frequently occur during exercise or postexercise.
- Orthostatic (postural): occurs with change in position, especially in elderly and diabetic individuals; individuals may have tachycardia. Occurs with hypovolemia, vasodilator, diuretic, and β-blocker medications
- Vasovagal: frequently preceded by stressful, painful experience; may be accompanied by tachycardia, nausea and vomiting

Treatment: Treat cause or refer as appropriate. Vasovagal episodes usually resolve spontaneously or by removing the precipitating factors. Increasing plasma volume may help patients experiencing orthostatic hypotension.

 Red Flag: Ensure airway patency. Place patient in supine position, elevate legs, loosen constricting clothing, and monitor vital signs.
Follow-up: See patient as indicated by cause of symptom. See patient until problem resolves.

Sequelae: Possible complications depend on cause of symptom.

Prevention/prophylaxis: Prevention strategies depend on cause of symptom. Encourage patient to follow a healthy lifestyle and to avoid factors or situations leading to syncopal episode. Instruct the patient with orthostatic hypotension to change positions slowly, sleep with the head of the bed elevated, and dangle legs and do leg exercises before getting out of bed.

Referral: Refer to or consult with appropriate specialist as indicated by cause of symptom.

Education: Explain cause of symptoms, tests or procedures used to determine the cause, and symptomatic treatment, if any. Advise patient when to seek medical care.

URINARY INCONTINENCE

Incontinence of urine	ICD-9-CM: 788.3
Incontinence, overflow	ICD-9-CM: 788.39
Incontinence, stress (female)	ICD-9-CM: 625.6
Incontinence, urge	ICD-9-CM: 788.31

Description: Urinary incontinence is the involuntary loss of urine. Stress incontinence is intermittent urine leakage occurring as a result of activities that increase intra-abdominal pressure, such as laughing, coughing, or sneezing. Urge incontinence is the inability to suppress a sudden urge to urinate. Mixed incontinence is a combination of stress and urge incontinence. Overflow incontinence is due to chronic urinary retention allowing urine to dribble out of the bladder. Reflex, or unconscious, incontinence is continual incontinence.

Etiology: Caused by any injury or dysfunction of the midbrain or descending spinal pathways, resulting in loss of coordination of the urinary bladder, sphincter, and detrusor muscle. Neurologic problems, such as cerebrovascular disease, Parkinson's disease, brain tumors, multiple sclerosis, severe dementia, and prior cranial or spinal procedures, may cause incontinence. Other problems that may cause incontinence include anatomic defects of the lower urinary tract, decrease in bladder tone, outlet dysfunction as seen with prostatic enlargement, loss of detrusor tone (associated with tabes dorsalis, diabetes mellitus, and hypermotility of the bladder neck), prolapse of pelvic organs (cystocele, rectocele, uterine prolapse, and weakening of the pelvic support structures), and urinary tract infection.

Occurrence: Affects about 13 million Americans or 10% to 35% of adults. About 35% of postmenopausal women, 53% of homebound older adults, and 50% of nursing home residents are incontinent.

Age: Incidence increases with age.

Ethnicity: No significant ethnic predisposition.

Gender: Occurs more in women than in men.

Contributing factors: Increasing age, estrogen deficiency in women, immobility, smoking, fecal impaction, high-impact physical activity, multiparity, medications that affect the bladder and voiding such as diuretics and caffeine, pregnancy (usually transient incontinence). The mnemonic *DIAPERS* can be used to identify quickly contributing factors:

*D*elirium/dementia/drugs

*I*nfection

*A*trophy/atrophic vaginitis

*P*rostate/psychological/pharmaceuticals

*E*ndocrine

*R*etention/restricted mobility

*S*tool impaction

Signs and symptoms:

History

Obtain information about the onset, frequency, timing, amount, and duration of symptoms; daily fluid intake; bowel and bladder habits; and current medications.

Associated Signs and Symptoms

The presence of symptoms such as frequency, nocturia, and dysuria and urinary incontinence may indicate bladder dysfunction, infection, or an inflammatory process. Obstruction is suggested by hesitancy, straining to void, changes in stream, or inability to empty the bladder completely. Precipitating events, such as coughing, sneezing, laughing, lifting, or any sudden increase in intra-abdominal pressure, may indicate stress incontinence. A strong urge to void that is unrelated to position or activity and is associated with inflammation, infection, or neurologic bladder disorder suggests urge incontinence. Constant dribbling and chronic retention of urine suggest overflow incontinence.

Physical Examination

Assess the patient's cognitive and functional levels. Focus the physical examination on identifying neurologic deficits. Assess the back for spinal deformities and costovertebral angle tenderness. Evaluate the abdomen for distention, pain, and masses. Palpate and percuss the suprapubic area for pain and distention. Skin in the genital area may show signs of excoriation or fungal infection from the incontinence. A rectal examination is needed to assess sphincter tone, for the presence of a fecal impaction, and for an evaluation of prostate size and consistency. A vaginal examination may reveal a pelvic prolapse. Ask the patient to bear down during the examination. Reproduction of the activity that produces the urine loss is important because direct observation of urine loss can confirm a diagnosis of stress incontinence.

Diagnostic tests:

Tests	Results Indicating Disorder	CPT Code
Urinalysis	Especially for urge incontinence to determine infection; WBCs, bacteria, and nitrates in urine suggest infection	81001
Urine culture and sensitivity	If urinalysis positive for infection, determine organism and antibiotic treatment	87088
BUN/creatinine ratio	Increased in prerenal azotemia	84520, 82565
Serum glucose	Increased levels suggest diabetes mellitus	82947
Post residual voiding	Increased residual amount of urine suggests overflow incontinence	51798
Renal and pelvic ultrasound	Determine kidney and pelvic masses and obstruction	75770, 76856
Intravenous pyelogram	Determine renal pathology or other urodynamic obstruction	74400
Voiding cystourethrogram	Determine bladder and urethral pathology	51600

Differential diagnosis:

- Stress incontinence: loss of urine with activities that increase intra-abdominal pressure; no leakage in supine position; multiparity
- Urge incontinence: strong urge to void; unrelated to position or activity; associated with inflammation, infection, or neurologic disorder
- Overflow incontinence: retention and dribbling of urine
- Incontinence (stress, urge, overflow): caused by physiologic or psychological problems

Treatment: Treat cause or refer as appropriate.

Pharmacologic

Evaluation and changing of medications or times of medication administration may eliminate incontinence.

Urge incontinence: Anticholinergic agents, such as oxybutynin, 2.5 to 5 mg three or four times daily, or propantheline, 7.5 to 30 mg three or four times daily, or tricyclic antidepressants, such as dicyclomine, 10 to 20 mg three times daily; imipramine, 25 to 100 mg at bedtime; doxepin, 25 to 100 mg every HS; desipramine, 25 to 100 mg every HS; or nortriptyline, 25 to 100 mg once a day (owing to sedative effects).

Stress incontinence: α-Adrenergic agents, such as phenylpropanolamine, 25 to 100 mg twice daily, or pseudoephedrine, 15 to 30 mg three times daily. Use with caution in hypertensive patients.

Stress or mixed incontinence: Estrogen replacements, such as conjugated estrogen orally, 0.3 to 1.25 mg once a day or vaginally, 2 g once a day.

Physical

Behavioral interventions, including a toileting schedule, bladder training, and pelvic muscle exercises, may be successful in controlling incontinence. Other measures that may be used for incontinence include intermittent and indwelling catheters, suprapubic catheters, external collection systems, penile compression devices, pelvic organ support devices, pads, and protective undergarments.

Surgical

Surgical intervention may be necessary to remove obstructions or to correct abnormalities.

Follow-up: See patient as indicated by cause of symptom.

Sequelae: Possible complications depend on cause of symptom. Complications of chronic urinary incontinence include urinary tract infections, skin breakdown, hydronephrosis, renal failure, and possibly death. There is also a tremendous psychosocial impact on the patient and family.

Prevention/prophylaxis: Prevention strategies depend on cause of symptom. For women, encourage the patient to perform daily Kegel exercises to strengthen pelvic muscle tone.

Referral: Refer to or consult with appropriate specialist as indicated by cause of symptom. If the patient has anatomic defects or obstructions, refer to a surgeon for possible surgical interventions.

Education: Explain cause of symptoms, tests or procedures used to determine the cause, and symptomatic treatment, if any. Advise patient when to seek medical care.

WEIGHT LOSS, UNINTENTIONAL

| Weight loss, unknown | ICD-9-CM: 783.21 |

Description: Unintentional weight loss is weight loss of >5% of usual body weight within 6 to 12 months and may reflect a physical or psychological illness.

Etiology: The mechanisms of pathologic weight loss include decreased intake, decreased absorption, and accelerated metabolism. Most serious illnesses are accompanied by anorexia. Many illnesses increase the basal metabolic rate.

Occurrence: Occurs frequently as a presenting symptom for many underlying pathologic conditions.

Age: Becomes more common with increasing age.

Ethnicity: No significant ethnic predisposition.

Gender: Occurs in both genders. More common in women with eating disorders and in men with HIV.

Contributing factors: Caused by many medical conditions, including cancer, especially GI tract and lymphoma or leukemia; endocrine and metabolic dysfunction (hyperthyroid or hypothyroid, diabetes mellitus); infection (tuberculosis, HIV, subacute bacterial endocarditis); medications; GI disease (malabsorption syndromes, enteritis, peptic ulcer, GERD, cholelithiasis, constipation); cardiac disorders (heart failure); respiratory disorders (emphysema, chronic bronchitis); renal disorders (uremia); connective tissue diseases (rheumatoid arthritis, systemic lupus erythematosus); oral disorders (absence of teeth, dysphagia, pain with eating); neurologic disorders (dementia, Parkinson's disease, costovertebral angle); and psychiatric and behavioral problems, such as depression, anxiety, bereavement, alcoholism, and anorexia nervosa. Psychosocial conditions, including social isolation; economic hardship; poor dentition; loss of sense of taste or smell; and recent lifestyle changes such as death of spouse, divorce, and loss of job, also may result in weight loss.

Signs and symptoms:

History

Confirm actual weight loss because it cannot be substantiated in 50% of patients. Poor dentition, oral lesions or irritation, and infection can precipitate weight loss. Obtain a complete history, including a diary of dietary intake, history of cigarette and alcohol use, active medical problems, medication use, and previous surgeries.

Associated Signs and Symptoms

Changes in bowel habits, nausea, vomiting, and abdominal pain with weight loss may indicate a GI disturbance. Weight loss, polyuria, polydipsia, polypepsia, heat intolerance, and exophthalmus may suggest an endocrine imbalance. Weight loss with fever and other GI complaints may be associated with infection, including opportunistic infections and possibly HIV. Excessive weight loss, dental caries and enamel erosion, cold intolerance, amenorrhea, loss of hair, hypotension, and constipation are seen in anorexia nervosa.

Diagnostic tests:

Tests	Results Indicating Disorder	CPT Code
CBC with differential	Increase in lymphocytes suggests viral infection; increase in WBC count with left shift suggests bacterial infection; increase in monocytes may suggest tuberculosis, CMV, lymphoma, metastatic cancer; increased eosinophils associated with drug reaction, allergy, lymphoma	85004
Serum electrolytes	Determine electrolyte and acid-base balance	80053
Glucose	Increased level suggests diabetes mellitus	82947
TSH	Increased level suggests hypothyroidism; decreased level suggests hyperthyroidism	84443

(Continued)

Tests	Results Indicating Disorder	CPT Code
ESR	Increased level suggests infection, inflammation, neoplasm	85652
Stool for occult blood	Positive results suggest GI bleeding, neoplasm	82270
AST, ALT	Increased levels suggest hepatocellular damage or inflammation; ALT more specific for liver disease; ALT levels more elevated than AST levels suggest viral hepatitis; AST levels at least twice ALT levels suggest liver injury from alcoholism	80053
Alkaline phosphatase	Increased levels suggest cholestasis or infiltrative liver disease; also may be elevated with bone and intestinal problems	80053
Bilirubin, total	Increased levels suggest liver injury, biliary obstruction, hemolysis	80053
Bilirubin, direct	Increased levels suggest biliary obstruction/cholestasis ($\geq$50% conjugated bilirubin)	80053
Bilirubin, indirect	Increased levels suggest hemolysis of RBCs (>80% of total bilirubin level)	82247
Serum albumin/total protein	Decreased levels suggest liver disease	80053
Urinalysis	Determine urinary infection, renal disease	81001

Differential diagnosis:
- Physical cause: can be found in approximately 65% of patients
- Psychiatric cause: can be found in about 10% of patients
- No identifiable cause: is found in about 25% of patients

Treatment: Treat cause or refer as appropriate. If patient has nutritional deficiency, treat as appropriate. Appetite stimulants also may be helpful in some patients, such as megestrol, 800 mg/day, for patients with HIV-associated anorexia and weight loss.

Follow-up: See patient as indicated by cause of symptom. If no cause is found, reevaluate patient in 1 to 2 months.

Sequelae: Possible complications depend on cause of symptom; usually none in the healthy patient.

Prevention/prophylaxis: Prevention strategies depend on cause of symptom. Encourage good nutritional habits as appropriate.

Referral: Refer to or consult with appropriate specialist as indicated by cause of symptom. If indicated, refer to a nutritionist, social worker, or psychologist.

Education: Explain cause of symptoms, tests or procedures used to determine the cause, and symptomatic treatment, if any. Advise patient when to seek medical care.

REFERENCES

General

Barker, LR, et al (eds): Principles of Ambulatory Medicine, ed 5. Williams & Wilkins, Baltimore, 2001.

Dains, JE, et al: Advanced Health Assessment and Clinical Diagnosis in Primary Care. Mosby, St Louis, 1998.

Dambro, M: Griffith's 5 Minute Clinical Consult. Williams & Wilkins, Baltimore, 2002.

Ferri, F: Practical Guide to the Care of the Medical Patient, ed. 5. Mosby, St Louis, 2001.

Noble, J (ed): Textbook of Primary Care Medicine, ed 3. Mosby, St Louis, 2001.

Pfenninger, JL, and Fowler, GC: Procedures for Primary Care Physicians. Mosby, St Louis, 1994.

Rakel, R: Manual of Medical Practice. WB Saunders, Philadelphia, 2000.

Sellers, R: Differential Diagnosis of Common Complaints, ed 4. WB Saunders, Philadelphia, 1999.

Tierney, LM, et al: Current Medical Diagnosis and Treatment 2002. McGraw-Hill, New York, 2001.

US Preventive Service Task Force: Clinician's Handbook of Preventative Services, ed 2. 1998. Contact: http://www.ahrq.gov/clinic/ppiphand.htm.

Back Pain

AHCPR: Acute low back pain in adults. Clinical Practice Guideline No. 14, AHCPR Publication No. 95-0642. Agency for Health Care Policy and Research, Rockville, Md., 1994.

Borenstein, D: A clinician's approach to acute low back pain. Am J Med 102(Suppl A), 1997.

Chest Pain

Anderson, J, and Kessenich, CR: Women and coronary heart disease. Nurse Practitioner 26:9, 2001.

Bennet, J: Esophagus: Atypical chest pain and motility disorders. BMJ 323:44, 2001.

Douglas, P, and Ginsburg, G: The evaluation of chest pain in women. N Engl J Med 334:1311, 1996.

Milner, KA, et al: Symptom predictors of acute coronary syndromes in younger and older patients. Nurs Res 50:4, 2001.

Constipation

Mollen, RMHG: The evaluation and treatment of functional constipation. Scand J Gastroenterol 32(suppl 223):8, 1997.

Cough

Irwin, RS, and Madison, JM: Symptom research on chronic cough: A historical perspective. Ann Intern Med 134(9 Suppl), 2001.

Diarrhea

Covington, C: Diarrhea, a review of common and uncommon issues. Adv Nurse Pract 10:77, 2002.

IInyckyj, A: Clinical evaluation and management of acute infectious diarrhea in adults. Gastroenterol Clin North Am 30:401, 2001.

Schiller, LR: Diarrhea. Med Clin North Am 300, 2000.

Dizziness

Hoffman, RM: Evaluating dizziness. Am J Med 107, 1999.

Sloan, PD: Dizziness: State of the science. Ann Intern Med 134 (9 Suppl):550, 2001.

Weinstein, B, and Devons, C: The dizzy patient: Step wise work up of a common complaint. Geriatrics 6:42, 1995.

Fatigue

Lee, P: Recent developments in chronic fatigue syndrome. Am J Med 105(Suppl 3A):1S, 1998.

Fever

Mackowiak, PA: Concepts of fever. Arch Intern Med 158:1871, 1998.

Headache

Blumenthal, HJ, and Rapoport, AM: The clinical spectrum of migraine. Med Clin North Am 42:334–337, 2001.

Evans, RW: Diagnositic testing for headache. Med Clin North Am, 2001.

Purdy, RA: Clinical evaluation of a patient presenting with headache. Med Clin North Am 2001.

Spierings, ELH: Mechanism of migraine and action of antimigraine medications. Med Clin North Am 2001.

Hearing Loss

US Department of Health and Human Services, Public Health Service, Office of Disease Prevention and Health Promotion: Clinicians' Handbook of Preventive Services, ed 2. US Government Printing Office, Washington DC, 1998.

Hoarseness

Hanson, DG, and Jiang, JJ: Diagnosis and management of chronic laryngitis associated with reflux. Am J Med 108(Suppl 14a), 2000.

Spiegal, JR, et al: Acute laryngitis. Ear Nose Throat J 7:488, 2000.

Insomnia

Harvard Health Letter: Sleep Disturbance: A Special Report. Harvard Medical School Health Publication Group, Cambridge, Mass., 1999.

Morin, C: Insomnia: Psychological Assessment and Management. Guilford Press, N.Y., 1996.

Jaundice

Beckingham, IJ, and Ryder, SD: Investigation of liver and biliary disease. BMJ 322, 2001.

Hass, PL: Differentiation and diagnosis of jaundice. AACN Clinical Issues 10:4, 1999.

Palpitations

Barsky, AJ: Palpitations, arrhythmias, and awareness of cardiac activity. Ann Intern Med 134(9 part 2), 2001.

Peripheral Edema

Powell, AA, and Armstrong MA: Peripheral edema. Am Fam Physician 55, 1997.

Pruritus

Beltrani, VS: Allergic dermatosis. Med Clin North Am 1998.

Schwarzenberger, K: The essentials of the complete skin examination. Med Clin North Am 1998.

Syncope

Grub, BP, and Dosinski, DJ: Syncope resulting from autonomic insufficiency syndromes associated with orthostatic intolerance. Med Clin North Am 2001.

Schnipper, JL, and Kapoor, WN: Diagnositic evaluation and management of patients with syncope. Med Clin North Am 2001.

Urinary Incontinence

Maloney, CM, and Cafiero, M: Achieving bladder control, treatment in the primary care setting. Adv Nurse Pract 10: 37, 2002.

US Department of Health and Human Services: Managing acute and chronic urinary incontinence. AHCPR Publication No. 96-0686. Agency for Health Care Policy and Research, Rockville, Md., 1996.

Weight Loss, Unintentional

Lankisch, P, et al: Unintentional weight loss: Diagnosis and prognosis. The first prospective follow-up study from a secondary referral center. J Intern Med 249: 99, 2001.

Chapter 3
SKIN DISORDERS

ACNE

SIGNAL SYMPTOMS ▶ erythematous papules and pustules without pruritus (*acne vulgaris*); flushed face (*acne rosacea*)

Acne vulgaris	ICD-9-CM: 706.1
Acne rosacea	ICD-9-CM: 695.3

Description: Acne vulgaris, a chronic inflammation of the skin of the face, trunk, and back, is a potentially disfiguring skin disease. Acne rosacea refers specifically to adult acne that occurs on the skin of the face, usually the cheeks and the nose. Both are commonly seen disorders in the primary care setting.

Etiology: The exact cause is unknown; however, the disorder tends to be familial. In acne vulgaris, the production of androgens in adolescence is theorized to stimulate the turnover of keratin in the sebaceous glands. The keratin plug, visible as a comedo, causes an increased accumulation of sebum. These comedones may be closed (whiteheads) or open (blackheads). In some cases, the presence of *Propionibacterium acnes,* a normal skin resident and principal component of the microbial flora of the pilosebaceous follicle, may stimulate an inflammatory response (the intensity of which is thought to be genetic) to the sebum. This response may result in the papule and pustule formation commonly called *cystic acne.*

Acne rosacea is a vascular disorder of unknown etiology.

Occurrence: Acne vulgaris is common; virtually 80% to 90% of all adolescents (approximately 50 million) experience some form of acne; approximately 15% seek medical attention. Acne rosacea affects approximately 13 million people in the United States.

Age: Acne vulgaris occurs most commonly from early to late puberty, although it may persist into the 20s and 30s. Acne rosacea is common in adults ≥30 years old.

Ethnicity: Acne vulgaris occurs in adolescents of all ethnic backgrounds; however, incidence and severity are lower in blacks and in Asians. Acne rosacea more commonly occurs in people of northern European and Celtic heritage.

Gender: Acne vulgaris occurs slightly more often in men than in women; men also may be more severely affected. Acne rosacea affects women more than men, but men may be more severely affected.

Contributing factors:

Acne vulgaris: Use of androgenic steroids, lithium, phenytoins, bromides, and iodides; hot, humid climates; use of oily cosmetics; occlusion of the skin surface, such as from wearing sports helmets, using the telephone, or touching the face; age; male sex.

Acne rosacea: Thyroid disturbances, stress. Drinking hot liquids; eating spicy foods; exposure to heat or cold, wind; however, none of these risk factors are proven.

Signs and symptoms:

Acne vulgaris: Lesions most commonly occur on the face, upper back, neck, and shoulders; may present as comedones (open or closed), pustules, pimples, pitted scars, or nodulocystic lesions, with or without erythema. Pathologic sequence may be as follows: papules to pustules to nodules to cysts. All forms may be present at any one time, although symptoms usually are classified as follows: mild (noninflammatory), moderate (papulopustular), or severe (cystic).

Acne rosacea: Skin flush and redness that most commonly affects the cheeks, nose (specifically the lower half), chin, and forehead; comedones (rare); papule, pustule, or nodule/cystic acne lesions. Telangiectatic vessels account for the erythematous flush. Also may be present on earlobes, neck, and chest. Ocular rosacea is a major cause of red eye and dry eye. It may present with blepharitis, conjunctivitis, chalazia, keratitis, or iritis.

Diagnostic tests: Usually none needed for diagnosis.

Differential diagnosis:

- Skin eruptions caused by certain drugs, such as steroids, iodides, and bromides or by occupational or cosmetic exposures
- Gram-negative folliculitis
- Seborrheic dermatitis
- Lupus

Treatment: Depends on severity of the condition (Table 3–1).

Comedones and mild, noninflammatory acne vulgaris: Treat topically. Have patient cleanse face twice daily with a mild, nonirritating soap. Topical tretinoin may be applied to dry skin at bedtime, beginning with 0.025% cream. Gel (0.01%) is also available and is more drying, making it a better choice for

Table 3–1 Treatment of Acne

Type of Acne	Treatment	Special Considerations
Mild acne	Benzoyl peroxide	Start at 5% applied to dry skin at bedtime
	Topical retinoid preparations (tretinoin)	Apply to dry skin at bedtime Begin with 0.025% cream; increase to 0.05–0.1%, if no response after 6 wk
	Topical antibiotics	Clindamycin, 1% solution (Cleocin T) Erythromycin, 1.5–3% benzoyl peroxide (Benzamycin) Minocycline, 50–100 mg bid for 6 wk
Moderate acne	Oral antibiotics	Tetracycline, 500 mg orally bid or 250 mg qid for 6 wk; then taper by 250 mg every 6 wk until lowest effective dose is achieved Erythromycin, if tetracycline not effective
Severe acne	Hormonal treatment	For women only; oral contraceptives used
	Isotretinoin	0.5–1.0 mg/kg/day in 2 doses for 12–16 wk; LFTs must be monitored.

shoulder and back lesions. Caution patient that there may be an initial flare of lesions with this treatment.

 Clinical Pearl: Retinoids are extremely teratogenic (check for pregnancy and birth control) and photosensitive (patient should avoid sunlight).

If the patient does not respond to treatment after a 6-week trial, gradually increase the concentrations to 0.05% to 0.1% of the cream, or 0.025% of the gel.

If patient has papules or pustules as well as comedones, benzoyl peroxide starting at 5% may be applied to dry skin at bedtime.

Papulopustular or moderate acne: Treat as for mild acne. Also may use a combination of tretinoin and benzoyl peroxide, to a maximum concentration of 10%. If this proves ineffective after a 6-week trial or too irritating, substitute a topical antibiotic, such as clindamycin, 1% to 2% solution, or topical erythromycin, 1.5% to 3%, in combination with benzoyl peroxide. Oral antibiotic therapy also may be used. Minocycline (Minocin), 50 to 100 mg twice daily, is the most effective, but most expensive, of the acne medications. Tetracycline, 500 mg orally twice daily or 250 mg four times daily, is given for approximately 6 weeks, then tapered by 250 mg every 6 weeks until the lowest effective dose is achieved. For second-line or third-line treatment, trimethoprim and sulfamethoxazole (TMP/SMX) can be used. Give TMP/SMX (Bactrim DS) one tablet daily for 1 month. Oral contraceptives also may be considered, especially contraceptives with low adrenergic activity.

Nodular or severe cystic acne: The patient most likely will be referred. Isotretinoin, 0.5 to 1.0 mg/kg per day in two doses, given for 15 to 20 weeks, with a second course for an 8-week interval, may help a patient who is refractory to all other treatments. Adjust dosage for side effects. This treatment is indicated only for severe, recalcitrant, nodulocystic acne. The agent is highly teratogenic, and its use in women of childbearing age requires written consent and negative pregnancy test before starting and highly effective contraception during therapy. Isotretinoin has numerous side effects, including cheilitis, myalgias, epistaxis, impaired hearing, decreased night vision and corneal opacities, liver function elevation, hyperlipidemia, and leukopenia. Frequent liver function tests (every 2–4 weeks), triglycerides testing, and complete blood count (CBC) are advised. Isotretinoin also has been implicated in the onset of depression and psychosis.

 Clinical Pearl: Avoid alcohol and UV rays or sunlight and donating blood for 1 month after discontinuation of therapy.

Acne rosacea: Treat with low-dose oral tetracycline, 500 to 1000 mg/day, and topical metronidazole, 0.75% gel each morning and night; avoid topical steroids. Artificial tears are indicated for ocular rosacea.

Surgical

Cosmetic surgery such as dermabrasion may be used to remove unsightly scars. Laser peels also may be used.

Follow-up: See patient a minimum of three times over 8 to 12 weeks to establish success of regimen and adjust as needed. Good record keeping concerning changes is important.

 Clinical Pearl: Explain that it may take 1 to 3 months for improvement, depending on treatment regimen, and that the condition may worsen initially before improving.

Sequelae: Possible complications include scarring, both physical and psychological, and severe, confluent inflammatory acne with systemic symptoms (acne conglobata).

 Clinical Pearl: Acne is usually more significant to the patient than to the health care provider and often provides a point of entry to the health care system to address other concerns, such as contraception, stress, and lifestyle advice.

Prevention/prophylaxis: Prevention strategies include advising the patient to avoid oil-based cosmetics, to cleanse skin daily, to wash hair frequently, to keep hair and hands off face, to avoid picking or squeezing comedones (may worsen condition and contribute to secondary infection) or rubbing skin, and to avoid resting face in hands. Sunlight (in moderation) may be helpful. For male adolescents who are shaving, use a clean, disposable razor each time.

Referral: Refer to, or consult with, a dermatologist if the patient has severe or refractory acne or a physician if patient is being treated with isotretinoin. May require referral to an ophthalmologist for ocular rosacea.

Education: Explain disease process, signs and symptoms, and treatment (including side effects of medications). Discuss prevention strategies. Explain rationales behind treatment modalities, why they take time to work, and the importance of keeping to a regimen after beginning it. Provide reassurance. Explain that most cases resolve over time with no sequelae, but occasional flare-ups are to be expected. Reassure patient that acne is not caused by sex, masturbation, dirt, or foods. Teach how to cleanse oily skin: gently massage with unscented, antibacterial soap for 3 to 5 minutes while avoiding touching the sorest areas. (An astringent might be indicated to remove oil.) Rinse off soap for 1 to 2 minutes. Use a fresh washcloth every day. Educational resources are available from the American Academy of Dermatology, 930 N. Meacham Road, PO Box 4014, Schaumber, IL 60168 (708-330-0230), and the National Rosacea Society, 220 S. Cook Street, Suite 201, Barrington, IL 60010. Websites include: Acne, www.acne-site.com; rosacea, www.rosacea.org.

BITES: ANIMAL/HUMAN

SIGNAL SYMPTOMS▶ teeth marks on skin; redness

Open wound(s) of unspecified site without complications	ICD-9-CM: 879.8
Hand, open wound	ICD-9-CM: 882.0
Face, open wound, without complications	ICD-9-CM: 873.40

Description: An animal bite is a bite wound to humans from dogs, cats, or other animals, including humans. The integrity of the skin is disrupted by puncture wounds, possible lacerations, and perhaps crush injuries. All bites, regardless of the source, are considered to be contaminated and to have a substantial risk for infection.

Etiology: Caused by bite from an animal, including humans; most are from a domestic pet known to the victim. Dogs inflict >80% of bites, commonly causing puncture wounds and crush injuries; bites to the hand (65% of bites), face (25%), and lower extremities (10%); and an overall infection rate of 15% to 20% (commonly from *Staphylococcus aureus, Pasteurella multocida* [25% of bites], *Streptococcus viridins, Bacteroides,* and *Fusobacterium*). Cats inflict 3% to 15% of bites, commonly causing puncture wounds, with an infection rate around 50%

(commonly *P. multocida* and mixed bacteria, including several species of aerobic and anaerobic organisms). The third most common cause of bites is from humans, with infection rates of >50%, commonly from *S. aureus, Bacteroides,* and *Eikenella corrodens*. Infection from bites is essentially an inflammatory reaction to the oropharyngeal flora of the biting animal or human.

Occurrence: There are approximately 3 million animal bites per year in the United States, and approximately half of all Americans are bitten by an animal at some point in their lifetime. Dog and cat bites are responsible for 1% of all emergency department visits: dog bites, 1200/100,000; cat bites, 160/100,000 (approximately 10% of all bites).

Age: Occurs in all ages, most commonly in children. Bite injuries from fights ("fight bites," i.e., one person striking another with a clenched fist) are common in teenagers and alcohol-intoxicated men age 30 to 35.

 Clinical Pearl: Elderly patients are at increased risk for infection.

Ethnicity: No significant ethnic predisposition.

Gender: Occurs more in men than in women.

Contributing factors: Most bite wounds are from a domestic pet known to the victim. Large dogs are the most common source. Dog bites are more common in early afternoon and in hot weather and are more likely to occur from male dogs. Clenched fist injuries are usually human bites that occur during a fistfight and are associated with alcohol use. Risk of bite wound infection depends on the wound location, tissue damage, patient characteristics, time elapsed before treatment, and biting animal. Patients at high risk for infection include those with any of the following: bites from domestic cats, primates, pigs, and humans; bites in the hand, wrist, foot, or over a joint; fight bites; puncture wounds or nondébridable crush injuries; age >50; prosthetic joints or valves; long-term corticosteroid therapy; asplenia; chronic alcoholism; diabetes mellitus; altered immune status; or peripheral vascular disease.

Signs and symptoms: History of bite, injury, or fight. Presence of wound with teeth marks, redness, lacerations, punctures, soft tissue injury, scratches, swelling, crush injury, or devitalized tissue. Depending on extent and location of injury, vascular status, motor and sensory nerve function, and range of motion may be compromised. Signs and symptoms of infection may be seen, such as fever, erythema, drainage, and swelling. *Inquire about tetanus status.*

Diagnostic tests: Diagnosis usually is made by history and physical examination.

Test	Result Indicating Disorder	CPT Code
X-ray of affected area	Detects fracture or presence of foreign body	70000; choose specific area for code
CBC	Indicates infection: increased WBCs, neutrophils, monocytes, lymphocytes, and bands	85025
Gram stain	Detect infection and offending organism	87205
Culture and sensitivity	Detect infection and offending organism	87070 culture 87187 sensitivity
Aerobic and anaerobic cultures	Detect infection and offending organism; perform on high-risk wound	87076 anaerobic 87071 aerobic
Complete chemistry: electrolytes, glucose, BUN, creatinine	Indicated if patient is seriously ill with a bite wound infection. Any changes from normal need to be treated	80050 includes CBC 80048 (basic)
Prothrombin time and partial thromboplastin time	Indicated if patient is seriously ill with a bite wound infection. Any changes from normal need to be treated	85611 85732

WBCs, white blood cells; BUN, blood urea nitrogen.

Differential diagnosis: None; diagnosis is straightforward.

 Clinical Pearl: Judging the risk to the patient and the risk of infection is crucial. Signs of infection in cat bites are usually evident in 12 hours; in human bites and dog bites, in ≤24 hours. Infection also may be predicted by presentation >8 hours after the bite, older age, and puncture wounds. Puncture wounds may be associated with septic arthritis, tenosynovitis, or abscess.

Treatment: Low-risk bites in nonimmunocompromised patients may not require prophylactic antibiotics.

Pharmacologic

 Clinical Pearl: Culture all wounds before beginning antibiotic therapy.

Antimicrobial therapy: For fresh bite (dog, cat, human) wounds (≤12 hours), administer antibiotic prophylaxis with amoxicillin-clavulanate, 250 to 500 mg orally three times daily × 3 to 5 days.

For infected wounds, antibiotic therapy is guided by aerobic and anaerobic culture results. For mild, local wound infections secondary to dog, cat, pig, or human bites, give amoxicillin-clavulanate, 500 mg orally three times daily × 10 days; if parenteral therapy is necessary, give cefuroxime, 1.2 g intravenously (IV) every 12 to 24 hours; ampicillin-sulbactam, 1.5 to 3 g IV every 6 hours; or ticarcillin-clavulanate, 3.1 g IV every 4 to 6 hours. For penicillin-allergic patients, use doxycycline, 200 mg every 12 hours × 10 days (do not use in children <9 years old or in pregnant or lactating women), or ceftriaxone or erythromycin in dog and cat bites; for human bites, use doxycycline or cefoxitin, 80 to 160 mg/kg per day given in three to four divided doses. Fluoroquinolone and TMP/SMX are additional alternatives.

Use tetanus toxoid in individuals previously immunized, but >5 years since last dose. Consider tetanus immune globulin in patients without a full primary series of immunizations. Rabies prophylaxis is needed for bites by carnivorous wild animals, such as skunks and raccoons, and, in some cases, unvaccinated dogs and cats. Refer to local health department or infectious disease specialist for rabies prophylaxis. If postexposure rabies prophylaxis is indicated, human diploid cell rabies vaccine (or rabies vaccine, adsorbed) and rabies immune globulin should be given as soon as possible. Discontinue vaccine if fluorescent-antibody tests for rabies of the sacrificed animal's neural tissue are negative. (Contact specialist for specific dosing and schedule.)

Analgesia: Give agents for pain relief as appropriate.

Physical

Wound cleansing: Cleanse with povidone-iodine and copious irrigation of the wound with sterile normal saline via a catheter tip (decreases risk of infection). Then, if the bite wound was caused by a wild animal, irrigation with 1% benzalkonium chloride (has been shown to be capable of killing the rabies virus).

Positioning: Elevate injured area for several days; for bites over joints, immobilize for 3 to 5 days in proper position. Splint hand if indicated.

Surgical

Wound débridement: Remove foreign material, devitalized tissue, and eschar. Débridement of puncture wounds is not recommended. Consider surgical closure if bite is <12 hours old.

Wound closure: Puncture wounds and human bite wounds should be left open. Dog bites to the hand, wrist, and foot also should be left open. Bites to the facial area or other areas with excellent blood supply that appear clinically unaffected may undergo primary closure. Close wounds without signs of inflammation after thorough wound cleansing and preparation. For bites >24 hours old and all high-risk wounds, use delayed primary closure and apply a layer of fine-mesh gauze to wound, pack open, dress, and follow closely; in 3 to 5 days, if there is no purulence or wound margin erythema, wound closure may be performed.

Follow-up: See patient within 24 to 48 hours for evaluation of wound healing and signs of infection.

Sequelae: Possible complications include infection, cellulitis, abscess, osteomyelitis (especially in cat bites with puncture wounds that may get near bone), septicemia, tenosynovitis, pyarthrosis, rabies, loss of the injured body part, bubonic plague, cat-scratch disease, rat-bite fever, leptospirosis, tularemia, tetanus, and sporotrichosis.

Prevention/prophylaxis: Prevention strategies include advising patient how to prevent subsequent infections, by ensuring that bitten extremity is appropriately immobilized and elevated and to contact health care provider if signs of fever, redness, swelling, increased pain, foul odor, or increased drainage occur.

Referral: Refer to, and consult with, physician if patient needs to be hospitalized (patients with severe cellulitis; systemic manifestations of infection; failure to respond to appropriate outpatient treatment within 48 hours; or bite wound infections that involve a bone, joint, tendon, or nerve). Obtain early infectious disease consultation if needed. Septic arthritis, osteomyelitis, and closed-fist injuries ("fight bites") require orthopedic consultation. Refer to plastic surgeon for face wounds.

Education: Explain disease process, signs and symptoms, and treatment (including side effects of medications and adverse drug reactions). Discuss prevention strategies. Dog bites occur most commonly in summer and late afternoon. Counsel patients about this. For animal bites, advise concerning the need to have animal checked for rabies.

BITES AND STINGS: INSECTS

SIGNAL SYMPTOMS▶ pruritic, erythematous papules or pustules, isolated and scattered

Insect sting (venomous)	ICD-9-CM: 989.5
Insect sting (nonvenomous)	ICD-9-CM: 919.4
Injury superficial by site	ICD-9-CM: 910-919
Injury (infected)	ICD-9-CM: 919.5

Description: Insect bites and stings involve penetration of the skin by some part of the insect with release of venoms that cause local or systemic symptoms. Insects such as ticks also can transmit disease.

Etiology: Caused by bite or sting of an insect with release of venom. Venoms produced by venomous insects and other arthropods can be classified as follows: venoms that produce blisters (vesicating toxins), such as from blister beetles, certain stinging caterpillars, and millipedes; venoms that attack the central nervous system (neurotoxins), such as from black widow spiders and Hymenoptera (bees, wasps, hornets, yellow jackets); venoms that destroy tissue (cytotoxic and hemolytic), such as from Hymenoptera, fire ants, ground scorpions, mites, and brown recluse spiders; and toxins that prevent blood from clotting (hemorrhagic), such as from lice, fleas, and ticks.

Occurrence: Common; millions of people in the United States are injured by or die from venoms produced by insects and other arthropods each year.

Age: Occurs in all ages; more common in children than in adults.

Ethnicity: No significant ethnic predisposition.

Gender: No significant gender differentiation.

Contributing factors: Warm weather in spring and summer, lack of protective measures, areas of heavy insect infestations, previous exposure (can predispose to anaphylaxis). Perfumes, colognes. Children and elderly are at greater risk.

Signs and symptoms: Local reactions usually on exposed areas, such as arms, legs, or feet. Look for puncture wound from insect bite or sting; skin eruption varies with species of insect and may include local pain and swelling, erythema, papules, and pustules.

- Bees, wasps, and yellow jackets: Painful red wheal with central punctum; the wheal fades in hours. A persistent local reaction with intense swelling around the bite area may arise.
- Ants: Fire ant stings produce wheals with two hemorrhagic puncta; they usually evolve into pustules within hours.
- Mosquitoes: Pruritic wheals develop within hours of bites.
- Fleas: Grouped urticarial papules, some with puncta, frequently on leg.

Systemic reactions or signs and symptoms of anaphylaxis may occur depending on species of insect and history of previous exposure; may include urticaria, rash, fever, chills, malaise, nausea, vomiting, edema, pain, headache, lymphadenopathy, muscle spasms and rigidity, paresthesias, numbness, joint pain, hyperreflexia, ptosis, diplopia, nystagmus, diaphoresis, arrhythmias, hypotension, hypertension, wheezing, laryngeal edema, bronchospasm, agitation, confusion, seizures, and psychosis.

Diagnostic tests: Diagnosed by history and physical findings (if possible, determine exact time of injury and species of insect). Diagnostic tests may be performed to assess for complications and systemic involvement and may include blood type and crossmatch, coagulation studies, CBC, electrolytes, BUN, creatinine, urinalysis, arterial blood gases (ABGs), pulse oximetry, and antibody titer. A biopsy also may be performed to help confirm the diagnosis if in question.

Test	Result Indicating Disorder	CPT Code
Biopsy	Anthropod bite	11100

Clinical Pearl: An inexpensive, hand-held ×30 illuminated microscope is a good office instrument for tick identification. Be aware of local insect distribution.

Differential diagnosis:

- Punctures or trauma (patient history)
- Drug reactions (new medications or vitamins)
- Arthus reactions (usually 8–13 days after exposure to drug or blood products)
- Streptococcal necrotizing fasciitis, focal cutaneous necrosis, various infections, local thromboses

Treatment: Varies with extent of injury and species of insect. Insect or stinger or both should be removed from skin.

 Clinical Pearl: Scrape it out; do not grasp or pull insect because this usually causes more venom or toxin to be released.

Contact local, regional, or national poison control center for specific treatment. Hospitalize for severe systemic reactions with threatened airway obstruction, bronchospasm, hypotension, or severe angiodermatitis. Use antinuclear antibody (ANA) kit and over-the-counter antihistamines until able to get patient to emergency department for treatment.

- For all, appropriate tetanus prophylaxis; analgesics for pain relief
- Local treatment, such as cleansing site and applying antiseptic, application of ice packs (10 minutes on and 10 minutes off), cold compresses
- Phenolated calamine lotion as a soothing agent
- Corticosteroids, parenteral or oral (methylprednisolone [Medrol Dosepak]—begin at 40 mg orally and taper down to 5 mg) or topical (apply mid-potency steroids [Triamcinolone 0.1%] to high-potency steroids [betamethasone dipronpionate 0.05% cream or ointment] twice daily for 2 weeks)
- Antibiotics as necessary: Cephalexin (Keflex), 500 mg orally every 12 hours (2 times a day) for 7 to 10 days
- If swelling occurs, elevate affected part (if possible)
- Rest the affected area to avoid spreading poison
- Débride ulcers as necessary and drain abscesses
- EpiPen for future home use

Follow-up: Follow-up varies with type of bite, patient reaction, and treatment required. Patients with mild or local reactions can be treated and sent home; patients with large or infected wounds or with scorpion stings, or who show signs of a systemic reaction, should be hospitalized. Patients bitten by a black widow spider should be observed for 12 to 24 hours because hypertension and muscle spasm commonly recur. Patients with compromised cardiovascular or respiratory systems should be admitted to the intensive care unit.

Sequelae: Possible complications include infection, abscess formation, cellulitis, anaphylaxis, sepsis, and generalized systemic reactions with hemolysis, thrombocytopenia, hemolytic anemia, and death.

Clinical Pearl: Identification of ticks in the primary care setting allows for increased awareness and detection of tick-borne diseases transmissible by identifiable vectors for each infectious syndrome.

Prevention/prophylaxis: Prevention strategies include advising patient with known sensitivity to wear medical identification tags, carry anaphylactic kits, or consider desensitization to allergen. Advise topical application of agent. Use insect repellant, such as DEET.

 Clinical Pearl: Permethrin applied to clothes is better against ticks than DEET.

Referral: Refer to, or consult with, physician, surgeon, or allergist, depending on type of bite, patient reaction, treatment required, extent of patient's wound, need for skin grafting, or need for desensitization. If needed, consult with experts from local, regional, or national poison control centers.

Education: Explain disease process, signs and symptoms, and treatment (including side effects of medications). Discuss prevention strategies. Teach patient methods to avoid insect bites and stings, as follows: stand still if a stinging insect is nearby; if it attacks, brush it off (do not slap at it) to prevent a sting. Advise patient to seek health care immediately and contact the local poison control center. If possible, capture insect for identification. Be aware of possible diseases that may emerge related to disease transmission from tick/insect.

BURNS

SIGNAL SYMPTOMS▶ erythema, swelling, possibly blistering or whitish hardening of skin; may or may not have pain

Burn, unspecified	ICD-9-CM: 949.0
Burn, first-degree	ICD-9-CM: 949.1
Burn, second-degree	ICD-9-CM: 949.2
Burn, third-degree	ICD-9-CM: 949.3

Description: Burns are tissue injury resulting from physical agents. The extent of the injury (depth of the burn) results from the intensity of the heat source and the duration of exposure. Partial-thickness burns may be first-degree, involving the superficial layers of the epidermis, or second-degree, involving the epidermis and the dermis, usually with blister formation. Full-thickness, or third-degree, burns involve the destruction of all skin elements.

Etiology: Caused by exposure to heat or cold, chemicals, or electrical or radioactive agents, usually the result of accident or trauma. Open flames, scalding liquids, and steam are the most common causes of burns. In electrical burns, there is sometimes significant injury with little visible damage to skin. Excess sun exposure can cause first-degree burns. Caustic chemicals and acid also may cause burns.

Occurrence: Approximately 2 to 5 million burns occur per year requiring assistance; 1 million per year require hospitalization; 12,000 deaths occur from burns every year; however, 95% of all burns can be managed in the primary care setting.

 Clinical Pearl: Burns are the third leading cause of accidental death, after motor vehicle accidents and firearm accidents.

Age: Occurs at any age.

Ethnicity: No significant ethnic predisposition.

Gender: Trauma usually occurs more frequently in men than in women.

Contributing factors: Carelessness with burning cigarettes, sometimes secondary to alcohol or drug intoxication; unsafe heaters in homes; faulty wiring; and hot-water heaters placed in high or unsafe areas; workplace exposure to chemicals, electricity, or irradiation; stress and fatigue; excessive sun exposure.

Signs and symptoms:

- First-degree burns: erythema, hyperemia, tenderness, pain; no vesicles or blisters; skin blanches with pressure; history of injury
- Second-degree burns: erythema, hyperemia, pain, vesicles, blisters; raw, moist surface; history of injury
- Third-degree burns: whitened or charred tissue; initially may be hard and leathery but later begins to ooze; usually not painful or tender unless mixed with first-degree or second-degree burns; history of injury

Diagnostic tests: Diagnosis arrived at by history and physical examination. Additional diagnostic tests depend on degree of burn. First-degree burn usually requires no diagnostic tests. Second-degree burn depends on the extent and whether any signs of infection are noted. Third-degree burn usually requires testing; type and amount depend on the individual case.

Test for Third-Degree Burns	Result Indicating Disorder	CPT Code
CBC	Indicates infection or inflammatory response. Hemoglobin and hematocrit may be altered in severe burns, owing to third spacing	85025
Complete chemistry	May show alterations in values depending on severity of burn. Treat as necessary cautiously owing to third spacing.	80050 includes CBC and albumin 80053 includes albumin
Albumin	May be low in severe burns	82040
ABGs (if smoke inhalation)	Metabolic acidosis	82803 82805 (oxygen saturation)

The rule of nines is used to estimate the percentage of body surface area affected (head and both upper extremities together represent 9%; the face, front of trunk, and back of trunk are 18% each; each lower extremity is 18%; and the perineum is 1%, for a total of 100%) (Fig. 3–1).

ABGs to assess for smoke inhalation may be helpful.

Differential diagnosis:

- First-degree burns: dermatitis or allergic reaction caused by distribution
- Third-degree burns: Stevens-Johnson syndrome

 Clinical Pearl: Consider abuse or neglect in elderly.

Treatment: For all burns, administer tetanus toxoid, 0.5 mL intramuscularly, if not up-to-date; use Hyper-Tet for patients who have not been immunized. The first step in treating burns is to stop the burn process with cool water. May apply cold, wet towels. May need to apply warm blankets to rest of body to prevent hypothermia.

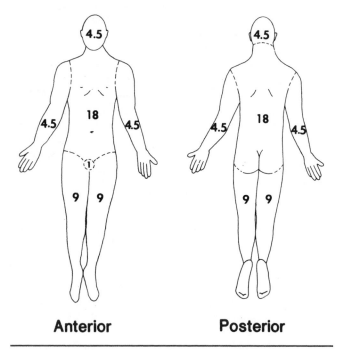

Anterior   **Posterior**

Figure 3–1. Rule of nines for calculating total burn surface area. (From Richard, R, and Staley, M: Burn Care and Rehabilitation. FA Davis, Philadelphia, 1994, p 109.)

First-degree burns: Submerge in cold water. Mild analgesics, topical anesthetic, a covering, or an emollient (for pain). Usually heals spontaneously in 3 to 4 days and requires little or no treatment except keeping area clean with soap and water. Avoid sun exposure.

Second-degree burns: Cleanse with mild soap and water. Anesthetic ointments or mild analgesic (i.e., acetaminophen [Tylenol]). Antibiotic or antiseptic ointment or cream, such as bacitracin, applied to area; silver sulfadiazine (Silvadene) 1% ointment for large or deep burns. Do not open blisters. Hospitalization or antibiotic therapy may be required. Nonadherent gauze and bulky sterile dry dressing.

Third-degree burns: Immediate prehospital emergency care; hospitalization with referral to burn center; evaluate and treat as indicated for airway intervention, fluid replacement, pain management, and prevention of infection or sepsis. Depth of tissue damage determines the need for skin grafting.

Follow-up: Outpatient follow-up care can be managed for the following patients: patients with first-degree burns; patients with superficial second-degree burns of about 5% to 6% of total body surface area (TBSA) that do not affect areas of function or cosmesis; patients with selected, deeper second-degree burns if not on the lower extremities, hands, face, or genitals and do not affect areas of function or cosmesis and do not cover >1% to 2% of TBSA. See patient as needed depending on extent of injury and treatment; for first-degree burns, no follow-up may be necessary unless complications occur; for second-degree burns, patient may need daily follow-up for dressing changes until the patient shows signs of healing. For all burns, re-epithelialization should occur in 10 to 14 days; monitor for signs of secondary infection.

 Clinical Pearl: Report suspicion of abuse/neglect.

Sequelae: Possible complications include secondary infections, temporary immobilization, disability, pain, financial difficulties, emotional distress, permanent scarring or disfigurement, and brain damage from hypoxia.

Prevention/prophylaxis: Prevention strategies include advising patient how to prevent burn injuries and accidents, such as by isolating household chemicals, safeguarding access to electrical outlets and wires, using household smoke detectors, preparing a family or household evacuation plan, having a fire extinguisher available, and knowing how to use and store flammable substances. For patients with burns, use sterile techniques for dressing changes or reverse isolation to prevent infection and sepsis.

Referral: Refer to, or consult with, physician or burn center if patient has deep second-degree or third-degree burns; burns of face, hands, feet, perineum, or over a joint, or circumferential burns; electrical or lightning burns; inhalation burns; chemical burns; burns resulting from child or adult abuse; and serious secondary infection, such as toxic epidermal necrolysis syndrome. Hospitalization or burn center referral is necessary for all burns >10% of TBSA in patients ≤10 years old and ≥50 years old; for burns >20% TBSA in all other patients; and for all third-degree burns.

Education: Explain disease process, signs and symptoms, and treatment (including side effects of medications). Discuss prevention strategies. Teach patient how to monitor for signs of secondary infection and how to keep burn area clean. The patient may soak in tub or use lukewarm compresses once a day. To help prevent edema, prop burn area higher than rest of body if possible. Discuss need for physical therapy, especially if burn overlies a joint; full range-of-motion exercises may be needed at least three times a day. Educational resource materials are available from the National Burn Victim Foundation, 3234 Scotland Road, Orange, NJ 07050 (201-676-7700). Burn Survivor Resource Center: www.burnsurvivor.com.

BURNS: SUNBURN, SUN POISONING, AND CONTACT PHOTODERMATITIS

SIGNAL SYMPTOMS ▶ mild erythema to red rash with itching; blistering or fever may develop

Burn due to solar radiation (sunburn)	ICD-9-CM: 692.71
Burn due to other specific agents	ICD-9-CM: 692.89

Description: *Sunburn* is a first-degree or superficial partial-thickness (blisters) burn. *Sun poisoning* (phototoxicity) is a systemic reaction to or overexposure to the sun or sensitization to light exposure related to medication ingestion. *Contact photodermatitis* is an acute or chronic inflammatory skin reaction caused by photosensitization of the skin by certain drugs or chemicals.

Etiology: Sunburn is caused by prolonged exposure to the sun (by 12–24 hours after exposure, skin changes from sunburn are maximal). Sun poisoning (phototoxicity) is caused by exposure to the sun or UV light, usually in conjunction with sunburn. Contact photodermatitis is caused by contact with perfumes, antiseptics, and other chemicals.

Occurrence: Common; sunburn and sun poisoning are most likely to occur during hot seasons when UV light is strongest.

Age: Occurs in all ages; elderly and children at highest risk for sun poisoning.

Ethnicity: Occurs more in people with fair skin, blue eyes, and red or blond hair.

Gender: Occurs equally in men and in women.

Contributing factors:

- *Sunburn/poisoning:* Prolonged exposure to sun or UV light.
- *Photodermatitis:* Prolonged exposure to sun or UV light may be complicated by use of medications that cause photosensitivity, such as oral contraceptives, tetracycline antibiotics, amoxicillin, sulfa drugs, and thiazide diuretics; underlying infection; metabolic disorders such as diabetes mellitus or thyroid disease; previous episodes of sun poisoning; use of immunosuppressive drugs; medical disorders such as discoid lupus erythematosus, systemic lupus erythematosus, or porphyria; exposure to industrial light sources, such as welding arcs; use of oral antidiabetic agents, nonsteroidal anti-inflammatory drugs (NSAIDs), antibiotics, phenothiazines, sulfones, chlorothiazides, and griseofulvin. Exposure to certain chemicals, para-aminobenzoic acid (PABA) in sunscreen lotion; perfumes; dyes.

Signs and symptoms:

- *Sunburn:* mild erythema with subsequent blistering; history of sun or UV light exposure; pain; pruritus may be present.
- *Sun poisoning:* may have rash or blisters accompanied by edema, chills, fever, gastrointestinal symptoms, or malaise; history of sun or UV light exposure.
- *Contact photodermatitis:* reaction usually delayed; itchy; red skin rash in area where chemical was applied and sun exposure occurred.

Diagnostic tests: Usually diagnosed by history and physical examination. Diagnostic tests performed may include photopatch testing (identifies photoallergic causes) and urinalysis (in contact photodermatitis may show proteinuria, casts, and hematuria).

Test	Result Indicating Disorder	CPT Code
Patch testing	Erythematous papules over area tested	95044

Differential diagnosis:

- Contact dermatitis (affecting non–sun-exposed areas)
- Erythropoietic protoporphyria (complains of burning pain with immediate sun exposure)
- Systemic lupus erythematosus (SLE) ("butterfly" pattern on face)
- Pellagra, porphyria cutanea tarda (new and resolving blisters on the hands and lower arms)

Treatment:

For relief from pain or itching: Saline-soaked dressings, calamine lotion, remedies with benzocaine or lidocaine, aspirin or NSAIDs.

For severe burns: Corticosteroids, such as triamcinolone acetonide, 0.1% topically, or systemic corticosteroids, such as prednisone, 40 mg orally to start with dose tapered over 3 to 5 days.

Antihistamines, such as hydroxyzine, 25 to 50 mg orally four times daily, for pruritus.

Follow-up: See patient as needed depending on extent of injury and response to treatment; if large blisters develop, see patient in 2 to 3 days to ensure secondary infection has not developed; patient may need hospitalization for severe or extensive burns.

Sequelae: Possible complications include recurrence of the rash and other symptoms when exposed to the sun even for short periods, especially in spring and summer; skin cancer, including malignant melanoma; keratoses; premalignant skin lesions; premature wrinkling; loss of skin elasticity; temporary delirium (in worst cases, from sun poisoning).

Prevention/prophylaxis: Prevention strategies include advising the patient to use regularly a sunscreen containing PABA or dioxybenzone and with a sun protective factor (SPF) of at least 30 before exposure (sunscreens with PABA may cause photosensitivity dermatitis; Photoplex broad-spectrum sunscreen lotion or sunscreens containing titanium dioxide, zinc oxide, or talc may be beneficial for patient experiencing photosensitivity); to avoid prolonged sun exposure, especially for persons with fair, sensitive skin (remind patient that a great deal of UV light is reflected off water, sand, snow, and sidewalks and is not screened out by thin clouds on overcast days); to condition the skin by grading exposure and wearing protective clothing; to stay out of the sun during the hours of strongest UV light (10 A.M. to 2 P.M.); and to notify health care provider if pain and fever persist >48 hours.

Referral: Refer to, or consult with, dermatologist as needed.

Education: Avoid photosensitizing drugs. Explain disease process, signs and symptoms, and treatment (including side effects of medications).

CELLULITIS

SIGNAL SYMPTOMS ▸   redness, streaking, swelling

Cellulitis	ICD-9-CM: 682.9

Description: Cellulitis is an acute, rapidly spreading infection of the skin and subcutaneous tissues. The infection may spread via the lymphatics and bloodstream and may be life-threatening unless promptly and reliably treated. It is most common in the extremities, but it may be seen in the scalp, face, and perianal area. Recurrent cellulitis of the leg is seen after saphenous venectomy. It is characterized by hyperemia, swelling, and leukocyte infiltration.

Etiology: Caused by bacteria entering the bloodstream via a disruption in the skin integrity, usually after a bite, laceration, abrasion, blister, burn, or puncture wound, or may be an extension from a contiguous focus, such as an abscess or a metastatic dissemination from bacteremia. The pathogen invades the compromised area, overwhelming the immune response and affecting the surrounding tissue. Group A β-hemolytic streptococci and *S. aureus* are responsible for most cases. Other agents include gram-negative rods, such as *Serratia, Proteus,* and *Enterobacter,* and fungi such as *Cryptococcus neoformans* (in immunocompromised patients) and *Erysipelothrix rhusiopathiae* (in patients handling fish, meat, and poultry). Facial cellulitis in adults most commonly is caused by *Haemophilus influenzae* type B.

Occurrence: Unknown.

Age: Occurs in all ages.

Ethnicity: Not significant.

Gender: Not significant.

Contributing factors: Diabetes mellitus, pedal edema, venous and lymphatic compromise such as post–coronary artery bypass in patients whose saphenous veins have been removed, immunocompromised status, prior trauma, underlying skin lesions such as a furuncle or boil, poor nutritional status, compromised living conditions, burns, intravenous drug use, recent infection, and surgery.

Signs and symptoms: History of trauma (usually) followed by local tenderness, pain, erythema, swelling (sometimes), chills, high fever, malaise, and regional lymphadenopathy. Progression of symptoms may be rapid. Involved area is red, hot, and swollen; borders not demarcated or elevated. Lower extremity is most common site.

Diagnostic tests:

Test	Result Indicating Disorder	CPT Code
Culture	Aspirates from point of maximum inflammation yield a 45% positive culture rate compared with 5% from leading-edge culture; bacteriologic diagnosis difficult unless open lesion is present	87070 87187
Blood cultures	Isolates potential pathogens in only 25% of patients	87040
CBC	Usually shows a mild leukocytosis with a shift to the left, which assists in gauging severity of infection and hematologic response	85025
ESR	May be elevated	85652

ESR, erythrocyte sedimentation rate.

Differential diagnosis:

- Erysipelas (superficial cellulitis involving skin but not soft tissue; streaking is prominent, and often the face is involved), deep vein thrombosis

Clinical Pearl: Common in elderly patients with cellulitis—symptoms of pain and cordlike structure on palpation help to differentiate; also the skin is usually normal and cool.

- Necrotizing fasciitis (systemic symptoms much more severe; the patient is very ill; bullae may form on the skin)
- Toxic shock syndrome (malaise, fever, chills, nausea, vomiting)
- Osteomyelitis

 Clinical Pearl: If crepitus, fluctuance, or divitalization present, order x-ray to look for gas production in soft tissue, indicative of gangrene; also order x-ray of for diabetic or immunocompromised patients or cases of previous injury to assess for underlying osteomyelitis.

Treatment:

Pharmacologic

- Generally empirical.
- Uncomplicated cases in the primary care setting, treat with phenoxymethylpenicillin, 500 mg four times daily, 1 hour before meal and at bedtime.
- Monitor closely for 48 to 72 hours; if unable to monitor, or no resolution, prescribe penicillinase-resistant penicillin (e.g., amoxicillin [Augmentin], 500 mg orally four times daily for 10 days).
- If penicillin-allergic (type I hypersensitivity), treat with erythromycin, 500 mg orally four times daily for 10 days.
- If allergy to penicillin not well documented, consider first-generation cephalosporin, such as cephalexin, 500 mg orally four times daily for 10 days.
- Reserve fluoroquinolones, such as ciprofloxacin, for gram-negative cellulitis. Only moderate antistreptococcal and antistaphylococcal activity in vitro; use with caution in cellulitis.
- If anaerobes suspected, use fluoroquinolone plus clindamycin or metronidazole.
- Give 0.5 mL tetanus toxoid intramuscularly to patients with open wound but without tetanus booster in past 10 years.
- Give antipyretics and analgesia as indicated.

Physical

- Use indelible pen to mark borders of lesion to track progress of lesion.
- Sterile saline dressings (decreases local pain); cool Burow's compresses are sometimes effective for pain relief.
- Moist heat (localizes infection). Warm Epsom salt soaks also effective.
- Bed rest with the affected area elevated (if possible).

Follow-up: See patient in first 24 to 48 hours to monitor for changes; worsening can occur rapidly, which may require hospitalization.

Sequelae: Possible complications include immobilization, pain, disruption of activities of daily living (short-term), permanent scarring, osteomyelitis, gangrene, and possible loss of limb (long-term). Potentially life-threatening in immunosuppressed patients. Monitor for sepsis.

Prevention/prophylaxis: Prevention strategies include advising the patient to avoid skin damage; to wear protective clothes as indicated, such as when gardening or fishing; to avoid swimming with open lesions; and to use support hose if patient has peripheral edema. Advise patient on the proper care of skin and wounds by cleansing with soap and water and using antibiotic ointment if breaks in skin occur. For early detection, advise patient to have area evaluated at the first sign of symptoms.

Referral: For orbital or periorbital involvement, refer to, or consult with, plastic surgeon and ophthalmologist.

Education: Explain disease process, signs and symptoms, and treatment (including side effects of medications). Explain importance of taking entire course of antibiotics. Discuss prevention strategies. Advise patient to rest; to finish entire course of antibiotics; and to report continued fever, blistering, drowsiness, lethargy, nausea, and vomiting.

CONTACT DERMATITIS

SIGNAL SYMPTOMS▶ erythematous papules with scaling; itching

| Dermatitis, contact | ICD-9-CM: 692.9 |
| Dermatitis, drug-related | ICD-9-CM: 693 |

Description: Allergic contact dermatitis is an eczematous eruption of the skin resulting from contact with an irritating substance or allergen. It sometimes is called "housewife's eczema." Secondary bacterial infection can occur, producing worsening inflammation and honey-colored exudate.

Etiology: Caused by contact with an irritating substance or allergen. Types include irritant contact dermatitis (most common), in which the epidermal reaction is usually immediate and commonly is caused by contact with substances such as soap, solvents, and urine, and allergic contact dermatitis, which represents a type IV delayed hypersensitivity reaction that affects individuals who have been previously exposed. This reaction usually takes several hours to manifest fully and commonly is caused by contact with substances such as chemicals; plants such as poison ivy, poison oak, and poison sumac; nickel, rubber, and latex.

Occurrence: Allergic contact dermatitis accounts for approximately 7% of all occupation-related illnesses in the United States and approximately 30% of dermatitis of the hand.

Age: Occurs in all ages.

Ethnicity: No significant ethnic predisposition.

Gender: Not significant because variations are caused by differences in exposures to offending substances.

Contributing factors: Varies depending on offending substances and length of exposure; includes, but not limited to, jewelry, cosmetics, travel, hobbies, and certain occupations, such as healthcare worker.

Signs and symptoms: Pruritus, stinging, burning, and pain (primary presenting symptoms). Extent of the response varies with the patient's susceptibility and amount of exposure; patient may or may not be aware of the noxious substance that has precipitated the skin eruption, including history of new medication.

Physical examination reveals an eczematous process of the skin with varying degrees of inflammation and erythema accompanied by vesicles and scaling. Secondary bacterial infection also may be noted.

Diagnostic tests: Usually diagnosed by careful history of what has touched the patient's skin. Patch test of suspected substances may be performed (re-elicits the reaction so that the patient will know what substances to avoid in the future). Potassium hydroxide (KOH) preparation test may be done (rules out tinea). Culture and sensitivity also can be done to rule out a bacterial infection.

Test	Result Indicating Disorder	CPT Code
Culture	Presence of bacteria	87070
Sensitivity	Sensitivity to specific antibiotics	87187
KOH	Branching, filamentous structures that are uniform in width	87220

Differential diagnosis:

- Tinea (central clearing, red painful scaly skin, usually in warmer areas of the body; may be itchy)
- Psoriasis (well-defined erythematous lesions with silvery scales; pruritus may or may not be present)
- Seborrheic dermatitis (greasy, yellowish scales involving face/scalp; nonpruritic)
- Nummular eczema (well-defined, coin-shaped erythematous lesions)

Treatment: Removal of irritating substance or irrigation after exposure. Evaluate all drug therapies and Interactions.

Pharmacologic

- High-potency topical steroids, such as fluocinonide (Lidex), 0.05% ointment three or four times daily.
- Methylprednisolone (Medrol Dosepak), 60 mg/day, tapered over 5 days, may be needed.
- Cephalexin, 500 mg orally two times daily, for 7 to 10 days if secondary infection present.
- Antihistamines, such as hydroxyzine, 25 to 50 mg four times daily, or diphenhydramine, 25 to 50 mg four times daily, as needed may be

effective in controlling itch and promoting sleep *or* nonsedating antihistamines, such as loratadine, 10 mg orally daily, or fexofenadine, 180 mg orally daily.

- Calamine lotion may be used topically for its soothing effect.

 Clinical Pearl: Avoid similar preparations that contain topical diphenhydramine, which may cause sensitization and result in increased itching.

Physical

- Cool, moist compresses—try $1/2$ milk and $1/2$ water *or*
- Burow's solution diluted to 1:40
- Cool tub baths with colloidal oatmeal may be helpful during the inflammatory, blistering phase

Follow-up: See patient until symptoms subside; perform patch testing if offending substance has not been identified.

Sequelae: Possible complications include secondary bacterial infection, more generalized skin eruptions, and worsening of reactions and symptoms.

Prevention/prophylaxis: Prevention strategies include advising patient to use gloves for housework and gardening to prevent hand rash reoccurrences, to keep affected part as clean and dry as possible (wash with mild soaps without a lot of perfumes and pat skin dry), and to keep a list of offending agents. Patient also may be a candidate for possible desensitization of the offending substance.

Referral: Refer to, or consult with, physician or dermatologist if patch testing is needed or if symptoms persist despite treatment.

Education: Explain disease process, signs and symptoms, and treatment (including side effects of medications). Discuss prevention strategies, methods to avoid offending substances, and need to be aware of secondary sources of infection, such as nails and clothing.

CORNS AND CALLUSES

SIGNAL SYMPTOMS ▶ hard nodules usually over bony areas

Corns and calluses	ICD-9-CM: 700

Description: A corn (heloma) is a horny induration and thickening of the outer layer of the skin, usually occurring over bony areas, such as toe joints. Often painful, the corn may be hard (heloma durum) or soft (heloma molle), depending on its location. A callus is a circumscribed, hyperkeratotic plaque of skin that may form on any part of the body, such as the hands, feet, or knees, exposed to repeated pressure or irritation. It is usually not painful.

Etiology: Corns and calluses form to protect the skin from injury caused by repeated irritation. Persistent friction or pressure, such as from ill-fitting shoes and wear and tear related to activity, causes a buildup of keratin. A layer of skin forms when dead cells move from deeper layers of the skin to the surface. Calluses may precede the development of corns and may serve a protective function.

Occurrence: Common.

Age: Incidence usually increases with age but also can happen in adolescents, depending on risk factors.

Ethnicity: No significant ethnic predisposition.

Gender: No significant gender differentiation. Corns usually occur more in women than in men because of high heels and tight-fitting shoes; however, they can occur more in men when occupation is a contributing factor. Calluses are more frequent in men related to manual labor.

Contributing factors: Any activity that causes repetitive pressure and irritation, such as shoveling, gardening, writing, playing sports, wearing ill-fitting shoes; structural deformities, such as hammer toes or abnormal bony prominences.

Signs and symptoms:

Corns: Patient reports pain when foot is in a tight-fitting shoe or pain on weight bearing (plantar corns). Hard corns are seen commonly on the lateral aspect of the fifth toe; soft corns are seen in the web spaces between the fourth and fifth toes. Plantar corns occur on the balls of the feet.

Calluses: Often painless. Sometimes the patient reports pain on weight bearing, burning sensation, and pruritus. The soft surfaces of the hands and feet are common sites for calluses.

Diagnostic tests: None. Diagnosed by appearance, clinical findings, and location.

Test/Treatment	CPT Code
Paring or cutting	11055

Differential diagnosis:

- Warts (circumscribed skin elevations, may have black dots)
- Foreign body granuloma with secondary keratosis (chronic inflammation around a foreign body)
- Calcaneal spurs (exostotic growth on the calcaneus bone)
- Plantar fasciitis (pain in heel or arch of foot, often worse in the morning)

Treatment: Refer if patient has diabetes mellitus. Remove source of pressure if possible.

Corns

- Analgesia as indicated.

- Peel the upper layers of the corn; apply a nonprescription, 5% to 10% salicylic ointment (Compound W, DuoFilm, Mediplast, Sal-Acid); cover to help soften and wear down corn.
- Pad bony prominences; recommend appropriate footwear, orthotics; lamb's wool between toes.
- Débridement of excessive buildup of epidermis—can be scraped or pared by provider with a No. 15 blade scalpel (leave depression in center of callus); usually no anesthetic needed.
- Soft corn infections—warm soaks twice daily and topical antibiotics, such as mupirocin.

Calluses

Soften calluses in a warm soak. Peel or rub the thickened area (do not cut) weekly, using a pumice stone or emery board. Take care not to disrupt healthy epithelium; leave a small amount of callus to provide protection. Pad area around pressure points with moleskin. A painful callus may need surgical débridement, or surgical correction of structural defects may be required for painful calluses; topical keratolytic therapy also may be required.

Follow-up: See patient as needed for treatment of symptoms; advise patient to call at the first signs of any infection.

Sequelae: Possible complications include recurrence and infection.

Prevention/prophylaxis: Prevention strategies include advising the patient to perform good foot care on a regular basis; to wear properly fitting shoes; and to remove sources of pressure or friction or use products such as inner soles, foam rubber pads, or moleskin to minimize pressure or friction. Teach patient that the cause is often faulty weight distribution from poor-fitting shoes or foot problems; metatarsal bars or orthotic inserts can be designed to correct the imbalance.

Referral: Refer to, or consult with, orthopedist or podiatrist if the patient has diabetes mellitus or needs surgical correction of defects, reduction of bony prominences, or other procedures to lessen excessive pronation.

Education: Explain disease process, signs and symptoms, and treatment (including side effects of medications). Discuss prevention strategies.

ECZEMA

SIGNAL SYMPTOMS Signs and symptoms start in infancy (1 month old) with generalized skin dryness and roughness; progresses to erythema, papules, pruritus, scaling, fissures

Dermatitis, atopic	ICD-9-CM: 691.8

Description: *Eczema* and *atopic dermatitis* are synonymous terms for chronic skin irritation that occurs cyclically. It is characterized by abnormally dry skin and a lowered itch threshold that leads to an itch-scratch-rash cycle. It may present in one of three stages: acute, subacute, or chronic (Table 3–2).

Etiology: Cause unknown; genetic factors have been implicated. According to one study, when both parents have atopic dermatitis, the offspring have an 80% chance of developing this condition. The integrity of the skin is impaired in atopic dermatitis. Changes in the lipid content cause increased water loss from the epidermis, reducing the water content and pliability of the skin. The skin is chronically dry, leading to a higher risk of penetration by a variety of irritants.

Occurrence: Occurs commonly; affects 10% of the U.S. population at some point in their lives. The prevalence has tripled over the last 30 years.

Age: Occurs in all ages; most common in infants to young adults. Condition usually improves in early childhood or before age 25 (40–75% of patients).

Ethnicity: No significant ethnic predisposition.

Gender: Occurs equally in men and in women.

Contributing factors: Childhood history of eczema, skin disorders, emotional stress, irritating clothing and chemicals, excessively hot or cold climate, exposure to tobacco smoke, hay fever, asthma. Associated with family history of atopy (asthma, allergic rhinitis, atopic dermatitis) in 50% to 60% of cases.

Signs and symptoms:

- Intense itching (cardinal symptom)
- History of generally dry skin (xerosis)
- History of involvement in skin creases in the folds of elbows, behind the knees, fronts of ankles, or around the neck
- Frequent cutaneous infections
- History of asthma or allergic dermatitis
- Chronic or relapsing dermatitis

There may be secondary infections, including herpes simplex (eczema herpeticum) and dermatophytosis. There may be associated facial erythema or pallor and conjunctivitis (see Table 3–2).

Table 3–2 Stages of Eczema: Signs and Symptoms

	Stage		
	Acute	Subacute	Chronic
Degree of itching	Intense	Slight to moderate	Moderate to intense
Appearance of lesions	Color: very red Lesions: vesicles or blisters	Color: red Lesions: fissured, parched, or scalded skin	Color: variegated Lesions: fissured, thickened, or lichenified skin, excoriations

Diagnostic tests: No specific diagnostic tests.

Test	Result Indicating Disorder	CPT Codes
Serum IgE level	Increased in 80–85% population	82785
Skin testing	Positive for allergen	95004

Differential diagnosis:
- Psoriasis (scaling, silver skin)
- Other dermatitis (new eruption; no history of atopy)
- Drug eruptions (new medications with new eruption)
- Nummular eczema (usually show different distribution patterns)

Treatment:

Pharmacologic

Topical corticosteroids (effective in >90% of patients). Use a short course of higher potency topical corticosteroids for flare-ups, such as betamethasone dipropionate 0.05% cream or ointment twice daily for 2 weeks; reduce to lower potency drug (creams preferred) for control, such as triamcinolone 0.1% twice daily for several weeks. Lower potency agents should be used in thin skin areas, such as face and skin folds.

 Clinical Pearl: Chronic use of potent fluorinated corticosteroids may cause striae or atrophy.

Apply corticosteroids in direction of hair growth to cover the affected areas; hydration of the skin increases penetration.

 Clinical Pearl: A general rule is that 30 g of medication covers the average adult body one time.

Coal tar preparations, such as tar-oil baths, or topical application of tar at bedtime may prove effective in certain cases.

Systemic corticosteroids for severe flare-up: Start at 40 mg orally and taper until 5 mg every other day until complete.

Oral antibiotics, such as cephalexin (Keflex), 500 mg orally two times daily for 7 to 10 days, if secondary infection occurs.

Antihistamines, such as hydroxyzine, 25 to 50 mg as needed and at bedtime (helps control itching). Also, nonsedating antihistamines, such as loratadine (Claritin) 10 mg orally daily, or fexofenadine (Allegra), 180 mg orally daily, can be used for acute attacks or maintenance therapy.

Newer classes of topical immunomodulators, such as tacrolimus (Protopic) 0.03% to 0.1% ointment to affected areas, can be used for extended periods. Treatments such as this that are steroid sparing are new-line regimens that avoid steroid use and possible toxicity and side effects.

Cyclosporine, 5 mg/kg per day, may produce a rapid clearing of lesions.

Physical

Wet wraps may be used in conjunction with topical corticosteroids. Wet, occlusive dressings can increase dramatically the penetration of the corticosteroids; they also may help reduce pruritus.

Wet (use warm water), cotton-blend pajamas may be worn underneath dry pajamas (the wet must be next to the skin); likewise, warm, wet tube socks may be worn with dry tube socks on top.

Teach stress reduction techniques.

 Clinical Pearl: Phototherapy can be used in recalcitrant cases; UV light therapy or psoralens phototherapy (PUVA) may be effective.

Follow-up: See patient as needed until treatment regimen is established and control achieved; follow-up is individualized and frequent. If disorder is resistant to treatment, consider a coexisting contact dermatitis.

Sequelae: Possible complications include secondary infections; eczema herpeticum; psychological issues related to body image.

 Clinical Pearl: The skin of >90% of patients with atopic dermatitis is colonized with *S. aureus* compared with only 5% of people without the disease.

Prevention/prophylaxis: Prevention strategies are individualized according to the causative agent, organism, or condition. Advise patient to avoid any irritating agent; take lukewarm, not hot, baths; use superfatted soaps; lubricate skin with oil baths, moisturizers (should be applied three to four times per day to prevent dryness); avoid stress and nervous tension (can worsen the condition), clothing that irritates the skin (wear loose, nonrestrictive clothing), and certain foods if associated with allergies (10% of patients). Caution patient that cold weather can cause fissures. Hot weather can cause severe flare-ups; use air conditioning when possible. House dust, mites, animal dander, and pollen all have been identified as potential triggers of exacerbation. Fingernails should be kept short and clean. Encourage the patient to consider joining a support group of peers to help deal with psychological issues of disease.

Referral: Refer to, or consult with, dermatologist if patient's condition worsens or is uncontrollable.

Education: Explain disease process, signs and symptoms, and treatment (including side effects of medications). Discuss prevention strategies and potential causes of secondary infection, such as nails and clothing. Advise patient that the goal of treatment is control, not cure. Educational resource materials are available from the American Skin Association, Inc, 150 East 58th Street, 32nd floor, New York, NY 10155–0002

(212–753–8260), and the Eczema Association for Science and Education (E.A.S.E.), 1221 SW Yamhill, Suite 303, Portland, OR 97205 (503–228–4430) (website: www.eczema-assn.org). National Eczema Society: www.eczema.org.

HERPES ZOSTER INFECTION

SIGNAL SYMPTOMS▶   unilateral dermatomal vesicular rash with pain

Herpes zoster infection	ICD-9-CM: 053.9

Description: Herpes zoster infection, also known as *shingles,* is a cutaneous viral infection characterized by a unilateral, painful, vesicular eruption distributed along the dermatome of an infected nerve root. The thoracic and cervical spinal dermatomes are most commonly affected, although the facial roots also may be affected.

Etiology: Caused by the reactivation of the varicella-zoster (chickenpox) virus, which has been lying dormant in the dorsal root ganglia of the dermatome.

Occurrence: Occurs in 10% to 20% of people at one time or another; 215 cases per 100,000 population per year. Active herpes zoster, 23.9/100,000; postherpetic neuralgia, 86/100,000.

Age: Occurs at any age; however, it is more common in adults >40 years old. Incidence increases with age.

Ethnicity: No significant ethnic predisposition.

Gender: No significant gender differentiation.

Contributing factors: Increasing age, stress, immunocompromised status, underlying malignancy.

Signs and symptoms:

Prodromal phase: Usually tingling, itching, and pain over involved dermatome before eruption.

Acute phase: Characterized by erythema and a maculopapular rash along the involved dermatome; rapidly evolves into grouped vesicles; vesicles become pustular or hemorrhagic in 3 to 4 days; dry crusts form in 7 to 10 days; resolution of outbreak takes about 2 to 3 weeks; scarring may result.

Malaise, fatigue, low-grade fever, headache, and weakness also may occur.

Diagnostic tests: Laboratory tests are rarely necessary.

Test	Result Indicating Disease	CPT Codes
Viral cultures	Indicates herpetic virus	87531 (herpes) 87253 (general viral culture)

(Continued on following page)

Test	Result Indicating Disease	CPT Codes
Tzanck's smear	Shows presence of multinucleated giant cells, but does not distinguish between varicella-zoster and herpes simplex virus	88199

TORCH, toxoplasmosis, rubella, cytomegalovirus, herpes simplex.

Differential diagnosis:

- Herpes simplex virus (recurrent in same area)
- Contact dermatitis (usually scattered and nonpainful)

 Clinical Pearl: Burning, painful sensations have caused some patients to think that they were having heart attacks or appendicitis when in fact they had herpes zoster.

Treatment:

Pharmacologic

- Antiviral agents (if initiated within 48 hours of outbreak, may help ease symptoms and speed resolution), such as acyclovir (Zovirax) capsules, 800 mg orally five times a day for 7 to 10 days (in severe cases, may need to be given IV); famciclovir (Famvir), 500 mg orally three times daily for 7 days; valacyclovir (Valtrex), 1 g orally three times daily for 7 days.
- Antipyretics as indicated.
- Analgesics such as acetaminophen, codeine, and NSAIDs. Avoid acetylsalicylic acid.
- Silver sulfadiazine (Silvadene) or mupirocin (Bactroban) topically for secondarily infected rash.

Physical

Soothing baths with baking soda added; topical compresses with Burow's solution 5% applied for 30 to 60 minutes four to six times a day; calamine lotion (may provide symptomatic relief).

Follow-up: See patient as needed.

Sequelae: Possible complications include cutaneous dissemination (ocular involvement could occur with facial zoster), secondary bacterial infection, pain, disfigurement, immobilization, lack of energy, postherpetic neuralgia, permanent scarring, recurrences. Consider underlying human immunodeficiency virus (HIV) infection in an otherwise healthy young patient with herpes zoster.

Prevention/prophylaxis: Prevention strategies include advising patient not to pick or scratch lesions. Other strategies are individualized, for example, seizure precautions when infection involves the fifth cranial nerve. Strict isolation for hospitalized patient because virus may be transmitted to susceptible people.

Referral: Refer to, or consult with, physician if patient is immunosuppressed or has underlying malignancies; refer immediately to an ophthalmologist if patient has lesions affecting the eyes; refer to dermatologist if needed.

Education: Explain disease process, signs and symptoms, and treatment (including side effects of medications). Discuss prevention strategies. Reassure patient. Advise patient to report visual changes or pain. Explain the infectious nature of the disorder and advise patient to avoid pregnant women, neonates, people who are immunosuppressed, and anyone who has not had chickenpox.

ONYCHOMYCOSIS

SIGNAL SYMPTOMS▶   yellowish, whitish coloring of nail, with pitting; nail may be brittle or thick

| Dermatophytosis of nail | ICD-9-CM: 110.1 |

Description: Onychomycosis, also called *tinea unguium,* is a fungal infection of the fingernail or toenail.

Etiology: Caused by a fungus. Dermatophytes that invade normal keratin include *Trichophyton rubrum* (most common), *Candida albicans,* and molds such as *Scopulariopsis brevicaulis.*

Occurrence: Common; occurs in approximately 15% to 20% of adults.

Age: Not common until after puberty. Age varies with type; for example, mold is more common in adults >60 years old.

Ethnicity: No significant ethnic predisposition.

Gender: Men are more likely to have one or more thickened toenails, whereas women are more likely to have fingernails affected.

Contributing factors:

T. rubrum: Warmth and moisture, such as from tennis shoes or ill-fitting, tight shoes; peripheral vascular disease; and immunosuppression.

C. albicans: Chemical or mechanical damage to the cuticles; maceration; occlusion; direct contamination from perianal itching; and underlying systemic conditions, such as diabetes, malnutrition, and altered circulation to the hands such as in Raynaud's phenomenon.

Signs and symptoms:

- Yellow or white discoloration that usually begins at edge of nail; brittle, crumbly, or thick nail (more often seen in toenails than in fingernails); nail may separate partially from nail bed; nail erosion; nail pitting. (In cases of rapid spread, consider immunodeficiency or chronic metabolic disease.)
- Secondary infection may occasionally be seen

Diagnostic tests:

Test	Result Indicating Disorder	CPT Code
Biopsy	Periodic acid–Schiff stain positive for fungus	11755
10% KOH	May confirm hyphae typical of *Trichophyton*; also may show budding or microspores	87220
Cultures of nail and debris on Sabouraud's agar*	Shows organism	87101

*For culture sample, collect scales from the stratum corneum beneath the nail if possible, or collect part of the crumbling nail. Discontinue all topical medications several days before collecting specimen.

Differential diagnosis:

- Psoriasis (well-defined erythematous lesions with silvery scales; pruritus may or may not be present)
- *Candida* or bacterial infection (black or dark green discoloration)
- Herpetic whitlow (associated vesicles)
- Drug or chemical exposure (possible black discoloration lateral poles)

Treatment: A cure is difficult; fingernail involvement has better prognosis.

Pharmacologic

- Topical antifungals, such as clotrimazole or miconazole.
- Systemic therapies include itraconazole, 200 mg orally every 12 hours for 1 week, then 3 weeks off (*phase therapy*). Repeat two cycles for fingernail involvement or three cycles for toenail involvement. Take medication on a full stomach, and monitor liver function tests. Terbinafine, 250 mg daily for 6 weeks (fingernail) or 12 weeks (toenail). Limit alcohol intake.

Surgical

Nail removal is recommended for certain recalcitrant forms. This is rarely curative, but may be used in combination with one of the other therapies for best results.

Follow-up: If on systemic therapy, see patient every 2 to 3 months to obtain CBC and liver function tests to follow for possible side effects. All treatments require lengthy follow-up: 9 months (fingernails), 12 months (toenails), or 12 to 24 months (great toe involvement).

Sequelae: Possible complications include secondary infections with progression to cellulitis or osteomyelitis, permanent disfigurement of nails, and recalcitrant nature of the disorder.

Prevention/prophylaxis: Prevention strategies include advising the patient to avoid tight, occlusive footwear; to wear absorbent cotton socks; to avoid wool and synthetic fibers; to change towels and clothes frequently; and to keep affected area clean and dry. Advise patient to dry hands and feet thoroughly without cross contamination from feet to hands.

Referral: Refer to, or consult with, dermatologist or podiatrist as needed or requested by patient.

Education: Explain disease process, signs and symptoms, and treatment (including side effects of medications). Discuss prevention strategies. Teach how to avoid secondary infection from picking or removing nails and avoid putting hands or fingers in the mouth.

PEDICULOSIS

SIGNAL SYMPTOMS▶   itching

| Pediculosis, unspecified | ICD-9-CM: 132.9 |

Description: Pediculosis is infestation of a human host by lice. Two species infest humans: (1) *Pediculus humanus* has two subspecies—*capitis,* which affects the head, and *corporis,* which affects the body. (2) *Phthirus pubis* affects the pubis.

Etiology: Caused by ectoparasites (lice) that feed solely on human blood by piercing the skin, injecting saliva, and sucking blood. Lice and their eggs (nits) are transmitted by close personal contact, by contact with personal items such as clothing, or through poor hygiene (*P. corporis,* or body lice); by contact with personal objects such as combs, hats, clothing, or bed linen (*P. capitis,* or head lice); or by sexual contact (*Ph. pubis,* or pubic or "crab" lice).

Occurrence: Common.

Age: Pubic lice most common in adults; head lice most common in children.

Ethnicity: No significant ethnic predisposition.

Gender: Occurs in women more than in men.

Contributing factors:

   Head lice: Contact with affected personal items.

   Body lice: Poor hygiene, unsanitary conditions, crowded living conditions.

   Pubic lice: Sexual contact, concomitant sexually transmitted diseases.

Signs and symptoms:

   P. capitis (head lice): Itching (most often on the back of the head and neck and behind the ears); secondary infections from scratching.

   P. corporis (body lice): Itching (most common symptom); occasionally secondary infection.

P. pubis (pubic lice): Pruritus in the pubic area, usually first noticed at night (may have no symptoms during the 30-day incubation period). Lice may be visible; resemble sea crabs, with large, widespread claws on the second and third legs. There may be secondary infection, groin inflammation, and regional lymphadenopathy; infestation may spread to the hair around the anus, abdomen, axillae, and eyebrows and eyelashes.

Diagnostic tests:

Test	Result Indicating Disorder	CPT Code
Wood's light	Identification of lice and nits on clothes and body Live nits—fluoresce white Empty nits—fluoresce gray	Included in the examination code for the visit
Magnification or microscope	Identification of lice or nits	88348

Differential diagnosis: None; diagnosis is definitive.
Treatment:
  Pharmacologic: Pediculicides
  The prescription preparation lindane (Kwell, Scabene), over-the-counter preparations (shampoo and lotion), synergized pyrethrins/piperonyl butoxide (RID), and 1% permethrin (Nix) (treatment of choice for all infestations except eyelash infestations) are available. The shampoo should be left on for 5 to 10 minutes before rinsing. After treatment, nits remain and should be removed with a fine comb (a nit comb). The lotion and cream should be applied over the entire affected area, washed off after 10 minutes, and repeated in 7 to 10 days. Lindane should be avoided in infants and pregnant women. When the eyelashes are involved, careful manual removal is necessary. Petroleum jelly application three to four times a day for 8 to 10 days along with manual removal of lice and nits for eyelash infestations is indicated.
  Malathion 0.5% (Ovide) lotion is an alternative for refractory pediculosis. It has ovicidal activity and is applied to the affected area and washed out 8 to 12 hours later.

Follow-up: See patient as needed.
Sequelae: Possible complications include itching, secondary infection, and reinfestation. With proper treatment, cure rate is 90%.
Prevention/prophylaxis: Prevention strategies include advising patient to treat entire family and sexual contacts; not to share hair care items with other people; to machine wash all linens, towels, and clothing in hot water and steam clean upholstery; to soak all hair care items in pediculicides; to cut hair if needed; and to store clothes or nonwashable items

for 30 days (lice die in about 10 days if they cannot feed; nits can be destroyed by drying for 24 minutes at high heat).

Referral: Not usually necessary.

Education: Explain disease process, signs and symptoms, and treatment (including side effects of medications). Discuss prevention strategies. Educational resource materials are available from the Mayo Foundation for Medical Information and Research, Section of Patient and Health Education, Sieber Subway, Rochester, MN 55905 (507-284-8140) and www.headlice.org.

PSORIASIS

SIGNAL SYMPTOMS ▶ erythema; thickening; silvery plaques, itching

Psoriasis	ICD-9-CM: 696.1

Description: Psoriasis is a persistent skin disease that received its name from the Greek word meaning "itch." The skin is characterized by erythema, thickening, and silvery plaques. Psoriasis is characterized by periods of partial remission and exacerbation.

Etiology: Cause unknown; however, many of the skin changes can be explained by an extremely rapid turnover of the epidermis.

Occurrence: 1000 to 2000/100,000 in the United States.

Age: Peaks of onset are between ages 16 and 22 and ages 57 and 60.

Ethnicity: Occurs in 1.5% to 3% of whites. Incidence is higher in cold areas.

Gender: No significant gender differentiation.

Contributing factors: Cold weather, seborrheic dermatitis of the scalp, areas of previous injury, infection, hormonal changes, stress, alcohol use, steroid withdrawal, antimalarials, lithium, β-blockers, indomethacin (Indocin); 30% have family history.

Signs and symptoms: Itching and classic lesions (sharply demarcated, silvery colored, scaly plaques and papules); most often seen on the scalp, elbows, knees, lower back, and buttocks; may be mild or may cover large areas of the body. In approximately 25%, psoriasis spreads to the fingernails, producing small indentations and yellow or brown discolorations. In severe cases, the accumulation of thick, crumbly debris under the nail causes it to separate from the nail bed.

Other common signs and symptoms include stippled nails and pitting, positive Auspitz sign (underlying pinpoints of bleeding after scraping), Koebner's phenomenon (psoriatic response in previously unaffected area 1–2 weeks after skin injury), and arthritis symptoms.

Diagnostic tests: Diagnosed by physical examination of the skin, nails, and scalp.

Test	Result Indicating Disorder	CPT Code
Biopsy, skin	Thickened stratum corneum, hyperplasia of the epidermis, and a little inflammation	11100 (single) 11101 (multiple)
Serum uric acid	Elevated in 10–20% of patients	84550
ESR	May be elevated	85652
CBC	Occasionally leukocytes, anemia may be present in some cases	85025
Vitamin B$_{12}$	May be decreased	82607 62608 (binding capacity)
Folate	May be decreased	82746
Iron	May be decreased	83540

Differential diagnosis:
- Seborrheic dermatitis (greasy, scaly, itchy skin)
- Eczema (erythematous patches)
- Tinea (red, painful, scaly skin, usually in warmer areas of the body; may be itchy)
- Drug eruptions (new medications or vitamins)
- Lichen planus (distribution and shapes of lesions differ)

Treatment:

Pharmacologic: Topical Therapy
Start treatment with aqueous creams twice daily to soften scales (may use petroleum jelly, although this is not an aesthetically appealing approach). Follow with topical corticosteroid creams and ointments of medium to high strength three or four times daily. Overnight occlusion with plastic wrap hastens resolution. Taper topical steroids to prevent rebound. Switch from one product to another when efficacy diminishes. Alternate with coal tar; use tar shampoos for treatment of scalp lesions.

Physical
Sunlight; UV A and B exposure for mild disease. Oatmeal baths for itching. Wet dressings may decrease pruritus. Apply an occlusive ointment, such as petroleum jelly, salicylic acid preparations, or preparation containing urea, then use soft brush to dislodge the scales.

Others
Other treatments include coal tar, vitamin D, light therapy (PUVA), retinoids, methotrexate, and anthralin. The use of cyclosporine is currently under investigation.

Follow-up: See patient as necessary for laboratory work according to therapy prescribed; during periods of acute flare-ups, see patient frequently for supportive care.

Sequelae: Possible complications include secondary bacterial infection, psychological or emotional distress, and continuous chronic flare-ups.

Prevention/prophylaxis: Prevention strategies include advising the patient to avoid alcoholic beverages, irritating or stimulating drugs, and antimalarial compounds. Sunlight may help in small amounts. Advise patient of risk factors and need to reduce risks. A desert climate may be favorable for some patients.

Referral: Refer to, or consult with, dermatologist specializing in UV therapy.

Education: Explain disease process, signs and symptoms, and treatment (including side effects of medications). Discuss prevention strategies. Reassure patient that disease is not contagious. Instruct about UV therapy and need for eye examination before the start of therapy. Educational resource materials are available from the National Psoriasis Foundation, Suite 300, 6600 SW 92nd Avenue, Portland, OR 97223 (503-244-7404, 800-723-9166) (website: http://www.psoriasis.org).

SCABIES

SIGNAL SYMPTOMS▶   generalized nocturnal pruritus

Scabies	ICD-9-CM: 133.0

Description: Scabies is a communicable skin disease characterized by diffuse rash and itching, especially at night.

Etiology: Caused by an arachnid (the itch mite, *Sarcoptes scabiei*). Impregnated female mites burrow in the stratum corneum and deposit eggs and fecal pellets, which hatch in 4 to 8 days, reach maturity in about 14 days, mate, and repeat the cycle. Transmission occurs by close personal contact; the incubation period in people without previous exposure is 4 to 6 weeks.

Occurrence: Common; incidence worldwide is 300 million cases per year.

Age: Occurs in any age. In young adults, it may be sexually transmitted.

Ethnicity: No significant ethnic predisposition.

Gender: Occurs equally in men and women; in men, genitalia are often involved.

Contributing factors: Personal, skin-to-skin contact, such as sexual contact; crowded, poor, unsanitary living conditions; institutional settings such as prisons, nursing homes, and shelters; exposure to infested clothes, towels, dogs (canine scabies); immunocompromised status; atopic dermatitis.

Signs and symptoms: Generalized nocturnal pruritus (hallmark symptom). Primary lesions are burrows (difficult to see, obscured by itching), vesicles, and papules. Secondary lesions, usually caused by scratching, are often present with erythema and scaling. Common sites are the hands (90%), specifically the finger webs and wrists; axillary folds; belt line; navel; and penis, scrotum, and areola. Nodules may appear in covered areas, and there may be atypical infestations in immunosuppressed patients.

Physical examination with a magnifying glass may reveal the typical burrows, gray or skin-colored ridges a few centimeters in length, in finger webs, flexor of wrist, and penis. Dark point at the end of the burrow is the mite, which can be extracted with a 25-gauge needle and examined microscopically.

Diagnostic tests:

Test	Result Indicating Disorder	CPT Codes
Microscopic on slide with immersion in oil and examined on low power	Scrapings from under fingernails are often positive for mite visualization	88348
KOH wet mount	Scrapings from under fingernails are often positive for mite visualization	87220
Ink stain	If burrows are not obvious, apply ink to a suspicious area of rash. After washing off the ink with alcohol, any area that remains stained represents a burrow. The area can be scraped and examined	Included in the examination code for the visit

Differential diagnosis:
- Pediculosis (visible parasites)
- Urticaria (large wheals that can come and go)
- Impetigo (honey-crusted plaques)
- Eczema (erythematous patches)
- Secondary infection (redness, swelling, fever)
- Scabies dermatitis (rash secondary to underlying scabies)

Treatment: Therapeutic trial usually is indicated even if mite cannot be seen. All family members and contacts must be treated.

Pharmacologic

Permethrin (Elimite) cream (treatment of choice). Apply cream from the neck down and leave on for 8 to 14 hours; then thoroughly wash off; 30 g is usually adequate for an adult. A repeat application 7 to 10 days later is usually necessary.

Antihistamines or topical or oral corticosteroids (for intense itching and inflammation).

Physical

Wash all clothing, bed linens, and towels in normal wash cycle with hot drying cycle. Items that cannot be laundered should be placed in plastic storage bags for at least 1 week. Mites do not live for longer than 3 to 4 days away from the host.

Follow-up: Follow-up usually is not needed unless problem continues. Contact patient by phone to ensure all instructions were followed to prevent reinfestation. Recheck patient at weekly intervals only if rash or itching persists.

Sequelae: Possible complications include persistent or lingering itching, secondary infection caused by scratching, and eczema.

Prevention/prophylaxis: Prevention strategies include advising the patient that the entire family and contacts be treated and educating on good personal hygiene.

Referral: Refer to, or consult with, dermatologist if patient has a persistent problem.

Education: Explain disease process, signs and symptoms, and treatment (including side effects of medications). Discuss prevention strategies. Advise patient that itching may persist days to weeks because of lingering allergic reaction to the mite.

SEBORRHEIC DERMATITIS

SIGNAL SYMPTOMS▶ greasy, scaly itchy skin

Dermatitis, seborrheic	ICD-9-CM: 690

Description: Seborrheic dermatitis is an inflammatory skin disease occurring in areas of the body with a high concentration of sebaceous glands.

Etiology: Cause unclear; seems to be inherited.

Occurrence: Common; higher frequency of occurrence in patients with HIV, Parkinson's disease, and quadriplegia.

Age: Occurs at any age.

Ethnicity: No known ethnic predisposition.

Gender: Occurs equally in men and in women.

Contributing factors: Other skin disorders, stress, depression, obesity; worsens in the fall and winter and improves in spring and summer.

Signs and symptoms: Greasy, red scaling of the involved area accompanied by itching, flaking, and erythema. Common on the scalp; also may affect other areas, such as the eyebrows, eyelid margins, nasolabial folds, ears, retroauricular folds, presternal area, and mid upper back. There is usually a chronic waxing and waning course, with minimal pruritus.

Diagnostic tests: Usually diagnosed by clinical examination.

Test	Result Indicating Disorder	CPT Code
KOH wet mount preparation	Rules out tinea; negative for hyphae	87220

Differential diagnosis:
- Atopic dermatitis (generalized skin dryness and roughness; progresses to erythema, papules, pruritus, scaling, fissures)

- Psoriasis (well-defined erythematous lesions with silvery scales; pruritus may or may not be present)
- Tinea (red painful scaly skin, usually in warmer areas of the body; may be itchy)

Treatment:

Pharmacologic

> Shampoos such as selenium sulfide 2.5%, pyrithione zinc 2%, or ketoconazole 2% used two to three times per week are the principal mode of treatment. Shampoos have cytostatic and antimycotic effects. Some sources recommend alternating shampoos.

> Topical steroids or ketoconazole 2% cream (for nonhairy areas) if shampoos fail.

> Remove thick scales by applying warm mineral oil for several hours and washing off with mild detergent and soft-bristle brush.

Follow-up: See patient every 1 to 2 months initially to establish an effective, individual treatment strategy; follow more closely during periods of exacerbation.

Sequelae: This is a chronic, recurring condition; it does not cause permanent hair loss or baldness, unless skin or hair becomes grossly infected.

Prevention/prophylaxis: Prevention strategies include advising the patient of the chronic and seasonal nature of the disease (worsens in cold weather, probably because of low humidity and lack of sunlight) and planning to treat each exacerbation. Advise patient to reduce stress (stress worsens condition); not to pick or peel infected areas (can cause secondary infection); to dry skin folds thoroughly after bathing; and to wear loose, ventilated clothes. Shampoo frequently with a nondrying, moisturizing, nonperfumed soap and avoid cosmetics. Men should shave regularly.

Referral: Refer to, or consult with, dermatologist if patient's condition worsens, if the patient has severe secondary bacterial infection, or if alopecia develops.

Education: Explain disease process, signs and symptoms, and treatment (including side effects of medications). Discuss prevention strategies and provide emotional support. Teach patient proper method of applying shampoo: apply to all affected areas, follow directions, leave shampoo on for 3 to 5 minutes to penetrate scalp, and loosen scales with fingernails while shampooing and scrub at least 5 minutes.

SKIN CANCER

SIGNAL SYMPTOMS ▶ changes in skin; moles that are new or changing in size or color

Melanoma of the skin, site unspecified	ICD-9-CM: 172.9
Basal cell carcinoma, site unspecified	ICD-9-CM: 173.9
Face	ICD-9-CM: 173.3
Scalp/neck	ICD-9-CM: 173.4
Trunk	ICD-9-CM: 173.5
Upper limb	ICD-9-CM: 173.6
Lower limb	ICD-9-CM: 173.7

Description: Skin cancer is cancer occurring in the skin and includes basal cell carcinoma, squamous cell carcinoma, and malignant melanoma.

Etiology: Basal cell carcinoma is caused by a malignant tumor arising from the basal cell layer of the epidermis; squamous cell carcinoma, by a malignant tumor arising from keratinizing cells of the epidermis; and malignant melanoma, by the malignant transformation of epidermal melanocytes (Table 3–3).

Occurrence: Basal cell carcinoma is the most commonly occurring cancer in the United States, with squamous cell carcinoma the second most common cutaneous malignancy. Malignant melanoma is on the rise, with approximately 38,000 new cases each year, or 4.5/100,000 in the United States. Approximately 700,000 Americans develop skin cancer every year, with an estimated 2300 deaths from nonmelanoma skin cancer and 6700 deaths from malignant melanoma annually.

Age: Basal and squamous cell carcinomas are more frequent after middle age; malignant melanoma has a median age of 53, with 50% of all cases occurring between ages 20 and 40.

Ethnicity: Occurs more commonly in whites than in people with dark skin.

Gender: Occurs more in men than in women.

Contributing factors: Overexposure to sunlight, especially when it results in sunburn and blistering; repeated x-rays; scarring from disease or burns; occupational exposure to compounds, coal, arsenic; previous sunburns, blistering, excessive sun exposure; having fair skin and blue eyes; sunburning easily; previous pigmented lesions; family history or heredity. Previous melanoma is an increased risk factor for recurrence and increased numbers of nevi.

Signs and symptoms: Changes in the skin, especially changes in moles, such as new appearance, color, shape, discolorations, scaly areas, or sores; scaliness; oozing; bleeding; bumps; nodules; spread in pigmentation; nonhealing lesion.

Diagnostic tests:

Test	Result Indicating Disorder	CPT Code
Biopsy (curetted, electrodesiccated, saved)	Confirms diagnosis	11100 (single) 11101 (multiple)
Full-thickness total excisional biopsy	Confirms diagnosis with suspicion of melanoma	11600–11646 (dependent on area and size)

Table 3–3 Comparing Three Common Types of Skin Cancer

| | Type of Cancer | | |
Characteristic	Basal Cell Carcinoma	Squamous Cell Carcinoma	Malignant Melanoma
Cause	Excessive sun and exposure (including x-rays); some types of nevis; genetic skin type	Frequently occurs on previously damaged skin	Neoplastic growth of melanocytes
Prognosis	Slow-growing; invades local tissue Metastasis is rare	Treated; high cure rate Untreated: may metastasize to regional lymph nodes	Potential invasion and widespread metastases; spreads by local extension, regional lymphatic vessels, and bloodstream Poor prognosis
Common sites	Face, scalp, pinnae, earlobes	Sun-exposed areas such as face, hands, ears	Back (men/women) Chest and lower legs (women)
Signs and symptoms	Small, semitranslucent, slowly enlarging papule; overlying telangiectasia; center is eroded. ulcerated, or depressed. May bleed Superficial lesion: erythematous, sharply defined, multinodular plaques with varying scaling and crusting	Early lesion;opaque, firm nodules with nondistinct borders; scaling; ulceration Late: lesion covered with scale with firm margins	Irregular color, surface, and border; variegated; 6mm
Treatment	Surgical removal (excisional)	Surgical removal	Surgical removal (wide excision; full-thickness) Adjuvant therapy for lesions ≥ 1.5 mm or more in depth

Clinical Pearl: With suspicion of melanoma, a full-thickness total excisional biopsy must be sent for pathologic specimen and should never be curetted, electrodesiccated, or shaved.

Differential diagnosis:

- Actinic keratosis (single or multiple dry, rough, scaly lesions caused by sun exposure; can lead to squamous cell carcinoma)
- Basal cell carcinoma (translucent, white papule, "pearly" in appearance; may have central ulceration; scaly patch with crust; telangiectasia; face and upper back)
- Benign mole (nonchanging; no bleeding, itching, or burning)
- Hyperpigmentation (new pigmented lesion)

Treatment:

> *Nonmelanoma skin cancer:* Careful selection of initial treatment offers the best cure rate and the best cosmetic results. When deciding treatment, evaluate anatomic area, histologic type, whether lesion is recurring, and age of patient. Choices include surgical excision, electrodesiccation and curettage, cryosurgery, radiotherapy, and chemotherapy. Topical 5-fluorouracil cream may be used for basal cell carcinoma.

> *Melanoma:* Treatment depends on staging. Stage II has a 36% 5-year survival rate; stage III has a 5% 5-year survival rate. Treatment may include surgery, chemotherapy, radiation therapy, or any combination thereof as well as supportive care.

Follow-up:

> *Nonmelanoma:* See patient every 3 months for the first year, then once or twice a year for 5 years.

> *Melanoma:* See patient every 3 to 6 months for total body examination for any abnormal-appearing or changing nevi; do a chest x-ray and bone scans yearly. Advise patient to report any new skin changes immediately.

Sequelae: Possible complications include scarring, recurrence (with nonmelanoma), metastases, and death (with melanoma).

Prevention/prophylaxis: Prevention strategies include advising the patient how to guard the skin against known causes, for example, avoiding sun, limiting exposure by covering up and using sunscreens (at least 30 SPF), wearing long-sleeve shirts, and wearing a hat with a brim to protect the face.

Referral: Refer to dermatologist if patient has any suspicious skin changes.

Education: Explain disease process, signs and symptoms, and treatment (including side effects of medications). Discuss prevention strategies. Teach patients to become familiar with their bodies and any moles they may have so that if a change occurs, it will be noticed (the patient is usually the one to find the problem area). Early detection is the best preventive method. Most skin cancers are curable. Encourage the patient with a history of melanoma to have frequent examinations for any abnormal-appearing or changing nevi. Website: www.melanoma.com.

STASIS ULCER

SIGNAL SYMPTOMS nonhealing ulcer on lower leg, usually without pain

| Stasis ulcers | ICD-9-CM: 454.0 |

Description: Stasis ulcers are poorly healing breaks in the skin, classically defined as affecting the lower extremities.

Etiology: Commonly caused by minor trauma to the extremity; however, healing often is complicated by chronic arterial or venous insufficiency (or both).

Occurrence: Common; 80% to 90% occur from venous insufficiency; 5% from arterial insufficiency; 2% from diabetes; 3% from other causes.

Age: Incidence increases with age.

Ethnicity: No significant ethnic predisposition.

Gender: Occurs more in women than in men.

Contributing factors: Cigarette smoking (major risk factor), stasis dermatitis (a chronic noninflammatory edema of the lower leg is a major contributing factor), varicosities, arterial or venous insufficiency, diabetes mellitus, history of venous thrombosis, connective tissue diseases, poor hygiene, unsanitary living conditions, alcoholism, poor nutritional status, immobility, obesity, dry skin.

Signs and symptoms: Classic presenting symptom is a nonhealing ulceration of the lower leg; usually painless, but some patients complain of aching discomfort when leg is dependent, with pain relief on elevation of the leg. There also may be pruritus if the ulcer develops on top of a stasis dermatitis.

On inspection, venous ulcers tend to have irregular borders with a classic brown or brown-red color to the surrounding skin; most common location is the malleoli. Ulcers caused by arterial insufficiency or neuropathic or diabetic pathology usually present on pressure sites, with lesions having a "punched-out" appearance, hair loss in the surrounding skin, and no associated pigmentation. Evaluate for dependent rubor. Untreated ulcers may have a purulent exudate related to secondary infection with concomitant tenderness and redness.

On palpation, compromise in peripheral pulses and capillary refill suggests arterial cause; alterations in touch and vibratory sensation suggest neuropathic cause. Peripheral pulses are more likely to be normal in venous ulcers, and these ulcers are more likely to have underlying edema and occasionally stasis dermatitis. Cool skin is more likely to indicate arterial compromise, whereas warm skin is more consistent with venous derangement.

Diagnostic tests:

Test	Result Indicating Disorder	CPT Code
Culture of exudate	If systemic infection or cellulitis is suspected to isolate offending organism	87070
Doppler studies	Assess vascular status	93965

(Continued on following page)

Test	Result Indicating Disorder	CPT Code
X-ray of extremity	If underlying osteomyelitis is suspected	73000–73225 (choose area of upper extremity) 73500–73725 (choose area of lower extremity)
CBC	Elevated WBCs, neutrophils, monocytes, bands, lymphocytes in infection	85025
ESR	May be elevated with inflammatory response	85652
Glucose	Elevated in diabetes	82947
Albumin	Decreased in malnutrition	82040

Differential diagnosis: To treat adequately, it is necessary to distinguish between arterial, venous, neurologic, and orthopedic causes. Occasionally, malignancies, such as Kaposi's sarcoma and metastatic tumors, may present as an ulceration.

Treatment:

For ulcers resulting from venous insufficiency: Stage ulcer; compression to resolve edema; antibiotics if indicated for infection; débridement if necrotic tissue is present; moist dressings; nutritional support as indicated.

For ulcers resulting from arterial insufficiency or neuropathic or diabetic pathology: Refer to physician or surgeon.

Follow-up: See patient in 7 days to evaluate treatment; if patient is responding to treatment, follow-up every 2 weeks until healed; if patient is not responding to treatment, refer with possible consideration given to hospitalization.

Sequelae: Possible complications include cellulitis, systemic infections, recurrence of ulcers, scarring, problems associated with immobility, and amputation (especially possible in patients with diabetes).

Prevention/prophylaxis: Prevention strategies include advising the patient to stop smoking; to avoid recurrence of edema by elevating legs when possible such as using blocks to elevate the foot of the bed, wearing support or compression stockings, not sitting with legs crossed, not standing for prolonged periods, and avoiding constrictive clothing; to stay active such as by walking; to lose weight if overweight; to inspect feet and legs daily and report changes; to avoid thermal trauma to extremities by not using heating pads, hot water bottles, cold solutions, and ice; and to use moisturizers such as Eucerin or Keri to prevent dry skin.

Referral: Refer to, or consult with, physician or surgeon if patient is not responding to treatment or if débridement is necessary.

Education: Explain disease process, signs and symptoms, and treatment (including side effects of medications). Discuss prevention strategies. Advise patient to report changes in color, temperature, pain, sensation, odor, or drainage.

TINEA

SIGNAL SYMPTOMS red painful scaly skin, usually in warmer areas of the body. May be itchy.

Tinea cruris	ICD-9-CM: 110.4
Tinea pedis	ICD-9-CM: 110.3

Description: *Tinea* refers to a fungal infection of the skin that can involve any part of the body. *Tinea pedis,* commonly known as *athlete's foot,* is a fungal infection of the foot. *Tinea cruris,* commonly known as *jock itch,* is a fungal infection of the groin.

Etiology: Caused by fungus. Superficial fungal infections include dermatophytoses and cutaneous candidiasis. Dermatophytes are aerobic organisms that parasitize the keratin of the skin, hair, and nails and include *Microsporum* (generally infects the hair), *Trichophyton* (generally infects the hair, skin, and nails), and *Epidermophyton* (generally infects the groin or feet). Deeper penetration usually occurs with local or systemic immunosuppression. *C. albicans* invades the mucosal epithelium or stratum corneum in areas of maceration or in patients with decreased cell-mediated immunity.

Occurrence: Common; tinea pedis the most common.

Age: Varies with type of fungus.

Ethnicity: No significant ethnic predisposition.

Gender: Occurs equally in men and in women.

Contributing factors: High heat and humidity, occlusive footwear, immunosuppression, obesity, wet clothing, multiple layers of clothes, tight clothes.

Signs and symptoms:

> *Tinea pedis:* May be pruritic. Three forms may be seen: common interdigital type, with macerated, red, scaly toe web spaces, most frequently the fourth web space; vesicular type, with erythema and vesicles; and moccasin type, with dry, scaling skin on the soles of the feet, especially the sides.

> *Tinea cruris:* Erythematous plaques with sharp margins; papules, vesicles, or pustules may stud the border. Seen in the groin area with the scrotum and penis usually unaffected.

Diagnostic tests:

Test	Result Indicating Disorder	CPT Code
KOH preparation of skin scrapings from the leading border	May show translucent branching, rod-shaped hyphae	87220

(Continued on following page)

Test	Result Indicating Disorder	CPT Code
Cultures of skin scrapings or hair plucks from involved area on Sabouraud's dextrose agar or dermatophyte test medium	Shows fungus; use of antifungals may alter test results	87070
Wood's light examination from active border	Reveals yellow or green-yellow fluorescence on hair shafts	Included in the examination code for the visit

Differential diagnosis:
- Erythema (generalized, pink)
- Psoriasis (well-defined erythematous lesions with silvery scales; pruritus may or may not be present)
- Candidiasis infection (white plaque)

Treatment:

Terbinafine (Lamisil) is a topical fungicide, allowing for cure in 7 days of treatment. Approved for 4 weeks of treatment.

Topical antifungals, such as clotrimazole (Lotrimin), ketoconazole (Nizoral), or tolnaftate (Tinactin), twice daily for at least 3 weeks and no more than 6 weeks if they contain corticosteroids (treatment of choice in uncomplicated cases).

Oral antifungals, such as griseofulvin ultramicrosize, 500 mg daily with food for 3 to 4 weeks; ketoconazole, 200 mg daily for 3 to 4 months; or fluconazole (Diflucan) (for resistant cases with symptom discomfort; requires baseline liver function tests and CBC, with liver function tests monthly).

Antifungal absorbent powder may help to avoid excess moisture.

Follow-up: See patient in 1 or 2 weeks or as needed to monitor progress.

Sequelae: Possible complications include secondary bacterial infection, reoccurrence, and striae or atrophy (with long-term use of medications with corticosteroids).

Prevention/prophylaxis: For tinea pedis, prevention strategies include advising the patient to dry feet well and to dry feet last after bathing, to wear cotton socks and nonrestrictive shoes, and to change socks frequently. For tinea cruris, advise patient to dry groin area well, to dry groin before drying feet to help prevent further spread, and to wear nonrestrictive undergarments, changing them frequently. Put socks on before underwear. For both types, if activity is associated with pain, advise patient to rest until healing occurs.

Referral: Refer to, or consult with, dermatologist if condition is not resolving with treatment.

Education: Explain disease process, signs and symptoms, and treatment (including side effects of medications). Discuss prevention strategies and need to complete treatment because infection may recur if treatment is stopped before completed. Advise patient that contagiousness is minimal.

URTICARIA

SIGNAL SYMPTOMS▶ red itchy welts

Urticaria	ICD-9-CM: 708.9

Description: Urticaria, also called *hives,* is a condition involving single or multiple superficial, raised, pale macules with red halos. Urticaria may be acute, arising and subsiding rapidly and spontaneously, or chronic and recurrent.

Etiology: Caused by an allergic response. A massive histamine release from mast cells in the superficial dermis leads to dilation of the blood vessels with extravasation of fluid and edema in the interstitial lesions. May be an idiopathic process in some people.

Occurrence: Occurs in 15% to 20% of the population at least once in their lifetime; some sources report higher incidence.

Age: Occurs at any age.

Ethnicity: No significant ethnic predisposition.

Gender: Occurs equally in men and in women; chronic form occurs more in older women.

Contributing factors: Medications (either from allergy or idiosyncrasy) such as acetylsalicylic acid, NSAIDs, penicillins, and other antibiotics; transfusion reactions; insect bites or stings; physical trauma; heat or cold; emotional stress; food allergies or additives; infection; and collagen vascular disease such as SLE.

Signs and symptoms: Intensely pruritic, single or multiple raised, blanched, central wheals (1–2 mm to ≥ 15–20 cm) surrounded by red flare that occur anywhere on body. Onset usually rapid; may resolve spontaneously in 24 to 48 hours. May occur alone, with generalized anaphylactic response, or with angioedema.

Diagnostic tests: Diagnosed by history and physical examination (accurate history important).

Test	Result Indicating Disorder	CPT Code
Skin (RAST) testing	Determine allergen	95065
CBC	May show increased eosinophils	85025
ESR	May be elevated	85652
Thyroid panel	Hyperthyroidism–chronic urticaria may be exacerbated secondary to this disease	84443 (TSH) 84479 (T_4) 84480 (T_3)
ANA	May be elevated	86038

RAST, radioallergosorbent test; TSH, thyroid-stimulating hormone; T_4, thyroxine; T_3, triiodothyronine.

Differential diagnosis:

- Insect bites (history—ask patient about recent travel, exposure; entry point on plaques)
- Drug ingestion (new medication; history)
- Contact dermatitis (red, scaly, dry, pruritic plaques)
- Vasculitis (often have systemic symptoms, such as fever/chills, fatigue, malaise)
- SLE (butterfly facial pattern, increased ESR)

Treatment: Avoid offending agent. Lesions usually subside spontaneously.

Pharmacologic

Epinephrine if patient has anaphylaxis or laryngeal edema.

Antihistamines, such as hydroxyzine or diphenhydramine, 25 to 50 mg orally every 4 to 6 hours, to treat pruritus. If recalcitrant to treatment, the addition of an H_2 blocker to the antihistamine (H_1 blockers) may be effective.

Steroid therapy, such as prednisone, 40 mg orally daily for 5 to 7 days, then taper, occasionally may be warranted to decrease inflammation.

Follow-up: No follow-up is necessary if symptoms subside without incident. See patient for frequent follow-up if symptoms persist or recur.

Sequelae: Possible complications include severe systemic allergic reaction (bronchospasm, anaphylaxis); 70% of patients are better in 72 hours; 30% of patients develop chronic condition.

Prevention/prophylaxis: Prevention strategies include advising patient to avoid offending agents.

Referral: Refer to, or consult with, physician if patient has chronic condition or anaphylaxis.

Education: Explain disease process, signs and symptoms, and treatment (including side effects of medications). Discuss prevention strategies. Teach patient to have antihistamine available if accidentally re-exposed to offending agent; may have to have injection kit near at all times. Resource materials are available from American Academy of Allergy, Asthma and Immunology (telephone: 800-822-2762; website: www.aaai.org).

WARTS

SIGNAL SYMPTOMS painless lesions on skin, may be skin colored and rough

Warts	ICD-9-CM: 078.10

Description: Warts, or verruca vulgaris, are painless, circumscribed areas of cutaneous elevation resulting from hypertrophy of the papillae and epidermis.

Etiology: Caused by the human papillomavirus (HPV); passed on by direct contact with an infected person or from recently shed virus kept in a dark and moist place. There are >60 different types of HPV, and different types are associated with different clinical manifestations, although they often overlap. The wart virus is located within the epidermal cell nucleus.

Occurrence: Occurs in 7% to 10% of the population.

Age: Occurs primarily in children and young adults.

Ethnicity: No significant ethnic predisposition.

Gender: Occurs more in women than in men.

Contributing factors: Atopic dermatitis, skin trauma, health clubs and locker rooms, immunosuppression.

Signs and symptoms: Painless papule or cluster of papules that are usually skin-toned in color and otherwise asymptomatic. The hands are the most common sites.

There are five documented types, with a black punctum frequently seen in all types: (1) common warts, or verruca vulgaris (1–2 mm to 1 cm in size; usually firm, nontender, and solid with a hyperkeratotic, corrugated surface; clusters may be dense and matted, are most common on the distal extremities and occasionally occur on the face); (2) flat warts, or verruca plana (smooth and flat-topped; appear on the extremities and face, specifically the eyelids, but may be less noticeable than common warts); (3) plantar warts (covered by a thick callus; show a hemorrhagic spot or root; painful; occur on the soles of the feet, often on pressure points such as the heel); (4) venereal warts, or condylomata acuminata (thin, flexible, high papules without the visible or palpable keratin of other warts; may resemble cauliflower); and (5) epidermodysplasia verruciformis (flat, reddish lesions found on the hands and shoulders; occur during childhood with lifelong persistence; one third progress to malignancy).

Diagnostic tests: Diagnosis usually made on clinical appearance.

Test	Result Indicating Disorder	CPT Code
Biopsy for lesions resistant to treatment	Identifying type of organism	11100
Pap smears	If HPV-associated histology of the cervix is suspected. HPV cannot be cultured	88141

Differential diagnosis:

- Plantar corns (raised hyperkeratotic thickening of skin, usually over bony prominences)
- Premalignant lesions (growths in varied sizes; no punctum)
- Epidermal nevi (biopsy)
- Herpes simplex virus type 2 infection (vesicles usually found on mucous membrane)

Treatment: Most warts resolve within 12 to 24 months without treatment; watch and wait may be the best approach for most asymptomatic warts that do not dramatically alter the patient's appearance. Otherwise, a wide range of treatment options exists, all with side effects and none with a guaranteed cure.

For flat warts: Chemotherapeutic approaches, including topical retinoids, such as tretinoin twice daily for 4 to 6 weeks.

For common warts: Salicylic acid transdermally (Trans-Ver-Sal) daily for about 6 weeks, or salicylic acid in propylene gel (Keralyt) rubbed into warts each night; occlusion (inexpensive method) by covering the wart with waterproof tape, leaving on for 1 week, removing and leaving open for 12 hours, then retaping if wart still present (environment under tape does not foster viral growth).

For plantar warts: 40% salicylic acid plasters (Mediplast), which are cut to size and applied over wart, then removed after 48 hours, peeling off part of wart and using a pumice stone to wear away at rest, followed by repeated applications until entire wart is removed. Usually takes 6 to 8 weeks, although pain relief may occur early.

Wart recurs unless entire wart is removed; may need referral for cryosurgery or laser ablation.

Follow-up: See patient as needed.

Sequelae: Possible complications include scar formation, recurrences, and pain. One third of warts of epidermodysplasia may become malignant.

Prevention/prophylaxis: Prevention strategies include advising the patient to use own footwear for sports and in locker-room settings and to cover warts under treatment to prevent self-inoculation and transmission to others.

Referral: Refer to, or consult with, physician or surgeon if patient has periungual warts, deep and painful plantar warts, or warts that severely interfere with appearance or function; may need cryosurgery or laser ablation.

Education: Explain disease process, signs and symptoms, and treatment (including side effects of medications). Discuss prevention strategies and infectious nature of warts.

WOUNDS

SIGNAL SYMPTOMS ▶ open cut; bleeding; object protruding out of skin

Unspecified upper extremity: uncomplicated	ICD-9-CM: 884.0
Unspecified lower extremity: uncomplicated	ICD-9-CM: 894.0
Unspecified trunk: uncomplicated	ICD-9-CM: 879.6
Unspecified head: uncomplicated	ICD-9-CM: 873.8

There are many other codes that depend on site, cause, and complications or infection.

Description: A wound is a break in the continuity of the skin or soft tissue. Usually caused by violence or trauma, there are many types of wounds, depending on the location and cause of the wound. Common types include an incision (a sharp, clean wound); a laceration (unclean wound with a jagged edge); a penetrating wound (skin is broken, and the agent that caused the wound is embedded inside); a perforating wound (agent that caused the wound entered and emerged from the body); a puncture wound (wound caused by a sharp-pointed instrument); and a tunnel wound (wound has a small entrance and exit). A contusion is a wound in which the skin is not broken, but injury occurs to the underlying tissue.

Etiology: Caused by trauma, violence, accidents, occupational hazards, postsurgical procedures without proper healing.

Occurrence: Common.

Age: Occurs at any age.

Ethnicity: Not significant.

Gender: Varies, although men (especially young men) usually have a higher incidence of trauma and violence than women.

Contributing factors: Accidents, drug or alcohol use, fatigue, stress, risk-taking behavior, high-risk environments or occupations, domestic violence.

Signs and symptoms: Break in the integrity of the skin; may be associated with other signs and symptoms such as pain; bleeding; blistering; drainage; protrusion of fatty tissue, bone, or tendon; and signs and symptoms of infection. Appearance varies depending on type or cause of wound. Assess for domestic violence.

Diagnostic tests: Diagnosis usually made by history and physical examination.

Differential diagnosis: Usually none.

Treatment:

Wounds

The first priority is to follow advanced cardiac life support (ACLS) standards and to prevent the loss of life (as in excessive bleeding) or the loss of limb (as in absence of pulse or circulation). When this priority has been met, additional treatment usually is indicated and may include the following:

Tetanus prophylaxis as indicated. A tetanus toxoid booster if patient has not received one within the last 10 years; tetanus toxoid immune globulin (250 U intramuscularly for a moderate wound or 500 U intramuscularly for a severe wound) if patient has not been previously immunized (Table 3–4).

Table 3–4 Tetanus Prophylaxis: Guidelines for Routine Wound Management

Previous Tetanus Vaccinations	Clean, Minor Wounds	All Other Wounds
Uncertain of $<$ 3	Administer Td ° to adults and children age $\geq$ 7; or DTP † (or DT ‡ if pertussis vaccine is contraindicated) to children age $\leq$ 7	Administer Td to adults and children age $\geq$ 7; or DTP (or DT if pertussis vaccine is contraindicated) to children age $\leq$ 7 *and*
$\geq$ 3	Administer a booster if last vaccination was $\geq$ 10 years earlier	Administer TIG § Administer a booster if last vaccination was $\geq$ 5 years earlier

° Td = tetanus and diphtheria toxoids absorbed.
† DTP = diphtheria and tetanus toxoids and pertussis vaccine absorbed.
‡ DT = diphtheria and tetanus toxoids absorbed.
§ TIG = tetanus immune globulin.
Source: Adapted from Advisory Committee on Immunization Practices (ACIP): Diphtheria, Tetanus, and Pertussis: Guidelines for Vaccine Prophylaxis and Other Preventive Measures. MMWR: 34: 1–17, 1985; and Diphtheria, Tetanus, and Pertussis: Recommendations for Vaccine Use and Other Preventive Measures. MMWR: 40: 1–28, 1991. ACP Task Force on Adult Immunization and Infectious Disease Society of America: Guide for Adult Immunization, ed 3. American College of Physicians, Philadelphia, 2002.

Thorough inspection of wound to ensure proper functioning of all underlying tendons, nerves, and blood vessels.

Wound irrigation (usually with copious amounts of normal saline solution) to remove foreign bodies and debris.

Thorough cleansing of wound (usually with soap and water or antiseptic solution).

Wound closing as indicated. This may be by dressing or suturing; most wounds should be closed within 4 to 8 hours after injury.

Wound dressing with sterile dressing; splint, shield, or other devices may be applied to facilitate healing and prevent reopening of wound.

Antibiotics as indicated (if wound shows evidence of contamination, a 5- to 7-day course is indicated).

Contusions

Ice, cold compresses, elevation, and rest. After 48 hours, heat may be applied.

Follow-up: See patient in 2 days or as indicated if wound has been sutured or there is a high suspicion of infection; follow-up wound checks as indicated. Suture removal guidelines: face, 4 to 7 days; trunk, 10 to 12 days; extremities, 10 to 14 days.

Sequelae: Possible complications include bleeding, pain, discomfort, immobilization, loss of sensation, scarring, disfigurement, gangrene, loss of limb, and death.

Prevention/prophylaxis: Prevention strategies include advising the patient how to avoid accidents or trauma, such as by avoiding drugs, alcohol, and hazardous situations and maintaining proper gun control, and advising the patient of the importance of maintaining proper immunizations, such as for tetanus and hepatitis.

Referral: Refer to physician or surgeon patients with wounds that have damage to nerves or joints or that are contaminated, infected, or contain surrounding tissue damage and patients who have underlying medical conditions, such as diabetes, circulatory impairment, or immunosuppression or who have a tendency to scar. Refer patients with facial wounds to a plastic surgeon.

Education: Explain disease process, signs and symptoms, and treatment (including side effects of medications). Discuss prevention strategies and signs and symptoms to watch for and report, such as swelling, redness of wound, fever, chill, odor or drainage, bleeding, increased pain, and opening of wound.

REFERENCES

General

ACP Task Force on Adult Immunization and Infectious Disease Society of America: Guide for Adult Immunizations, ed 3. American College of Physicians, Philadelphia, 2002.

Dambro, M (ed): Griffith's 5 Minute Clinical Consult. Williams & Wilkins, Baltimore, 2002.

Dunphy, LM, and Winalnd-Brown, JE (eds): Primary Care: The Art and Science of Advanced Practice Nursing. FA Davis, Philadelphia, 2001.

Goroll, A, and Mulley, A (eds): Primary Care Medicine, ed 4. Lippincott-Raven, Philadelphia, 2000.

Habif, TP, et al: Skin Diseases: Diagnosis and Treatment. Mosby, St. Louis, 2001.

Hurst, JW (ed): Medicine for the Practicing Physician. Appleton & Lange, Norwalk, Conn., 2000.

Lin, TL, and Rypkema, SW (eds). The Washington Manual of Ambulatory Therapeutics. Lippincott Williams & Wilkins, Philadelphia, 2002.

Noble, J (ed): Primary Care Medicine, ed 2. Mosby, St. Louis, 2000.

Pfenninger, JL, and Fowler, GC: Procedures for Primary Care Physicians. Mosby, St. Louis, 2000.

Running, A, and Berndt, A: Management Guidelines for Nurse Practitioners Working in Family Practice. FA Davis, Philadelphia, 2003.

Sellers, R: Differential Diagnosis of Common Complaints, ed 4. WB Saunders, Philadelphia, 2000.

Swartz, M: Textbook of Physical Diagnosis. WB Saunders, Philadelphia, 2000.

Taylor, RB (ed): Manual of Family Practice, ed 2. Lippincott Williams & Wilkins, Philadelphia, 2002.

Uphold, C, and Graham, MV: Clinical Guidelines in Family Practice, ed 3. Barmarrae Books, Gainesville, Fla., 1998.

Woolf, J, et al (eds): Health Promotion and Disease Prevention in Clinical Practice. Lippincott Williams & Wilkins, Baltimore, 2000.

Acne

Goodheart, H: Acne and related disorders in women: Part 3. Treatment modalities for acne. Womens Health Prim Care 3:167, 2000.

Goodheart, H: Acne and related disorders in women: Part 5. Rosacea. Womens Health Prim Care 3:499, 2000.

Webster, G: Combination azelaic acid therapy for acne vulgaris. J Am Acad Dermatol 43:S47, 2000.

Psoriasis

Goodheart, H: Psoriasis. Womens Health Prim Care 3:147, 2000.

Chapter 4

HEAD AND NECK DISORDERS

ARTERITIS, TEMPORAL (Giant Cell Arteritis, Cranial Arteritis, Vasculitis, Granulomatous Arteritis)

SIGNAL SYMPTOMS▶   unrelenting unilateral headache; eye pain usually unilateral

| Temporal Arteritis | ICD-9-CM:446.5 |
| Giant Cell Arteritis | ICD-9-CM:446.5 |

Description: Temporal arteritis (giant cell vasculitis [GCV], cranial arteritis) is a chronic (at times, inflammatory) autoimmune disorder of vascular collagen commonly affecting medium- to large-sized cranial blood vessels. It may involve other blood vessels of the aortic and occipital branches, particularly the temporal arteries. Left untreated, irreversible blindness can result. It is frequently associated with polymyalgia rheumatica (PMR).

Etiology: A cell-mediated autoimmune etiology is suspected. The histopathology of the affected arteries and the infiltrates demonstrate primarily either mononuclear cells or granulomas with giant multinucleolar cell elastic lamina.

Occurrence: More common in northern latitudes with approximately 15 to 30/100,000 people older than 50 years of age; vs. 2/100,000 in southern latitudes, primary white.

Age: Commonly ranges from age 50 to 85; average onset is age 70 but rarely under age 50.

Ethnicity: More often seen in people of Northern European descent, particularly those of Nordic heritage and within family clusters.

Gender: Female-to-male ratio is 2:1 in older adults. A genetic predisposition seems linked

Contributing factors: The presence of PMR significantly increases the risk of GCV with greater than 10% of people with PMR presenting symptoms. Approximately 50% of people with GCV also have PMR. GCV and PMR may be related because they often occur simultaneously. Because GCV primarily occurs in older adults, the suggestion has been made that there may be a relationship to the process of aging.

The headaches may produce a tender scalp that becomes worse at night with the recumbent position and direct contact with the mattress and pillow. Exposure to cold may also exacerbate headache pain.

Signs and symptoms:

- Abrupt onset of insidious or unilateral unrelenting headaches with visual disturbances.
- Flulike symptoms including mild fever <101°F and malaise.
- Suspect temporal arteritis if any patient older than age 50 complains of sudden, new-onset headaches and diplopia, blurred vision, or other unilateral visual disturbances.
- Jaw or tongue claudication can occur.
- Scalp tenderness occurs on the affected side surrounding the affected artery in the temporal (50% of cases), periorbital, or occipital portions of the cranium.
- The headache may be dull, or explosive in nature, superimposed with jabbing or jolting pains or progressive dull to boring head pain increasing in intensity and in debility.
- Transient partial or total visual loss may occur if central retinal artery becomes occluded.

Other signs and symptoms may include:

- Pain and difficulty in chewing, weakness, fatigue, malaise, morning stiffness, low fever, sweats, appetite loss, and weight loss.
- Symptoms of polymyalgia rheumatica are characterized by stiffness and diffuse pain in the neck, lower back, shoulders, hips, or thighs.
- Physical examination may reveal swollen, nodular, erythematous, tender, indurated, pulseless, and noncompressable temporal arteries; and tender or painful temporal scalp areas.
- Ophthalmoscopic examination may show a swollen optic disk with hemorrhage if the central retinal artery is occluded.

Diagnostic tests:

Test	Result indicating disorder	CPT code
ESR	>50 although 10% of patients may be normal.	85652
Complete blood count (CBC)	May show increased leukocytosis with a positive normochromic or mild to moderate normocytic anemia	85025
Biopsy of the temporal artery or affected muscle	Reveals lymphocytes, monocytes, neutrophils, and giant cells that confirm the diagnosis; serial sectioning recommended	37609

ESR, erythrocyte sedimentation rate.

Laboratory

Findings confirming an inflammatory process, but not specific for this disease process, may include a mild leukocytosis or thrombocytosis, with or without elevated liver enzymes, specifically both the alkaline phosphatase and aspartate aminotransferase.

Differential diagnosis:

- Migraine headache (unilateral, pulsating, photophobia and phonophobia, prodrome, nausea and vomiting, moderate to severe in intensity)
- Trigeminal neuralgia (tic douloureux, tender facial points, can have violent muscle spasms that are unilateral and painful)
- Myofascial pain syndrome (chronic, recurrent pain in facial muscles; distinguishing feature one or more trigger points)
- Temporomandibular joint (TMJ) dysfunction (jaw and/or ear pain, "clicking," pain on palpation at TMJ joint)
- Infectious disorders affecting the cranial musculature (increased leukocytes, fever, headache, stiff neck)
- Transient ischemic attacks (TIA) (lasts 5 to 20 minutes, weakness, numbness, aphasia, vision loss)
- Sinusitis (concurrent nasal drainage, possible fever, congestion)
- Retinal detachment or other causes of loss of vision (flashing lights followed by floaters)

Treatment:

Pharmacologic

For pain: Mild analgesics such as acetaminophen, nonsteroidal, anti-inflammatory drugs (NSAIDs), or aspirin, if not contraindicated, orally every 4 to 6 hours. For the primary inflammatory disorder, corticosteroid therapy is used to provide an anti-inflammatory effect while awaiting biopsy results. Give prednisone 60 mg orally daily for 6 weeks, then begin a slow taper by 5 mg weekly if the patient is asymptomatic and the erythrocyte sedimentation rate (ESR) is decreasing, while recognizing that the ESR may never normalize. Continue the taper until 10 to 15 mg is the daily dose for several months and possibly years, with attempts every 2 months to taper by 1 to 2 mg. Symptoms and ESR guide the tapering process. The goal of the therapy is that the patient has no relapse and is symptom free.

Physical

Warm compresses may relieve symptoms of headaches and muscle pain. Massage therapy may help but may also increase pain.

Rest in a quiet and a soothing environment along with attention to pain relief foster the comfort, and therefore, the compliance of the patient to the regimen.

Acupuncture may be a valuable tool for resolution and pain control.

Surgical

The diagnostic confirming biopsy of the temporal artery often relieves and resolves the headache pain. The biopsy must be performed within 96 hours of the institution of corticosteroids for an accurate diagnosis. If the results are negative, one should consider biopsy of the contralateral artery that may increase the confirmation of the diagnosis by 10% to 14%.

Follow-up: During the acute phase, see patient weekly until the ESR is decreasing and to assess the patient compliance with treatment plan. Because ESR may signal any inflammatory process within the body, significant care should be taken to monitor symptoms and patient well-being. Early identification and treatment are the cornerstones to success, including the preservation of vision.

 Clinical Pearl: The better patient and family education and the more involvement in the treatment plan, the less likely you will receive calls daily. Patients are truly fearful and see temporal arteritis as life-threatening with uncontrollable pain.

Sequelae: Usually, there are no complications if the condition is treated promptly and effectively. Failure to treat may lead to ischemic optic neuritis and blindness (50% of cases). Other possible complications include coronary artery disease (CAD); cerebrovascular accident (CVA); liver function abnormalities; and peripheral vascular disease of the extremities or bowel, leading to gangrene. Long-term corticosteroid therapy may lead to significant side effects, including osteoporosis and peptic ulcer disease. The average time from first symptom to disease to remission is 3 to 4 years, with a range of 1 to 10 years. Monitor the serum glucose because prednisone may cause it to become elevated. Adrenal suppression could occur with prolonged prednisone use. Careful monitoring for infections and concomitant treatment of diabetes, congestive heart failure, and systemic fungal infections are of prime importance.

Prevention/prophylaxis: There are no known preventive measures.

Patient Education: Warn the patient about the long-term use of steroids and the increased risk of osteoporosis. Inform the patient on a tapering dose of the corticosteroid that an exacerbation may occur with the dosage adjustment. Be proactive to prevent medication-induced problems.

Referral: Refer to vascular surgeon immediately to confirm diagnosis. Refer to an ophthalmologist if patient has acute blockage of blood flow to the ophthalmic (ocular pain, acute visual loss) or refer to a gastroenterologist if the intestinal (bloody stools, severe abdominal pain) vessels are involved; this is a medical emergency.

Education: Explain disease process, signs and symptoms, and treatment (including side effects of medications). Dietary consultations include limiting salt intake and carbohydrates, monitor glucose levels and to ingest adequate calcium 1500 mg/day all of which are in response to the side effects of prednisone, which must be used. Educational resource materials are available from the Arthritis Foundation, 1314 Spring St. Northwest, Atlanta, GA 30309 (800-283-7800). Websites include: American College of Rheumatology: *http://www.rheumatology.org*

CANDIDIASIS, ORAL (THRUSH, PARASITIC STOMATITIS)

SIGNAL SYMPTOMS painful, burning, itching, tongue, mouth and throat

Candidiasis, mucocutaneous	ICD-9-CM: 112.9
Candidiasis of mouth	ICD-9-CM: 112.0
Candidiasis, disseminated	ICD-9-CM: 112.5

Description: Oropharyngeal candidiasis is an abnormal overgrowth in the oral cavity of the yeastlike fungus *Candida albicans* and less commonly, *Candida tropicalis*. Also known as thrush and parasitic stomatitis, candidiasis is readily treatable but often recurs in immuno-compromised patients. Oral candidiasis may present as one of four types: (1) pseudomembranous candidiasis (the most common form), (2) hyperplastic candidiasis, (3) atrophic candidiasis, and (4) angular cheilitis. Gastrointestinal candidiasis including gastritis and even ulcers are associated with thrush. Candida esophagitis is usually associated with an immunosuppressive host.

Etiology: Candida species colonize human mucocutaneous surfaces, and most infections are endogenously acquired from this reservoir when stressed by external or internal forces. Although a part of the normal oral flora, overgrowth on the tongue and oral mucosa occurs when balance is disrupted. Host immunosuppression, antibiotic-related disruption of the natural oral microbial flora, and breaks in the natural mucosal immunity barrier of the mouth, neutropenic states, and infant prematurity are all recognized causes of candida.

Occurrence: Rare in otherwise healthy adults; reflective of an underly-ing immunocompromised state; one of the 10 most common clinical complications of HIV-infected, immunocompromised patients, common in infants, especially those who are premature.

Age: Occurs in immunocompromised patients of any age; most com-monly seen in newborns (vertical transmission at birth) and older patients (age-related immunocompromised).

Ethnicity: There is no significant ethnic predisposition.

Gender: Occurs equally in men and in women.

Contributing factors: Immunosuppression, such as that related to HIV infection, granulocytopenia, malignancy, chronic metabolic diseases such as diabetes, cancer chemotherapy, head and neck radiotherapy, selective immunoglobulin A deficiency compromising mucosal immunity, and age-related decreases in natural immunity; prolonged antibiotic therapy; corticosteroid use; superimposed bacterial or viral infections; alcoholism; drug abuse; malnourishment; oral lesions; trauma to the oral mucosa; ill-fitting dentures.

Symptoms:

- White, painless exudative patches with an erythematous base are easily scraped from buccal mucosa, tongue, posterior pharynx.
- Esophagitis causing dysphagia, odynophagia, and retrosternal pain.
- Excessive dryness of the mouth, foul halitosis, and a burning sensation
- Minor to severe oral pain (particularly if lesions have been scraped)
- Constitutional symptoms such as fever, malaise, and headache, which may be secondary to systemic infection.

Physical examination may reveal a tender, edematous, often-rough appearing, fire engine red oral mucosa. Anterior cervical or jaw lymphadenopathy may be felt. Pseudomembranous candidiasis presents with white to creamy yellow, slightly raised, 3- to 10-mm plaques resembling milk curds on an erythematous base on the dorsal and lateral areas of the tongue, buccal mucosa, palate, gingival, tonsils, larynx, and pharynx that can be scraped off. Hyperplastic candidiasis shows white plaques on the lateral borders of the tongue and buccal mucosa. If scraped with a tongue blade, denuded lesions appear erythematous, become painful, and may bleed. Atrophic candidiasis presents as marked erythema (flat, red lesions without visible exudates) of the mucosa of the hard and soft palate; usually a sign of more advanced disease. Angular cheilitis causes fissuring and cracking of the angles of the mouth.

 Clinical Pearl: Beware of fluoride toothpaste sensitivity, especially in persons with dental braces; the angular cheilitis mimics candidiasis.

Diagnostic tests:

Test	Results indication disorder	CPT code
Gram stain and 10% potassium hydroxide (KOH) wet mount of lesion scrapings	Demonstrates budding yeast forms indicating candidal fungal infections.	87205
Slide preparation	Reveals hyphae or pseudohypha	87205
Barium Swallow	Esophageal candidiasis may show a "cobblestone" appearance with a barium swallow	74246
Esophagogastroduodenoscopy (EGD)	Reveals fistulas and plaques that are readily available for biopsies.	43202

Differential diagnosis:

- Leukoplakia or hairy leukoplakia (white lingual patches, precancerous)
- Advanced invasive squamous cell carcinoma (usually appears with nodular growths)

- Lichen planus (thin, bluish, white spider web lines)
- Nicotinic stomatitis (irritation with exposure)
- Geographic tongue (circular areas of bright red denuded epithelium surrounded by rings of light yellow piled-up cells)

Treatment:

Pharmacologic

Type of Treatment	Medication	Directions
Oropharyngeal treatment	Clotrimazole (Mycelex)	10-mg troche slowly dissolved in the mouth five times daily for 7 to 10 days, preferably over 20 minutes.
	Nystatin pastille	1–2, qid for 7–14 days (48 hours after disappearance of thrush)
	Oral nystatin suspension (100,000 units/mL)	Children apply 5–10 mL qid for 10 days and for adults; it is used as a rinse and then swallowed. Mild angular cheilitis and lesions found under dentures may be treated topically with nystatin ointment.
	Amphotericin B (Fungizone)	Oral suspension 100 mg/ml . 1 ml qid × 7 days, swish and swallow between meals. Beware of the serious side effects!
Esophagitis treatment:	Ketoconazole (Nizoral)	200–400 mg 1 daily for 14–21 days
	Itraconazole (Sporanox)	Oral solution 20 mg qd without food × 7 days
	Fluconazole (Diflucan)	200 mg than 100 mg qd × 10–21 days
Gastrointestinal (GI) treatment	Fluconazole	200 mg tabs PO × 14–21 days
	Amphotericin B	IV 50 mg tid in resistance cases (0.3–0.5 mg/kg /day) × 14 days. Warrants consult ID or GI

ID, infectious disease specialist.

Physical

Symptomatic treatment includes rinsing the mouth with half-strength 3% hydrogen peroxide (1:1 with water) four times a day (relieves discomfort). Parenteral fluids may be given for supportive therapy to prevent dehydration. Xylocaine viscous 1 tbsp mixed with Maalox may decrease severe discomfort of oral lesions and aid in hydration, allowing the patient to swallow fluids. If the cause is ill-fitting dentures, the only answer is to replace them, therefore, preventing chronic reoccurrence.

 Clinical Pearl: To correct the underlying cause is the aim of treatment. Restore microbial balance. Eating active culture yogurt helps.

Follow-up: See patient as needed until all lesions have resolved; uncomplicated oral infections will typically clear in 3 days if treated appropriately; however, recurrence is likely. Encourage the patient to perform self-examination to recognize lesions early and self-care after notifying the health care provider.

Sequelae: Possible complications include dehydration; malnutrition; systemic spread to the vagina, skin, larynx, gastrointestinal tract, or respiratory system. In the immunocompromised person severity of complications is dependent on the degree of compromise. In a person with a CD4 count less than 100, thrush lends to systemic infection, particularly kidney involvement. Esophageal candidiasis may occur concurrently with another infection, that is, herpes simplex virus or cytomegalovirus esophagitis.

Prevention/prophylaxis: Prevention strategies include encouraging proper oral hygiene (prevents fungal overgrowth and other types of oral infections) and cautious discriminatory use of antibiotic and corticosteroid therapy.

Referral: Consult an infectious disease specialist for a patient who has disseminated candidiasis, fever, or secondary bacterial infection demonstrated by fever or increased pain, erythema, edema, and tenderness of the oral mucosa.

Education: Explain disease process, signs and symptoms, and treatment (including side effects of medications). Discuss the importance of proper oral hygiene (brushing teeth twice daily with a soft-bristled toothbrush and daily flossing); proper balanced nutrition; need for increased fluid intake during treatment; and avoiding hot, spicy, salty, or acidic foods and beverages that irritate. Advise patient to drink through a straw if lesions are particularly painful.

CHALAZION

SIGNAL SYMPTOMS ▶ red, elevated mass on eyelid

Chalazion	ICD-9-cm: 373.2

Description: A chalazion is a mass on the eyelid margin resulting from a granulomatous infection, inflammation of a meibomian (oil-secreting) gland of the upper or lower eyelid. Meibomian glands lubricate the lid margins.

Etiology: Blockage in a duct leading to the eyelid surface from the gland or obstruction of a meibomian gland results in inflammation, the formation of a hard mass, and/or infection (usually from *Staphylococcus*).

Occurrence: Common.

Age: Occurs at any age.

Ethnicity: There is no significant ethnic predisposition.

Gender: Occurs equally in men and in women.

Contributing factors: Previously unresolved blepharitis, poor eyelid hygiene, contact lens wearers, application of makeup, immunosuppression, skin conditions such as acne rosacea or seborrheic dermatitis.

Signs and symptoms:

- Slow-developing, painless to painful lump, eye irritation, hard mass with infection of the meibomian gland and possible involvement of the surrounding tissue.
- Physical examination with eversion of the eyelid reveals a red, elevated mass that may become quite large and press against the eye, causing pain and possible nystagmus.

Diagnostic tests:

Tests	Results indicating disorder	CPT code
Visual acuity examination	Rules out other problems	99172
Culture of drainage	If incision and drainage is done; a C & S reveals causative organism.	87070
Biopsy of recurrent chalazion	Rules out malignancy	67810

C&S, culture and sensitivity.

Differential diagnosis:

- Foreign body (foreign body sensation and tearing)

 Clinical Pearl: Use of a magnet to remove metal chips is preferred.

- Hordeolum ("sty," inflammation of eyelash follicle)
- Blepharitis (inflammation of eyelids)
- Sebaceous cell carcinoma (rare, suspect if intractable blepharitis)

Treatment:

Pharmacologic

Sulfacetamide sodium 10% ophthalmic ointment four times a day for 7 days thinly applied to the lid margin with a cotton-tipped applicator. Antibiotic eye drops may be used (prevents secondary bacterial infection in other parts of the eye).

Oral antistaphylococcal penicillin for internal meibomian glands.

Physical

Eyelid hygiene daily with baby shampoo and rinsing well may prevent recurrent infections. Warm compresses to the area four times a day reduces inflammation, hastens healing and stimulates the potential for spontaneous drainage.

Surgical

Refer to ophthalmologist for incision and drainage if no response to medication and topical treatment.

Follow-up: See patient in 1 week for evaluation of treatment.

Sequelae: May take several weeks to months for complete resolution. Recurrences are common.

Prevention/prophylaxis: Prevention strategies include advising the patient to perform proper lid hygiene (helps prevent recurrence) by gently scrubbing lids with diluted baby shampoo daily or by directly applying baby shampoo with cotton-tipped applicator and then rinsing. When hand washing do not share towels or washcloths because infection may spread to other members of the family. Wash hands frequently. Also advise the patient to apply warm wet compresses several times a day at the first sign of eyelid irritation or if chalazion starts to return. Use a clean cloth for each warm compress to each eye. Hypoallergenic eye cosmetics should be used. Discard all used eye makeup. Remove all eye makeup thoroughly. Discontinue eye cosmetics if the problem recurs. Avoid fumes and smoke.

Referral: Refer to, or consult with, an ophthalmologist if patient has a visual change, increasing pain, or impairment to the eye or if chalazion does not heal spontaneously in 6 weeks.

Education: Explain disease process, signs and symptoms, and treatment (including side effects of medications). Discuss prevention strategies.

CONJUNCTIVITIS

SIGNAL SYMPTOMS conjunctival hyperemia, tearing, burning, exudate and matting

Conjunctivitis	ICD-9-CM: 372.30
Viral conjunctivitis	ICD-9-CM: 077.99
Conjunctival degeneration, unspecified	ICD-9-CM: 372.50
Other chronic allergic conjunctivitis	ICD-9-CM: 372.14

Description: Conjunctivitis is an inflammation of the conjunctiva the palpebral or bulbar conjunctiva that covers the exposed surface of the sclera. "Pink eye" refers to non-*Neisseria* bacterial conjunctivitis. Types of conjunctivitis include:

- Infectious either bacterial or viral to include chlamydial inclusion
- Allergic conjunctivitis, both seasonal and perennial
- Toxic conjunctivitis, either chemical or irritative

Etiology: The most common cause is contact with bacteria (commonly *Staphylococcus aureus, Streptococcus pneumoniae, Haemophilus influenzae, Neisseria gonorrhoeae,* or *Neisseria meningitidis);* viruses (commonly adenoviruses, herpes simplex, or herpes zoster); or allergens (linked to a humoral response and some autoimmune disorders such as Sjögren's syndrome and Wegener's granulomatosis). Other causes include chlamydia (inclusion conjunctivitis); association with certain systemic diseases, such as thyroid disorders and Reiter's syndrome (idiopathic conjunctivitis); and the chronic use of eye medications over a long period of time (noninfectious conjunctivitis).

Occurrence: Very common; most common eye disease.

Age: Occurs in all ages.

Ethnicity: There is no significant ethnic predisposition.

Gender: Occurs equally in men and in women.

Contributing Factors: Numerous factors such as wind, trauma from heat and cold, various chemicals and environmental stressors, and foreign bodies.

Signs and symptoms:

- Conjunctival hyperemia
- Lacrimation (excessive uncontrollable tearing)
- Burning eyes
- Green yellow exudate and matting
- Pruritus (itching) affected by the causative organism, from mild to severe.

 Clinical Pearl: Remember always to wear gloves when examining near the eye and eye exudate. Tissues with wet exudate can cause infections.

General: Burning and/or sandy feeling in the eye and may have itching tearing, lid matting, and exudate. Physical examination reveals a diffusely injected conjunctiva, "cobblestoning."

Infectious Causative Agent:

Bacterial: Minimal pruritus, moderate tearing, and mucopurulent exudates and matted lids in mornings; usually begins unilaterally, and then evolves into a bilateral process. Most common gram-positive pathogens are *Streptococcus pneumoniae, Haemophilus influenzae,* and *Staphylococcus aureus,* and less frequently, gram-negative *Moraxella* species, *Escherichia coli,* and *Pseudomonas* species.

Viral or chlamydial inclusion: Usually bilateral, with copious serous or mucoid tearing and minimal pruritus. Systemic viral symptoms such as preauricular adenopathy, fever, and malaise may also be present. Chlamydia, virus, and bacteria are transmissible by eye-hand contact.

Noninfectious Causative Agent:

Allergic or dry eye: Presents bilaterally with severe itching, stinging, redness, and serous or mucoid (stringy or ropy) discharge.

Toxic or chemical: Photosensitivity, swollen eyelids (usually develops 5 to 10 days after exposure).

Diagnostic tests:

Test	Result indicating disorder	CPT code
Culture and sensitivity of any exudate	Identifies bacterial pathogen and indicates appropriate antibiotic therapy	87070 culture 87184 sensitivity
Gram and Giemsa stains of conjunctival scrapings	Usually shows monocytes, if cause is viral; neutrophils, if bacterial; eosinophils, if allergic	87205
Frei Test	For lymphogranuloma venereum.	86729
Bovin fixation and Papanicolaou stain	For multinucleated giant cells of herpes simplex.	88314 (Other cytology) 88143 (Pap)
Use cell culture, direct fluorescent monoclonal antibody staining of smears, enzyme immunoassays, DNA hybridization assays and a polymerase chain reaction test to identify chlamydial antigens.	To identify chlamydial infections	87206 Fluorescent stain 87320 immunoassay 87486, 87491 assay 83898 PCR test

Clinical Pearls: Always refer to an ophthalmologist for a full ocular assessment a patient with chronic unilateral conjunctivitis, pain, photophobia, and blurred vision that fails to clear with a blink. Chlamydial or gonococcal infection of the conjunctiva may be suggested by the patient's sexual history. A history of collagen vascular disease or the use of diuretics or antidepressant medications may promote dry eye syndrome.

Differential Diagnosis:

- Foreign body (foreign body sensation and tearing, visible on examination)

Clinical Pearl: Use of a magnet to remove metal chips is preferred.

- Abrasions (painful tearing, use fluorescin paper and blacklight to diagnose)
- Herpes simplex (crater appearance; caked yellow exudate, pain, usually more than one lesion)
- Acute glaucoma (extreme ocular pain, vision loss, dilated pupil)
- Keratitis (inflammation of the cornea)
- Iritis (uveitis) (pain, decreased vision, photophobia, tearing, iris swollen, throbbing pain)
- Choroiditis (inflammation of uveal tract extending also to choroid)
- Iridocyclitis (inflammation of uvea, iris extending to ciliary body)
- Blepharitis (inflammation of eyelids, edema of all levels of severity)

- Lacrimal duct obstruction (acute inflammation with tenderness beside the nose, swelling may extend to eyelid)
- Scleritis (associated with autoimmune diseases, severe deep boring pain, area appears purple in daylight)
- Episcleritis (milder form of scleritis; lesion appears as a salmon-colored nodule or with a diffuse salmon-pink color)
- Corneal disease (diagnosed by an ophthalmologist)

Treatment:

General

- Record visual acuity for both eyes.
- Fluorescin staining to detect ulcer keratitis.
- No patch, no topical steroids.
- Warm compresses with single-use clean cloth; no cotton balls.
- Cold compresses for allergy or irritation.
- Giant papillary allergic conjunctivitis requires discontinuation of contact lens use.
- Strict hand washing and the avoidance of cross-contamination among family members.

Pharmacologic

BACTERIAL

- Hyperacute bacterial conjunctivitis, frequently caused by *N. gonorrhea* and *Neisseria meningitidis,* usually presents in a neonate 3 to 5 days old and in sexually active young adults. In adults, the organism is usually transmitted form the genitalia to the hands, and then to the eyes. Left untreated, rapid and severe corneal involvement, ulceration, perforation, and profound and sometimes permanent loss of vision. The treatment is immediate with systemic antibiotics and saline irrigation to prevent serious sequelae.

OPHTHALMIC ANTIBIOTICS

- Aminoglycosides, such as 0.3% tobramycin (TobraDex) solution or gentamicin (Garamycin) as drops 1-2 instilled in both eyes every 4 hours while awake for 5 days, always cleansing with warm water or saline first. The gram-negative coverage is good, whereas the coverage of the causative microorganisms that are gram positive is poor, including the *Streptococcus* and *Staphylococcus* species.

 Clinical Pearl: Neomycin ophthalmic preparations can cause oculocutaneous allergic reactions and, therefore, should be avoided as first-line therapy.

- Ophthalmic 10% sodium sulfacetamide (Bleph-10), gtt 1 to 2 every 4 hours while awake for 5 days ou (both eyes).
- Tetracycline and erythromycin ophthalmic ointment 1 inch four times a day to both eyes for 7 days

- The fluoroquinolones, which include ciprofloxacin (Ciloxan), ofloxacin (Ocuflox), and norfloxacin (Chibroxin), are usually reserved for moderate to severe cases owing to the cost and the potential for resistance from overuse.

VIRAL/CHLAMYDIAL

- Ocular *Chlamydia trachomatis* can occur in two different forms: trachoma (associated with serotypes A through C) and inclusion conjunctivitis (associated with serotypes D through K)
- Trachoma, a chronic keratoconjunctivitis, is the most common cause of ocular morbidity and preventable blindness throughout the world. Although endemic to Africa, Asia, and the Middle East, with travel mobility today the rise in cases seen is increasing
- Inclusion conjunctivitis is a common, primarily sexually transmitted disease that occurs in newborns and the most frequent cause of conjunctivitis in neonates.
- Treatment consists of a 2- to 3-week course of oral tetracycline, doxycycline, minocycline (Minocin), or erythromycin. Oral doxycycline 100 mg twice a day for 3 weeks for inclusion conjunctivitis.
- A single 1-g dose of azithromycin (Zithromycin) is recommended for adults with lower genital tract infection, but a longer course may be necessary in patients with chlamydial conjunctivitis.
- Adenovirus, the most common cause of viral conjunctivitis, is treated by universal precautions and careful monitoring in the community and schools, especially hand washing and symptom treatment with topical vasoconstrictors and cold compresses.
- Ocular herpes simplex and herpes zoster are managed with topical or systemic antiviral agents.
- Trifluridine (Viroptic) 1 gtt ou topical ophthalmic solution given every 3 hours may be helpful.
- Acyclovir (Zovirax) oral tablets for herpetic lesions 400 mg three times a day for 10 days. Also Valacyclovir (Valtrex) 1 g three times a day for 7 days and famciclovir (Famvir) 500 mg every 8 hours for 7 days may be ordered.

ALLERGIC:

- Seasonal allergic rhinoconjunctivitis is an immunoglobulin E (IgE)–mediated hypersensitivity reaction precipitated by small airborne allergens.
- A topical vasoconstrictor or antihistamine combination such as 0.05% naphazoline or antazoline (Albalon-A, Vasocon-A).
- Oral antihistamines help relieve symptoms.
- Topical cromolyn (Opticrom) 4% four times a day starting 2 weeks before allergy season for mast cell stabilization
- Systemic treatment for *Neisseria* species as other sites.

- Ciprofloxacin, norfloxacin ophthalmic 1 to 2 drops four times a day for 10 days.
- Allergic conjunctivitis is successfully treated with topical nonsteroidal anti-inflammatory agents such as ketorolac tromethamine (Acular) and diclofenac sodium (Voltaren).

Follow-up: See patient as needed, which may be in 24 hours for severe cases and 2 to 3 days for moderate cases. For nonresolving or worsening cases, refer the patient to an ophthalmologist.

Sequelae: Possible complications include blindness (if not treated properly).

Prevention/prophylaxis: Prevention strategies include advising the patient that the disorder is transmitted by contaminated towels and washcloths or from the patient's own hands, and advising the patient of methods to use to prevent transmission. Avoid noxious fumes and smoke. Do not use contact lenses or eye makeup; only hypoallergenic eye makeup may be used.

Referral: Refer to an ophthalmologist, especially if an eye ulcer, keratitis, or suspected herpes worsens after 24 hours of treatment.

Education: Explain disease process, signs and symptoms, and treatment (including side effects of medications). Discuss prevention strategies. Demonstrate eye drop techniques, that is, to instill eye drops in the inner canthus. Demonstrate ointment application techniques.

 Clinical Pearl: The conjunctiva can hold only 2 drops of medication at a time, more is a waste. Eye ointment causes blurry vision and can be frightening if patient is not informed of this effect before use.

Refer to Figure 4–1 for comparison in the differential diagnosis of conjunctivitis.

EPISTAXIS

SIGNAL SYMPTOMS▶   blood in the nares, unilateral or bilateral; taste of blood

Epistaxis	ICD-9-CM: 784.7

Description: Epistaxis, commonly called a "nosebleed," is a hemorrhage of the nasal mucosa, resulting from the traumatic or spontaneous rupture of superficial capillaries, veins, or arteries. Epistaxis may be classified as anterior (bleeding from the front of the nasal cavity; commonly along the anterior septum) or posterior (bleeding from the back of the nasal cavity; commonly just under the posterior half of the inferior nasal turbinate or roof of the nasal cavity).

Etiology: The condition is idiopathic in most cases. More than 90% caused by local irritation related to trauma or inflammation. Trauma to

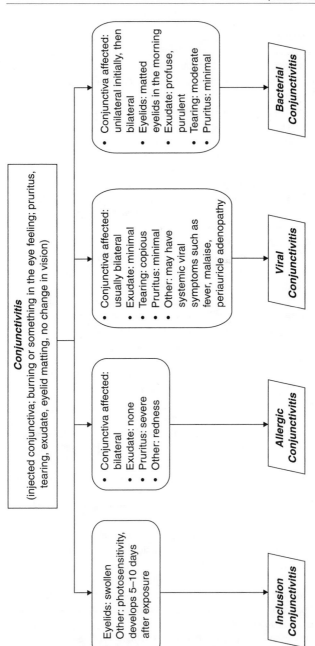

Figure 4–1. Differential diagnosis: conjunctivitis.

Conjunctivitis
(injected conjunctiva; burning or something in the eye feeling; pruritus, tearing, exudate, eyelid matting, no change in vision)

- Eyelids: swollen
- Other: photosensitivity, develops 5–10 days after exposure

Inclusion Conjunctivitis

- Conjunctiva affected: bilateral
- Exudate: none
- Pruritus: severe
- Other: redness

Allergic Conjunctivitis

- Conjunctiva affected: usually bilateral
- Exudate: minimal
- Tearing: copious
- Pruritus: minimal
- Other: may have systemic viral symptoms such as fever, malaise, periauricle adenopathy

Viral Conjunctivitis

- Conjunctiva affected: unilateral initially, then bilateral
- Eyelids: matted eyelids in the morning
- Exudate: profuse, purulent
- Tearing: moderate
- Pruritus: minimal

Bacterial Conjunctivitis

any nasal polyps and nasal mucosa is the most common direct cause, particularly from picking of the nose (epistaxis digitorum) or forcible injury related to blunt trauma. Other causes of injury include foreign bodies lodged in the nasal airways, spontaneous rupture of the nasal vessels from chronic sinusitis, upper respiratory infection, or rhinitis; and malignant growths in the nasal cavity or paranasal sinuses. Nosebleeds are also common in patients with coagulation defects. Vascular abnormalities may cause bleeding such as sclerotic vessels of age, hereditary hemorrhagic telangiectasias and arteriovenous malformation. Less than 10% are caused by neoplasm or coagulopathy.

Occurrence: Common; approximately 10% of the population experiences at least one significant nosebleed in a lifetime.

Age: Most common in children under age 10 and adults over age 50.

Ethnicity: No significant ethnic predisposition.

Gender: Occurs equally in men and in women.

Contributing factors:
- Excessive dryness of the nasal mucosa in poorly humidified environments or at high altitudes;
- Septal deviation; arteriovenous nasal malformations;
- Chronic disorders, such as cirrhosis, renal disease, cancer (especially Hodgkin's disease), and hypertension; vascular diseases,
- Hereditary hemorrhagic telangiectasia, coagulopathies;
- Use of medications that prolong bleeding time, such as warfarin or aspirin;
- Cocaine abuse; prolonged use of nose drops or nasal sprays;
- Nutritional deficiencies, including scurvy;
- Febrile infectious disorders;
- Rheumatic, scarlet, or typhoid fever.

Signs and symptoms: Usually only one bleeding site exists; however, if multiple sites or a diffuse ooze is evident, an underlying systemic bleeding disorder is likely.

Patient with significant blood loss may demonstrate pallor, particularly in the face; signs and symptoms of hypovolemia (lightheadedness, shortness of breath, tachycardia); or melena (blackened stools) from clotted, swallowed blood.

Anterior epistaxis: May present with a history of several minor nosebleeds over several weeks. Physical examination may reveal bleeding or clotted blood along the anterior septum; if the patient is actively bleeding, the blood is typically bright red.

Posterior epistaxis: The patient may be asymptomatic or present with hemoptysis, nausea, hematemesis, or melena. Physical examination may reveal bleeding from the posterosuperior nasal cavity and pharynx; if the patient is actively bleeding, the blood is typically a darker red. Clotted blood and brown to red throat discoloration may also be seen.

Epistaxis is diagnosed by physical examination.
Diagnostic tests:

Test	Result indicating disorder	CPT code
Partial prothrombin time Thromboplastin time (PT/PTT)	Helps determine platelet-related coagulopathies and clotting factor disorders. Look for clotting irregularities such as thrombocytopenia or decreased clotting time.	85611 PT 85730 PTT
CBC	Helps determine chronicity of the condition. (Monocytes may be increased and lymphocytes decreased with thrombocytopenia)	85025
Radiographs or imaging of the nasal cavity and paranasal sinuses	Identifies masses, foreign bodies, and sinusitis and malformations and abnormalities of nasal cavity	70160 (nasal) 76080 (sinus)
Nasal endoscopy	To locate and cauterize bleeding vessel	31238

CBC, complete blood count.

Differential diagnosis:

- Posterior versus anterior epistaxis (anterior: front of nasal cavity; posterior back of nasal cavity)
- Hemoptysis (coughing up blood from the airway, could appear as bloody sputum, look for source)
- Hematemesis (vomiting blood, could be mixed with stomach contents, look for source other than nares)
- Chronic sinusitis (pain at sinus points, concurrent nasal drainage, pressure in sinus areas, headache)
- Nasopharyngeal or paranasal sinus tumors (obstruction by mass, CT scan necessary)

Treatment: After stopping the bleeding, treat the underlying cause as appropriate.

Anterior Epistaxis

Apply firm, continuous pressure for 10 to 15 minutes to both sides of the nose, immediately superior to the nasal cartilages. Have the patient sit upright with head non-angulated and breathe through the mouth.

If bleeding persists, you may use vasoconstricting agents or chemical cauterization: For vasoconstriction, place nasal pledget soaked in a topical vasoconstricting agent such as 0.25% phenylephrine, 1:1000 epinephrine, 0.1% xylometazoline, or 4% cocaine solution to the nasal vestibule; press against the bleeding site for 5 to 10 minutes.

An ice pack may also be placed over the nose. Almost all anterior venous nosebleeds are stopped in this manner, but treatment may need to be repeated. For chemical cauterization, after anesthetizing the mucosa with a cotton ball soaked in either 4% cocaine, 4% lidocaine, 2% lidocaine viscous preparation, or 2% lidocaine jelly, apply a bead of either chromic acid, 25-50% trichloroacetic acid solution, or silver nitrate stick directly with firm pressure onto the bleeding vessels for 30 seconds. Thermal or bipolar electrocautery may be required in cases of deeper lesions involving larger vessels.

Anterior nasal packing (if bleeding does not stop after using the treatments listed above [CPT code 30905]): Use layers of petroleum jelly $^1/_2$ × 72-inch ribbon gauze to fill the entire nasal fossa. The gauze may also be impregnated with an antibiotic cream or ointment to minimize bacterial growth and reduce odor. If infection is suspected, administer prophylactic oral antibiotics. Remove packing in 24 to 36 hours. If leukemia or another source of bone marrow immunosuppression is suspected as a causative factor, avoid nasal packing because of the increased risk of infection. Instead, use topical thrombin or hemostatic substances (Oxycel cotton or Gelfoam).

Posterior Epistaxis:
Refer to specialist. Treatments include posterior nasal packing (gauze or balloon), sphenopalatine ganglion nerve block, and surgical ligation of the compromised vessels.

Follow-up: Usually no follow-up is needed for minor cases caused by local trauma or inflammation. See patient as indicated to monitor for effectiveness of therapy if patient has recurrent epistaxis; severe cases resulting in hemodynamic instability and blood loss may require hospitalization.

Sequelae: Possible complications include anemia, hypovolemia, vasovagal episodes, and syncope. Possible complications from treatment include cocaine or lidocaine toxicity, sinusitis or infection, septal hematoma, abscess, or perforation; external nasal deformities; mucosal pressure necrosis; and airway obstruction.

Prevention/prophylaxis:

- Prevention strategies include advising the patient to avoid blowing the nose or sneezing for at least 12 hours after an acute episode to prevent dislodging the protective blood clot
- Increase environmental humidity in the home, especially during the winter months
- Apply petroleum jelly to the nares to help prevent mucosal drying
- Avoid nasal probing with the fingers
- Avoid vigorous blowing of the nose
- Advise the patient to avoid taking medications that contribute to increased bleeding, such as aspirin. If the patient is taking anticoagulants, reinforce all the nasal hygiene above.

Referral: Refer to a specialist or clinical emergency department if patient has posterior epistaxis, recurrent anterior epistaxis (especially with severe blood loss or refractory to vasoconstrictive or cauterization therapy), or epistaxis with the comorbidity of coagulopathy or malignancy. Refer to surgeon for arterial ligation for intractable bleeding.

Education:

- Explain disease process, signs and symptoms, and treatment (including side effects of medications).
- Discuss prevention strategies such as moisturizing the mucous membrane.
- Demonstrate proper nasal pinching techniques. Advise the patient with minor bleeding to sit upright, minimize physical activity, keep the head elevated 45 to 90 degrees even at night.
- Avoid blood swallowing or talking during episodes of active bleeding (may inhale blood into the trachea and bronchi or cause nausea and vomiting).
- Advise patient not to drink alcohol or hot liquids after an acute attack.

GLAUCOMA

SIGNAL SYMPTOMS▶   **progressive vision loss, especially night vision**

Glaucoma	ICD-9-CM: 365.9
Primary angle-closure glaucoma, unspecified	ICD-9-CM: 365.20
Borderline glaucoma, anatomical narrow angle	ICD-9-CM: 365.02
Primary open-angle glaucoma	ICD-9-CM: 365.11
Glaucomatous atrophy (cupping of optic disc)	ICD-9-CM: 377.14
Low-tension glaucoma	ICD-9-CM: 365.12

Description: Glaucoma is an abnormal increase in intraocular pressure (IOP) caused by inadequate drainage of aqueous fluid from the anterior chamber of the eye. Glaucoma is classified as developmental (congenital), open-angle, or angle-closure (classically referred to as closed-angle). Open-angle glaucoma is the more commonly seen and is characterized as a chronic form of the disorder with an excellent prognosis if treated early and appropriately. Angle-closure glaucoma may have subacute and chronic components, but it is most associated with acute episodes that, if untreated, will cause loss of vision. Glaucoma is the second-leading cause of blindness.

Etiology:

Open-angle: Results from inadequate drainage of aqueous humor into the trabecular meshwork of the eye, a phenomenon often associated with aging.

Angle-closure: Results when there is an obstruction in the outflow of aqueous humor caused by a shallow anterior chamber of the eye. This is usually a structural defect caused by a predisposing ocular anatomy. If this obstruction occurs acutely, it is an ophthalmic emergency.

Occurrence: Open-angle: Most prevalent form; with >90% being primary open-angle glaucoma (POAG); affects approximately 4% of the population older than age 40. Angle-closure: Not as common; affects approximately 1% of the population. Primary angle-closure occurs in 100/100,000 of the population; 500/100,000 in blacks and Asians; more common than in whites. Polygenic inheritance for primary angle-closure glaucoma first-degree relatives have a 2% to 5% lifetime risk.

Age:

Open-angle: Usually occurs in patients older than age 40, but can occur at any age.

Angle-closure: Usually occurs between ages 55 and 70 years.

Ethnicity:

Open-angle: Higher incidence in blacks.

Angle-closure: Higher incidence in blacks, Asians, and people with Eskimo heritage. Blindness from glaucoma is six to eight times more common in blacks than in whites, especially in those older age 35 years.

Gender:

Open-angle: Occurs equally in men and women.

Angle-closure: Female > male.

Contributing factors: Use of steroids, amphetamines, and chlorpromazine (can increase IOP).

Open-angle: Increasing age, family history, diabetes.

Angle-closure: Small cornea, hyperopia, use of antidepressant or anticholinergic medications, emotional stress. Cataracts, shallow anterior chamber, iris and ciliary body cysts.

Signs and symptoms:

Open-angle: Gradual onset with slow, painless bilateral peripheral vision loss, and poor night vision. Frequent changes in refractory prescription may be a common presenting symptom. Later stages may include rainbow halos around lights and further visual loss. The physical examination is most likely be unremarkable. In later stages, the eyeball may be hardened. Visual acuity may or may not be affected. Visual field abnormalities to confrontation are present only in very late, profound cases. A Marcus Gunn pupillary defect (afferent pupillary defect) may be present. The earliest findings on funduscopic examination are an increased cup-disk ratio related to atrophy, and asymmetry on comparison with the other eye.

Angle-closure: Normal IOP 10 to 23 mm Hg in and around eye, enlarged pupil that may change to oval shape. Rapid onset with unilateral pain and pressure, blurred vision, rainbow halos around lights, photophobia, followed by loss of peripheral vision, followed by central vision loss. Frontal headache and possibly nausea and vomiting may be present. The physical examination may reveal a pupil that is semidilated and immobile. The conjunctiva may be injected, and the cornea may have a "steamy" appearance. Visual acuity is severely affected, because visual field defects are common. On palpation, the affected eye usually feels harder than the other. The funduscopic examination shows a pale optic disk with excavated cupping and a shallow anterior chamber. There may be aqueous turbidity.

 Clinical Pearl: Pathological findings on examination would include corneal stromal and epithelial edema, endothelial cell loss, optic disc congestion, or optic nerve atrophy.

Diagnostic tests:

Test	Result indicating disorder	CPT code
Optic nerve topography	Open-angle- A Marcus Gunn papillary defect (afferent papillary defect) may be present Angle-closure—pupils semidialated and immobile	92120
Visual fields	Open-angle—may or may not be affected, but late profound cases will show abnormalities to confrontation Angle-closure—loss of peripheral vision, followed by central loss, acuity is severely affected	92081
Funduscopic exam	Open-angle—increased cup-disc ratio compared with the other eye Angle-closure—pale optic disk with excavated cupping and a swallow anterior chamber	92014
Tonometry Measures intraocular pressure	Chronic open-angle, pressure may be normal (10–23 mm Hg) or elevated; Chronic angle-closure, pressure may or may not be elevated Acute exacerbation of angle-closure, pressure may be between 40–80 mm Hg	92100
Gonioscopy Determines the angle of the eye's anterior chamber; differentiates between open-angle and angle-closure glaucoma	Angle is normal in open-angle glaucoma Narrows with aging	92020

Differential diagnosis:

- Conjunctivitis (conjunctival hyperemia, tearing, burning, exudate, and matting)
- Anterior uveitis (intraocular inflammation of the iris alone or the iris and ciliary body)
- Vascular occlusive disease (indication of embolism in the retinal arteries, visible on funduscopic examination)

- Neovascular glaucoma (changes in peripheral vision in open-angle/eye pain with acute angle)
- Severe anemia (low Hct, low Hgb)
- Cerebral neoplasia

Treatment:

> *Open-angle:* Treatment of COAG is directed at lowering the IOP so that a <23 mm Hg. OP is obtained in order to decrease pressure on the optic nerve. Traditionally, open-angle glaucoma is managed pharmacologically for as long as possible, with laser or surgical treatment reserved for medically uncontrolled glaucoma. Goal of therapy is to control the disease sufficiently to decrease IOP sufficiently to protect the optic nerve from progressive damage and ultimate visual damage and visual loss. Medications to decrease and control IOP include the following:

- Beta-adrenergic–blocking agents, adrenergic agents, carbonic anhydrase inhibitors, and topicals to increase aqueous humerous outflow (cholinergic agents), direct-acting cholinergic agents, prostaglandin analog (e.g., Xalatan)
- If medications do not control the pressure, laser trabeculectomy may be performed.

> *Angle-closure:* Hospitalization with ophthalmology consult and bed rest. Acute angle-closure glaucoma requires emergency treatment, or total blindness follows in 2 to 5 days. (Use of mydriatic drops, exposure to a darkened room, or use of anticholinergic agents in susceptible people, such as those with a shallow anterior chamber, may precipitate an acute attack.) A combination of hyperspasmotic agents and carbonic anhydrase inhibitors may be used. Medications such as:

- Acetazolamide (Diamox) and intravenous (IV) mannitol with a topical miotic such as dorzolamide 2% eye drops every 8 hours are administered to lower IOP enough to permit intraocular penetration so that surgical intervention (Argon or Nd: YAG laser iridotomy) can occur.
- Beta-blockers. Timolol (Timpotic) 0.5% every 72 hours or levobunolol (Betagan) 0.5% every 12 hours, betaxolol (Betoptic) 0.5% every 12 hours,
- Miotics: pilocarpine 2% to 4% one dose,
- Corticosteroid-prednisolone acetate (Pred Forte) 1% every 4 to 6 hours or other apraclonidine (Lopidine) 0.5% or 1% every 8 hours,
- Atanoprost (Xalatan) 0.005% every 24 hours.

Follow-up: Patients should be followed by an ophthalmologist. Lifelong follow-up is required for all patients with glaucoma.

Contraindications: With a history of recent intraocular surgery, the possibility of malignant glaucoma is increased and miotics may be contraindicated. Precautions: Timolol, levobunolol, and betaxolol are used cautiously with congestive heart failure (CHF) and chronic obstructive pulmonary disease (COPD). Mannitol is used cautiously in persons with chronic heart failure or renal failure. Diamox should be used cautiously with nephrolithiasis or metabolic acidosis. Diamox may cause hypokalemia and metabolic acidosis in patients on other diuretics.

Sequelae: Possible complications include loss of vision and possible blindness if not diagnosed and treated promptly and consistently. Check tonometry and gonioscopy initially every 3 months after laser iridotomy, follow visual fields every 6 to 12 months. CBC q6 months while on acetazolamide (Diamox). Recurrence is quite rare following peripheral iridotomy or iridectomy and implies a rare variant know as the iris plateau syndrome.

Prevention/prophylaxis: Prevention strategies include advising the patient to have annual eye examinations with tonometry readings, especially after age 40, and to seek medical attention for any visual changes. Prophylactic laser treatment of second eye is recommended.

Referral: Refer all patients with suspected or diagnosed glaucoma to an ophthalmologist.

Education: Explain disease process, signs and symptoms, and treatment (including side effects of medications). Discuss prevention strategies, need for annual eye examinations, and medications that may interfere with treatment. Advise patient when to seek medical attention. Provide support and counseling. Educational resource materials are available from the Foundation for Glaucoma Research Foundation, 490 Post St., Suite 1427, San Francisco, CA 94102 (415–986–3162;) and the American Academy of Ophthalmology, 655 Beach St., Box 7424, San Francisco, CA 94120 (415–561–8500).

HERPES SIMPLEX INFECTION

SIGNAL SYMPTOMS▶ burning, itching, pain prodrome along the vermillion line of the upper lip

| Herpes simplex (of the lips or oral cavity) | ICD-9-CM: 054.9 |
| eczema herpeticum any site, | ICD-9-CM: 054.0 |

Description: Herpes simplex of the lips or oral cavity refers to a secondary or recurrent herpes simplex virus (HSV) infection caused by endogenous reactivation of the virus in a latently infected host, which may take one of two forms. Secondary herpetic gingivostomatitis (characterized by erythema and vesicular or ulcerative lesions of the oral mucosa) and herpes labialis (characterized by recurrent clusters of external vesicular or ulcerative lesions surrounding the facial lips and are commonly called fever blisters or cold sores).

Etiology: Caused by HSV type 1, the initial infection usually occurs in infancy or childhood. The virus may lie dormant for many years until it is reactivated by reinfection with HSV, environmental triggers, or generalized immunosuppression. HSV type 2 is primarily associated with genital lesions. HSV is transmitted in adults primarily by person-to-person sexual contact through ulcerative lesions or through infected saliva, stools, urine, or ocular discharge.

Occurrence: Widespread; occurs in approximately 20,000 to 70,000/100,000 people. 29.2/100,000 office visits per year; 0.65-20% of adults may be excreting HSV1 or HSV2 at any given time.

Age: Secondary herpetic gingivostomatitis and herpes labialis occur commonly in young to middle-aged adults; primary herpetic gingivostomatitis occurs primarily in children younger than age 5 years.

Ethnicity: There is no significant ethnic predisposition.

Gender: Occurs equally in men and women.

Contributing factors: Previous HSV infection, immunosuppression, aging, fever, physical and emotional stress, excess sun exposure, menstruation, common colds, GI upset, dental work, HIV infection, malignancy, chemotherapy, and chronic metabolic diseases such as diabetes.

Signs and symptoms:

General

- The patient may complain of excessive dryness of the mouth
- Foul halitosis
- Minor to severe oral pain
- Fever, malaise, and headache, which may be secondary to systemic HSV infection
- A tender or edematous oral mucosa
- Anterior cervical or jaw lymphadenopathy.

Secondary Herpetic Gingivostomatitis:

- The patient may report a 24- to 48-hour prodrome of burning or tingling pain sensations in the oral mucosa before the appearance of vesicular lesions.
- Found primarily on the gingivae, hard palate, buccal mucosa, and tongue, the erythematous vesicular or ulcerative lesions appear individually or in groups and are commonly 1 to 2 mm in size.
- If observed in a later stage of healing (4 to 10 days following vesicle formation), the lesions may appear ulcerated and crusted with a yellow exudate.

Herpes Labialis:

- The patient may report a prodrome of burning, pain, tingling, or itching before the appearance of the lesions along the vermilion border of the lips.

- Found primarily in the labial area, particularly at the mucocutaneous border surrounding the facial lips, the clusters of open vesicular or ulcerative lesions have erythematous bases and possibly crusting, (yellow to pale amber color) if in an advanced stage of healing.

Diagnostic tests:

Test	Result indicating disorder	CPT code
CBC	Reveals signs of viral infection (Increased monocytes and lymphocytes)	85025
Giemsa- or Wright-stained Tzanck smear of scraped lesion	Confirms herpetic stomatitis	87205
HSV viral cultures	Confirms diagnosis	87528 (probe) 87530 (quant.)
Immunoglobulin-G titers	Rules out primary HSV infection	86001

CBC, complete blood count; HSV, herpes simplex virus.

 Clinical Pearl: Be sure the viral cultures are appropriate for the laboratory used. In some cases, the culture swab must be refrigerated before use.

Differential diagnosis:

- Aphthous stomatitis; stomatitis caused by allergies or nutritional deficiencies;
- Chemical irritation; thermal or mechanical injury to the mucosa, such as from hot beverages,
- Frostbite, ill-fitting dentures, or rough tooth surfaces
- Syphilitic lesions
- Impetigo; systemic or local vasculitis
- Oral neoplasia
- Measles or chickenpox
- Infectious mononucleosis
- Warts
- Prodromal primary HIV infection

Treatment:

- Both conditions call for a high fluid intake (parenteral fluids may be required in severe cases) to counteract dehydration secondary to oral pain
- Antiseptic mouthwashes to prevent secondary bacterial infection.

Secondary Herpetic Gingivostomatitis

- Drinking cool liquids and sucking on frozen juice bars may reduce discomfort.
- Ice cubes applied for an hour to newly formed lesions may assist in healing.

- Non-narcotic analgesics or anti-inflammatories such as acetaminophen, 600 mg every 4 to 6 hours or ibuprofen 600 mg every 8 hours with food may relieve minor pain.
- For mild attacks, oral rinses with half-strength 3% hydrogen peroxide solution (1:1 with water) or with liquid antacids and aluminum or magnesium hydroxide qid.
- Equal amounts of antihistamine elixirs such as diphenhydramine may be mixed with liquid antacids (1:1) to reduce inflammation. Flavorings (e.g., cherry) may make this formula more palatable.
- A viscous solution of 2% lidocaine may be applied to oral lesions every 3 hours as a topical anesthetic or used as a gargle and swallow, 15 mL every 3 hours.
- For severe attacks, topical gel-based triamcinolone acetonide is applied at bedtime and, if needed, twice a day or three times a day after meals.
- Anti-inflammatory oral steroid bursts may be appropriate.
- For the immunocompromised patient, a combination of both oral and systemic medication may be ordered, that is, oral acyclovir, 400 mg three times a day for 10 days, and topical treatments such as penciclovir (Denavir) every 2 hours or more often for comfort.

Herpes Labialis

- Gentle scraping of the vesicular lesion to open vesicle and then apply application of Campho-Phenique.
- Intermittent cool, moist dressings with Burrow's solution (an aqueous preparation of aluminum sulfate, acetic acid, calcium carbonate) or Domeboro (aluminum subacetate) as an antiseptic.
- Penciclovir (Denavir) 1% cream every 2 hours while awake for 4 days;
- Oral medications: Valacyclovir (Valtrex) 1 g for 5 to 10 days; famciclovir (Famvir) 250 to 500 mg twice a day for 5 days.

Follow-up: See patient with severe secondary herpetic gingivostomatitis or herpes labialis within 2 to 3 days to assess effectiveness of treatment. Although most cases tend to be self-limiting and resolve within 7 to 14 days with symptomatic treatment only, recurrences are common; therefore, follow patients once a week until all oral lesions and systemic manifestations resolve.

Sequelae: Possible complications include dehydration, malnutrition, secondary bacterial infections, impaired mastication or swallowing (from recurrent scarring), and disseminated HSV infection, along with its associated complications.

Prevention/prophylaxis:

- Prevention strategies include advising the patient to refrain from behaviors that put one at risk for HSV infection;
- Use safe sex practices, including those pertaining to oral sex;
- Perform proper and frequent hand washing; to seek early medical treatment;

- Wear zinc oxide–containing sunscreens on the lips and face to prevent herpes labialis flare-ups when exposed to excessive sunlight.
- Emphasize the contagious nature of the infection; advise the patient to avoid contact with infants and immunocompromised persons because they are particularly susceptible to HSV infection.

Referral: Consult with physician to evaluate usefulness of oral steroid burst and oral acyclovir as pharmacotherapy, if secondary bacterial infection develops, or if patient has signs of disseminated infection.

Education: Explain disease process, signs and symptoms, and treatment (including side effects of medications). Discuss prevention strategies and the importance of proper oral hygiene and healthful nutritional habits. Encourage increased fluid intake; advise drinking through a straw if oral lesions are particularly painful. A liquid diet may be helpful, such as milk, liquid gelatin, yogurt, ice cream, and custard; avoid hot, spicy, salty, or acidic foods and alcoholic or carbonated beverages.

HORDEOLUM

SIGNAL SYMPTOMS▶   bump on eyelid

Hordeolum	ICD-9-CM: 373.1

Description: A hordeolum, commonly known as a stye, is a small, pus-filled abscess involving the hair follicle of the eyelashes (external hordeolum) or meibomian glands (internal hordeolum)

Etiology: Usually caused by staphylococcal infection; may be a secondary infection.

Occurrence: Common.

Age: Most common in children and adolescents.

Ethnicity: No significant ethnic predisposition.

Gender: Occurs equally in men and in women.

Contributing Factors: Recurrent blepharitis, makeup, contact lens, poor eyelid hygiene, eye irritation from smoking.

Signs and symptoms:

- Styes may be accompanied by erythema, swelling, itching, scaling, and discharge on the lid. Physical examination (using gloves) reveals the head of the stye on the outside of the lid, or when the eyelid is everted, on the underside.

Diagnostic test:

Test	Result indicating disorder	CPT code
If drainage is present, culture may be done	Determines causative agent	87070

Diagnosed by physical examination including visual examination.

Differential diagnosis:

- Chalazion (redness of eyelid margin, scaling, discharge)
- Eyelid neoplasms (positive cytology)
- Blepharitis (inflammation of eyelids)

Treatment:

Pharmacologic

Erythromycin ophthalmic ointment thinly applied to the area with a cotton-tipped applicator three times a day. Try gentamicin ophthalmic ointment if the lesion is refractive to treatment.

Physical

Warm, moist saline compresses to the eyes several times a day. Allow stye to open and drain spontaneously; do not squeeze. (Pain decreases when stye opens and drains.)

Follow-up: See patient in 2 to 3 weeks for evaluation or sooner if unresolved.

Sequelae: Possible complications include cellulitis of the eyelid and repeated styes (if these occur, evaluate for diabetes mellitus).

Prevention/prophylaxis:

- Prevention strategies include advising the patient to perform good eyelid hygiene by washing the lids daily with diluted baby shampoo,
- Do not rub the eyes
- Do not squeeze the stye
- Apply warm compresses
- Frequent hand washing
- Using a fresh cloth and towel after touching eye
- Using hypoallergenic makeup and practicing careful and thorough removal of makeup.

Referral: Refer to ophthalmic surgeon if patient needs surgery to drain the abscess.

Education: Explain disease process, signs and symptoms, and treatment (including side effects of medications). Discuss prevention strategies.

IRITIS (ANTERIOR UVEITIS)

SIGNAL SYMPTOMS▶   decreased visual acuity, acute onset; deep eye pain; unilateral

Iritis, unspecified   ICD-9-CM: 364.3

Description: Uveitis is a global term referring to an intraocular inflammatory disorder. Iritis (anterior uveitis) is an intraocular inflammation of the iris alone or iris and ciliary body (iridocyclitis) and is the most frequently seen form of uveitis. The inflammation may be acute or chronic, mild or severe. With iritis, the iris, ciliary body, and anterior choroid are usually all involved because of a common blood supply. With posterior uveitis, inflammation is usually confined to the posterior choroid, which quickly spreads to the sensory retina, resulting in potential destruction of vision.

Etiology: Infectious process results from viral, bacterial, parasitic or fungal etiologies. Autoimmune inflammatory process postulated in association with systemic, especially rheumatologic, disorders. Other causes include trauma such as lacerations, punctures, contusions, and chemical burns. About 25% are idiopathic. Iritis affects 50% to 70% of persons who are HLA-B27 positive.

Occurrence: Incidence rate is approximately 8/100,000 per year. Anterior uveitis is the most common type and is four times more prevalent than is posterior uveitis.

Age: Most common in adults.

Ethnicity: There is no significant ethnic predisposition.

Gender: Men and women are affected equally by the condition. An exception is HLA-B27 anterior uveitis wall, in which the female-to-male ratio is 2.5:1)

Contributing Factors: Systemic diseases such as ankylosing spondylitis, sarcoidosis, systemic lupus erythematosus (SLE), and Reiter's syndrome.

Signs and symptoms:

- Varies depending on the structures affected as well as the underlying organism.
- With acute iritis, the patient may present with sudden onset of unilateral, dull, deep eye pain; photophobia; blurred vision; and tearing.
- With varicella zoster infection or infectious mononucleosis comorbidity, the patient may also have fever and malaise.
- With posterior uveitis, the patient may present with blurred vision and "floaters" (floating spots). More common bilaterally and more insidious onset.
- Physical examination may reveal a unilateral "red eye," sensitivity to light, a constricted (miotic) pupil that does not react to light, and an iris that may change colors.
- There may also be a skin or eyelid rash. It may be difficult to open the lid for examination.
- Retinal patches may be seen on funduscopic examination.
- Slit lamp (binocular microscope) examination may reveal milkiness of the aqueous humor and inflammatory cell particles on the back of the cornea, a pattern resembling light passing through smoke.

Diagnostic tests:

Test	Result indicating disorder	CPT code
Giemsa stain of corneal or skin lesion scrapings	To detect multinucleated giant cells	87205
C&S if discharge present	To determine causative agent	87070 culture 87184 sensitivity
Slit lamp examination, chest radiograph	Rule out sarcoidosis, histoplasmosis, or tuberculous lymphoma	92499 (other) 71035 CXR
CBC, BUN/creatinine	Interstitial nephritis (Decreased lymphocytes, Increased WBCs)	85025 (CBC) 84520 (BUN) 82565 (creatinine)
HLA-B27 typing	Ankylosing spondylitis, Reiter's syndrome	86812
ANA, SS-A	SLE, Sjögren's syndrome	86038 (ANA) 86235 (SS-A)
VDRL, FTA	Syphilis	Missing 80090 (TORCH) panel (VDRL) 88346 (FTA)
Lyme serology	Lyme disease	86617

ANA, antinuclear antibodies; BUN, blood, urea, nitrogen; CBC,: complete blood count; FTA, fluorescent treponemal antibody; C&S, culture and sensitivity; SS-A, Sjögren's syndrome antibodies; TORCH; toxoplasmosis, rubella, cytomegalovirus, herpes simplex; VDRL, Venereal Disease Research Laboratory; WBCs, white blood cells.

- Diagnosis is made on history and physical examination. If systemic disease is present, a complete work-up may be necessary, because it may be autoimmune in nature.
- If there is a discharge, C&S may be done.

Differential Diagnosis

- Acute angle-closure glaucoma (mild aching of eyes, headache, photophobia, blurring of vision, loss of peripheral vidian, decreased visual acuity that increases at night. Halos around lights, gradual loss of vision over years that leads to tunnel vision)
- Conjunctivitis (conjunctival hyperemia, tearing, burning, exudate and matting)
- Foreign body (foreign body sensation and tearing)
- Scleritis (associated with autoimmune diseases, severe deep boring pain, area appears purple in daylight)
- Keratitis (inflammation of the cornea)
- Cataracts (progressive, painless loss of visual acuity)
- Closed-angle glaucoma (severe unilateral eye pain and pressure, decreased visual acuity, blurred vision, diplopia, tearing, May have nausea and vomiting due to IOP. **THIS IS AN OPHTHALMIC EMERGENCY**)

Treatment: Immediate ophthalmologist referral is necessary because aggressive management may be required. More severe cases may require systemic corticosteroids, with careful monitoring of the IOP. Treatment also includes analgesics for pain, bed rest, and decreased activity until the episode resolves, and treatment of the underlying cause.

Pharmacological

Homatropine hydrobromide (Isopto 2%) ophthalmic solution 2 gtts to the affected eyelid or as often as every three hours, if necessary; plus prednisone acetate 1% ophthalmic suspension 2 gtts to the affected eye every hour initially, tapering to once a day with improvement. Contra-indications: Hypersensitivity, glaucoma patients (no cycloplegia), and topical corticosteroid therapy secondary to infectious etiologies.

Precautions: Homatropine hydrobromide may produce adverse systemic autoimmune effects. Topical corticosteroids may increase IOP. Prolonged use may cause cataract formation and exacerbate existing herpetic keratitis, which may masquerade as iritis.

Follow-up: Ophthalmologist sees patient for follow-up.

Sequelae: Possible complications include progression to posterior uveitis (especially if untreated), which involves some residual vision loss and markedly blurred vision, and may lead to cataracts, glaucoma, retinal detachment. Uveitis resulting from local infection tends to resolve with eradication of the underlying infection. Uveitis associated with seronegative anthropathies tends to be acute less than 3 months and frequently recurrent.

Prevention/prophylaxis: Prevention strategies include advising the patient of the importance of early treatment and follow-up care.

Referral: Immediate referral to an ophthalmologist.

Education: Explain disease process, signs and symptoms, and treatment (including side effects of medications). Discuss prevention strategies. Instructions on administration of eye drops. Wear dark glasses if photophobic.

MÉNIÈRE'S DISEASE *(Ménière's Syndrome, Endolymphatic Hydrops)*

SIGNAL SYMPTOMS▶ spontaneous attacks of vertigo with 20 minutes to several hours of hearing loss; low- frequency range and may fluctuate with ear fullness.

Ménière's disease   ICD-9-CM: 386.00

Description: Ménière's disease (Ménière's syndrome, endolymphatic hydrops) is an inner ear disorder (labyrinthine) characterized by an increase in volume and pressure of the endolymph.

Etiology: The cause of the condition is unknown. Theories relate to an inner ear responsive to a variety of stressors such as reduced middle ear pressure, allergy, endocrine disease, lipid disorder, vascular, viral, and most recently, intracranial compression of balance nerve by blood vessel.

Occurrence: Prevalence is estimated at 1150 per 100,000, with the severity and frequency diminishing over the years, but with increasing loss of hearing.

Age: Age of onset ranges from age 20 to 60 years, with most cases developing during the fifth decade of life; the condition is rare in young children and adults older than age 70 years.

Ethnicity: Some studies indicate whites of European descent are at an increased risk. Whites are at a higher risk.

Gender: Men and women are equally affected.

Contributing factors: Stress, allergies, smoking, high salt intake, prolonged exposure to high noise levels, chronic serous otitis media.

Signs and symptoms:

- Acute episodes last anywhere from 20 minutes to 3 hours and are characterized by sudden attacks of nausea, emesis, pallor, diaphoresis, dizziness (spatial disorientation), vertigo, roaring tinnitus, and increased pressure, fullness, and hearing loss in the affected ear.
- Rapid movement aggravates all proprioceptive symptoms,
- Patients often report a history of falls or accidents during acute episodes.
- The frequency and severity of attacks may decrease over time, and hearing may improve immediately following an acute attack. However, some episodes have been known to last for over 24 hours. Overall, low-frequency hearing loss is typically progressive, with bilateral involvement in 10% to 50% of cases.
- Between acute attacks, patients may also experience motion-related imbalance without vertigo.
- Complete hearing loss in advanced cases is associated with a cessation of vertiginous episodes.
- Physical examination may reveal spontaneous nystagmus after preventing eye fixation by having the patient wear 40-diopter glasses (Fresnel lenses) during the period of observation.
- Otoscopic examination typically reveals no apparent abnormalities.
- Weber and Rinne tests elicit findings characteristic of a sensorineural hearing defect with sound lateralization to the nonaffected ear (Weber test) and air conduction superior in duration and volume to bone conduction (positive Rinne test).

Diagnostic tests:

Test	Result indicating disorder	CPT code
Serological Tests: Specific for *Treponema pallidum* (FTA, MHA); thyroid and lipid studies	To rule out other disease processes: FTA-ABS–positive (syphilis) TSH, T_3, free T_4 (thyroid disease) Lipid profile with high cholesterol, HDL, LDL, or triglycerides (hypercholesteremia)	88346 (FTA) 84443 (TSH) 84480 (T_3) 84479 (T_4 uptake) 80061 (lipid profile)
Audiometry	Demonstrates low-frequency sensorineural hearing loss, as well as impaired speech discrimination	92588
Otoscopy with air pressure applied to the tympanic membrane	Movement of membrane and fluid status in inner ear. Also check for cerumen impaction	92599 (other)
Tuning fork test (Weber and Rinne)	To confirm validity of audiometry. Air conduction less than bone conduction	92553

FTA, fluorescent treponemal antibody; FTA-ABS, fluorescent treponemal antibody absorption test; HDL, high-density lipoproteins; LDL, low-density lipoproteins; MHA, microhemagglutination assay; T_3, triiodothyronine; T_4, thyroxine; TSH, thyroid-stimulating hormone.

Ménière's disease is a diagnosis of exclusion; disorders that mimic its clinical picture must first be ruled out.

Differential diagnosis:

- Multiple sclerosis; otitis media; vestibular neuronitis; secondary or tertiary syphilis; acute viral or bacterial infection of the labyrinth (extreme weakness and fatigue, inability to maintain standing position)
- Discrete lesions of the central nervous system (magnetic resonance imaging (MRI) of central nervous system (CNS) with neurological referral)
- Degenerative nervous disorders (referral to neurologist if suspected)
- Hypothyroidism (diagnosed by blood tests and thyroid nuclear scan with contrast)
- Benign positional vertigo (tilt test)
- Presbycusis (hearing loss due to wear and tear, worse with aging)
- Hypoglycemic disorders; anemic conditions; lipid disorders; transient ischemic attacks; vertebrobasilar ischemia; subclavian steal syndrome; iatrogenic drug-induced ototoxicity (unexplained attacks of metabolic disorders)
- Sedative side effects of many medications; multidrug interactions
- Acoustic neuroma (growth on the acoustic nerve)
- Psychiatric illnesses, such as depression, anxiety, panic attacks, somatization disorders; alcoholism; and other forms of substance abuse (diagnosed by exclusion of all other causes; screening tools for depression and anxiety, unexplained attacks of metabolic disorders)

- Associated conditions include cochlear hydrops (hearing problem only), vestibular hydrops (balance problem only) and drop attacks (excludes by audiologists and ear, nose, and throat (ENT) referral; unexplained attacks of metabolic disorders)

Treatment:

Pharmacological

Pharmacotherapy is directed at symptomatic relief of vertigo and nausea, because no medications are known to affect the disease process. For an acute attack, a combination of antimuscarinics or anticholinergics and vestibulosuppressive histamine blockers from various classes may be prescribed. Anxiolytics may be used to sedate patients during severe episodes. Maintenance therapies may include an antihistamine such as meclizine (Antivert, Bonine) 25 to 100 mg orally either at bedtime or in divided doses up to four times a day. Diazepam 2 mg twice a day for relief of muscle spasms and anxiety. Ergotamine-belladonna-phenobarbital (Bellergal) 1 mg every 12 hours may be used. Caution with atropine use especially with patients diagnosed with supraventricular tachycardia and other dysrhythmias. During acute attacks, adult doses are indicated, such as atropine 0.2 to 0.4 mg IV, diazepam (Valium) 5 to 10 mg IV slowly, and transdermal scopolamine applied to skin surface behind the ear for 3 days. Alternative drugs include droperidol, promethazine, diaphane, hydramine are used for acute attacks. For maintenance therapy, alternative drugs may include dimenhydrinate (Dramamine), promethazine (Phenergan) or diphenidol (Vontrol). Streptomycin therapy for bilateral Ménière's disease when conventional management has failed. Streptomycin may be administered over a period of several days or weeks intentionally to damage the neuroepithelium of the balance centers and reduce their function. This procedure can be done only under the care of an otolaryngologist.

Physical

Acute attacks are best treated by calm bed rest with the eyes closed and protection from falling for attacks rarely last longer than 4 hours.

Surgical

New procedures include administering gentamicin through the tympanic membrane into the inner ear space. Disabling symptoms may require surgical intervention (5% to 10% of all cases). For patients with normal hearing, decompression of the endolymphatic sac or intracranial transection of the vestibular nerve may be performed. For the patient whose hearing ability has degenerated and is deemed unsalvageable, the cochlea itself may be decompressed (cochleocentesis) or directly perfused with streptomycin. A more radical surgery is labyrinthectomy of the affected ear, which entirely ablates vestibular function.

Follow-up: The otolaryngologist is the director of the patient's care. See patient in 3 to 6 weeks if symptoms do not worsen. If disabling symptoms such as tinnitus, vertigo, nausea, or emesis persist, immediate re-evaluation is indicated. Hearing loss must be carefully monitored for progression, because this is a telltale sign of an underlying, potentially life-threatening, acoustic neuroma.

Sequelae: Possible complications include progressive bilateral hearing loss, chronic tinnitus, deafness, disabling vertigo, accidental injuries related to vestibular dysfunction, increasing inability to function productively at home or at work. Also, clinical failure to diagnose acoustic neuroma.

Prevention/prophylaxis: Prevention strategies include encouraging the patient to stop smoking, reduce stress, reduce salt intake to 1 g/day, avoid ototoxic medications and polypharmacy, and protect ears from loud noises.

Referral: Consult with otolaryngologist for second opinion and monitoring.

Education: Explain disease process, signs and symptoms, and treatment (including side effects of medications). Discuss prevention strategies, the importance of follow-up care, and when to report symptoms. In order to avoid accidental injuries and minimize symptoms, advise patient to avoid driving, climbing ladders, working near dangerous machinery, walking without assistance, reading, or looking at glaring lights during acute episodes. To lessen nausea and vomiting, advise patient to reduce food intake during acute attacks.

ORAL CANCER

SIGNAL SYMPTOMS ▶ new or increasing painless growth in the oral cavity

| Malignant neoplasm of the mouth, unspecified | ICD-9-CM: 145.9 |

Description: Oral cancers include all those occurring on the lip, tongue, floor of mouth, pharynx, salivary glands, inside of cheeks, gums, and palate. The lower lip is the most common site and has the best prognosis.

Etiology: Ninety percent are squamous cell carcinomas, which may result from immune alterations such as local imbalances in T-cell function and Epstein-Barr virus.

Occurrence: Incidence is about 11/100,000; accounts for about 2% of all cancer deaths.

Age: Occurs primarily in adults over age 60 (75% of all cases).

Gender: Occurs in men more than in women.

Ethnicity: Incidence highest in African-American men; also a high incidence in Asians.

Contributing Factors: Use of tobacco including chewing tobacco and snuff, cigarettes, cigars, and pipes; heavy alcohol use, especially when combined with the use of snuff; exposure to ultraviolet light, especially in light-skinned persons; nutritional deficiencies, specifically riboflavin or iron-deficiency anemia; poor dentition and oral hygiene; HIV infection; environmental exposure to wool dust; oral trauma.

Signs and symptoms:

- Classic presentation is the persistence of a lump or sore within the oral cavity.
- General symptoms include a mild soreness when eating, a lesion or lump in the mouth, and problems with articulation.
- Late symptoms may include pain, bleeding, foul breath, excessive salivation, loose teeth, change in speech, or a hard neck mass.
- Physical examination may reveal a red, velvety patch on the mouth or tongue (erythroplakia) or a white patch on the mucosa of the mouth, tongue (leukoplakia), or lips, sometimes called "smoker's patch."
- There may also be areas of brownish or black pigmentation, masses or ulcers on the oral mucous membrane.
- Parotid enlargement, facial deformities, and an asymptomatic neck mass (30% of patients) may also be seen.
- Palpation might reveal a palpable mass, usually painless, and lymphadenopathy.
- An oral mass or ulcer that is malignant is usually hard with indurated margins that extend beyond the mass or ulcer itself.

Diagnostic tests:

Test	Result indicating disorder	CPT code
Liver function tests	Rules out metastasis if liver function studies (SGOT, SGPT are within normal limits)	80076
Imaging: Appropriate to symptom; may include mandible films, dental films, panoramex films of the teeth, CT with bone windows, CT or MRI of the neck, and CXR	Rules out metastases if masses or growths absent CPT-# indicates without contrast for first number or changing last digit to the "-#" for with contrast	70480-1 CT orbits/ears 70486-7 CT maxillary facial 70490-1 CT neck 70540-1 MRI neck 71020 CXR Pa & Lat
Biopsy (punch biopsy most common)	Any lesion present for more than 4 to 6 weeks (confirms diagnosis) and direct treatment therapy	11100

CT, computed tomography; CXR, chest x-ray study; Lat, lateral; MRI, magnetic resonance imaging; Pa, posteroanterior; SGOT, serum glutamic-oxaloacetic transaminase; SPGT, serum glutamate pyruvate transaminase.

Differential Diagnosis:

- Benign lesions of the oral cavity (biopsy of lesions to confirm)
- Leukoplakia (thin, white lesions, wrinkles, pearly white lingual patches)
- Erythroplakia (red, elevated lesions, well demarcated)

- Mouth ulcers, such as aphthous ulcers and canker sores (lingual ulcer, small vesicles, painful small round ulcers, white floor, yellow margins)
- Oral candidiasis (pruritic eroded area in mouth, positive culture)

Treatment: The treatment varies depending on the location and staging of the tumor.

Surgical

Wide resection, with or without radiation therapy and/or chemotherapy, is usually the treatment of choice. For unresectable tumors, radiation or chemotherapy are performed for palliative care. Small lesions of the mouth can be removed surgically without long-term impairment of speech or aesthetics.

Radiotherapy

Small or larger lesions and the draining lymphatics can be irradiated over about 7 weeks using external beam and interstitial implants to the local area (results in a cure rate of about 95%). Chemotherapy may be used to sensitize the tumor during radiation.

Follow-up: See patient monthly until side effects of treatment have diminished; then every 3 months.

Sequelae: Fifty-three percent of oral cancers have spread to regional or distant structures at the time of diagnosis; overall survival rate is 52%. Most deaths occur within 3 to 4 years of diagnosis. Possible complications of untreated oral cancers include disfiguring, necrotic, and ulcerating lesions, another form of oral cancer, and death. Possible complications of treated oral cancers include functional or cosmetic disabilities proportional to the degree of surgery and stage of disease and persistent dysphagia; problems with articulation, nutrition, and candidiasis (secondary to treatment).

Prevention/prophylaxis: The essential prevention strategy is encouraging the patient to stop smoking or using chewing tobacco (snuff) and to decrease alcohol use. Other prevention strategies include annual oral and dental examinations for a patient at high risk and teaching the patient to perform a self-oral examination.

Referral: Refer to the multidisciplinary team, including physician, surgeon, medical oncologist, radiation oncologist, dentist, nutritionist, social worker, and speech or occupational therapist, as appropriate.

Education: Explain disease process, signs and symptoms, and treatment (including side effects of medications). Discuss prevention strategies, treatment options, lifestyle changes, the importance of maintaining good nutrition, and the importance of dental (at least three times a year) and medical follow-up care. Also discuss methods to help the patient stop smoking and refrain from drinking alcohol. Educational resource materials are available from the American Cancer Society (800-4CANCER). Website *www.acs.org*

OTITIS EXTERNA

SIGNAL SYMPTOMS ▶ excruciating ear pain (otalgia), loss of hearing, rumbling noise.

| Otitis externa, infectious otitis externa. | ICD-9-CM: 380.10 |

Description: Otitis externa is an inflammation of the membranous lining of the auditory canal and/or contiguous structures of the outer ear. The term refers to a wide spectrum of both acute and chronic inflammatory processes that may be diffuse, localized, or invasive in nature. Invasive otitis externa (malignant necrotizing eczematous otitis externa accompanies externa), typical atopic eczema or other primary skin condition) is a potentially life-threatening disease, if it is left untreated.

Etiology: Most commonly caused by microbial infection; bacterial agents include *Pseudomonas aeruginosa*, 67% are caused by Staphylococcus aureus, and group A *Streptococcus pyogenes*; if a fungal microbe causal agent 90% are *Aspergillus niger, Phycomycetes, Actinomyces, Rhizopus* and yeast. Other causes include hyperkeratotic processes such as eczema, psoriasis, and contact or seborrheic dermatitis; local skin maceration; and traumatic injury. Chronic otitis externa may result from inadequately treated acute disease, untreated underlying dermatologic conditions, or chronic otitis media.

Occurrence: Occurs 10 to 20 times more during the warmer summer months than during cooler seasons.

Etiology: Unknown: Most prevalent in the summer or with adults swimming year round. Skin disorders may predispose persons to developing chronic condition.

 Clinical Pearls: Persons with access to private swimming pools develop otitis externa early in the season and usually culture *Pseudomonas* organism possibly related to the pool acid-base balance. Always refer a unilateral recalcitrant draining ear to the ENT specialist for further evaluation.

Age: Adults over age 50 are at greatest risk for invasive otitis externa. Necrotizing otitis media, diabetes mellitus, and debilitating diseases increase risk, especially in elderly population. Children and teens require immediate attention and pain relief.

Ethnicity: No significant ethnic predisposition.

Gender: Men and women are equally affected.

Contributing factors:

- Immunocompromised status
- Environmental changes such as an increase in temperature or humidity
- Change in the pH of the auditory canal from acidic to alkaline

- Excess moisture from any cause
- Inadequate cerumen production
- Seborrheic dermatitis
- Manual picking of the ear; foreign bodies in the auditory canal
- Prolonged use of ear plugs, hearing aids, or cotton swabs
- Previous ear infections; skin allergies, particularly those to hair sprays and dyes that may enter the ear canal.

Signs and symptoms

- Acute, often severe otalgia (ear pain) of sudden or gradual onset, usually unilateral but may be bilateral, may worsen at night and disturb sleep
- Exacerbated by pulling the pinna or earlobe, applying pressure to the tragus, or, in severe cases, by chewing.
- In its early stages, the affected ear may feel full or obstructed, and a temporary conductive hearing loss is common if edema is severe.
- The affected ear may also be pruritic.
- Otoscopic examination typically reveals an edematous and erythematous disruption of superficial lining of the auditory canal, with accumulations of fluid or drainage (copious green exudate with *Pseudomonas* infection; yellow crusting in the middle of a purulent exudate with staphylococcal infection; a fluffy, white or black, malodorous carpet of growth with fungal infections; and scaly, cracked, or weepy tissue with allergic reactions).

Diagnostic tests:

Usually diagnosed by history and physical examination.

Test	Result indicating disorder	CPT code
Culture and sensitivity of fluid or exudate from the ear	Identifies causative organism	87071 culture 87184 sensitivity
ESR	May be elevated	85652
CT scans, MRI, plain films, or gallium or technetium-99 bone scans	Detect soft tissue or bony involvement in malignant disease	70480 CT without contrast 70481 CT with contrast 70540 MRI without contrast 70541 MRI with contrast 78305 Bone scan multiple areas 78300 Bone scan limited areas

CT, computed tomography; ESR, erythrocyte sedimentation rate; MRI, magnetic resonance imaging.

Differential diagnosis:

- Cranial nerve palsy (VII, IX to XII) (caused by infections, viral or bacterial, inability to move parts of face, tongue)
- Otitis media (infection of middle ear, suppuration)

- Sinusitis (infection of sinuses, pain over sinus areas)
- TMJ dysfunction (clicking with pain when opening and closing mouth)
- Dental disease (halitosis, infection, abscess of teeth and gums)
- Neurologic disorders such as trigeminal and glossopharyngeal neuralgia
- Parotitis secondary to mumps (paramyxovirus infection, obstruction or inflammation of parotid; lemon or dill pickle causes increased pain)
- Tumors of the middle ear and auditory meatus (rare, referral to ENT)
- Chondrodermatitis nodularis, chronica helicis (referral to ENT)
- Impetigo (cratered lesions, usually *Staphylococcus* infection)
- Herpes zoster infection (papular crusted lesions along dermatome; pain)
- Insect bites (inflammatory symptoms with injection site)
- Mastoiditis (pain behind ear; swelling, MRI to confirm)
- Meningitis (irritation of meninges, headache with severe neck pain, inability to move head to chest)
- Temporal bone fracture (history of trauma)
- Invasive tumor (biopsy)
- Primary skin and cartilage disorders such as sarcoidosis, discoid lupus, and trauma-related perichondritis of the pinna
- Cerumen impaction (hearing loss, new onset of buzzing, change in sound with mouth open and shutting)
- Gouty tophi; tuberculous otitis (rare); leprosy (rare); and syphilitic otitis (rare) (presence of lesions and positive biopsy)

Treatment: Treatment generally involves three basic steps: Gentle cleansing of ear canal to remove all cerumen, exudate, and epidermal debris; irrigation with isotonic saline; evaluation of otic discharge and edema of the auditory canal and tympanic membrane; and selection of an appropriate pharmacotherapy. Use of a cotton pledget or wick may be too painful but is the most effective. Pain may be relieved with a warm compress over the affected ear or nonprescription pain relievers such as aspirin or acetaminophen, 300 to 600 mg orally every 4 hours and anti-inflammatory agents. Narcotics may be required for pain relief. Occasionally, the pustules or furuncles associated with localized otitis externa may require surgical drainage before pharmacotherapy is administered. An ear wick is required to relieve a nearly occluded ear canal so medication can be instilled and auditory canal can be kept open.
Prevention: Use ear plugs for swimming to prevent swimmer's ear.

 Clinical Pearl: The use of topical otic solution such as benzocaine (Americaine) will allow placement of the wick if the drops are instilled before the procedure. The ear holds 5 to 8 gtts without waste

Acute and Chronic Bacterial Otitis Externa:

- Treat empirically with propylene glycol preparations such as Cortisporin Otic Suspension (polymyxin B, Oflox 0.3% solution twicea day, 4 gtt four times a day for 10 days, neomycin, and hydrocortisone).

- VoSol HC (2% nonaqueous acetic acid and hydrocortisone), 4 drops in the affected ear four times a day for 7 to 10 days.
- If luminal occlusion prevents the passage of otic preparations, insert an absorbent 1-inch cotton wick or sponge; place drops on the wick for 2 to 3 days (until swelling subsides); then place drops directly into the ear canal.
- Ciprofloxacin (Cipro) 500 mg twice a day for 10 to 21 days depending on the clinical response especially in the treatment of a *Pseudomonas* infection.
- Dicloxacillin 500 mg four times a day for 10 days.
- For chronic otitis externa usually secondary to seborrhea, add selenium sulfide shampoo or bacteriostatic shampoo. Recurrence is decreased or prevented by drying with drops (1/3 white vinegar, 2/3 rubbing alcohol after swimming), then antibiotic drops or 2% acetic acid solution.
- Acute malignant otitis externa, with or without diabetes are treated with imipenem (Primaxin) 0.5 g every 6 hours IV, or meropenem 1.0 g IV every 8 hours or Cipro 400 mg every 12 hours or 750 mg orally every 12 hours for 14 days depending on the size of the patient and the type and duration of infection before treatment.
- Parenteral antibiotics for necrotizing otitis externa are antistaphylococcus and antipseudomonal treatment for 4 to 6 weeks.
- Surgical débridement may be required of the affected area (drains abscesses and removes sequestered collagen), is usually required followed by 4 to 6 weeks of IV antibiotic (antipseudomonal) therapy.
- CT or an MRI scan is more sensitive than an x-ray study if bone is involved or suggested.

Fungal Infections:

After cleaning the auditory canal, apply a single dusting of sulfanilamide powder, followed by an otic suspension, such as VoSol (2% nonaqueous acetic acid) or Otic Domeboro (2% acetic acid), 4 drops in each affected ear four times a day for 7 to 10 days. Topical fungicide preparations containing nystatin or clotrimazole every 3 hours may also be used. If warranted, parental antifungal therapy with amphotericin-B is given. Patients with Ramsey-Hunt syndrome facial nerve weakness are treated with acyclovir IV.

Follow-up: In managing a patient with acute otitis externa, see the patient in 48 hours to assess effectiveness of treatment (acute otitis externa is commonly cured after 7 to 10 days of treatment) and then at the end of treatment promptly. See daily in hospital rounds for necrotizing otitis externa.

Sequelae: Possible complications include dermatitis medicamentosus (common); severe furunculosis (boil formation); cellulitis (deep tissue infection) within the ear canal; invasive otitis externa (potentially life-threatening complication of poorly treated diffuse and localized disease); serious cranial infections including meningitis, mastoiditis, parotitis, and osteomyelitis of either the temporal bone or the base of the skull; cranial nerve palsies (20% to 30% of patients with invasive disease).

Prevention/prophylaxis: Prevention strategies include advising the patient to avoid getting water in the ears for at least 4 to 6 weeks after symptoms subside, because moisture from any source can trigger a recurrent episode, to wear shower caps or soft sponge when bathing, and to avoid swimming for at least 1 month following an acute episode.

Referral: Refer to ENT specialist, otorhinolaryngologist if patient has invasive otitis externa, cellulitis, bony involvement, complicating cranial infections, refractory disease or is immunocompromised.

Education: Explain disease process, signs and symptoms, and treatment (including side effects of medications). Discuss prevention strategies, proper methods of cleaning the ears and auditory canal, and the importance of keeping the ear canals dry for at least 4 to 6 weeks after an acute episode.

OTITIS MEDIA

SIGNAL SYMPTOMS▶ Ear pain, fever

Otitis media, acute	ICD-9-CM: 382.0
Otitis, chronic serous	ICD-9-CM: 382.9
Otitis media, acute suppurative	ICD-9-CM: 381.10

Description: Otitis media is an inflammation of the structures within the middle ear. Serous otitis media involves the transudation of plasma from middle ear blood vessels leading to effusion. Acute otitis media (also known as suppurative or purulent otitis media) is an inflammation secondary to infection, typically of bacterial origin, that may present with or without effusion. Recurrent acute otitis media (three or more AOMs in 6 months or four or more AOMs in 1 year) is characterized by the clearance of middle ear effusions between acute episodes of otic inflammation. Chronic otitis media occurs when inflammation persists for more than 3 months and is typically related to tympanic membrane perforation with either intermittent or persistent otic discharge (Fig. 4–2). Otitis media with effusion (OME) is persistent inflammation manifested as symptomatic middle ear fluids with or without prior AOM.

Etiology: The main bacterial causes of AOM are *Streptococcus pneumoniae,* nontypable *Haemophilus influenza,* and *Moraxella catarrhalis.* Viral infections are the most common. Chronic otitis media may occur with or without cholesteatoma.

Serous otitis: Brought about by a transudation of plasma fluid from engorged blood vessels resulting from the loss of eustachian tube

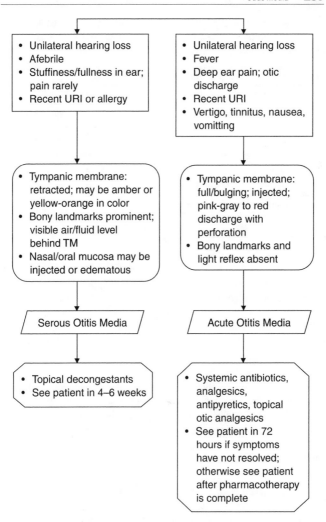

Figure 4–2. Differential diagnosis and treatment: otitis media.

patency, caused by either the swelling of its membranous lining or direct anatomic blockage.

Acute otitis media: Results when bacterial infection by nasopharyngeal microorganisms follows eustachian tube dysfunction, most commonly *Streptococcus pneumoniae* in adults. May be caused by beta lactamase producing bacterial strains which may be resistant to first-line antibiotics.

Chronic otitis media: May be caused by all of the listed bacteria and commonly by *Pseudomonas aeruginosa* and *S. aureus*.

Otitis Media: Causes

Acute-Bacterial	Acute-Viral	Chronic
Group A beta hemolytic	Rhinovirus	Likely noninfectious
	Adenovirus	Irritation PND discharge of
Streptococcal	Parainfluenzae virus	chronic allergic rhinitis or reflux
Neisseria gonorrhoeae	Coxsackie virus	Chemical irritation or smoking
Corynebacterium diphtheriae	Coronavirus	Neoplasm/vasculitides
Haemophilus influenzae	Echovirus	Trauma
Moraxella (Branhamella) catarrhalis	Herpes simplex virus	
Group C&G streptococcus	Epstein-Barr virus(mono) Cytomegalovirus RSV – Respiratory synctal virus	

PND, paroxysmal nocturnal dyspnea.

Occurrence: Peak incidence age range from 6 to 18 months; declines in adults, although relatively common with or after upper respiratory infection (URI) or airplane travel or scuba diving with URI.

Age: Occurs in all ages but is most common in young children.

Ethnicity: Higher incidence in Native Americans, particularly Navajos, and Alaskan Eskimos; also an increased rate is seen in light-skinned whites of European descent.

Gender: Men are affected > women.

Contributing factors: Recent or concurrent URI; allergies; sinusitis; smoking; rhinitis; pharyngitis; anatomic abnormalities, such as hypertrophy of the adenoids, cleft palate, deviated nasal septum, or nasopharyngeal tumors; perforation of the eardrum; certain genetic conditions such as Down syndrome; smoking; crowded or unsanitary living conditions; family history of otitis media.

Signs and symptoms

Serous otitis media: Recent history of viral URI or allergic or vasomotor rhinitis; stuffiness; fullness; loss of auditory acuity unilaterally in the affected ear; and popping, crackling, or gurgling sounds when chewing, yawning, or blowing the nose; very rarely, vertigo or ataxia.

Acute otitis media: Marked "deep" ear pain and fever, unilateral hearing loss, otic discharge, which often indicate tympanic membrane perforation; recent history of URI, dizziness (space disorientation), vertigo, tinnitus, vomiting, or nausea. Pain typically subsides if the tympanic membrane ruptures.

Chronic otitis media: History of repeated bouts of acute otitis media, followed by a period of continuous or intermittent otorrhea lasting more than 3 months.

Otoscopic examination may reveal a retracted tympanic membrane with prominent bony landmarks and possibly bubbles or a visible air-fluid level posterior to the membrane and usually inferior surface. In acute otitis media, the tympanic membrane is usually injected and pinkish-gray to fiery red; in acute serous otitis media, the membrane is dull, full, or bulging with absent or obscured bony landmarks and cone light reflex. Discharge from the middle ear may be present if the tympanic membrane has perforated; otorrhea may be purulent or mucoid. In chronic otitis media, the tympanic membrane may be perforated and draining, and have invasive granulation tissue. Chronic, foul-smelling otorrhea is typical of anaerobic bacterial infection, and a chronic, grayish-yellow suppuration may indicate cholesteatoma from the degenerative products of invasive epithelialization.

Physical examination with acute infection may reveal preauricular and posterior cervical node; lymphadenopathy is common and tenderness of the mastoid process may be present.

Diagnostic tests: Usually diagnosed by history and physical examination. Diagnostic tests are rarely needed if symptoms clearly fit the classic clinical picture.

Test	Result indication disorder	CPT code
Pneumatic otoscopy and tympanometry	Confirms diagnosis and shows little or no movement of the tympanic membrane.	92599 (other otoscopy) 92567 (Tympanometry)
CBC	Shows leukocytosis in acute otitis media	85025
Cultures and antibiotic sensitivity testing	Helps guide treatment by indicating causative agent	87071 culture 87184 sensitivity
Sinus x-rays and CT scans	Shows mucosal thickening and effusion	70130 X ray 70480 CT without contrast 70481 CT with contrast
Pure tone audiometry and Weber and Rinne tests	Evaluate hearing loss Bone conduction greater than air conduction. Tones unequal in affected ear	92553
Nasopharyngoscopy	If chronicity becomes a problem.	92511

CBC, complete blood count, CT, computed tomography.

Differential Diagnosis:

- Otitis externa (severe ear pain, loss of hearing, rumbling noise, discharge)
- Barotrauma (caused by barometric changes, e.g. diver's ear)
- Mastoiditis (ear pain, fever, may occur after otitis media)
- TMJ dysfunction (jaw or ear pain, "clicking")
- Dental abscesses (tooth pain, fever, possible drainage)

- Parotitis secondary to mumps or obstruction (parotic gland irritation or infection)
- Nasopharyngeal neoplasm (confirmed with CT scan and/or biopsy)
- Cerumen impaction (hearing loss, possible pain and itching)
- Tuberculous otitis (rare, diagnosed by biopsy by ENT referral)
- Leprosy (rare) (nasal discharge, hoarseness; nodules, papules, macules on forehead, cheeks, ears; lab results confirms diagnosis)
- Syphilitic otitis (rare, confirmed by positive results on the fluorescent treponemal antibody test [FTA-ABS])
- Tympanosclerosis (diagnosed by ENT, hardening of tympanic membrane)

Treatment:

Otitis Media with Effusion

Serous otitis: Topical decongestants (relieve negative pressure in the middle ear), such as nonprescription 0.25% to 0.5% phenylephrine nasal preparations, two sprays per nostril, repeated in 5 to 10 minutes, or if using a nasal solution, 3 to 4 drops instilled with head hyperextended, followed by 3 to 4 additional drops after turning the head laterally, with the affected side downward may be used. Discontinue topical decongestants after 3 days to avoid rebound hyperemia. Eustachian tube ventilation exercises such as yawning and induced Valsalva's maneuvers to make the ears "pop," equalizing pressure between the middle ear and nasal cavity. For severe serous otitis media, myringotomy (tympanotomy) and inserting middle ear ventilating tubes may be performed. Antibiotics may be needed, usually at half the dose prescribed for acute otitis media.

Acute Otitis Media:

- In severe AOM, infectious disease experts recommend as first-line therapy: Amoxicillin, 250 to 500 mg orally three times a day for 10 days (the initial treatment of choice).
- If symptoms fail to improve within 2 days, or in communities where resistant organisms are prevalent, or for an immunocompromised patient, beta-lactamase–resistant antibiotics, such as trimethoprim-sulfamethoxazole, one double-strength tablet 8 mg TMP/kg/day divided into two daily doses; or amoxicillin plus clavulanate (Augmentin), 500 mg twice a day or 875 mg twice a day with food for 10 days may be used.
- For penicillin allergic patients, erythromycin (E-Mycin) one 333-mg tablet every 8 hours with food for 10 days.
- Otalgia may be relieved by applying heat to the areas surrounding the affected ear or with nonprescription pain relievers such as aspirin, acetaminophen, or anti-inflammatory agents 600 mg every 4 hours.

Codeine, 15 to 60 mg orally every 4 to 6 hours, may help to control severe pain. Topical pain relievers such as benzocaine (Americaine or Auralgan Otic Solution), 4 to 5 drops every 2 to 4 hours, may also be prescribed. Cortisporin Otic Suspension (polymyxin B sulfate, neomycin, and hydrocortisone), 4 drops in the affected ear four times a day for 7 to 10 days, may be used to relieve inflammation.

Alternative drugs are indicated for a significant group of AOM patients:

- Patients with penicillin allergy
- Persistent symptoms after 48 to 72 hours of amoxicillin
- AOM within 1 month of amoxicillin therapy
- AOM due to *Chlamydia trachomatis* responds to macrolides and sulfonamides.
- AOM due to *Mycoplasma pneumoniae* responds to macrolides
- Clarithromycin is not effective against *Haemophilus influenzae*
- Both trimethoprim-sulfamethoxazole and erythromycin sulfisoxazole 40 mg/kg/day may be less effective in treating some strains of pneumococci (approximately 30%).
- For recurrent AOM, a single 75-mg/kg dose of sulfisoxazole may be used.
- If a perforated tympanic membrane fails to heal spontaneously within 2 months, microsurgical repair may be needed.

Follow-up: See all severe cases after 10 days of therapy to assess effectiveness of treatment. See the patient with serous otitis media 4 to 6 weeks after treatment for evaluation. See the patient with acute otitis media in 72 hours if symptoms have not resolved; otherwise, see patient several days after the completion of pharmacotherapy. See patient with chronic otitis media once a month to assess efficacy of treatment and monitor for recurrence, refer to otolaryngologist for further evaluation.

Sequelae: Possible complications include irreversible conductive hearing loss; chronic otitis media; otitis interna (labyrinthitis); vertigo; ataxia; or several acute, subacute, and chronic infections of adjacent cranial structures, including mastoiditis, meningitis, and epidural, subdural, or brain abscesses. Other complications include perforation of the tympanic membrane, cholesteatoma, facial nerve palsies, lateral sinus thrombophlebitis, and otitic hydrocephalus.

Prevention/prophylaxis: Prevention strategies include advising the patient to stop smoking or clear household of cigarette smoke; avoid swimming until infection clears; to keep ear canal dry; avoid putting cotton swabs or sharp objects in the ear; avoid flying; and avoid traumatic injuries to the middle ear. If the tympanic membrane is perforated, advise the patient to avoid blowing the nose or to blow it gently. Teach the patient how to clean the ear canal without using chemical agents, sharp objects, cotton swabs, or a finger.

Referral: Refer to, or consult with, a specialist or otorhinolaryngologist in the following instances: if a patient with serous otitis media has hearing loss that lasts longer than 6 weeks, extends bilaterally, or reaches more than 20 decibels; or if a patient with acute otitis media has vertigo or ataxia, has a ruptured tympanic membrane close, nonhealing has symptoms that worsen after 3 to 4 days of treatment, or has significant hearing loss that persists for more than 3 weeks; or if a patient with subacute, recurrent, or chronic otitis media fails to clear after two to three courses of antibiotics.

Education: Explain disease process, signs and symptoms, and treatment (including side effects of medications). Discuss prevention strategies. Encourage the patient to seek medical attention if symptoms have not been relieved after 48 hours of treatment, to complete the full regimen of antibiotic therapy, and to reduce activities or maintain bed rest if symptoms are severe.

PHARYNGITIS, TONSILLITIS

Pharyngitis and Tonsillitis

SIGNAL SYMPTOMS ▶ Sore throat, dysphagia

Acute pharyngitis	ICD-9-CM: 462.00
Acute tonsillitis	ICD-9-CM: 463.00
Chronic pharyngitis	ICD-9-CM: 472.10
Chronic tonsillitis	ICD-9-CM: 474.00
Streptococcal sore throat	ICD-9-CM: 034.00
Scarlet fever	ICD-9-CM: 034.10

Description: Pharyngitis and tonsillitis are generalized inflammatory processes involving the pharynx and pharyngeal tonsils, respectively, caused by an acute infection. Of greatest concern is the group A streptococcus due to the potential risk of rheumatic sequelae.

Etiology: Acute cases are caused by both bacteria and viruses. Chronic low-grade symptoms may be related to reflux disease or vocal abuse.

Occurrence: Occurs in colder months. About 12% to 25% of sore throats are responsible for outpatient visits. School-age children, about 11%, see their health care provider for pharyngitis.

Age: Occurs at any age; streptococcal infection has greatest incidence 5 to 18 years of age.

Ethnicity: There is no significant ethnic predisposition.

Gender: Men and women are equally affected.

Contributing Factors: Individuals with a positive family history of rheumatic fever show a higher risk of rheumatic sequelae following a contracted group A hemolytic streptococcal infection. Upper respiratory tract infection, immunocompromised status such as that with a chronic illness (e.g., diabetes mellitus and white blood cell dyscrasias such as agranulocytosis or acute leukemia), work-related stress, excessive alcohol consumption, close living quarters, person-to-person contact, history of receptive oral intercourse with an infected sexual partner, excessive antibiotic use. Tobacco and particularly marijuana smoking, exposure to allergens such as dust and pollen, past or family history of allergic reactions, low humidity, mouth breathing.

Signs and symptoms: Signs and symptoms vary and are those typically seen with the specific causative agent.

General: Most patients report mild to severe throat pain or the sensation of a "tickle" or pruritus in the throat. Other symptoms may include malaise, generalized aches and pains, and headache and irritability. With tonsillitis, the patient may have swollen lymph glands bilaterally between the fauces of the posterior pharynx with associated anterior neck pain. With severe tonsillitis, the patient may also have ear pain, dysphagia and tonsillar exudates. Temperatures > 101.5°F suggest a streptococcal infection. Characteristic erythematous-based clear vesicles are seen in herpes stomatitis. Scarlet fever rash is described as punctate erythematous macules with reddened flexor creases and circumoral pallor equal streptococcal pharyngitis. Gray pseudomembrane found in diptheria and, occasionally, mononucleosis is seen. Many patients describe their throats as feeling swollen with a "lump" in the back of the throat that persists despite repeated swallowing. With viral infections, the patient may also have laryngitis and cough as well as conjunctivitis (usually adenovirus). Anorexia is common with this infection. Physical examination may reveal edematous and erythematous pharyngeal mucosa and tonsils; soft palate petechiae; significant, tender, anterior cervical lymphadenopathy; conjunctivitis.

Chronic pharyngitis: Symptoms include persistent, clear postnasal drip; paroxysmal sneezing; itchy, watery eyes; rhinorrhea; and a mild sore throat that typically worsens with recumbency. Physical examination may reveal edematous pharyngeal mucosa and tonsils with minimal erythema of the pharynx. Also, symptoms may be associated with allergies.

Diagnostic tests: Diagnostic testing and identification of causative organisms through culture are usually unnecessary if the patient's clinical picture is consistent with influenza, the common cold, or irritant-induced throat inflammation. However, bacterial and viral cultures of throat swabs may be appropriate for more complicated or resistant cases. Tests performed include those specific to the suspected agent.

Test	Result indicating disorder	CPT code
Rapid strep test	To detect group A streptococcal antigens and diagnose infection	87650
Throat culture (throat swab), the gold standard test for diagnosis of streptococcal infection	Streptococcal organism present Perform for the patient with a sore throat and either a temperature above 38.7°C (101°F), tonsillar exudate, or anterior cervical lymphadenopathy,	87071
A CBC may be done for any patient with infectious pharyngitis	An increase in granulocytes indicates bacterial etiology; Lymphocytosis (50% lymphocytes with at least 10% of atypical morphology) indicates viral etiology.	85025
Gram stain	Eosinophils in nasal secretions strongly indicates noninfectious (allergic) pharyngitis	87205
CT scan of the neck	May indicate peritonsillar abscesses	70490 without contrast 70491 with contrast

CBC, complete blood count; CT, computed tomography.

Differential diagnosis: Includes all of the causes listed in the table

- Rhinitis (inflammation of nasal mucosa, sneezing, nasal discharge and obstruction, purulent nasal discharge)
- Peritonsillar abscess (uvula is not midline, tonsils asymmetrical, refer to ENT)
- Noninfectious (allergic) pharyngitis
- Sinusitis (concurrent nasal drainage, possible fever, congestion, tenderness and pain over sinus)
- Stomatitis (tender, ulcerated and/or bleeding gums, infection with fusospirochetal organism)
- Epiglottitis (child usually in tripod position, drooling, no speech, looks sick)
- Pharyngeal or tonsillar malignancy (confirmed by CT scan)

Treatment:

Symptomatic

For throat pain: Voice rest; ambient humidification, such as with a cool-mist ultrasonic humidifier; saline nasal sprays; viscous Xylocaine; various types of gargles, such as hot or cold double-strength tea or a warm salt-water solution (1 teaspoon salt in 8 ounces of warm water); nonpre-scription throat lozenges such as zinc lozenges with vitamin C and Echinacea; nonprescription analgesics, such as acetaminophen or aspirin, 650 mg every 4 to 6 hours (for mild pain); codeine preparations, 30 to 60 mg orally every 4 to 6 hours (for severe pain).

For enlarged, tender cervical lymph glands: Warm, moist compresses applied four times a day for 30 to 60 minutes at a time. For fatigue and malaise: Limit physical activity until symptoms have subsided; advise bed rest if fever is present. To maintain nutritional intake: Increase daily fluid intake (such as water or nonacidic juices) to 8 to 12 glasses. For dysphagia: A liquid or soft-food diet, such as milkshakes, soups, and high-protein diet drinks. Xylocaine viscous 2% gargle 1 tsp every 4 to 6 hours may be used.

Bacterial or Fungal Infections

Therapies for a full 10-day course include penicillin V potassium, 250 mg twice a day or four times a day for 10 days (25 to 50 mg/kg/day). If the patient is allergic to penicillin, erythromycin, 300 to 400 mg twice a day for 10 days (30 mg/kg/day), is recommended. For penicillin-resistant beta-lactamase–producing organisms, amoxicillin-clavulanate potassium, (Augmentin) 40 mg/kg per day PO in three divided doses; or erythromycin ethyl succinate, 50 mg/kg per day orally in three divided doses. Other therapies include ceftriaxone (for *Neisseria gonorrhoeae* infections); nystatin or clotrimazole (for candidal infections); and erythromycin, 250 mg twice a day or four times a day for 10 days (for *M. pneumoniae* or *Chlamydia* infections). Penicillin is the treatment most documented to prevent rheumatic sequelae but cephalosporins have lower rate of bacteriologic failure. The newer macrolides erythromycin and clarithromycin are also effective against streptococci pharyngitis but are more expensive. The chief advantage is patient compliance with a 5-day course with a 10-day effective duration. Also, cephalosporins are generally effective but also are more expensive then cephalexin. For chronic pharyngitis, minimize contact with the environmental irritant. Treat patient symptomatically with a combination of antihistamines and decongestants.

Surgical

Refer to otolaryngologist for evaluation for a tonsillectomy which is recommended if the patient has any of the following: airway obstruction; more than three occurrences per year; mild dysphagia; a history of rheumatic fever with heart damage; or if the tonsils remain chronically hypertrophied.

Complementary Therapy

Nutrients for the patient with influenza or tonsillitis (Table 4–1)

- ACES + ZN—Vitamins A, C, and E plus selenium and zinc
- Vitamin A plus natural beta-carotene or carotenoid complex
- Vitamin C with bioflavonoids
- Zinc lozenges
- Colloidal silver for viral infections and promotes healing
- Free form amino acid complex—repair tissue and control fever
- Maitake extract/shitake extract or reishi extract—boost immunity and fight viral infections
- Chlorophyll—used as a gargle
- Grape seed extract or pycnogenol—reduces inflammation

Table 4–1 Complementary therapy for colds, fever, flu, inflammation and/or infections including all types of coughs

Common Name	Scientific Name	Other Specific Uses
Angelica Root	Angelica archangelica	
Boneset Herb	Eupatorium perfoliatum	
Catnip Herb	Nepeta cataria	
Chamomile Flowers, German	Matricaria chamomilla	
Elderberry Flowers	Sambucus canadensis	Also helpful in treating sinusitis and hay fever
Elecampane Root	Inula helenium	
Eyebright Herb	Euphrasia officinalis	Treats congestion of nasal catarrh and sinusitis
Fenugreek Seed	Foeniculum vulgare	Eases bronchitis and sore throats
Garlic	Allium sativum	Also powerful preventative
Ginger Root	Zingiber officinalis	
Goldenrod Flowering Tops	Solidago canadensis/odora	
Goldenseal Root	Hydrastis canadensis	
Horseradish Root	Amoracia rusticana	Useful in sinusitis and laryngitis
Hyssop Flowering Herb	Hyssopus officinalis	
Licorice Root	Glycyrrhiza glabra	
Mullein Leaf and Flowers	Verbascum thapsus	
Myrrh Gum	Commiphora molmol	Effective in mouth infections sinusitis, laryngitis
Osha Root	Ligusticum porterii	
Peppermint Leaf	Mentha piperita	
Pleurisy Root	Asclepias tuberosa	
Red Clover Blossoms		Coughs and mild skin conditions, eczema
Sage Leaf	Salvia officinalis	Gingivitis, laryngitis, and tonsillitis
Thyme Leaf	Thymus vulgaris	Sore throats, laryngitis
Wild Cherry Bark	Prunus serotina	
White Pine Bark	Pinus strobes	
Wild Indigo Root	Baptisia tinctoria	

Follow-up: If symptoms do not improve in 2 to 3 days, see patient for further evaluation for sequelae and possible dehydration because most cases are usually self-limiting and symptoms tend to improve within this time frame. The usual course of streptococcal pharyngeal infection is a 5-day course with peak of fever at 2 to 3 days.

Sequelae: Possible complications include pneumonia, airway obstruction, epiglottitis, severe respiratory complications, mastoiditis, sinusitis and rhinitis, otitis media, cervical adenitis, peritonsillar abscess, scarlet fever, septicemia or autoimmune rheumatic fever, hematuria, and post-streptococcal glomerulonephritis.

Prevention/prophylaxis: Prevention strategies for infectious forms of pharyngitis and tonsillitis include advising the patient to avoid contact with persons with actively inflamed throats, particularly those with URIs; to avoid sharing personal items such as washcloths, food, and eating and drinking utensils during the active infection; to replace toothbrushes as soon as a sore throat develops and after treatment of infection; to keep all immunizations up to date; and to practice safe sex, especially if performing oral sex. For chronic pharyngitis, advise the patient to avoid environmental irritants such as tobacco and marijuana smoke, pollution, dust and other allergens, and low-humidity environments.

Referral: Refer to otolaryngologist as needed for evaluation for tonsillectomy or abscess drainage.

Education: Explain disease process, signs and symptoms, and treatment (including side effects of medications). Discuss prevention strategies.

Figure 4–3 for steps in the differential diagnosis of pharyngitis.

RHINITIS, ALLERGIC

SIGNAL SYMPTOM▶ Constant nasal drainage

Rhinitis, allergic	ICD-9-CM: 472.0

Description: Rhinitis (coryza) is an inflammation of the nasal mucosa that is usually accompanied by edema and a profuse nasal discharge. It may be acute or chronic and allergic or nonallergic.

Etiology: Viral rhinitis usually results from viral upper respiratory tract infections. Common viral agents include rhinovirus, influenza virus, parainfluenza virus, respiratory syncytial virus, coronavirus, adenovirus, echovirus, and coxsackievirus. Allergic rhinitis results from an immediate and delayed reaction to airborne allergens, beginning with antigen-responsive IgE antibody receptors on most cells of the nasal mucosa, followed by this infiltration into the reactive region of the eosinophils, neutrophils, basophils, and mononuclear cells. Vasomotor rhinitis is a chronic condition of unknown etiology. Rhinitis medicamentosa results from the chronic use or abuse of topical nasal decongestants. Atrophic rhinitis is thought to be caused by bacterial infection. The condition may be seasonal or perennial depending on climate and individual response and the offending antigens. Seasonal responses are usually to grasses, trees, and weeds. Perennial responses are usually house mites, mold antigens, and animal by products.

Occurrence: Common.

Age: Viral rhinitis occurs at all ages. Allergic rhinitis: Occurs in all ages, most commonly between ages 30 and 40 years; rare in adults older than

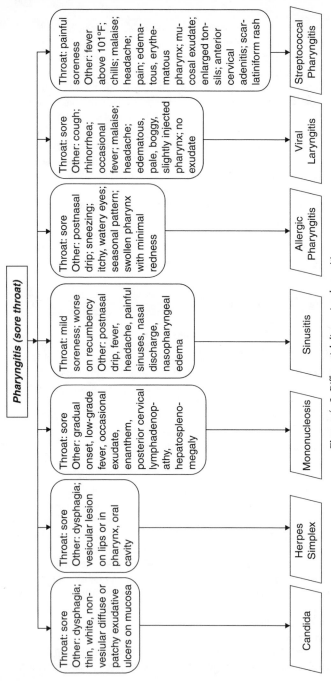

Pharyngitis (sore throat)

Candida
Throat: sore
Other: dysphagia; thin, white, nonvesicular diffuse or patchy exudative ulcers on mucosa

Herpes Simplex
Throat: sore
Other: dysphagia; vesicular lesion on lips or in pharynx, oral cavity

Mononucleosis
Throat: sore
Other: gradual onset, low-grade fever, occasional exudate, enanthem, posterior cervical lymphadenopathy, hepatosplenomegaly

Sinusitis
Throat: mild soreness; worse on recumbency
Other: postnasal drip, fever, headache, painful sinuses, nasal discharge, nasopharyngeal edema

Allergic Pharyngitis
Throat: sore
Other: postnasal drip; sneezing; itchy, watery eyes; seasonal pattern; swollen pharynx with minimal redness

Viral Laryngitis
Throat: sore
Other: cough; rhinorrhea; occasional fever; malaise; headache; edematous, pale, boggy, slightly injected pharynx; no exudate

Streptococcal Pharyngitis
Throat: painful soreness
Other: fever above 101°F; chills; malaise; headache; pain; edematous, erythematous pharynx; mucosal exudate; enlarged tonsils; anterior cervical adenitis; scarlatiniform rash

Figure 4-3. Differential diagnosis: pharyngitis.

age 50 years; onset of symptoms usually between ages 10 to 20 years. Vasomotor rhinitis: Usually manifests during the third and fourth decades. Rhinitis medicamentosa: Primarily affects young to middle-aged adults. Atrophic rhinitis: Primarily affects older adults, although onset of symptoms may begin as early as puberty.

Ethnicity: Most forms of rhinitis appear to have no significant ethnic predispositions; however, blacks and people of Hispanic and Asian heritage are particularly susceptible to atrophic rhinitis.

Gender: Viral and atrophic rhinitis occur in women more than in men; other forms occur equally in men and women.

Contributing factors: Viral rhinitis: Exposure to virus, URI. Allergic rhinitis: Exposure to offending allergens (commonly pollen and mold spores for seasonal form; dust, mites, tobacco smoke, and animal dander for perennial form); immunosuppression secondary to illness or medication use; family history of allergic diseases such as eczema and asthma. Vasomotor rhinitis: Low humidity, sudden temperature or pressure changes, cold air, strong odors, emotional stress, cigarette smoke, and other nasal irritants. Rhinitis medicamentosa: Use of nasal decongestants more frequently than every 3 hours or for periods longer than 3 weeks.

Signs and symptoms:

Viral rhinitis: Malaise, headache, substernal tightness or burning, and occasionally fever, sneezing, coughing, and a sore or burning throat. Physical examination may reveal a tender, erythematous external nose with a transnasal crease; enlarged nasal turbinates, palatine or pharyngeal tonsils (adenoids); friable, erythematous nasal mucosa; erythematous and edematous pharyngeal mucosa or vocal cords; and if complicated by a secondary bacterial infection, nasal discharge may be greenish-yellow.

Allergic rhinitis: Itching in the nasal passages, conjunctivae, and roof of the mouth; epiphora (stringy, watery ocular discharge); sneezing; coughing; and a sore or burning throat. Physical examination may reveal a tender, erythematous external nose with a transnasal crease; enlarged nasal turbinates, palatine, or pharyngeal tonsils (adenoids); a pale, boggy (edematous) nasal mucosa with a blue, yellow, gray, or erythematous hue; gray-blue to yellow-tan nasal polyps (with chronic perennial rhinitis); inflamed conjunctivae (allergic conjunctivitis) with the palpebral conjunctiva being particularly edematous (chemosis) and "cobblestoned" in appearance; dark circles under the eyes ("allergic shiners"); and excess wrinkles under the lower eyelid (Dennie lines).

Vasomotor rhinitis: Pronounced, watery, postnasal drip (watery rhinorrhea); rapid-onset, persistent nasal obstruction or congestion that may switch sides with each attack; nasal speech;

and forced mouth-breathing. Physical examination may reveal bright red to blue nasal mucosa and swollen nasal turbinates.

Rhinitis medicamentosa: Dry, rubbery nasal mucosa. Physical examination may reveal an injected and edematous nasal mucosa and an increased heart rate and blood pressure (because of the effects of sympathomimetic decongestants).

Atrophic Rhinitis: Nasal congestion, a thick postnasal drip, frequent clearing of the throat, anosmia, a constant foul odor in the nose, and severe epistaxis. Physical examination may reveal nasal mucosa crusted with dried mucus or blood and patent nasal passages.

Diagnostic tests: Diagnostic tests are not typically indicated for uncomplicated cases of viral rhinitis, allergic rhinitis, rhinitis medicamentosa (usually diagnosed by history), or vasomotor rhinitis (tends to be a diagnosis of exclusion), although intradermal skin testing of minute amounts of allergens may help diagnose allergic rhinitis. Corticosteroids will ablate eosinophils.

Test	Result indicating disorder	CPT code
Nasal mucosal biopsy and bacterial cultures of nasal secretions	To confirm diagnosis of atrophic rhinitis	30100
If an exudate is present, a Giemsa- or Wright-stained smear	Eosinophils in nasal secretions strongly indicates noninfectious (allergic) pharyngitis	87205
CBC	Leukocytosis or polymorphonuclear neutrophils usually indicate infectious disorder; Eosinophilia usually indicates allergic rhinitis.	85025
Nasal probe smear with cytologic exam	Positive for eosinophils	88160
IgE level	Increased	82785
RAST determinations	Determines specific suspected allergens	95065
Sinus films when indicated	Significant for opacity, fluid level and mucosal thickening.	70220

CBC, complete blood count; IgE, immunoglobulin E; RAST, radioallergosorbent test.

Differential diagnosis:

- Acute or chronic sinusitis (facial pressure and pain, maxillary toothache)
- Foreign bodies of the nose (may be visible, consider if treatment unsuccessful for other possible diagnoses)
- Nasal polyps (present during visual examination)
- Deviated nasal septum
- Cocaine, inhalant, and other forms of substance abuse (history of substance abuse)
- Chronic inflammatory conditions such as sarcoidosis (cough, wheezing, eye/skin changes, shortness of breath, fever, fatigue, weight loss)

- Hormonal changes associated with pregnancy and thyroid disorders
- Nonallergic rhinitis with eosinophilia syndrome (NARES) and IgA deficiency with recurrent sinusitis
- Chronic aspirin use and aldosterone-converting enzyme inhibitors are other diagnoses to consider.

Treatment:

Viral rhinitis: Treat symptoms. Fever and headache may be treated with acetaminophen, 325 mg, two tablets every 4 hours as needed. Rhinorrhea may be treated with decongestants such as pseudo-ephedrine 15 to 120 mg, phenylpropanolamine, 15 to 30 mg orally every 3 to 4 hours as needed; or 0.25 to 0.5% phenylephrine nasal spray, one to two sprays in each nostril every 3 to 4 hours for no longer than 3 to 4 days. Persistent cough may be treated with codeine preparations, 10 to 15 mg every 3 to 4 hours as needed, or dextromethorphan, 15 to 30 mg every 3 to 4 hours prn.

Allergic rhinitis: Advise patient to avoid or reduce exposure to offending allergens. To reduce inflammation, nonsedating antihistamines, such as loratadine, 10 mg orally every day (least sedative effects but monitor carefully for potential drug interactions); other classes of antihistamines such as triprolidine, 50 mg four times a day; promethazine, 12.5 to 25 mg four times a day; or hydroxyzine, 10 to 25 mg four times a day (moderate sedative effects); and cyproheptadine, 4 mg four times a day; or diphenhydramine, 25 to 50 mg four times a day (strongest sedative effects). To reduce nasal congestion, 0.25% to 0.5% phenylephrine nasal spray or drops, one to two sprays or 2 to 3 drops in each nostril every 3 to 4 hours for no longer than 3 to 4 days, may be initiated before antihistamines; a topical saline solution applied two to four times per day; or antihistamine-decongestant combinations. If antihistamine and antihistamine-decongestant combinations are ineffective, topical steroid-containing nasal sprays, such as beclomethasone, one spray in each nostril, two to four times per day; dexamethasone, two sprays in each nostril, two to four times per day; or flunisolide, two sprays in each nostril, two to three times per day, may be useful. However, steroid therapy may require up to 2 weeks of use before symptomatic relief is realized. Desensitizing immunotherapy may be an option for patients refractory to pharmacologic treatment.

Vasomotor rhinitis: Treat symptoms. A vaporizer or humidified central heating system for environmental humidification. Topical saline nasal sprays or powered devices such as a Grossan irrigator for congestion and to restore nasal patency. Topical ipratropium may also relieve symptoms. Systemic decongestants, such as pseudoephedrine, 60 mg three or four times per day; or phenylpropanolamine, 30 mg three times per day, for rhinorrhea. Intranasal steroid preparations may also be helpful if other treatments are ineffective.

Rhinitis medicamentosa: Immediately stop all topical decongestant use; condition typically resolves in 2 to 3 weeks. Oral antihistamine-decongestant preparations; short courses of topical nasal steroids; or systemic steroids, such as prednisone, 40 mg given orally tapered over 8 to 10 days provide symptomatic relief.

Atrophic rhinitis: Topical bacitracin ointment intranasally two to three times per day until the nasal crusting and foul odor are eliminated. Expectorants, such as guaifenesin, 200 mg/5 mL, 10 mL every 4 hours; physiologic saline solutions; or powered irrigators such as the Grossan irrigator provide symptomatic relief. Surgical restoration of nasal cavity patency should be used only as a last resort. Postmenopausal women may be helped by systemic estrogens.

Follow-up: See patient in 2 to 3 weeks for evaluation of the effectiveness of treatment.

Sequelae: Possible complications include serous otitis media, acute or chronic sinusitis, repeated or disseminated respiratory infections; restless sleeping, chronic fatigue, and asthma (allergic rhinitis); and physical addiction to topical nasal decongestants (rhinitis medicamentosa).

Prevention/prophylaxis: Prevention strategies include the following: Viral rhinitis: Advise the patient to avoid or limit exposure to persons with active URIs. Allergic rhinitis: Advise the patient to avoid exposure to environmental irritants and allergens; to take steps to reduce pollen exposure (such as by using air conditioners or high-efficiency particle air filters; by minimizing contact with pets or keeping pets outside; by avoiding being outside on excessively windy days; by keeping ambient humidity between 30% to 40%; use nasal lavage twice a day; by thoroughly cleaning or removing carpets, drapes, curtains, and fabric-covered or stuffed furniture, as well as damp mopping, floor waxing, and dusting of all surfaces with a damp cloth. To help prevent allergic flare-ups, advise the patient in the prophylactic use of 4% cromolyn sodium nasal spray, one spray in each nostril, three to six times per day at regular intervals; or ophthalmic cromolyn sodium preparation, 1 to 2 drops in each eye, four to six times per day. Vasomotor rhinitis: Advise the patient to limit exposure to environmental triggers. Rhinitis medicamentosa: Advise the patient to avoid topical nasal decongestant use or use only as directed.

Referral: Refer to, or consult with, allergist physician for allergen skin testing, immunotherapy, nasal irrigation, or diagnosis and treatment of certain sequelae such as chronic sinusitis or high fever. Refer to surgeon if patient has anatomic obstructions of the nasal cavity (e.g., nasal polyps, deviated septum). Also, a nasopharyngoscopy may be indicated.

Education: Explain disease process, signs and symptoms, and treatment (including side effects of medications). Discuss prevention strategies and when to seek medical attention.

Refer to Figure 4–4 for steps in the differential diagnosis of rhinitis.

SINUSITIS

Sinusitis

SIGNAL SYMPTOMS ▶ facial pressure and pain; maxillary toothache

Sinusitis (chronic)	ICD-9-CM: 473.9
Chronic maxillary sinusitis	ICD-9-CM: 473.0
Sinusitis (acute), frontal	ICD-9-CM: 461.10
Ethmoid	ICD-9-CM: 461.20
Maxillary sinusitis	ICD-9-CM: 461.0
Sphenoidal	ICD-9-CM: 461.30
Sinusitis (fungal)	ICD-9-CM: 117.9
Other acute sinusitis (pansinusitis)	ICD-9-CM: 461.80

Description: Sinusitis is an inflammation of the mucous membranes of one or more of the paranasal sinuses: frontal, sphenoid, anterior ethmoid, and maxillary, with the latter two sinuses most often affected. It may be classified as acute (<4 weeks' duration), characterized by an abrupt onset of infection; subacute (4 to 12 weeks, symptomatic), in which a purulent nasal discharge persists despite therapy; or chronic (>12 weeks), which occurs with episodes of prolonged inflammation.

Etiology: Causes may be infectious both viral and bacterial. *Streptococcus pneumoniae, H. influenzae,* and *Branhamella (Moraxella) catarrhalis* are the most common causative agents in acute sinusitis. The bacteria in chronic sinusitis may be *Staphylococcus aureus, Pseudomonas,* and other gram-negative and gram positive aerobes. *Aspergillus* is the most common fungal organism that cause sinusitis.

Occurrence: Common. Acute bacterial sinusitis accounts for 16 million clinical visits annually.

Age: Occurs in all ages.

Ethnicity: No significant ethnic predisposition.

Gender: Men and women are equally affected.

Contributing factors: URI; smoking; air pollution; persistent coughing; sneezing against a closed mouth; exposure to cold, damp outdoor weather or dry indoor heat; summer activities such as contact with airborne allergens and swimming in contaminated water; injury to the nose or sinuses from foreign bodies or trauma; chronic use of over-the-counter (OTC) or prescription decongestants; dental abscess; recurrent or persistent bacterial infection; allergic rhinitis; asthma; anatomic abnormalities such as a deviated septum and hypertrophy of tonsils and adenoids; mucosal IgA deficiency; immobile cilia syndrome (Kartagener's syndrome); cystic fibrosis; chronic inflammatory diseases such as sarcoidosis and Wegener's granulomatosis; immunocompromised status (severe invasive sinus disease).

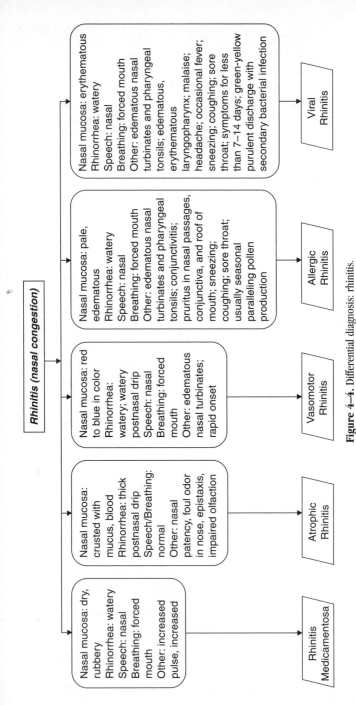

Figure 4–4. Differential diagnosis: rhinitis.

Rhinitis (nasal congestion)

Rhinitis Medicamentosa
Nasal mucosa: dry, rubbery
Rhinorrhea: watery
Speech: nasal
Breathing: forced mouth
Other: increased pulse, increased

Atrophic Rhinitis
Nasal mucosa: crusted with mucus, blood
Rhinorrhea: thick postnasal drip
Speech/Breathing: normal
Other: nasal patency, foul odor in nose, epistaxis, impaired olfaction

Vasomotor Rhinitis
Nasal mucosa: red to blue in color
Rhinorrhea: watery; watery postnasal drip
Speech: nasal
Breathing: forced mouth
Other: edematous nasal turbinates; rapid onset

Allergic Rhinitis
Nasal mucosa: pale, edematous
Rhinorrhea: watery
Speech: nasal
Breathing: forced mouth
Other: edematous nasal turbinates and pharyngeal tonsils; conjunctivitis; pruritus in nasal passages, conjunctiva, and roof of mouth; sneezing; coughing; sore throat; usually seasonal paralleling pollen production

Viral Rhinitis
Nasal mucosa: erythematous
Rhinorrhea: watery
Speech: nasal
Breathing: forced mouth
Other: edematous nasal turbinates and pharyngeal tonsils; edematous, erythematous laryngopharynx; malaise; headache; occasional fever; sneezing; coughing; sore throat; symptoms for less than 7–14 days; green-yellow purulent discharge with secondary bacterial infection

Signs and symptoms:

Acute sinusitis: Patient complains of gradual onset, recurrent or chronic dull, constant pain over the affected sinuses (because of expanding purulent inflammation). As sinusitis progresses, pain increases and becomes characteristically throbbing. The pain is exacerbated by coughing and sudden head movements. Frontal sinus pain may worsen with recumbency or flexion of upper body; maxillary sinus pain may worsen when erect; and ethmoidal sinusitis is associated with retro-orbital pain. Other symptoms include nasal congestion (stuffiness), mucopurulent rhinorrhea (runny nose), cough, sore throat, eye pain from ethmoid bone involvement, malaise, and fatigue. Acute sinusitis is strongly predicted by maxillary toothache, a poor response to nasal decongestants, and a colored nasal discharge. Other symptoms may include yellow-green or blood-stained rhinorrhea, voice nasality, anosmia caused by edematous nasal turbinates, early-morning periorbital edema, fever and chills (25% to 50% of cases), and headache that is worse in the morning or when bending forward. The patient may also sometimes report a nonproductive cough and disturbed sleep. Physical examination may reveal purulent nasal secretions, total opacification of affected sinuses on transillumination, and highly erythematous nasal mucosa.

The affected sinuses may be very tender to palpation: sphenoid sinusitis presents as tenderness over the vertex or mastoids; ethmoid sinusitis as retro-orbital or nasal bridge tenderness; maxillary sinusitis as cheek or dental tenderness; and frontal sinusitis as tenderness of the forehead.

Subacute or chronic sinusitis: Patient complains of a persistent cough or coldlike symptoms lasting from several weeks to several months, as well as a headache or pressure across the cranial midline; may be painless in some cases. Fever is less common, and most patients have a past history of responding poorly to sinusitis pharmacotherapy. Other symptoms include a thick postnasal discharge, "popping" ears, excessive tearing, toothache-like cheek pain, difficulty chewing, and halitosis.

Diagnostic tests: Usually diagnosed by history and physical examination.

Test	Result indicating disorder	CPT code
Sinus x-ray studies	Confirm diagnosis or response to treatment. Significant for opacity, fluid level, and mucosal thickening.	70220

(Continued)

Test	Result indicating disorder	CPT code
CT scan	Evaluates disease process, especially with chronic sinusitis	70480 upper facial without contrast 70481 upper facial with contrast 70486 maxillary without contrast 70487 maxillary with contrast
CBC	Detects infection. Increased WBCs. Increased lymphocytes, increased monocytes, increased bands, increased neutrophils	85025
Gram stain or cultures of sinus aspirates or nasal and throat secretions	Detects causative organism	87205
Allergy (RAST) testing	If allergic disease suspected	95065
Culture of sinus aspirates, sinus mucosal biopsy, or flexible fiberoptic rhinoscopy	Typically needed only for subacute or chronic sinusitis cases that are refractory to empiric pharmacotherapy in order to further differentiate the causative organism.	30100

CBC, complete blood count; CT, computed tomography; RAST, radioimmunosorbent assay test; WBCs, white blood cells.

Differential diagnosis:

- Myofascial pain (chronic, recurrent pain in facial muscles; distinguishing feature one or more trigger points)
- Dental abscess (tooth pain, possible drainage, fever)
- Migraine or cluster headache (cluster: eye pain, tearing; migraine unilateral, pulsating, photophobia and phonophobia, prodrome, nausea and vomiting, moderate to severe in intensity)
- Trigeminal neuralgia, allergic rhinitis, vasomotor rhinitis, rhinitis medicamentosa, mechanical nasal airway obstruction, acute upper respiratory tract viral infection (persistent viral rhinitis), chronic inflammatory conditions such as sarcoidosis or Wegener's granulomatosis.

Treatment: Antibiotic and symptomatic therapy is recommended for all forms of sinusitis to prevent disease progression and complications.

Pharmacologic

Analgesics: Acetaminophen, 600 mg every 6 to 8 hours; or acetaminophen, 300 mg, and codeine phosphate, 30 mg, combination.

Decongestants (corrects underlying edematous mucosa): Phenylephrine, one to two upright sprays in each nostril twice or four times a day for no longer than 1 week; or oxymetazoline, one to two upright sprays in each nostril twice or four times a day for no longer than 3 to 4 days. Oral alternatives include pseudoephedrine, 30 to 60 mg orally every 4 to 6 hours.

Expectorants (liquefy sinus secretions and facilitate drainage): Guaifenesin 100 mg/5 mL, 10-20 mL every 4 hours; or iodinated glycerol, 30 to 60 mg orally four times a day.

Topical steroids: Anti-inflammatory topical steroids in nasal spray preparations such as beclomethasone dipropionate, one to two sprays in each nostril twice a day, when sinusitis is secondary to allergic rhinitis.

Antibiotics:

- Empiric antibiotic therapy covering the most common etiologic agents should be instituted before the identification of the causative organism.
- For acute sinusitis, treat for a minimum of 10 days; if only partial response, treat for 14 to 21 days.
- Medications include trimethoprim-sulfamethoxazole twice a day double strength, amoxicillin 500 mg administered orally every 8 hours.
- For penicillin- and cephalosporin-resistant microorganisms, medications such as: cefaclor 500 mg PO every 6 hours; cefuroxime axetil (Ceftin) 250 mg PO every 12 hours; amoxicillin-clavulanate (Augmentin), 500 mg orally every 8 hours with food or clarithromycin (Biaxin), 500 mg orally twice a day. Penicillin- and cephalosporin-allergic patients may be given one double-strength tablet of trimethoprim (160 mg)-sulfamethoxazole (800 mg) orally every 12 hours.
- For immunocompromised patients, coverage against *S. aureus* with dicloxacillin sodium, 250 to 500 mg orally every 6 hours, and gram-negative bacteria, as well as empiric antifungal therapy. For treatment failure (no resolution of symptoms) change therapy for 10 to 14 days more. When there is a lack of response after 3 weeks of antibiotics, perform a Waters view film, limited coronal CT scan, or ENT referral.

Physical

Symptomatic treatment may include use of a cool-mist, ultrasonic humidifier or heated mist from a facial sauna, steam bath, shower, or hot, moist towels wrapped around the face and sinuses (may help relieve sinus and nasal pain and facilitate drainage by thinning and liquefying secretions); increasing fluid intake; and use of saline nose drops (improves sinus drainage).

Surgical

Maxillary sinus puncture and aspiration and washing may be needed to relieve pain that fails to subside following pharmacotherapy. Patient with subacute or chronic sinusitis may require surgery to remove damaged mucosal tissue or correct anatomic obstructions of the sinus ostia. Surgical intervention is necessary for massive nasal polyposes.

Acute complications: Subperiosteal or orbital abscess, frontal soft tissue spread of infection. Mucocele invasive or allergic fungal sinusitis also requires surgery. Cerebrospinal fluid rhinorrhea and an obstructing tumor require surgery also.

Follow-up: See patient in 2 to 3 days for evaluation of symptomatic improvement; then in 10 to 14 days from initial assessment for treatment evaluation.

Sequelae: Possible complications, although relatively uncommon, include visual impairments, ophthalmoplegia, orbital or facial cellulitis, severe fever, aphasia, abducens palsy (cranial nerve VI deficit), seizures, altered mental status, osteomyelitis of the frontal or maxillary bones, focal swelling over the frontal bone (Pott's puffy tumor), meningitis, subdural empyema, epidural abscess, cavernous sinus thrombosis, and other CNS complications.

Prevention/prophylaxis: Prevention strategies include advising the patient to seek prompt medical treatment for all respiratory infections (to help prevent acute sinusitis) and surgical interventions to correct anatomic blockages (to help prevent chronic sinusitis); to avoid contact with contributing factors such as cigarette smoke, airborne allergens, and side effects of OTC antihistamines; to use a humidifier and/or air conditioner (helps prevent recurrent attacks); to discard nose droppers or sprays after use; and to consider desensitization if inflammation is connected with an allergy.

Referral: Refer to, or consult with, a physician, an otolaryngologist, an appropriate specialist, or a surgeon if patient fails to respond to therapy after 3 to 4 weeks, disease is complicated, or surgical intervention is indicated.

Education: Explain disease process, signs and symptoms, and treatment (including side effects of medications). Discuss prevention strategies and when to seek medical attention.

STOMATITIS, APHTHOUS

SIGNAL SYMPTOMS ▶ Prodrome burning/tingling sensation in the oral mucosa; Pain in mouth

Stomatitis, aphthous	ICD-9-CM: 528.2
Stomatitis	ICD-9-CM: 528.00
Herpetic stomatitis	ICD-9-CM: 054.2
Vincent's stomatitis	ICD-9-CM: 101.00

Description: Aphthous stomatitis, also known as recurrent aphthous stomatitis (RAS), aphthous ulcers, or canker sores, is a recurrent, self-limiting condition characterized by painful ulcerative eruptions of the oral mucosa and tongue. It may involve either a portion of or the entire oral cavity. Recurrent aphthae may be divided into three classifications: minor (MiRAS), herpetiform or clusterform (CU), and major (MaRAS).

Etiology: The cause of the condition is unknown but is believed to involve an aberrant immune response triggered by any number of environmental or immune-related factors. Excessive dryness of the mucous membranes, mechanical or thermal injury to the oral cavity, food allergies, and chemical irritation may all be associated with aphthous stomatitis. Vitamin deficiency (riboflavin) causes angular stomatitis. Herpes simplex I and II, consackie A herpangina causes herpetic stomatitis.

Occurrence: Common; however, actual prevalence data have not been documented. Herpangina is fairly common as are nicotinic and denture related stomatitis.

Age: Occurs in adults of all ages; peak initial onset is between ages 10 to 19.

Ethnicity: There is no significant ethnic predisposition.

Gender: Women are affected $>$ men; herpetic—primary infections, children

Hand-foot and mouth disease—children

Vincent's stomatitis—teenagers and young adults

Contributing factors: Immunosuppression; smoking; ill-fitting dentures; recent dental work; poor oral or dental hygiene; contact with irritants or allergens including spicy, acidic, or salty foods, chocolate, peroxide-containing mouthwashes, toothpaste, and other dental care products, and excessively hot foods and beverages.

Signs and symptoms: Patient may complain of a 24- to 48-hour prodrome of burning or tingling sensations in the oral mucosa before the appearance of the ulcer. Oral mucosal pain may be so severe during the first 2 to 3 days that patient may alter normal eating or drinking habits and have difficulty speaking. Rate of recurrence is variable. Fever is rare.

Physical examination may reveal a tender and edematous oral mucosa. MiRAS lesions: Commonly appear singly or in groups of four to five, and located on the nonkeratinized oral mucosa (vestibular and buccal), tongue, soft palate, fauces (oropharyngeal opening), and floor of the mouth. Usually only two or three lesions appear during each attack, but it is not uncommon to see up to 10-15. The shallow, grayish, centrally necrotic ulcers are surrounded by a ring of hyperemia; may be as large as 0.5 cm (or larger in severe cases); usually begin as indurated papules; and are covered by a fibrinous yellow membrane. CU lesions: Characterized by multiple crops (frequently three or four dozen) of small, painful ulcers. Initially oval or round with a yellowish center, they often coalesce to produce large ulcers with irregular margins. MaRAS lesions: Tend to occur with frequency; are large and deep; may persist for several weeks; usually accompanied by severe pain, fever, and lymphadenopathy; may occur on the lips, soft palate, and fauces.

Diagnostic tests: Diagnosed by history and physical examination. Diagnostic tests may be performed to rule out differential diagnoses and may include

Test	Result indicating disorder	CPT code
Vitamin B$_{12}$, folate, and iron levels	Determine presence of nutritional deficiencies with decreases in these levels	82607, 82608 (B12) 83540 (iron) 82746 (folate)
CBC and differential	Rules out anemias and neutropenias.	85025

CBC, complete blood count.

Differential Diagnosis:

- Secondary herpetic stomatitis (development of herpetic lesion in mouth)
- Other bacterial, viral, or fungal infections (CBC and symptoms of infection, fever, chill,
- Self-induced vomiting from bulimia or anorexia (induced vomiting)

 Clinical Pearl: Check fingers for development of callus.

- Systemic or local vasculitis (inflammation of vascular system; hot, tender veins)
- Oral neoplasia (confirmed by biopsy)
- Measles (associated with fine, erythematosus lesions over trunk of body and later extremities)
- Viral infections including infectious mononucleosis, warts, prodromal primary HIV infection, and severe chickenpox.

Treatment: Treatment focuses on healing, prevention, and pain control.

Pharmacologic

Steroids and cytotoxic drugs for Behçet's disease.

Xylocaine viscous 2% for local discomfort.

For pain relief: OTC medications containing benzocaine (works best with MiRAS); apply to affected area three or four times per day. Liquid diphenhydramine swished and swallowed may be helpful. Antifungal ointment, for example, nystatin (Mycostatin) for candida complicating angular stomatitis..

To decrease inflammatory response and promote healing: Corticosteroids, such as fluocinonide cream, 0.05% four times a day (high-potency), or triamcinolone acetonide, 0.1% after meals and at bedtime (medium potency), applied to coat the ulcer with a thin film; most effective when instituted at the first signs of a lesion. Tetracycline syrup, 250 mg/10 mL for 14 days (for CU or MaRAS), along with dexamethasone elixir as a mouthwash, to be used for 2 minutes four times a day, then expectorated. Tell patient not to eat or drink for 20 minutes after using each of these medications. (This therapy will usually heal the lesions in 90% of patients within 7 to 10 days. Reinitiate this therapy at the first hint of recurrence, four times a day for 3 days. Patients with severe, recurrent, scarring aphthae may require systemic prednisone combined with tetracycline syrup.

Physical: General

Stop or correct behaviors or conditions contributing to lesion formation, such as smoking, eating spicy, salty, or hot foods, or wearing ill-fitting dentures. Treat any nutritional deficiencies as appropriate. Encourage consuming fluids (including cool, bland beverages such as milkshakes), ice cream, and custard, or a liquid diet, especially during the first 2 to 3 days if pain is severe and drinking through a straw if lesions are painful. Non-irritating gargles. Good, frequent oral hygiene; have patient brush teeth with a soft-bristled toothbrush at least twice daily and to floss regularly.

Follow-up: For severe cases, see patient within 2 to 3 days, then once a week until all lesions resolve (most resolve within 7 to 14 days with appropriate treatment).

Sequelae: Possible complications include impaired mastication or swallowing, dehydration, and malnutrition.

Prevention/prophylaxis: Prevention strategies include advising the patient to refrain from contributing behaviors such as smoking, eating hot or spicy foods, drinking alcohol, and practicing poor dental hygiene; to avoid exposure to affected persons, allergens, chemical irritants, or foods that seem to trigger attacks; to fit all dentures and dental prostheses properly to prevent mechanical injury of the oral cavity; and to seek early treatment of viral, bacterial, and fungal infections. For stomatitis cases related to bruxism (tooth grinding), a night-guard prosthesis with removable splints to reduce biting pressure on tooth surfaces may reduce damage to dentition and, in turn, prevent related stomatitis.

Referral: Refer to, or consult with, physician if patient has severe dehydration or disseminated infectious symptoms.

Education: Explain disease process, signs and symptoms, and treatment (including side effects of medications). Discuss prevention strategies and the importance of proper oral hygiene and proper nutrition. Reassure patient that ulcers are not contagious and cannot spread.

REFERENCES

General

The Allergy Report: Vol.1. Overview of Allergic Diseases, Vol. 2. Disease of Atopic Diatheses. American Academy of Allergy, Asthma and Immunology, Milwaukee, Wisconsin, 2000.

Balch P, and Balch J: Prescription for Healing. Avery, Penguin Putnam, Inc., New York, 2000.

Collins RD: Algorithmic Approach to Treatment. Williams & Wilkins, Baltimore, 2001.

Dambro M: Griffith's 5 Minute Clinical Consult. Williams & Wilkins, Baltimore, 2002.

Dunphy LM., and Winland-Brown JE: Primary Care: The Art and Science of Advance Practice Nursing, F.A. Davis, Philadelphia, 2001.

Fenstermacher K: Practice Guidelines for Family Nurse Practitioners, 2nd ed., WB Saunders, Philadelphia, 2000

Gilbert D, et al: Sanford Guide to Antimicrobial Therapy. Antimicrobial Therapy, Inc., Hyde Park, Vt., 2001.

Goroll A, May L, and Mulley A: Primary Care Medicine, ed 4. Lippincott-Raven, Philadelphia, 2000.

Hurst J. (ed): Medicine for the Practicing Physician, ed 5. Appleton & Lange, Norwalk, CT, 2001.

Naturopathic Handbook of Herbal Formulas: A Practical and Concise Herb User's Guide, ed 4.. Herbal Research Publications, Inc., New York, 1995.

Noble J (ed): Primary Care Medicine, ed 3. Mosby, St Louis, 2001.

Rakel, R. Textbook of Family Medicine, ed 6. WB Saunders, Philadelphia, 2002.

Sellers, R: Differential Diagnosis of Common Complaints, ed 4. WB Saunders, Philadelphia, 2000.

Uphold C, and Graham MV: Clinical Guidelines for Adult Nurse Practitioners in Family Practice, ed 2. Barmarrae Books, Gainesville, Fla., 1999.

Weiss B: Primary Care 20 Common Problems. McGraw-Hill, New York, 1999.

Woolf J, Jones J, and Lawrence R (eds): Health Promotion and Disease Prevention in Clinical Practice. ed 2. Williams & Wilkins, Baltimore, 2001

Conjunctivitis

Bielory L: Ocular allergy. Respiratory Digest 2:1–5, 2000.

Bielory L, and Friedlander M: Conjunctivitis and allergic eye diseases, In: Kaliner MA, ed: Current Reviews of Allergic Diseases. Current Medicine, Inc, Philadelphia, 2000, pp 207–214.

Morrow G, and Abbott R: Conjunctivitis, American Family Physician Website. *http://www.aafp.org/afp/980215ap/morrow.html.*

Ménière's Disease

Lucente FE, and Gady HE: Essentials of Otolaryngology, ed 4. Lippincott, Williams & Wilkins, Philadelphia, 1999, pp 116–125.

Otitis Media

Leibovitz E, and Dagan R: Otitis media therapy and drug resistance-Part 1: Management principles. Infect. Med 18:212–216, 2001.

Management of Acute Otitis Media. Summary, Evidence Report/Technology Assessment: Number 15, June 2000. Agency for Healthcare Quality and Research, Rockville, MD. *http://www.ahrq.gov/clinic/epcsums/otitissum.htm*

Rhinitis

Economides A, and Kaliner M: Allergic rhinitis. Curr Rev Allerg Dis 227–243, 2000.

Settipane R, and Settipane G: Nonallergic rhinitis. Curr Rev Allerg Dis 111–123, 2000.

Sinusitis

Kaliner, MA: Medical management of sinusitis. Curr Rev Allerg Dis 139-152. 2000.

Osguthorpe JD, and Hadley Jr: Rhinosinusitis: Current concepts in evaluation and management. Med Clin North Am 83:27-41, 1999.

Stomatitis, aphthous

Peterson M, and Baughman R: Recurrent aphthous stomatitis. Nurse Pract 5:36, 1996.

Chapter 5
CHEST DISORDERS

ANGINA, STABLE

SIGNAL SYMPTOMS ▶ Chest discomfort typically with exertion; may be bandlike heaviness, pressure; Dyspnea on exertion (DOE)

Angina	ICD-9-CM: 413.9

Description: Angina is pain that occurs when myocardial oxygen demand exceeds myocardial oxygen supply. Anginal patterns can be classified as stable or unstable. Stable angina is characterized by angina that is controlled with rest or medications and has a stable pattern of occurrence. Unstable angina is defined as new-onset ($<$ 2 months) angina that occurs at rest or low levels of activity; previously stable angina that is increasing in intensity or frequency; or recurrent angina within several days of a myocardial infarction (MI). Unstable angina is a medical emergency.

Etiology: The condition is primarily caused by narrowing of the coronary arteries because of atherosclerosis. Other causes include coronary artery thrombus, coronary artery vasospasm (variant angina or Prinzmetal's angina), aortic stenosis, aortic regurgitation (insufficiency), severe hypertension (HTN), idiopathic hypertrophic subaortic stenosis (IHSS), thoracic aortic aneurysm, or pericarditis.

Occurrence: Cardiovascular disease is the leading cause of death in the United States. Angina is the most common presenting symptom of ischemic heart disease. In the age range 45 to 59 years, 6% of men and 4% of women will present with angina; between the age of 65 and 74 years, it equalizes to 20% for both men and women.

Ethnicity: No significant ethnic predisposition; however, because of a higher prevalence of HTN, blacks may be at increased risk.

Gender: Middle-aged and older men and postmenopausal women are most at risk.

Contributing factors: Smoking, HTN, elevated blood lipids (the three greatest modifiable risk factors), family history of cardiovascular disease, advancing age, diabetes mellitus, obesity, and lack of exercise. For precipitating an attack: Physical activity, emotional stress, large meals, exposure to hot or cold, sexual intercourse, smoking, cocaine abuse.

Signs and symptoms: The classic symptom is chest discomfort, usually described as pressure, tightness (gripping and bandlike), burning, or heaviness. Anginal pain may radiate to the arms, back, neck, jaw, or teeth; or it may be in ONLY any one of these areas. It is sometimes mistaken for indigestion and may be accompanied by nausea or vomiting. The patient may also complain of DOE that is relieved with rest, with no other chest symptoms. Any of these symptoms may be accompanied by diaphoresis, palpitations, or presyncope.

 Clinical Pearl: Patients with coronary artery disease (CAD) may present with the complaint of fatigue *only;* suspect angina if there is new or worsened fatigue.

Chest pain may be:

1. Typical for angina if meets the following criteria:
   - characteristic quality and duration
   - provoked by exertion and/or stress
   - relieved by rest and/or nitroglycerin
2. Atypical for angina
   - if meets two of the above-mentioned criteria
3. Noncardiac
   - meets one or less of above criteria

Stable angina is normally relieved with rest or sublingual nitroglycerin. Pain unrelieved by these measures may indicate unstable angina or an acute MI, in which case, the patient should be transported to the hospital immediately. Pain that is pleuritic, localized to one finger, reproduced by movement or palpation of the chest wall, or is constant for days or lasts only a few seconds is unlikely to be angina.

Diagnostic tests:

Test	Result Indicating Disorder	CPT Code
CBC	Assesses for anemia, which can cause or exacerbate angina	85027
Lipid profile	Assessment of risk	80061
FBS	Assessment of risk	82947
Cardiac enzymes (CPK, LDH, troponins I and II)	Done if presentation is suggestive of unstable angina or MI and patient is admitted to the hospital; will be elevated with acute MI	82550 83615 84484
Nuclear stress test	Will be positive for ischemia in coronary artery disease	78465

(Continued)

Test	Result Indicating Disorder	CPT Code
Echocardiography	Assess chamber size, wall motion, valvular function, ejection fraction	93307 93320 93325
Chest X-ray	Assess heart size, pulmonary vasculature, aorta; rule out other pulmonary processes. Will be normal with angina.	71010 (PA), 71020 (PA& LAT)
Twelve-lead electrocardiogram (ECG)	Rules out acute MI; shows prior Q wave MI, LVH, ST-T changes consistent with ischemia, and establishes the cardiac rhythm	93000
Coronary angiography	Coronary angiography is the gold standard and should be performed in any patient who has a positive nuclear stress test (indicates ischemia), or in any patient with continuing symptoms suggestive of angina despite a negative stress test.	93510 93543 93545 93555 93556

CBC, complete blood count; CPK, creatine phosphokinase; LVH, left ventricular hypertrophy.

Differential diagnosis:

- Unstable angina (crescendo pattern; may occur even at rest)
- Acute MI (unrelieved after three sublingual nitroglycerine)
- Esophagitis (esophageal spasm)
- Peptic ulcer disease (pain may radiate to chest)
- Gastritis (pain may radiate to chest)
- Biliary colic (pain may radiate to chest)
- Costochondritis (sudden onset chest pain)
- Pericarditis (may cause chest pain, shortness of breath [SOB])
- Aortic dissection (can cause chest pain)
- Anxiety and panic disorders (can cause SOB)

Treatment: Immediate referral and transport to a clinical emergency department is indicated if the patient's pain is not relieved by rest or with sublingual nitroglycerin, or if the patient has unstable angina.

Acute Attack

Sublingual nitroglycerin, up to three tablets (usual dosage is 0.4 mg), 5 minutes apart, or nitroglycerin spray, up to three applications (dosage is 0.4 mg per application), with onset of chest pain. Rest is advised for the patient with an acute attack. Maximum of three doses in 15 minutes. If there is no relief, call 911. Nitroglycerin may also be given prophylactically 10 minutes before any activity that might induce angina, for example, sexual intercourse. Teach proper administration (take while sitting or lying) and storage (store in original dark container away from heat and light). Replace nitroglycerin every 6 months. Do not keep in a bottle with other pills.

Pharmacologic

The goal of treatment is to increase myocardial oxygen supply while decreasing oxygen demand. Pharmacologic treatment interferes with the neurohormonal axis (renin-angiotensin-aldosterone system {RAAS}) in order to prevent further myocardial deterioration. Medical management of stable angina includes the following:

- Aspirin, unless contraindicated, 75 to 325 mg per day)
- Beta blockers—all patients with prior infarct should be on a beta blocker. Those with angina should be started on a beta blocker unless contraindicated. (contraindications include abnormal ECG with conduction disease, chronic obstructive pulmonary disease (COPD) or asthma, intolerance of side effects such as fatigue, depression [use with caution], peripheral vascular disease)
- Calcium channel blockers—may substitute for beta blockers if beta blockers are not indicated. May use in addition to beta blockers for anginal control. Caution when using both, monitor cardiac rhythm with ECG for indication of development of conduction abnormalities. (Calcium channel blockers are not recommended if patient has low ejection fraction, or with pre-existing electrical conduction abnormalities such as first-degree block, Mobitz I or II, or bundle branch block).
- Nitrates—consider adding a long-acting nitrate (Imdur, Isordil, nitroglycerin patch) to the regimen if anginal symptoms occur despite using beta blockers and having an optimal blood pressure. (All anginal patients should have an optimal blood pressure). All anginal patients should have sublingual nitroglycerin (NTG SL) tablets or spray to use as directed as needed.
- Lipid-lowering therapy—if the patient is positive for CAD and the low-density lipoprotein (LDL) level is more than 130 (target LDL <100); or hyperlipidemia noted on lipid profile.

Physical

Measures are aimed at reducing CAD risk factors and factors that exacerbate the angina. These measures include lifestyle management with a low-fat, low-salt diet; treatment of HTN, anemia, hyperthyroidism, and congestive heart failure (CHF); and weight loss if overweight. Encourage participation in a cardiac rehabilitation program that provides for safe exercise and risk-factor modification education.

Follow-up: Generally, 5 to 6 months for stable and more frequent visits for changes in clinical status.

Sequelae: Thirty percent of patients with recent onset of angina will have a significant cardiac event within 1 to 2 years. A significant event may include progression to unstable angina, acute MI, CHF, cardiac arrhythmias, or sudden cardiac death.

Prevention/prophylaxis: Prevention strategies include advising the patient to modify CAD risk factors as appropriate, such as stopping smoking, controlling HTN, and maintaining a low-fat, low-cholesterol diet; and to adhere to activity limitations determined by exercise tolerance testing;

to use sublingual nitrates before activity expected to induce angina; and to avoid activity in cold weather or after heavy meals.

Referral: Refer to, or consult with, physician or cardiologist for continuing care and specialized testing such as cardiac catheterization, stress testing, echocardiogram.

Education: Explain disease process, signs and symptoms, and treatment (including side effects of medications). Discuss prevention strategies, importance of complying with therapy, risk factor modifications, importance of cardiac rehabilitation programs and support groups, and when to seek medical care.

ASTHMA

SIGNAL SYMPTOMS▶ SOB with wheezing; Chronic cough that may be worse at night

Asthma	ICD-9-CM: 493.9

Description: Asthma is a chronic lung disorder characterized by airway inflammation, increased airway responsiveness to a variety of stimuli (atopic and nonallergic), and airway obstruction that is at least partially reversible. Asthma is caused by an atopic stimulus and is referred to as extrinsic asthma. Asthma triggered by nonallergic stimuli is referred to as intrinsic asthma. Asthma is classified as:

Step 1: Mild, Intermittent
Step 2: Mild, Persistent
Step 3: Moderate, Persistent
Step 4: Severe, Persistent

Etiology: Underlying cause not completely understood. Asthma is triggered by an allergic stimulus, such as animal dander or pollen, or by a nonallergic stimulus, such as cold air or exercise. Although not all cases involve hereditary factors, two genetic influences are associated with asthma: the capacity to develop allergies and the tendency to develop reactive airway disease independent of allergies.

Occurrence: Affects 5% of the U.S. population (5% of adults; 7% to 10% of children); greatest prevalence in the southeastern states, with 5000 deaths in the United States attributed to asthma each year.

Age: Approximately 50% of cases develop in childhood, with another 33% occurring before age 40 years.

Ethnicity: No significant ethnic predisposition, but incidence among urban blacks and Hispanics is higher.

Gender: In children younger than age 10, the condition affects more boys than girls; at puberty, the incidence is about equal. Adult-onset asthma occurs more often in women than in men.

Contributing factors: Allergens (pollens, fungal spores, dust, dust mites, insect parts, animal danders, foods, drugs, vaccines, parasites); occupational factors (organic dusts, isocyanates, anhydrides, dyes, metal salts); medications (beta blockers, narcotics, aspirin, nonsteroidal anti-inflammatory drugs (NSAIDs), anesthetic agents, food additives); exercise (sports, sexual activity); irritants (odors, chemical fumes, air pollution, tobacco smoke, cold air, paint, perfume, hairspray, barometric pressure, humidity, aspiration, feather pillows); psychogenic factors (fatigue, anxiety, stress, laughter); viral infections (rarely bacterial); positive family history; coexistent illness (nasal polyps, hyperthyroidism, sinusitis, premenstrual state, vagal reflexes, gastroesophageal reflux); circadian rhythm (nocturnal exacerbation).

Signs and symptoms: Signs and symptoms vary in pattern and intensity.

 Clinical Pearl: Clinical appearance of SOB and wheezing may not correlate with the severity of the exacerbation; less wheezing may mean more severe obstruction and less air exchange.

Symptoms may be paroxysmal or continual. They may include SOB; chronic, persistent cough, especially at night; recurrent wheeze; or a feeling of tightness in the chest. The patient may complain of being awakened by nocturnal attacks.

Definition of symptoms by classification:

Classification	Frequency of Symptoms	Exacerbations	Nocturnal Symptoms
Step 1: mild, intermittent	No more than twice weekly	Brief; a few hours to a few days	< two times per month
Step 2: mild, persistent	More than twice weekly but < once daily	When occur may affect activity	More than twice per month
Step 3: moderate, persistent	Daily symptoms	Occur more than twice per week	More than once per week
Step 4: severe, persistent	Continuous symptoms	Frequent ; includes night symptoms	Frequent

The patient should be assigned to the classification of the most severe symptoms. Any patient may have mild, moderate, or severe exacerbations.

Physical examination may reveal wheezing that is usually precipitated by a stimulus and is louder over the lower airways. Hyperresonance may be present. Wheezing may increase at first, and then decrease as expiratory flow decreases; thus, diminished breath sounds in the dyspneic patient are an ominous sign. Other signs may include use of accessory respiratory muscles, tachycardia, cyanosis, pulsus paradoxus (from hyperinflation of the lungs), and Hoover's sign (an inward movement of the lower intercostal spaces with inspiration, which indicates flattening of the diaphragm and hyperinflation). Symptoms indicative of an emergency include peak flow < 50% of predicted normal, failure to respond to a beta agonist, severe wheezing/coughing, extreme anxiety due to breathlessness, gasping for air with diaphoresis or cyanosis, rapid deterioration, retractions or nasal flaring, and hunching forward.

Diagnostic tests: Primarily diagnosed by history, physical examination, and pulmonary function testing. Focus on environmental history and potential allergic/nonallergic triggers. Classify physical symptoms by intensity, duration, and frequency; and by their relationship to season, environment, and diurnal or circadian rhythm.

Test	Result Indicating Disorder	CPT Code
Chest x-ray study	Usually normal: hyperinflation may be seen in those with chronic symptoms	71010 (PA), 71020 (PA & LAT)
CBC with differential	Frequently reveals increased WBCs and eosinophils	85027
Blood chemistries (basic panel)	Usually normal	80049
Sputum culture	May show Curschmann's spirals and clumps of eosinophils	87083
ECG	May show P pulmonale and right axis deviation	93000
Allergy and immuno-deficiency testing	Screening	86005, 86003

CBC, complete blood count; ECG, electrocardiogram; LAT, lateral; PA; posteroanterior; WBCs, white blood cells.

Pulmonary Function Tests

Pulmonary function tests are used to diagnose asthma by documenting the severity and reversibility of airway obstruction. Objective assessments of pulmonary function are necessary for a diagnosis of asthma because medical history and physical examination are not always reliable. Additionally, there is often a lack of correlation between severity of obstruction and clinical symptoms. Spirometry is recommended for diagnostic purposes. Significant airflow obstruction reversibility is demonstrated if airflow improves by 12% or 200 cc forced expiratory volume (FEV) after short-acting bronchodilator is administered. Peak flow meters are designed as monitoring tools. Patients with moderate to severe, persistent asthma should learn how to monitor their peak expiratory flow (PEF) at home with a peak flow meter, once daily, in the morning. Likewise, peak flow monitoring is recommended during exacerbations for these patients. The 1999 Expert Panel Report does *not* recommend long-term daily peak flow monitoring for patients with mild intermittent or mild persistent asthma, except in cases in which it is useful in aiding treatment decisions. Remember that reference values are specific to each brand of peak flow meter and that these norms are not always available.

Mild, intermittent asthma: The forced expiratory volume in 1 second (FEV_1) or PEF rate is 80% of predicted or personal best. The PEF varies < 20% between readings and spirometry is normal.

Mild, persistent asthma: The FEV_1 or PEF is no more than 80% of predicted best, with a PEF variability of 20% to 30%.

Moderate, persistent asthma: The FEV_1 or PEF is more than 60% but <80% of the predicted maximum or personal best. The PEF variability is > 30%. Spirometry demonstrates an obstructive pattern with a > 12% or 200-cc improvement of FEV_1 after administration of short-acting bronchodilators.

Severe, persistent asthma: The FEV_1 or PEF is < 60% of predicted or personal best and the PEF variability is more than 30%. Spirometry reveals an obstructive pattern with > 12% or 200-cc improvement of FEV_1 after administration of short-acting bronchodilator.

Differential diagnosis:

- Pulmonary embolus (may cause sudden SOB and chest tightness)
- Hyperventilation (causes SOB)
- Anxiety (causes hyperventilation)
- Foreign body aspiration (may cause wheezing and SOB)
- Pneumothorax (sudden SOB)
- COPD (exacerbation may cause symptoms resembling asthma)

Treatment: The goals for successful management are to prevent chronic daily symptoms and acute exacerbations; to maintain a normal level of daily functioning, to maintain near-normal pulmonary function (PEF of 80% predicted or personal best and < 20% PEF daily variation), and to minimize adverse medication effects.

Physical

Lifestyle management includes allergy avoidance: Establish allergies by history and skin testing. Lifestyle management should include:

- Decrease exposure to house dust mites, pollens, animal danders; especially in bedrooms
- Encase mattress and bedding in plastic covers; use foam rubber pillows with hypoallergenic casings
- Remove carpets and treat floors with 8% tannic acid or benzoate powder, which kills mites
- Wash bed linen every 7 days in hot water
- Vacuum at least once per week; preferably use a vacuum with a high-efficiency particulate air (HEPA) filter
- Use air conditioner and dehumidifier as needed
- Use exterminator to eliminate cockroaches and keep pets outdoors (these are important sources of allergens)

- Once a month treat window frames, showers, bathrooms, and floors with a solution containing chloride, which kills mold
- Close windows and doors during season when plants are pollinating
- Avoid smoke in the environment
- Avoid beta blockers and sulfites
- Avoid outdoor exercise when pollution or pollen levels are high

Pharmacologic

Medications used to treat asthma include beta 2 agonists, corticosteroids, anti-inflammatory agents, and anticholinergics. The use of theophylline is controversial; current guidelines suggest its use only in the treatment of severe asthma; refer patient to a specialist. For a summary of drug treatment, see Table 5–1.

A stepwise approach to pharmacological therapy is recommended:

- The amount and frequency of medication is indicated by severity of symptoms and directed toward suppression of further airway inflammation.
- Initiate treatment at higher level at onset to get rapid control, then step down; use caution when stepping down
- Continual monitoring is essential

Table 5–1   Commonly Prescribed Drugs for Asthma

Drug Type	Drug
Short-acting beta$_2$ agonists	Albuterol (Ventolin) Pirbuterol (Maxair) Bitolterol (Tornalate) Terbutaline sulfate Brethaire (inhaler) Brethine (tablets)
Long-acting beta agonists	Salmeterol xinafoate (Serevent) Albuterol sulfate Proventil Repetabs
Anticholinergics	Ipratropium bromide (Atrovent)
Combination beta A$_2$ agonist and Anticholinergic	Combivent
Leukotriene Receptor Antagonist	Zafirlukast (Accolate) Zyflo (Zileuton) (5-lipoxygenase inhibitor)
Inhaled nonsteroidal anti-inflammatory agents	Cromolyn sodium (Intal) Nedocromil sodium (Tilade)
Inhaled corticosteroids	Beclomethasone dipropionate (Beclovent) Budesonide Turbuhaler (Pimicort) Turbuhaler Fluticasone propionate (Flovent) Triamcinolone acetonide (Azmacort)
Systemic corticosteroids	Methylprednisolone (Medrol) Prednisolone Prednisone (Deltasone)
Methylxanthine	Theophylline (Theo-Dur, Uni-Dur, Theo-24)

- Identify the minimum therapy needed in order to maintain control

Step 1 (Mild, Intermittent):

- No daily long-term medications are needed
- Short-acting $beta_2$ (such as albuterol, or terbutaline) agonist may be used prn for "rescue."
- Use of short-acting $beta_2$ agonist for over a 2-week period may mean that there is a need to add a long-acting $beta_2$ agonist for long-term treatment (such as salmeterol) to prevent bronchospasm

Step 2 (mild, persistent):

- Use daily inhaled, low-dose corticosteroid (fluticazone-salmeterol, triamcinolone, or budesonide), cromolyn, or nedocromil.
- Add a long-acting antiasthmatic drug like zafirlukast, one of the new leukotriene-receptor agonists (although position in treatment not fully established); 20 mg orally, twice a day, 1 hour before meals (AC) or 2 hours after meals (PC); or salmeterol.
- A short-acting $beta_2$ agonist should always be given for "rescue" or exacerbations

Step 3 (Moderate, Persistent):

- Long-term control used with inhaled steroid and/or long-acting $beta_2$ agonist
- Short-acting $beta_2$ agonist available for "rescue" or exacerbations

Step 4 (Severe, Persistent):

- Long-term control with inhaled anti-inflammatory agent
- Long-term control with long-acting inhaled $beta_2$ agonist
- Corticosteroid —(2 mg/kg/day; not to exceed 60 mg per day)
- Short-acting $beta_2$ agonist for "rescue"

A short course of oral corticosteroids (steroid burst) may be added as necessary at any step during exacerbations. Wash mouth out immediately after use of any corticosteroid inhaler to decrease risk of thrush. In addition, epinephrine may also be used for severe exacerbations (0.3 mg to 0.5 mg SQ every 20 minutes, up to three doses).

Avoid antihistamines with anticholinergic properties. May use newer, nonsedating antihistamines such as loratadine (Claritin), desloratadine (Clarinex), cetirizine (Zyrtec), and fexofenadine (Allegra).

Figure 5-1 provides management of asthma exacerbations through home treatment.

Follow-up: Emphasis on patient-provider communication and patient satisfaction. Monitor spirometry after initial treatment, as needed or yearly. See patient as needed for worsening of symptoms, complications, medication side effects, and evaluation of effectiveness of therapy.

Sequelae: Possible complications include pneumonia, atelectasis, and pneumothorax, as well as acute exacerbations of the disease; respiratory failure; may be fatal.

Home Treatment: Asthma

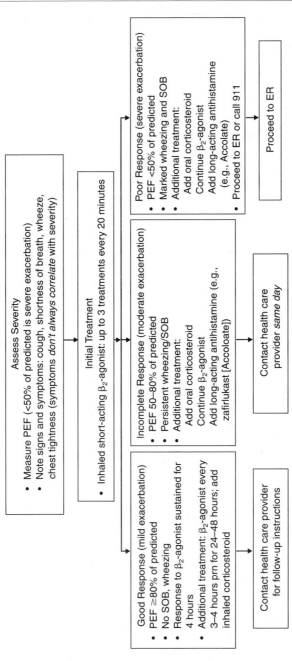

Assess Severity

- Measure PEF (<50% of predicted is severe exacerbation)
- Note signs and symptoms: cough, shortness of breath, wheeze, chest tightness (symptoms *don't always correlate with severity*)

Initial Treatment

- Inhaled short-acting β_2-agonist: up to 3 treatments every 20 minutes

Good Response (mild exacerbation)

- PEF ≥80% of predicted
- No SOB, wheezing
- Response to β_2-agonist sustained for 4 hours
- Additional treatment: β_2-agonist every 3–4 hours prn for 24–48 hours; add inhaled corticosteroid

Contact health care provider for follow-up instructions

Incomplete Response (moderate exacerbation)

- PEF 50–80% of predicted
- Persistent wheezing/SOB
- Additional treatment:
  - Add oral corticosteroid
  - Continue β_2-agonist
  - Add long-acting antihistamine (e.g., zafirlukast [Accolate])

Contact health care provider *same day*

Poor Response (severe exacerbation)

- PEF <50% of predicted
- Marked wheezing and SOB
- Additional treatment:
  - Add oral corticosteroid
  - Continue β_2-agonist
  - Add long-acting antihistamine (e.g., Accolate)
  - Proceed to ER or call 911

Proceed to ER

Figure 5–1. Home Treatment: Asthma. (From Bethesda [MD]: U. S. Dept. of Health and Human Services, Public Health Service, National Institutes of Health, National Heart, Lung and Blood Institute: Expert Panel Report 2: Guidelines for the Diagnosis and Management of Asthma. Jul. 1997 [update Mar. 1999].)

Prevention/prophylaxis: Prevention strategies include teaching patient to avoid asthma triggers and to use medications prophylactically. Yearly purified protein derivation (PPD), flu shot, pneumovax. Early treatment of asthma exacerbations is the best strategy for prevention. See Figure 5–1.

Referral: Consult with the appropriate specialist as indicated. Step 3 and step 4 need a pulmonologist.

Education: Explain disease process, signs and symptoms, and treatment (including side effects of medications). Instruct in the proper use and care of metered-dose inhalers and peak flow meters; teach use of spacers. Discuss methods to use to avoid cigarette smoking, secondhand smoke, and asthma triggers. Teach patients management of exacerbations, with clear, written instructions on when to go to emergency room. Encourage client to receive the pneumococcal and influenza vaccines. Educational resource materials are available from the American Lung Association (800-586-4872) and the Asthma and Allergy Foundation of America (8007-ASTHMA). Expert Panel Report II available Fall 1997 through the National Asthma Education and Prevention Program (301-251-1222), National Heart, Lung, and Blood Institute (NHLBI) Information Center, P.O. Box 30105, Bethesda, MD 20824-0105, http://www.nhlbi.nih.gov/nhlbi/lung/asthma/gp/ asthgdln.htm.

BRONCHITIS, ACUTE

SIGNAL SYMPTOMS Cough with sputum production; Fever, malaise

| Bronchitis | ICD-9-CM: 466.0 |

Description: Acute bronchitis is the inflammation of the tracheo-bronchial tree, trachea, bronchi, and bronchioles.

Etiology: Caused by infection from microbes such as the common cold viruses, influenza, mycoplasma pneumonia, *Chlamydia pneumoniae, Moraxella catarrhalis*, and secondary bacterial invasion with *Streptococcus pneumoniae* and *Haemophilus influenzae*, group b. Infection of the bronchial tree produces edema with an increased amount of bronchial secretions, which eventually results in destruction of the epithelium and impaired mucociliary activity.

Occurrence: Common; most often occurs after an acute URI.

Age: Occurs in all ages.

Ethnicity: No significant ethnic predisposition.

Gender: Occurs equally in men and in women.

Contributing factors: Chronic bronchopulmonary diseases, chronic sinusitis, bronchopulmonary allergy, tracheostomies, hypertrophied tonsils and adenoids, smoking, exposure to secondhand smoke and air pollutants, alcoholism, reflux esophagitis, immunosuppression.

Signs and symptoms: Cough (appears early in the course of the disease, increases in frequency and intensity). Slight fever, malaise, chills, sore throat, back and muscle pain (early in the course of the infection). Fever, mucopurulent sputum, substernal pain, dyspnea, and bronchospasm (if bronchitis is caused by bacterial infection). Physical examination may reveal rhonchi or wheezing on auscultation. No evidence of pulmonary consolidation.

 Clinical Pearl: Patients with COPD who have chronic crackles and/or rhonchi must have a chest x-ray study (CXR) for definitive diagnosis to rule out pneumonia.

Diagnostic tests: Usually diagnosed by history and physical examination.

Test	Result Indicating Disorder	CPT Code
Sputum culture and sensitivity	Identifies responsible organism and best antibiotic treatment	87070, 87181
CBC	May have elevated WBCs	85027
Chest x-ray study	Will be normal in bronchitis—may need to perform to rule out pneumonia	71010 (PA), 71020 (PA and LAT)

CBC, complete blood count; LAT, lateral; PA, posteroanterior; WBCs, white blood cells.

Differential diagnosis:

- Pneumonia (may have same clinical appearance as bronchitis)
- Pertussis (cough)
- Asthma (exacerbation may appear to be acute bronchitis)
- Allergic rhinitis (postnasal drip may cause cough)
- Chronic sinusitis (postnasal drip may cause cough)
- Retained foreign body (may cause wheezing and cough with SOB)
- Bronchiectasis (cough and sputum)
- Bacterial tracheitis (cough and sputum)

Treatment:

Pharmacologic

Because the etiology is most often viral, antibiotic therapy is usually not indicated. However, if acute bronchitis is complicated by secondary bacterial infection, broad-spectrum antibiotics may be used. These would include macrolides, fluoroquinolones, and sulfa as first choices. Cough suppressants may be prescribed if cough interferes with rest (for dry, nonproductive cough). Non-codeine cough suppressants would include Tessolon Perles or Humabid LA; try these preparations before resorting to use of codeine cough suppressants. If the patient has dyspnea, inhaled bronchodilators such as albuterol, two puffs as needed, may be used. Medrol dose pak should be used if patient has wheezing. Amantadine therapy is indicated in cases of influenza; initiate within 24 to 48 hours of symptom development. Antipyretic analgesics, aspirin, or acetaminophen every 4 to 6 hours may assist with symptom relief.

Physical

Increase fluids up to 3 to 4 liters per day (if not contraindicated, e.g. in CHF patients). Cool-mist vaporizers may assist in humidifying secretions, especially at night. Rest will assist with the recovery and should be continued until the fever subsides. The patient should avoid smoking and respiratory irritants.

Follow-up: Cough may persist for 1 to 2 weeks after acute infection or antibiotic therapy is finished; this may be due to bronchial irritation and will resolve. If discolored sputum or fever persists after the course of treatment is finished, see the patient again for evaluation.

Sequelae: Possible complications include bronchial pneumonia and acute respiratory failure. Serious complications are more likely to occur in the very young, elderly, or debilitated patient.

Prevention/prophylaxis: Prevention strategies include encouraging the patient to stop smoking, avoiding respiratory irritants, and avoiding people with acute URIs. Careful handwashing.

Referral: Refer to, or consult with, physician if patient shows no improvement or if patient has frequent episodes of acute bronchitis.

Education: Explain disease process, signs and symptoms, and treatment (including side effects of medications). Discuss prevention strategies. Advise patient that measures such as increasing fluids, getting rest, taking antipyretic analgesics, and using a cool-mist vaporizer may decrease symptoms. Educational resource materials are available from the American Lung Association, 1740 Broadway, New York, NY 10019 (212–315–8700).

CARDIAC ARRHYTHMIAS

SIGNAL SYMPTOMS *General supraventricular tachycardia (SVT):*
Palpitations and presyncope
Atrial fibrillation: Palpitations and DOE
Premature ventricular contractions (PVCs) and premature atrial contractions (PACs): None
Wenckebach: Asymptomatic
Mobitz II: Possible presyncope or syncope
Third-degree block: Presyncope and syncope

Cardiac arrhythmias	ICD 427.9

Description: Cardiac arrhythmias are disturbances in the normal electrical conduction of the heart. They are categorized by the site of origin of the impulse, heart rate, or mechanism of conduction. The etiology of any arrhythmia varies: it may be chemical (electrolyte imbalance), structural (damage to the conduction system), or abnormal automaticity or reentry phenomena.

Occurrence: Increases with age.

Signs and symptoms: Varies with the arrhythmia. May be asymptomatic; may have palpitations and racing heartbeat; may have presyncope or syncope; may have awareness of heartbeat but normal rate; **symptoms depend on the perfusion afforded by the arrhythmia.** Any rhythm that maintains normal blood pressure is more likely to be asymptomatic.

Diagnostic tests:

Test	Result Indicating Disorder	CPT Code
ECG. A standard 12-lead ECG study should be performed and, if necessary, a 24-hour Holter monitor should be used.	Will document NSR or suspected arrhythmia; if NSR should use a Holter to further investigate possible arrhythmia	93000

ECG, electrocardiogram; NSR, normal sinus rhythm.

Treatment: Treatment varies with the arrhythmia and includes symptomatic treatment of the patient and treatment of the underlying cause (Table 5-2).

Table 5–2   Selected Cardiac Arrhythmias

Sinus Bradycardia

EKG Criteria:
Rate: 40–60 beats per minute
    Rhythm: Regular
    P waves: Precede each QRS
    PR interval: Normal
    QRS: Normal
Comments: Many causes: increased vagal stimulation; increased intracranial pressure; overmedication with calcium blocker or beta blocker. Usually asymptomatic unless accompanied by hypotension. Rule out hypothyroidism.
Treatment: Usually none. If needed, adjust medication dosage (calcium or beta blocker) down; atropine if symptomatic.

Sinus Tachycardia

EKG Criteria:
Rate: 100–180 beats per minute
    Rhythm: Regular
    P waves: Precede each QRS
    PR interval: Normal
    QRS: Normal
Comments: Many causes: fever, pain, hypovolemia. Can lead to decreased cardiac output and hypotension.
Treatment: Treat cause; low-dose beta blocker.

Premature Atrial Contractions (PACs)

EKG Criteria:
Rate: 60–100 beats per minute
    Rhythm: Regular, except when PAC occurs → premature sinus beat with pause following.
    P waves (PAC): Often different morphology
    PR interval: Varies
    QRS: Normal; aberrant; or absent if nonconducted PAC
Comments: Atrial irritability. May be due to stress, caffeine, alcohol. Usually asymptomatic.
Treatment: None, unless symptomatic; treat cause.

(Continued)

Table 5–2 Selected Cardiac Arrhythmias *(Continued)*

Paroxysmal Atrial Tachycardia (PAT)

EKG Criteria:
Rate: 150 – 250 beats per minute
  Rhythm: Regular
  P waves (PAC): Different morphology than NSR baseline of patient
  PR interval: Shortened
  QRS: Normal or aberrant
Comments: Often abrupt onset with abrupt cessation. Often cardiac output palpitations and SOB. May be due to alcohol, caffeine, stress, smoking. May cause decreased cardiac output and pre-syncope or syncope.
Treatment: Valsalva maneuver; digitalis; beta-blocker; verapamil. To ER if persistent with hypotension.

Atrial Fibrillation (AF)

EKG Criteria:
Rate: Indistinguishable atrial rate; ventricular varies depending on AV conduction. May be slow ventricular rate (50 – 60) or rapid over 100.
  Rhythm: Irregularly irregular (hallmark of AF)
  P waves: None
  PR interval: None
  QRS: Normal to aberrant
Comments: Loss of atrial kick may cause hypotension. Symptoms may be palpitations, SOB, presyncope, DOE. May be asymptomatic entirely. Rule out hyperthyroidism.
Treatment: Betapace (by MD in hospital setting to initiate); digitalis; beta blocker; calcium blockers. If new onset, hospitalize for anticoagulation or cardioversion as applicable.

Junctional Rhythm

EKG Criteria:
Rate: 40–60 beats per minute
  Rhythm: Regular
  P waves: Absent, may be retrograde
  PR interval: None
  QRS: Normal to aberrant
Comments: May be due to number of causes; digitalis toxicity; over-medication with calcium or beta-blocker; acute MI. Rule out hypothyroidism.
Treatment: HOSPITALIZE.

First-Degree AV Block

EKG Criteria:
Rate: 60 – 100 beats per minute
  Rhythm: Regular
  P waves: Precede each QRS
  PR interval: Prolonged >.12 (normal .08–.12)
  QRS: Normal
Comments: May be due to digitalis toxicity; inferior wall MI; calcium blockers. Asymptomatic.
Treatment: Monitor; treat cause.

Second-Degree AV Block: Mobitz I Wenckebach

EKG Criteria:
Rate: 60–100 beats per minute
  Rhythm: May be irregular
  P waves: One for each QRS until dropped QRS seen
  PR interval: Progressive lengthening until QRS is dropped (hallmark of Wenckebach); then cycle repeats
  QRS: Normal
Comments: Due to conduction disease; acute MI; often asymptomatic.
Treatment: Monitor; treat cause.

(Continued)

Table 5–2   Selected Cardiac Arrhythmias *(Continued)*

Second-Degree A-V Block: Mobitz II

EKG Criteria:
Rate: 60–100 beats per minute
   Rhythm: May be irregular
   P waves: One for each QRS until non-conducted P wave dropped QRS. May have 2:1, 3:1, 4:1 Ps to QRSs.
   PR interval: Regular until dropped QRS
   QRS: Normal
Comments: Indicates higher degree of AV block than Wenckebach → highly likely to develop third-degree block. May be asymptomatic; after acute MI or sudden onset with history of conduction disturbance.
Treatment: Pacemaker

Third-Degree A-V Block (Complete Heart Block)

EKG Criteria:
Rate: Atrial 60–100 beats per minute; ventricular 40–60 beats per minute
   Rhythm: Regular
   P waves: Regular; marching through QRS with no association to QRS (not conducted)
   PR interval: None
   QRS: Morphology varies; dependent on escape mechanism pacing the heart; wider than normal
Comments: Symptoms depend on perfusion/blood pressure. Always an emergency.
Treatment: Atropine; pacemaker

Premature Ventricular Contractions (PVCs)

EKG Criteria:
Rate: 60–100 beats per minute
   Rhythm: Regular with occasional pause after PVC
   P waves (PVCs): Absent or retrograde
   PR interval (PVCs): None
   QRS: Wide and bizarre (hallmark of PVCs)
Comments: Due to increased irritability of ventricle and conduction system; hypoxia; ischemia; electrolyte imbalance. Symptoms may include palpitations, presyncope.
Treatment: Treat cause. May need no treatment if unifocal and asymptomatic; beta blockers if without success refer to MD.

CHRONIC OBSTRUCTIVE PULMONARY DISEASE (CHRONIC BRONCHITIS, EMPHYSEMA)

SIGNAL SYMPTOMS▶▶▶   *Chronic Bronchitis*
Chronic cough productive of sputum (for at least 3 months for 2 consecutive years); SOB

SIGNAL SYMPTOMS▶▶   *Emphysema*
DOE; Diminished breath sounds

| Chronic Bronchitis | ICD-9-CM: 491.20; 491.21 |
| Emphysema | ICD-9-CM: 492.8 |

Description: COPD includes a group of disorders characterized by airflow obstruction. The two most common disorders are emphysema and chronic bronchitis. These conditions occur alone or in combination.

Chronic bronchitis is an inflammation of the bronchial tubes character-ized by excessive tracheal-bronchial mucous production. It is defined by the presence of a cough for at least 3 months for at least 2 consecutive years. Emphysema is the permanent enlargement of the air spaces distal to the terminal bronchioles; alveolar membranes are destroyed. The onset of both conditions is gradual, slow, and progressive.

Etiology: Caused by inflammation of and damage to the lung, usually from an irritant. If the irritant is not removed, the damage is progressive. In chronic bronchitis, inflammation in the mucus-secreting mechanisms and thickened bronchial walls produces cough, airway resistance, nar-rowed airway lumina, and fibrosis. In emphysema, there is reduced gas exchange secondary to damaged alveoli, and decreased elastic recoil of the lungs, causing increased work of breathing.

Occurrence: Lung disease is the fourth leading cause of death in the United States. Chronic bronchitis is the most common obstructive pul-monary disease, followed by emphysema. COPD affects about 10 million people in the United States.

Age: Incidence increases with age. The onset of symptoms of chronic bronchitis usually occurs after age 35; symptoms of emphysema occur after age 50.

Ethnicity: Occurs more often in whites than in other races.

Gender: Overall, COPD is more common in men than in women; how-ever, chronic bronchitis is more common in women, and emphysema is more common in men.

Clinical Pearl: COPD is becoming more common in women and now is approaching equality with men due to the increased incidence of smoking in women.

Contributing factors: Cigarette smoking (primary factor), air pollu-tion, airway infection (i.e., severe viral pneumonia early in life), familial factors (including the genetic disorder, alpha$_1$-antitrypsin deficiency), occupational exposure (such as in fire fighting), passive smoking expo-sure (as especially in adults whose parents smoked), alcohol consump-tion, reactive airways disease.

Signs and Symptoms: Signs and symptoms are progressive. The patient with COPD often exhibits tachypnea, fatigue, and loss of libido.

Chronic Bronchitis

The chief complaint is a chronic productive cough with thick, mucopu-rulent or purulent sputum that is difficult to cough up. Cough must be present for 3 months in 2 consecutive years. Other complaints include progressive SOB and recurrent lung infections.

Symptoms are aggravated by upper and lower respiratory infections, fatigue, stress, and acute and chronic illnesses. Physical examination may reveal an overweight patient with varying degrees of central plethora, cyanosis, pedal edema, wheezes and rhonchi, diminished breath sounds, and use of accessory muscles of respiration.

Emphysema

The chief complaints are progressive DOE, SOB at rest, and weight loss. If a cough is present, it is often nonproductive. If the cough is productive, the sputum is usually clear mucoid sputum. The patient often has a history of occasional recurrent infections of the lungs and bronchial tubes. Symptoms are aggravated by upper and lower respiratory infections, fatigue, stress, and acute and chronic illnesses. During infections and exacerbations, the patient may experience severe DOE and SOB at rest; with advanced disease SOB may be present at rest. Physical examination may reveal an increased anteroposterior chest diameter (barrel chest), diminished breath sounds, hyperresonance lung fields on percussion, and use of accessory muscles of respiration.

Diagnostic tests:

Chest X-ray

The CXR is seldom diagnostic but may rule out other pathology. The CXR of a patient with more advanced chronic bronchitis may reveal increased bronchovascular markings and cardiomegaly. In contrast, the CXR of a patient with advanced emphysema is more likely to show a small heart, hyperinflation, and flat diaphragms.

Pulmonary Function Tests

The hallmark of COPD is an FEV_1 (forced expiratory volume in 1 sec.)/FVC (forced vital capacity) ratio that is below 70%. When treatment involves bronchodilators, there may be some reversibility, but it is more marginal than that classically seen with asthma (above 15%); this is one of the main ways to establish a diagnosis. The FEV_1/FVC is the most useful parameter in assessing severity of ventilatory impairment. Onset of DOE occurs after FEV_1 falls to below 50% of predicted. Residual volume (RV) and forced residual capacity (FRC) is almost always higher than normal due to air trapping. COPD is staged:

Stage	FEV_1/FVC	FEV_1	Symptoms
Stage 1 (mild)	< 70%	More than 80% of predicted	With or without chronic cough/sputum
Stage 2 (moderate)	< 70%	30% decrease or < 80% of predicted*	With or without chronic cough/sputum
Stage 3 (severe)	< 70%	< 30% predicted or < 50% predicted with right heart failure or respiratory failure	Cor-pulmonale: Right-sided heart failure to respiratory distress/failure

*IIA: 50% <FEV_1<80% predicted IIB: 30%<FEV_1<50% predicted

Arterial Blood Gases

Baseline values are useful to track progression and make decisions regarding oxygen therapy. Arterial blood gases may be normal during early stages of COPD; progression of disease may be documented by falling Pao_2 and increasing $Paco_2$ over the course of time. Acute changes in this respect represent acute respiratory failure and require hospitalization.

Serum Alpha₁-Antitrypsin

Evidence suggests that alpha₁-antitrypsin protects lung elastin from degradation. Alpha₁-antitrypsin deficiency is a genetic abnormality that should be considered in patients with COPD before the age of 45 with a strong family history and no risk factors. It is important to establish this diagnosis, as treatment is available. Intravenous alpha₁-antitrypsin may be given to slow or stop progression of this disease.

Differential diagnosis:

- Asthma (SOB, DOE, cough)
- CHF (SOB, DOE, fatigue, cough)
- Neoplastic lung disease (cough)
- Tuberculosis (TB) (cough, sputum)
- Bronchiectasis (cough, sputum)
- Bronchiolitis (cough, sputum)

Treatment: Treatment includes avoidance of contributing factors, prevention or early recognition and treatment of respiratory infections, bronchodilation, aggressive management of acute exacerbations, oxygen therapy, and lifestyle management, including active pulmonary rehabilitation.

Physical

Smoking cessation: Strongly encourage and support the patient to stop smoking. To prevent progression of disease, the patient must quit smoking. Various smoking cessation programs are available through the American Lung Association and the American Cancer Society. See new Agency for Health Care Policy and Research guidelines for smoking cessation: publication no. 09-0694. Bupropion HCl (Zyban) 150 mg orally each day for 3 days, then twice a day for 7 to 12 weeks. This is an effective adjunct therapy in smoking cessation. Avoid bedtime dosing. Maximum dose is 300 mg per day in divided doses. Patient should start this drug while still smoking, and stop smoking after a minimum of one week on the drug. If patient has not successfully stopped smoking after 7 weeks, discontinue. If patient successfully quits with using this drug it should be continued.

Prevention strategies: Encourage the patient to obtain annual influenza vaccinations and vaccinations against pneumonia. Advise the patient to avoid persons with infections and contact their health-care provider at the first signs of an infection. Antibiotic therapy for respiratory infections should provide broad-spectrum coverage and be started at the first sign of infection. Avoid the use of cough suppressants and antihistamines. If environmental factors are contributing to exacerbation or symptoms, perform a thorough environmental assessment. Air conditioning and the use of HEPA filters are recommended. If the patient lives in a climate with high air pollution or in a hot, humid climate, advise the patient to avoid outdoor activities when possible.

Chest physiotherapy: May be indicated for the patient who cannot effectively mobilize and clear secretions.

Pulmonary rehabilitation: Encourage the patient to participate in those programs that teach and reinforce the correct use of inhalers, use of pursed-lip breathing, lifestyle modifications to save energy, and measures to avoid respiratory inhalants and provide supervised methods of increasing exercise tolerance.

Nutrition: Nutritional replacement of calories and proteins in patients nearing end-stage disease can be important. These patients have high-energy requirements and are malnourished, with muscle wasting that contributes to inspiratory muscle weakness. In patients who retain CO_2, high-carbohydrate loads should be avoided because these lead to increased CO_2 levels.

Pharmacologic

Bronchodilators are the first line of treatment in COPD. Bronchodilation is usually accomplished with anticholinergic agents, beta-adrenergic agents, and theophylline.

Anticholinergic agents: Effective because of their slow onset and long duration. Using a metered-dose inhaler, inhaled ipratropium bromide (Atrovent) for example, 2 puffs four times per day on a regular basis; effective long-term control.

Beta$_2$ agonists: Short acting beta$_2$ agonists, such as albuterol 2 to 4 puffs every 4 to 6 hours, may be used for acute exacerbation. Combivent, a combination anticholinergic and beta-adrenergic agent, is also effective. Use 2 puffs four times a day (maximum 12 inhalations). A long-acting beta$_2$ agonist, Salmeterol (Serevent), provides significant long-term control.

Theophylline: If the patient does not significantly improve with both anticholinergic and beta$_2$ agonist, consider adding theophylline. Theophylline (Theo-Dur), 200 mg every 12 hours up to 900 mg/day, may provide effective bronchodilation and improve symptoms. Use with caution, with periodic measurement of serum theophylline levels (should be 10 to 20 mg/mL). Toxic levels of more than 20 mg/mL may have serious/lethal effects.

Corticosteroids: Oral steroids may be used for acute exacerbations of COPD. Prednisone, 40 mg orally daily or on alternate days, is usually used. If the patient improves on steroid therapy, gradually reduce dosage to the minimum necessary to provide relief; the goal being to wean off as exacerbation ends. If the patient does not improve in 14 days, refer the patient. Inhaled steroids may be used for long-term management but are only appropriate for patients with COPD who have shown documented obstruction reversal with spirometry. Beclovent, 2 puffs four times daily, can be used. Inhaled steroids are only for long-term management and are not helpful in acute exacerbations.

Oxygen therapy: Supplemental O_2 therapy at a low flow rate (2 liters/minute) by nasal cannula is indicated for the patient with significant hypoxemia (PO_2 of 55 or less, O_2 saturation of < 88%, hct. > 55, or cor pulmonale). Oxygen therapy of more than 15 hours per day has been shown to increase survival and decrease clinical symptoms; thereby improving quality of life.

Follow-up: See the patient as indicated by the stage of the disease. During an acute exacerbation or following an acute respiratory infection, the patient should be seen in the office every 2 to 3 days during the first week to ensure that treatment is effective. Figure 5-2 covers treatment of COPD.

Sequelae: Possible complications include chronic hypoxemia, pulmonary HTN, pneumonia, cor pulmonale, left ventricular heart failure, bullous lung disease, acute respiratory acidosis or respiratory failure requiring mechanical ventilation, death.

Prevention/prophylaxis: Prevention strategies include encouraging the patient to stop smoking, avoid secondhand smoke, avoid respiratory irritants and respiratory infection, and avoid temperature extremes. Advise the patient to receive annual influenza vaccinations and the pneumococcal vaccine. Check PPD once per year. Notify health-care provider of respiratory infection immediately. Patient may be taught to begin antibiotics on his or her own.

Referral: Refer to, or consult with, a respiratory specialist if the patient does not respond satisfactorily to treatment, if the patient's condition is rapidly declining, or if the patient has cor pulmonale.

Education: Explain the disease process, signs and symptoms, and treatment (including side effects of medications). Discuss prevention strategies and importance of compliance with therapy. Advise the patient when to seek medical care. Teach the patient the correct use and care of inhalers. Encourage participation in support groups and pulmonary rehabilitation programs. Provide support and encouragement. For the patient with advanced disease, discuss the issue of advanced directives. Educational resource materials are available from the American Lung Association, 61 Broadway, 6th floor, New York, NY 10006 (212–315–8700). Website: *www.lungusa.org*

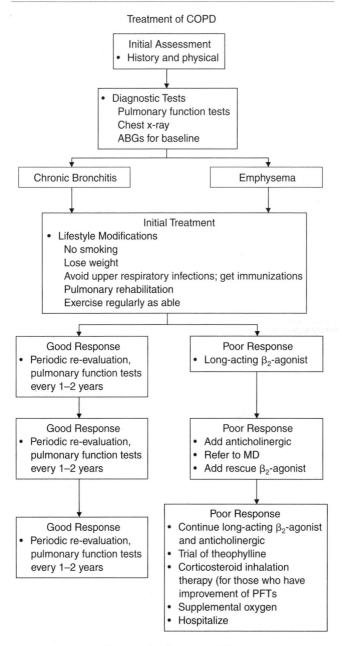

Figure 5–2. Treatment: COPD.

CONGESTIVE HEART FAILURE

SIGNAL SYMPTOMS Paroxysmal nocturnal dyspnea/orthopnea; Pedal edema

Congestive Heart Failure	ICD-9-CM: 428.0

Description: CHF is a state of altered cardiac function in which there is inadequate cardiac output to meet the oxygen demand of metabolizing tissues, leading to excessive retention of sodium and water. Determination of systolic versus diastolic dysfunction (or combination thereof) must be made to ensure the best course of treatment.

Etiology: Caused by any process that damages the heart. The most common causes are (1) ischemic heart disease and (2) hypertensive heart disease. Secondary factors that may aggravate or precipitate the condition include increased physical activity, increased sodium intake, anemia, renal failure, thyrotoxicosis, cardiac arrhythmias, concurrent illness such as pneumonia and emotional stress, and failure to take medications properly.

Occurrence: There are 4.7 million people with CHF in North America.

Age: Occurs primarily in people age 65 and older.

Ethnicity: No significant ethnic predisposition.

Gender: Occurs in men more than in women up to age 75, then occurs equally in men and in women.

Contributing factors: Coronary atherosclerosis, MI, rheumatic heart disease, idiopathic cardiomyopathy, hypertensive heart disease, aortic stenosis or regurgitation, volume overload, inappropriate use of calcium channel blockers, or other cardiac depressants. Fever, infection, hyperthyroidism, alcoholism.

Signs and symptoms: Signs and symptoms include DOE, which may progress to SOB at rest; orthopnea; paroxysmal nocturnal dyspnea; ankle swelling; nocturia; dry, hacking cough or wheezing, particularly at night; chronic fatigue; and weight gain, anorexia. Right-sided heart failure will predominate with pedal edema, hepatomegaly (even ascites), jugular venous distention (JVD). Left-sided heart failure will predominate with DOE, SOB at rest, paroxysmal nocturnal dyspnea (PND); if severe, pulmonary edema will result. There may be any combination of the above-mentioned conditions depending of presence of biventricular failure and other factors.

Physical examination may reveal resting tachycardia; JVD; crackles (rales), usually expiratory, particularly over the base of the lungs; presence of S_3; bilateral, dependent edema; and hepatomegaly with right upper quadrant (RUQ) discomfort (with severe heart failure). Abdominal bloating may be present. Patient may be tachypneic at rest.

Diagnostic tests:

Test	Result Indicating Disorder	CPT Code
Thyroid function tests	May be hidden cause of heart failure	80091
Chemistries; including Mg and Ca	Electrolyte disturbances may cause dysrhythmias and exacerbate heart failure	80054
CBC	Anemia can cause/exacerbate heart failure and ischemia	85027
Chest X-ray	Confirms diagnosis; assesses for presence of more severe pulmonary edema	71010 (PA), 701020 (PA & LAT)
ECG	Assess for rhythm and any changes indicative of ischemia/MI	93000
Echocardiogram (if not recently done)	To assess for structural changes; to assess ejection fraction	93307, 93320, 93325

Ca, calcium; CBC, complete blood count; ECG, electrocardiogram; LAT, lateral; Mg, magnesium; MI, myocardial infarction; PA, posteroanterior.

Differential diagnosis:

- Acute MI (may cause sudden heart failure)
- COPD (may lead to cor pulmonale and heart failure)
- Asthma (DOE, SOB, cough)
- Renal disease (fluid retention/overload)
- Liver disease (ascites, edema, fluid overload)
- Recurrent pulmonary emboli (SOB, pulmonary HTN, heart failure)

Treatment: Treatment goals involve (1) improvement of clinical symptoms and quality of life (decrease DOE and fatigue, increase exercise capacity, and prevent exacerbation), (2) interference with neurohormonal activity in CHF, specifically to decrease the influence of the sympathetic nervous system and the RAAS. Decreased tissue perfusion present in CHF causes overactivation of these systems and increases blood pressure, heart rate, sodium and water retention, and worsening CHF.

 Clinical Pearl: Once a diagnosis of CHF is made, in order to slow the progression of the disease, even patients who are asymptomatic should be on an angiotensin-converting enzyme (ACE) and a beta blocker; this approach counteracts RAAS.

Physical

Provide a low-sodium diet, initially 2 g sodium each day. Provide a low-fat diet as necessary, along with weight reduction. The patient may need fluid restriction; elevate feet to decrease pedal edema. Elevate head of bed and use antiembolic stockings to decrease edema. Encourage exercise as tolerated and as supervised by health professional; this is very important in maintaining physical strength and mental health.

Pharmacologic

The cornerstone of therapy is diuretic use. The following includes medical management of CHF:

- Diuretics (loop diuretics, e.g., furosemide [Lasix] or torsemide [Demadex]); monitor electrolytes and blood urea nitrogen (BUN)/creatinine
- Beta blockers—those approved for use in CHF include metoprolol (Toprol XL) and carvedilol (Coreg); monitor blood pressure and heart rate
- ACE inhibitors—there are many available; monitor electrolytes and BUN/ creatinine
- Angiotensin receptor blockers (ARBs)—use if patient is unable to take ACE inhibitor or in combination to suppress angiotensin effectively; valsartan (Diovan) is the only ARB approved for use in patients with CHF, but others are available; monitor electrolytes and BUN/creatinine
- Long-acting nitrates are recommended if etiology of CHF is ischemic or angina is present
- Digitalis if DOE persists despite use of above-mentioned treatment modalities
- Calcium channel blockers are contraindicated with low ejection fraction and may actually worsen CHF

Follow-up: See patient in 24 hours; then if patient has improved, see patient every week until patient is symptom free and dry weight is achieved. Then see patient every month for 3 months, and then every 3 months. Use the New York Heart Association classification to help gauge the patient's disease progression or improvement with therapy:

Class I: No limitation of physical activity. Ordinary physical activity does not cause undue fatigue, dyspnea, palpitations, or angina.

Class II: Slight limitation of physical activity. Patient is comfortable at rest. Ordinary physical activity may result in fatigue, dyspnea, palpitations, or angina.

Class III: Marked limitation of physical activity. Patient is fairly comfortable at rest. Less than ordinary physical activity will lead to symptoms.

Class IV: Inability to carry on any physical activity without discomfort. Symptoms of heart failure or angina are present even at rest. If any physical activity is undertaken, increased discomfort is experienced.

Figure 5-3 provides the differential diagnosis and treatment for CHF.

Sequelae: Possible complications include pulmonary edema, respiratory failure, lethal arrhythmias, electrolyte imbalances, hepatomegaly, ascites, peripheral edema, and digitalis toxicity. Once the CHF has occurred, the 6-year mortality rate for men is 80% and for women is

Treatment: CHF

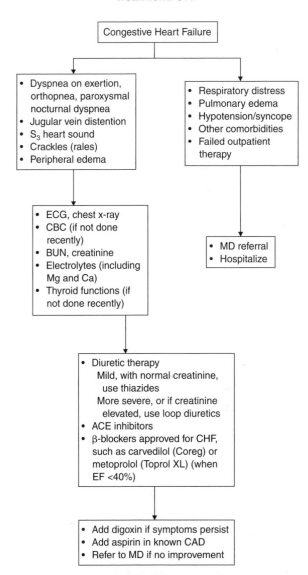

Figure 5–3. Differential Diagnosis and Treatment: CHF (From ACC/AHA Task Force Heart Failure Guidelines: Guidelines for the Evaluation and Management of Chronic Heart Failure in the Adult—A Report of the American College of Cardiology/American Heart Association Task Force on Practice Guidelines [Committee to Revise the 1995 Guidelines for the Evaluation and Management of Heart Failure], 2001.)

65%. It is the most frequent inpatient diagnosis for patients over the age of 65.

Prevention/prophylaxis: Prevention strategies include advising the patient to maintain a sodium (salt)–restricted diet (2 g/day), reduce weight if he or she is overweight, and incorporate rest periods into normal daily activities. Teach the patient and family how to read food labels for sodium content, and emphasize importance of adherence to medical regimen.

Referral: All patients with CHF, ischemic or otherwise, should be worked up by a cardiologist and have routine follow-up with him or her in conjunction with practitioner management.

Education: Explain the disease process, signs and symptoms, and treatment (including side effects of medications). Discuss prevention strategies, importance of compliance with therapy, and when to seek medical care (SOB, unusual fatigue, rapid weight gain, and an increase in pulse rate while resting; although the condition is secondary to beta blockade, the patient may not develop tachycardia as symptom). Instruct the patient to record his or her weight daily before breakfast and to report a rapid weight gain. Advise patient on methods to use to modify activities and to incorporate rest periods into daily activities. If needed, the patient may contact the American Heart Association, 7320 Greensville Ave., Dallas, TX 75231 (214-373-6300).

COSTOCHONDRITIS (TIETZE'S SYNDROME)

SIGNAL SYMPTOMS Sharp anterior chest pain; Pain that is reproducible with palpation of chest wall

Costochondritis (Tietze's syndrome)   ICD-9-CM: 733

Description: Costochondritis (Tietze's syndrome) is an inflammation of the cartilage of one or more ribs, most commonly the second or third ribs.

Etiology: Idiopathic, although trauma or overuse may precipitate the condition.

Occurrence: 10% of chest pain complaints; 15% to 20% of teenagers with chest pain.

Age: Occurs at any age; occurs more commonly in those younger than 40 years of age. In those patients older than 40, it tends to occur in the third, fourth, or fifth costochondral joint, and it occurs mostly in women.

Ethnicity: No significant ethnic predisposition.

Gender: Both sexes affected equally before the age 40; in patients who are older than the age of 40, the patients are mostly women.

Contributing factors: Trauma (usually rib fractures); unusual physical activity or stressful exercise; excessive coughing, such as from allergic responses or smoking; osteoporosis.

Signs and symptoms: Sudden, sharp, anterior chest wall pain (usually at the costochondral junction; however, some patients complain of radiation to other areas of the chest wall or to the arm) that usually worsens on deep inspiration, coughing, movement, or exercise. Patient may also complain of tightness in the chest and may have recently had a viral or bacterial respiratory infection or have been exposed to such illnesses.

Physical examination may reveal a patient in some distress (usually related to the pain), exhibiting signs of trauma such as ecchymosis or swelling in the chest wall area, pain on movement, and focal pain or tenderness on palpation of the area. The ability to reproduce the pain is highly significant in that, if the practitioner can reproduce the pain on palpation, then cardiac symptoms can be ruled out.

Diagnostic tests: Usually diagnosed by history and physical examination.

Test	Result Indicating Disorder	CPT Code
ECG	As adjunct in ruling out cardiac etiology	93000
Chest X-ray	Rule out rib fractures, pulmonary/cardiac etiology	71010 (PA), 71020 (PA & LAT)
Oxygen saturation	Hypoxemia may mean pulmonary embolus	94760-84762

ECG, electrocardiogram; LAT, lateral; PA, posteroanterior.

Differential diagnosis:
- CAD with angina (may cause chest pain)
- Hypertrophic cardiomyopathy (may cause chest pain)
- Mitral valve prolapse (may cause chest pain)
- Hyperventilation syndrome (causes SOB with or without chest pain)
- Esophageal disease (may cause chest pain)

Treatment:

Pharmacologic

Clinical Pearl: Nitroglycerin does not relieve the pain of costochondritis. Use anti-inflammatory/analgesics such as NSAIDs, (ibuprofen 400 mg every 4 to 6 hours for adults); if the patient is unable to use NSAIDs, he or she may use acetaminophen, two tablets orally every 4 hours as needed.

Physical
Apply local heat to the area. Rest.

Follow-up: Usually, no follow-up visit is necessary.

Sequelae: Usually, there are no sequelae related to costochondritis; however, respiratory complications related to decreased inspiratory volume may occur.

Prevention/prophylaxis: Prevention strategies include advising the patient to avoid excessive lifting, excessive exercise, or excessive coughing.

Referral: Referral or consultation is usually not necessary with a healthy patient with costochondritis.

Education: Explain the disease process, signs and symptoms, and treatment (including side effects of medications). Discuss prevention strategies. Advise patient to refrain from the activity that may have caused the condition until it resolves.

HYPERTENSION

SIGNAL SYMPTOMS▶ May be entirely asymptomatic; May have headache that is worse in A.M.

| Hypertension, essential | ICD-9-CM: 401.1; 401.0 |

Description: Hypertension (HTN) is defined as either prehypertension (120-139/80-89), or as hypertension when there is a sustained systolic blood pressure of >140 mm Hg or a diastolic blood pressure of >90 mm Hg, measured on at least three separate occasions. HTN may be classified as essential (primary) or secondary, and is a strong risk factor for cardiovascular disease.

Etiology: Essential (primary) HTN has no identifiable cause. Secondary HTN: Cause is identifiable and sometimes correctable, as in pheochromocytoma, renal artery stenosis, or fluid retention.

Occurrence: Occurs in about 20% of the population of the United States (about 50 million people).

Age: Often not detected until later in life; prevalence increases with age. Most common after age 60.

Gender: Occurs more often in men than in women.

Ethnicity: Highest incidence and greater severity in black Americans.

Contributing factors: Genetics; dyslipidemia; family history of premature heart disease; obesity; excess alcohol use; cigarette use; excess dietary sodium; stress; physical inactivity; renal diseases (glomerulonephritis, pyelonephritis, polycystic kidneys); endocrine diseases (diabetes, primary hyperaldosteronism, pheochromocytoma, hyperthyroidism, Cushing's syndrome); vascular diseases (coarctation, renal artery stenosis); chemical factors (use of oral contraceptives, NSAIDs, decongestants, antidepressants, sympathomimetics, corticosteroids, ergotamine alkaloids, lithium, cyclosporine, industrial chemicals).

Signs and symptoms: The 7th Report of the Joint National Committee on Prevention, Detection, Evaluation, and Treatment of High Blood Pressure (2003) recommends a good history and physical examination with emphasis on family history of HTN and cardiovascular disease; personal history of cerebrovascular disease, renal disease, diabetes, or risk factors for CAD; previous elevated blood pressure and treatments, history of weight gain, exercise activities, sodium intake, fat intake, and alcohol use; and psychosocial and environmental factors.

The patient is often asymptomatic (HTN is known as "the silent killer"). The patient may complain of a headache that occurs on awakening and is located in the occipital area (occurs with higher blood pressures). Assess for symptoms suggesting secondary HTN.

Obtain the patient's blood pressure in both arms; lying and standing; 2 minutes apart. Use the highest blood pressure measured. Obtain the patient's height, weight, and waistline girth. A waistline measurement of > 34 inches (86 cm) for women and > 39 inches (99 cm) in men is a predictor of comorbidity and coronary heart disease morbidity.

Physical examination may reveal retinopathy and an increased A_2 heart sound. Perform a funduscopic examination (may reveal arteriolar narrowing, arteriovenous compression, hemorrhages, cotton wool exudates, and papilledema), along with complete examination of the heart, peripheral pulses, and abdomen (for masses and bruits).

Diagnostic tests: Diagnosed by blood pressure measurement. Use proper technique each time blood pressure is taken (proper sized cuff, correct arm position). Blood pressure must be elevated on three separate occasions to make the diagnosis.

For the patient age 18 and older, blood pressure is classified as follows:

Optimal: Systolic equal to or < 120; diastolic < 80
Prehypertension: Systolic 120-139 or diastolic 80-89

Hypertension:

Stage I: Systolic 140 to 159; diastolic 90 to 99.
Stage II: Systolic equal to or >160 ; diastolic equal to or > 100

Diagnostic tests:

Test	Result Indicating Disorder	CPT Code
CBC	Anemia may contribute to development of hypertension	85022-85025
Urinalysis	May indicate renal pathology; renal disease may cause hypertension	81015
Chemistries	Abnormals may indicate renal disease; adrenal disease	80049
Lipid profile	Assess risk factors	80061
FBS	Assess risk factors	82950
Thyroid panel	Hyperthyroidism may cause hypertension	80091
Chest x-ray	Assess heart size and pulmonary vasculature	71010 (PA), 71020 (PA & LAT)

(Continued)

Test	Result Indicating Disorder	CPT Code
Echocardiogram	Assess heart function (ejection fraction), chambers, valves	93307, 93320, 93325
ECG	Assess rhythm, LVH indicates long-standing hypertension, presence of old MI	93000

* Further work-up depends on physical findings and the patient's response to treatment (e.g. abdominal bruit, perform renal arteriogram or magnetic resonance angiogram [MRA]).

Differential diagnosis: None.

Treatment: The goals of treatment are to lower systolic blood pressure to < 140 mm Hg and diastolic blood pressure < 85 mm Hg. Cardiovascular morbidity is considerably lower if systolic blood pressure is < 120 mm Hg and diastolic is < 80 mm Hg. In the presence of diabetes mellitus and chronic renal failure, it is especially important to control blood pressure to < 130 mm Hg systolic and 80 mm Hg diastolic. Throughout therapy, it is important to provide support and encouragement, to involve the patient and family, and to tailor the treatment program to the individual patient. See Figure 5-4 and Table 5-3.

Physical

Lifestyle modifications to help control HTN include advising the patient to lose weight to a body mass index of < 27, to maintain regular physical activity or exercise (aerobic activities such as walking), to reduce sodium intake, to reduce alcohol intake to no more than 1 oz of ethanol daily (10 oz of wine, 24 oz of beer, or 2 oz of whiskey), to limit caffeine intake, to stop smoking, and to take measures to reduce stress. It is important to note that lifestyle modifications must be instituted on **all** patients. Those with diabetes mellitus, target organ damage, or CAD must have the appropriate drug instituted immediately along with lifestyle modifications; those with high-normal or stage I HTN without diabetes, target organ damage, or CAD can try lifestyle changes alone for up to 1 year.

Pharmacologic

Therapy usually starts first with a thiazide diuretic, ACE, ARB, CCB or a beta blocker (unless contraindicated). If there is an inadequate response to the first drug chosen, add a second drug. Patients with Stage II hypertension should be started on two drugs, one of which should be a thiazide diuretic. If the patient continues to have an inadequate response after two drugs are titrated to a reasonable dose, add a third drug and titrate. If the blood pressure is not controlled on three different medications at maximal dosage, refer to a specialist.

Individualize therapy as much as possible. For example, give ACE inhibitors in patients with heart failure, diabetes mellitus, MI with systolic dysfunction, and renal disease. Angiotensin II receptor blockers are also effective with the above comorbidities; and may be given if ACE intolerant or with the ACE. The beta blockers are best in patients with post-MI,

Treatment: Hypertension

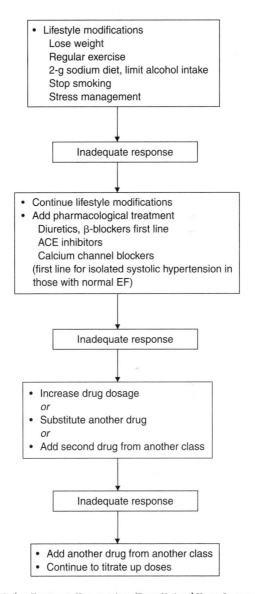

Figure 5–4. Treatment: Hypertension. (From National Heart, Lung, and Blood Institute: Seventh Report of the Joint National Committee on Prevention, Detection, Evaluation, and Treatment of High Blood Pressure. US Department of Health and Human Services, National Institutes of Health, Bethesda, Md, 2003.)

Table 5–3   Medications Used to Treat Hypertension

Diuretics	
Hydrochlorothiazide	12.5–25 mg qd
Furosemide (Lasix) – loop	20–240 mg qd
Torsemide (Demadex) – loop	5–20 mg qd
Bumetanide (Bumex) – loop	.5–2 mg qd
Ethacrynic acid (Edecrin) – loop	25–100 mg qd
Spironolactone (Aldactone) - K+ sparing	25–100 mg qd
Triamterene (Dyazide) – K+ sparing	50–150 mg qd
Beta Blockers	
Acebutolol (Sectral)	400–800 mg qd
Atenolol (Tenormin)	25–100 mg qd
Betaxolol (Kerlone)	5–40 mg qd
Bisoprolol (Zebeta)	2.5–20 mg qd
Metoprolol (Lopressor)	50–200 mg qd
Metoprolol (extended-release = Toprol LX)	50–400 mg qd
Nadolol (Corgard)	40–320 mg qd
Carvedilol (Coreg)	12.5–50 mg qd
Labetalol (Normodyne, Trandate)	200–1200 mg qd
Pindolol (Visken)	5–30 mg qd
Propanolol (Inderal)	40–240 mg qd in two doses
Timolol (Blocadren)	10–40 mg qd in two doses
ACE Inhibitors	
Benazepril (Lotensin)	10–40 mg qd
Captopril (Capoten)	25–300 mg qd
Enalapril (Vasotec)	2.5–40 mg qd
Fosinopril (Monopril)	5–40 mg qd
Lisinopril (Prinivil or Zestril)	5–40 mg qd
Quinapril (Accupril)	5–40 mg qd
Ramipril (Altace)	2.5–20 mg qd
ARBs (Angiotensin Receptor Blockers)	
Eprosartan (Teveten)	400–800 mg qd
Irbesartan (Avapro)	150–300 mg qd
Losartan (Cozaar)	25–100 mg qd
Valsartan (Diovan)	80–320 mg qd
Alpha-Adrenergic Blockers	
Doxazosin (Cardura)	1–16 mg qd
Prazosin (Minipress)	1–10 mg qd
Terazosin (Hytrin)	1–20 mg qd
Centrally Acting Alpha Agonists	
Clonidine (Catapres)	.1–1 mg qd in one or two doses
Guanabenz (Wytensin)	4–32 mg bid
Guanfacine (Tenex)	1–3 mg qd
Direct Vasodilators	
Hydralazine (Apresoline)	25–150 mg bid

patients with angina, migraine headache, and nonselective essential tremor. Alpha$_1$-adrenergic antagonists should be used in patients with benign prostatic hypertrophy. Elderly and black patients do well with long-acting calcium channel blockers, although each case should be evaluated selectively and the use of other agents should not be ruled out. First-line therapy for African-Americans is diuretic therapy. Long-acting calcium channel antagonists are effective for isolated systolic HTN; thiazide diuretics may be used for patients with this problem and osteoporosis, however, diuretics may worsen gout and diabetes. Beta blockers are usually contraindicated in reactive airway disease, heart failure, or heart block. Renovascular disease may be worsened by ACE inhibitors. Avoid calcium channel blockers with heart block or low ejection fraction.

Follow-up: The recommendations for follow-up for patients age 18 and older are as follows:

> Normal blood pressure (120 or less systolic or 80 or less diastolic): Recheck blood pressure in 2 years.
> Stage I (140 to 159 systolic or 90 to 99 diastolic): Confirm with three separate blood pressure checks within 2 months.
> Stage II (Systolic equal or $>$ 160 and diastolic equal or $>$ 100): Initiate therapy with two drugs, one of which should be a thiazide diuretic.

After initiating therapy, see the patient as indicated by blood pressure measurements. Once the blood pressure returns to an acceptable range, see the patient monthly for evaluation of effectiveness and compliance with therapy and continued assessment. Once he or she is stable, see the patient every 4 to 6 months for reevaluation.

 Clinical Pearl: Always suspect medication noncompliance when a patient who has been well controlled suddenly has uncontrolled HTN. A significant number of patients stop medications due to side effects or financial reasons and do not inform their health-care provider. Rule this out before making changes in the medical regimen.

Sequelae: Possible complications include left ventricular hypertrophy (LVH), CHF, renal failure, MI, cerebrovascular accident, peripheral arterial disease.

Prevention/prophylaxis: Prevention strategies include advising the patient to stop smoking, stop or decrease use of alcohol, lose weight if overweight, maintain a regular exercise program, and reduce stress. Encourage the patient to maintain compliance with therapy, including medication regimen. Stress consistent follow-up and compliance with regimen.

Referral: Refer to, or consult with, physician if the patient does not respond to therapy, especially if the patient is receiving the maximum allowable dosages of a combination of three different classes of medications.

Education: Explain the disease process, signs and symptoms, and treatment (including side effects of medications). Discuss prevention strategies, the importance of compliance with therapy, risk factors for CAD, and when to seek medical attention.

Educational resource materials are available from various sources, such as the American Heart Association; the Joint National Committee on Prevention, Detection, Evaluation, and Treatment of High Blood Pressure; the National Heart Lung Blood Research Institute; the National Institutes of Health (301-251-1222); the Agency for Health Care Policy and Research; the Centers for Disease Control and Prevention; the Health Resources and Services Administration; and the U.S. Public Health Services.

MITRAL VALVE PROLAPSE

SIGNAL SYMPTOMS▶ Chest pain; Palpitations

| Mitral valve disorders | ICD-9-CM: 424 |

Description: Mitral valve prolapse (MVP) is an anatomic abnormality of the mitral valve leaflets causing them to prolapse, or buckle back, into the left atrium during systole. Some patients are asymptomatic; others experience a constellation of cardiac and noncardiac symptoms.

Etiology: The cause is often unknown; the condition may be secondary to rheumatic heart disease or collagen tissue disorders. Redundancy of the mitral valve leaflets occurs with myxomatous degeneration of the mitral tissue. The posterior leaflet is usually affected more often than the anterior leaflet. The mitral valve annulus is enlarged, and the chordae tendineae may be elongated.

Occurrence: Occurs in about 5% of the population.

Age: Uncommon before adolescent growth spurt; most commonly diagnosed between the ages of 14 and 30 years.

Ethnicity: No significant ethnic predisposition.

Gender: Women younger than age 20 have higher incidence; equal incidence in men and women after age 20.

Contributing factors: Familial predisposition, cardiomyopathy, mitral commissurotomy, stress, fatigue, hormonal fluctuations (women), strenuous activities.

Signs and symptoms: Chest pain of a recurrent nature and occurring in the precordial and substernal areas, fatigue, dyspnea, syncope, lightheadedness, palpitations, migraine headaches, exercise intolerance, anxiety, and panic attacks all have been associated with this disorder. Many patients are asymptomatic.

Physical examination reveals a mid- to late systolic click or late systolic murmur on auscultation over the apex of the heart (hallmark sign). Patients are often thin, with arm span > height. Often abnormal thoracic cage or spine, such as pectus excavatum. Often high-arched palate.

Diagnostic tests

Test	Result Indicating Disorder	CPT Code
Echocardiogram (test of choice)	Demonstrates mitral valve prolapse; detects and quantifies mitral regurgitation	93307, 93320, 93325
Chest X-ray	Usually normal	71010 (PA), 71020 (PA & LAT)
ECG	Usually normal; may have biphasic or inverted T waves in inferior leads (II,III, AVF); PACs/PVCs possible	93000
Nuclear stress test	Rule out ischemia; assesses rate and rhythm with exercise	78465
Holter monitor	Assesses for abnormal rhythms; MVP may cause tachyarrhythmias, increased PACs/PVCs	93224

AVF, arteriovenous fistula; ECG, electrocardiogram; LAT, lateral; MVP, mitral valve prolapse; PA, posteroanterior; PACs, premature atrial contractions; PVCs, premature ventricular contractions.

Differential diagnosis:

- Hypertrophic cardiomyopathies (may cause arrhythmias and palpitations, chest pain)
- Papillary muscle dysfunction (may cause abnormal valvular function)
- CAD or spasm (may cause chest pain)
- Anxiety disorders (may cause palpitations)
- Congenital cardiac anomalies

Treatment:

Physical

There is no medical treatment to correct the valve abnormalities associated with MVP. Symptomatic management includes lifestyle changes, such as starting an aerobic exercise program (reduces plasma catecholamine, lowers heart rate, decreases stress, increases cardiac output and blood volume); avoiding caffeine, decongestants and products containing ephedrine, alcohol, chocolate, and cheeses; and drinking at least eight glasses of water a day (prevents dehydration). Focus on patient self-control of the disorder by encouraging the patient to maintain a diary to monitor symptoms and document effective management.

Pharmacologic

Beta blockers may be ordered for control of palpitations; however, because fatigue is already a problem for many of these patients, it may be exacerbated by this drug. Advise the patient to exercise caution in taking over-the-counter (OTC) drugs that may contain ephedrine. Endocarditis antibiotic prophylaxis (Table 5-4) is recommended for the patient with systolic murmur (mitral regurgitation) or thickened mitral leaflets on echo-Doppler.

Surgical

Occasionally, mitral valve replacement may be indicated for patients with severe mitral regurgitation and corresponding symptoms.

Table 5–4 Endocarditis: Antibiotic Prophylaxis

To prevent bacterial endocarditis, antibiotic prophylaxis is recommended for certain patients undergoing dental or operative procedures.

Recommended conditions	Aortic or mitral valve prolapse with valvular regurgitation.
	Rheumatic and other acquired valvular dysfunction, including after valve surgery.
	Most congenital cardiac malformations.
	Previous bacterial endocarditis, even without cardiac disease.
	Hypertrophic cardiomyopathy.
	Prosthetic cardiac valves.
	Surgically constructed systemic-pulmonary shunts.
Recommended standard antibiotic prophylaxis	Amoxicillin, 2 g orally 1 hour before the procedure.
	For the patient who cannot take amoxicillin or penicillin:
	Clindamycin, 600 mg orally 1 hour before the procedure; or
	azithromycin or clarithromycin 500 mg 1 hour before procedure.
	May be instituted if unexpected bleeding occurs, no later than 4 hours after the procedure.

Follow-up: See the patient who has mild to moderate symptoms requiring drug treatment and newly diagnosed patient in 2 weeks. with routine follow-up every 6 months. Patients with severe symptoms must be seen by cardiologist. Echocardiograms in stable patients should be repeated every 3 years.

Sequelae: Possible complications include mitral regurgitation (25%), arrhythmias, transient ischemic attacks (TIAs), cerebrovascular accident,, and infectious endocarditis (especially if the patient does not take prophylactic antibiotics before dental, surgical, or other invasive procedures).

Prevention/prophylaxis: Prevention strategies include advising patient to follow antibiotic prophylaxis and to integrate healthy lifestyle changes to control symptoms. Acetylsalicylic acid (ASA) may be indicated for TIA when no other cause detected.

Referral: Refer to cardiologist for initial diagnosis and as needed for follow-up.

Education: Explain disease process, signs and symptoms, and treatment (including side effects of medications). Discuss prevention strategies. Advise patient of support groups available. Educational resource materials are available from the American Heart Association, 7320 Greenville Avenue, Dallas, TX 75231 (214-373-6300).

PLEURISY

SIGNAL SYMPTOMS▶ Knifelike chest pain worsened with inspiration; Abrupt onset

Pleurisy	ICD 511.0

Description: Pleurisy is an inflammation (pleuritis) of the pleural surfaces, which may be primary or secondary, unilateral or bilateral, or localized. It may be acute or chronic, fibrinous, serofibrinous, or purulent. If the condition is left untreated, it may lead to pleural effusion and atypical chest pain.

Etiology: Caused by inflammatory or infectious processes, such as from bronchitis, pneumonia, TB, pulmonary infarction, viruses, or neoplasms, or by diseases outside the chest, such as rheumatoid arthritis, or subphrenic abscess.

Occurrence: May occur more frequently in patients with history of bronchitis or URIs.

Age: Occurs at any age, depending on underlying pathology.

Ethnicity: No significant ethnic predisposition.

Gender: Occurs equally in men and in women.

Contributing factors: Recent respiratory infection, bronchitis, rib trauma. Pleuritic pain exacerbated by sudden movements of the thorax, deep inspiration, sudden coughing, or sneezing.

Signs and symptoms: Abrupt onset of severe, knifelike, localized chest pain aggravated by inspiration; cough; dyspnea. Pleural pain is usually localized to the affected region rather than diffuse, but pain may be referred to ipsilateral neck or shoulder. (Inflammation of the intercostal nerves that supply the parietal pleura and periphery of the diaphragm causes pleuritic chest pain. Inflammation of the central diaphragmatic tendon, which is innervated by the phrenic nerve, causes pain that is referred to the ipsilateral shoulder.)

Physical examination may reveal shallow, rapid respirations and splinting on inspection; superficial chest tenderness on palpation; dullness, if there is underlying fluid in the pleural space on percussion; pleural friction rub (classic sign), as well as crackles (rales), rhonchi, and wheezing on auscultation.

Diagnostic tests:

Test	Result Indicating Disorder	CPT Code
CBC	Elevated WBC indicates acute bacterial infection	85027
ESR	Elevated with acute inflammatory or metastatic process	85651
BUN/creatinine	Rule out uremia	84520, 82565
Sputum C&S	If acute URI present with productive cough	87070
Chest X-ray	Rule out pneumonia, neoplasm, trauma	71010 (PA), 71020 (PA & LAT)
Ventilation-perfusion scan	Rule out pulmonary embolus	78596
CT scan of chest	Rule out neoplasm – if CXR indicates abnormality	71250 (without contrast), 71260 (with contrast)

BUN, blood urea nitrogen; CBC, complete blood count; C&S, culture and sensitivity; ESR, erythrocyte sedimentation rate; LAT, lateral; PA, posteroanterior; WBC, white blood cell.

Differential diagnosis:

- Pneumonia (may cause chest pain, pleurisy)
- Primary or metastatic lung cancer (may cause chest pain, pleural effusion with pleurisy)
- Pulmonary embolism (may cause chest pain and pain with deep breath)
- Uremia (may cause pleural effusion with pleurisy)
- Chest wall trauma (history of trauma, physical examination, x-ray study)
- Spontaneous pneumothorax (SOB sudden in onset with deep breath)

Treatment: Treat underlying process, if known.

Pharmacologic
Broad-spectrum antibiotics may be indicated for infectious processes. Analgesics and antipyretics as indicated.

Physical
Symptomatic management includes encouraging the patient to find and maintain a body position in which motion of the affected area is limited; to limit physical activities, including lifting or straining; to rest frequently; and to increase fluid intake. Deep breathing and coughing every 1 to 2 hours. Warm soaks may relieve symptoms.

Surgical
If pleural effusion is present, aspiration of pleural fluid or biopsy may be needed to define the underlying disease process.

Follow-up: Depends on the underlying diagnosis. Monitor the patient's response to the antibiotic. See patient in 1 week; then again in 1 month if the patient has exacerbation of pain or dyspnea.

Sequelae: Empyema; pleural effusion. Possible complications include heightened susceptibility to infectious processes, fatigue, and difficulty completing activities of daily living secondary to pain.

Prevention/prophylaxis: Prevention strategies are related to prevention of underlying causes and include advising the patient to use good hand-washing techniques and to avoid people with infectious respiratory disorders such as bronchitis or pneumonia.

Referral: Refer to, or consult with, an internist or pulmonologist if the CXR is abnormal or symptoms persist.

Education: Explain the disease process, signs and symptoms, and treatment (including side effects of medications). Advise the patient to report any increase in intensity, duration, or position of chest pain or fever, and to see practitioner immediately if the patient has difficulty breathing. Educational resources are available from the American Lung Association, 61 Broadway, 6th floor, New York, NY 10006 (212–315–8700) or local branch. Website: *www.lungusa.org*

PNEUMONIA

SIGNAL SYMPTOMS▶ Cough; usually productive of purulent sputum;
Crackles or rhonchi on auscultation

| Bacterial pneumonia | ICD-9-CM: 482.9 |
| Viral Pneumonia | ICD-9-CM: 481 |

Description: Pneumonia is an infection of the pulmonary parenchyma caused by bacterial species, mycoplasmas, chlamydiae, viruses, fungi, and parasites. Four major types of pneumonia are (1) bacterial (50% of all cases, with two thirds of these caused by *Streptococcus pneumoniae* or *Haemophilus influenzae* and about 15% by *Pseudomonas* or *Staphylococcus*); (2) *Mycoplasma* (leading cause in school-age children and young adults, about 130 cases/100,000 people); (3) *Pneumocystis carinii* pneumonia (PCP) (about 43% of all opportunistic infections in immunocompromised patients); and (4) viral.

Etiology: Caused by the aspiration of organisms, commonly aerobic gram-positive cocci and anaerobes, from the oropharynx, and the inhalation of infected particles, hematogenous spread, and contiguous spread from another infected site. Sixty percent of hospital-acquired pneumonia is due to gram-negative rods such as *Pseudomonas* or gram-positive rods from *Staphylococcus* (14.5%).

Occurrence: Accounts for about 10% of hospital admissions. Approximately 4 million persons per year; sixth leading cause of death and primary cause of death from infectious disease.

Age: Occurs at all ages. Bacterial form is the most common type found in older adults; *Mycoplasma* most common in children age 5 to 15; the viral type is most common in children.

Ethnicity: No significant ethnic predisposition.

Gender: Tends to occur equally in men and women, although PCP and *Mycoplasma* pneumonia have a higher incidence in men.

Contributing factors: Concurrent viral infection, hospitalization, immobility, alcoholism, HIV or other immunosuppression, renal failure, cardiovascular disease, functional asplenia, COPD, diabetes mellitus, malnutrition, malignancy, general anesthesia, mechanical ventilation, altered level of consciousness, travel history, pet exposure, exposure to others who are ill, occupation, age, presence or absence of teeth, season of the year, geographic location, smoking, HIV status, alterations in the normal protective mechanisms, depressed mucociliary transport.

Signs and symptoms: Signs and symptoms include fever, cough (with or without sputum; sputum may be green, thick, or bloody), dyspnea, pleuritic chest pain, rigors, myalgias, headache, diarrhea, and sudden onset of chills.

Physical examination may reveal chest dullness, decreased or bronchial breath sounds, crackles (rales), tachypnea, tachycardia, coarse rhonchi that may or may not clear with cough.

Signs and symptoms specific to causative organism are as follows:

Pneumococcal and *Haemophilus influenzae*: Signs and symptoms commonly include a sudden onset of high fever, shaking chills, productive cough (purulent or rusty), headache, and prostration. Pneumococcal is often seen in the previously healthy patient or after a URI. *Haemophilus* is often seen in older adults, in patients with COPD, or in patients who have had influenza or smoke.

Moraxella catarrhalis: Signs and symptoms are commonly mild, without chills, myalgias, or chest pain; often seen in patients with COPD or a chronic illness.

Gram-negative bacilli: Rarely seen in healthy adults; has a 20% to 30% mortality rate. Mainly hospital acquired.

Mycoplasma and *Chlamydia*: Signs and symptoms include hacking cough, fever, malaise, and headache; more common in patients younger than 35 years of age; commonly a mild, self-limited course; however, it may for last 6 weeks, despite treatment.

Legionella: Signs and symptoms are usually more severe and include confusion, headache, nausea, diarrhea, hematuria, hyponatremia, and elevated serum transaminase; the mortality rate is 10% to 30%.

Viral: Signs and symptoms are milder, but with a more prolonged prodromal phase, and include fever; chills; dry, hacking cough; pharyngitis; less elevated white blood cell count (WBC) and a CXR that shows no lobar distribution of infiltrate or pleural effusion.

Diagnostic tests

Test	Result Indicating Disorder	CPT Code
CBC	May show leukocytosis with infection	85007
Chemistries	Elevation of BUN/creatinine may show dehydration; rule out electrolyte abnormality	80049, 82565
Sputum C&S	Identify causative organism	87070
Oxygen saturation	Rule out hypoxia	82805, 82810
Chest x-ray	Look for air bronchogram; lobar or segmental consolidation; number of infiltrates	71010 (PA), 71020 (PA & LAT)

BUN, blood urea nitrogen; C&S: culture and sensitivity; CBC, complete blood count; LAT, lateral; PA, posteroanterior.

Patients should be admitted to the hospital for inpatient management if:

• History of a comorbid disease (CHF, COPD, liver or renal disease)
• Altered mental status
• Heart rate > 125 at rest

- Respiratory rate > 30
- Temperature < 95 or >104
- Systolic blood pressure < 90
- Oxygen saturation < 90
- More than one infiltrate on the CXR

Differential diagnosis:

- TB (cough, hemoptysis)
- CHF (cough, sputum, SOB)
- Atelectasis (SOB)
- Neoplasm (may cause repeated cases of pneumonia)

Treatment:

Pharmacologic

Antibiotic therapy: In clinical practice, you are primarily diagnosing and treating empirically. Antibiotics of choice for suspected and/or confirmed pneumonia:

For a patient with an onset of illness with a frank shaking chill, the most likely pathogen is *Streptococcus pneumoniae* and antibiotics of choice are (1) penicillin, (2) cephalosporin, (3) fluoroquinolone, or (4) macrolide

For a younger patient presenting with a less productive but prominent cough, the most likely pathogen is *Mycoplasma pneumoniae*. Antibiotics of choice are (1) doxycycline, (2) macrolide, (3) fluoroquinolone

Beta-lactamase production, which confers resistance to penicillin and oxacillin, is common in *M. catarrhalis* and occurs in a reasonable number of *H. influenzae* strains and occasionally *K. pneumoniae* strains. Vancomycin remains the drug of choice to eliminate these resistant strains, along with some of the newer macrolides. The quinolone antibiotics have relative inactivity against *S. pneumoniae* and should be used with caution.

Pseudomonas pneumonia may be treated with (1) aminoglycoside (check BUN/creatinine) (2) cephalosporin, or (3) fluoroquinolone

Cough suppressant use remains controversial. Dextromethorphan (DM) and codeine are effective suppressants that may be indicated when cough interferes with sleep. If codeine allergic or intolerant, benzonatate (Tessalon Perles) or guaifenesin (Humibid L.A.) are good alternatives.

Albuterol inhaler, two puffs four times a day for wheeze, if needed. Wheeze may also be ameliorated with a Medrol dose Pak for treatment of acute inflammation.

Others: Analgesia for fever and discomfort. Check and record temperature at least twice a day. Avoid overuse of cough suppressants (Fig. 5-5).

Outpatient Treatment: Pneumonia

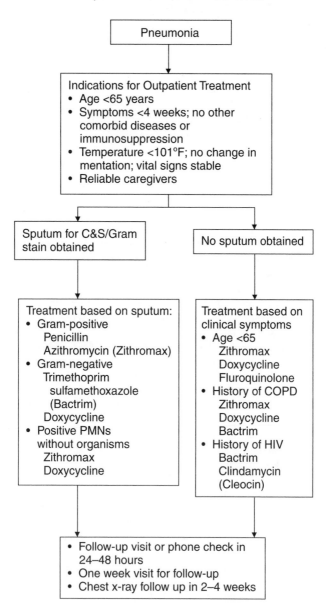

Figure 5–5. Outpatient treatment: pneumonia

Physical

Chest physiotherapy to aid in the expectoration of residual sputum. Adequate nutrition and hydration (at least 2000 mL daily, unless contraindicated). A soft diet is usually recommended during the acute phase. Bed rest or reduced physical activity are recommended during the acute phase. Encourage patient to stop smoking and stop or decrease alcohol intake.

Follow-up: May assess patient's progress daily through telephone contact. See patient in 1 week for re-evaluation. If no improvement in 72 hours, see the patient immediately. Consider hospitalization.

 Clinical Pearl: Repeat CXR 1 to 2 weeks after finishing antibiotics to establish resolution of pneumonia or rule out other underlying disease processes (such as neoplasm).

Sequelae: The usual course is acute. In otherwise healthy patients, improvement is usually seen and fever reduced in 72 hours. Pneumonia is exacerbated or prolonged by alcoholism, use of tobacco, diabetes mellitus, renal or liver disease. The overall mortality rate is about 5%. The poorest prognosis is noted in very young or very old patients and those with positive blood cultures, low WBC, comorbidities, and underlying immunosuppression.

Possible complications include empyema, pulmonary abscess, purulent pericarditis, pleurisy, pleural effusion, lung necrosis, superinfection, multiple organ dysfunction syndrome (MODS), and acute respiratory distress syndrome (ARDS). Continual symptoms, like fatigue, malaise, and cough, may persist for several weeks.

Prevention/prophylaxis: Prevention strategies include advising the patient to obtain pneumococcal and influenza vaccines, especially if patient is at high risk (older than age 65; has chronic heart, lung, or renal disease, sickle cell anemia, or diabetes mellitus; or is a resident of a chronic care facility). Also, advise the patient to avoid people with respiratory infections, maintain adequate nutrition and fluid intake, stop smoking, and decrease or stop alcohol use. For the postoperative or bedridden patient, encourage coughing and deep breathing exercises and turning at least every 2 hours.

Referral: Refer to, or consult with, physician or pulmonary specialist if patient is older than age 65 or has an HIV infection, a chronic disease, severe dyspnea, hemoptysis, or toxic pneumonia. Home health care referral may be indicated if patient is receiving outpatient treatment.

Education: Explain the disease process, signs and symptoms, and treatment (including side effects of medications). Discuss prevention strategies and when to seek medical attention (continued fever, dyspnea, drowsiness).

SLEEP APNEA, OBSTRUCTIVE

SIGNAL SYMPTOMS▶ Excessive daytime sleepiness; Snoring

| Sleep apnea | ICD-9-CM: 306.1 |

Description: Obstructive sleep apnea (OSA) is a chronic disorder characterized by repetitive episodes of upper airway obstruction during sleep, usually with hypoxia. OSA most commonly occurs during rapid eye movement (REM) sleep but can also occur during non–rapid eye movement (NREM) sleep. Nearly always associated with snoring.

Etiology: The obstruction is caused by upper airway narrowing, which may be caused by obesity, enlarged tonsils or uvula, low soft palate, hypertrophic soft palate, a large or posteriorly located tongue, or craniofacial deformities.

Occurrence: Occurs in 4% to 8% of adults in the United States.

Age: Occurs in middle-aged and older adults; frequency appears to increase with age and after menopause in women; uncommon in children.

Ethnicity: No significant ethnic predisposition.

Gender: Occurs more often in men than in women.

Contributing factors: Obesity; nasal obstruction caused by polyps; deviated septum; rhinitis; hypothyroidism; macroglossia, micrognathia, and acromegaly; HTN; cardiovascular disease; or alveolar hypoventilation; may be familial, but hereditary factors are not known.

Signs and symptoms: Excessive daytime sleepiness (EDS) (hallmark symptom). Other symptoms include loud snoring, disrupted sleep, repeated awakenings with transient sensation of SOB, fatigue on morning awakening, impaired memory, irritability, poor concentration, morning headaches, decreased libido, depression, and systemic and pulmonary HTN. Sleep apnea is almost always associated with snoring, and episodes of apnea often end with a snort or gasp. Family reports witnessed apneic episode.

Physical examination may reveal hypoxemia during episodes, and elevated end-tidal CO_2. Cardiac arrhythmias, usually sinus bradycardia, sinus arrest, and occasionally, second-degree heart block, also frequently accompany sleep apnea. The overall ECG pattern is one of bradycardia, followed by tachycardia. Increases in systemic and pulmonary pressures are also associated with apneic episodes.

Diagnostic tests:

Test	Result Indicating Disorder	CPT Code
CBC	Polycythemia may be seen as a result of nocturnal hypoxemia	85027
Thyroid function tests	Rule out hypothyroidism	80091,92

(Continued)

Test	Result Indicating Disorder	CPT Code
ABGs	Daytime elevations of CO_2 may be seen	82803, 82805-10
Serum calcium	Rule out hypocalcemia	82331
MRI, CT, or endoscopic examination of the upper airway	Assesses for airway abnormalities	76536
Sleep study (polysomnogram) that includes an assessment of oxygen saturation and CO_2 levels during the patient's normal sleep time	Indicated to diagnose sleep apnea. Abnormal results consistent with sleep apnea include repetitive episodes of cessation or marked reduction in airflow despite continued respiratory efforts. Apneic episodes must last at least 10 seconds and occur 10–15 times per hour to be considered significant. The polysomnogram shows the degree of hypoxemia, sleep disruption, cardiac arrhythmias, and elevated end-tidal CO_2 levels associated with sleep apnea.	95808-95811
Multiple sleep latency testing	Provides an objective measure of daytime sleepiness	95811
Cephalometric measurement obtained from lateral head and neck x-ray studies	Assesses craniofacial abnormalities	70260

ABGs, arterial blood gases; CBC, complete blood count., CT, computed tomography; MRI, magnetic resonance imaging.

Differential diagnosis:

- Narcolepsy (no snoring)
- Idiopathic daytime hypersomnolence (no snoring)
- Inadequate sleep (history)
- Depression (increased daytime somnolence with poor night sleep pattern)
- Gastroesophageal reflux (GERD) (sudden reflux with cough, awakening)
- Asthma (nocturnal exacerbations)
- COPD (pulmonary HTN)
- CHF (paroxysmal nocturnal dyspnea (PND) with sudden awakening)
- Sleep-associated seizure

Treatment: Treatment is dependent on the severity of obstructive sleep apnea.

OSA: Pharmacologic therapy may include protriptyline, 20 to 30 mg once daily at bedtime (HS).

If the sleep apnea occurs only when the patient is supine, physical therapies intended to prevent the patient from sleeping on the back may be undertaken. These include such measures as sewing a tennis ball into the back of the patient's pajamas or having the patient wear a fanny pack of tennis balls at the back.

Mild to moderate OSA: Weight loss; avoid alcohol; avoid sleeping in supine position; improve nasal patency; dental appliances.

Moderate to severe OSA: May be treated with surgery (tonsillectomy or uvulopalatopharygoplasty, which is effective only 50% of the time). May be treated with biphasic positive airway pressure (BiPAP or continuous positive airway pressure [CPAP]). Craniofacial surgery or tracheostomy may be indicated for severe OSA not controlled by other measures.

Follow-up: See patient as needed for evaluation of and compliance with treatment plan. Return of snoring, EDS, or sleep disruption may indicate inadequate control of apnea.

 Clinical Pearl: Include significant other in follow-up visits (not just during work-up) in order to assess efficacy of treatment.

Sequelae: Possible complications include pulmonary HTN, ventricular arrhythmias, cor pulmonale, and CHF. Severe HTN may occur during apneic episodes. Death from OSA is usually caused by arrhythmias, cardiac ischemia, complications of acute HTN, or motor vehicle accidents.

Prevention/prophylaxis: Prevention strategies include advising the patient to lose weight, if the patient is overweight, because obesity can be the cause of the sleep apnea. Recommend that the patient not drive or operate equipment until treatment is initiated because of the high risk for injury brought on by sleepiness or inability to be attentive. Also, advise the patient not to take sedatives.

Referral: Refer to, or consult with, physician or pulmonologist as needed.

Education: Explain disease process, signs and symptoms, and treatment (including side effects of medications). Discuss prevention strategies.

TUBERCULOSIS

SIGNAL SYMPTOMS Night sweats and weight loss with cough as a later symptom

Tuberculosis	ICD-9-CM: 010.8

Description: Pulmonary TB is a chronic, necrotizing bacterial infection. It most commonly affects the lungs, but other organs may be involved. TB is spread primarily by respiratory droplets. About 10% of infected people go on to develop active disease.

TB infection is usually asymptomatic and is detected primarily by a positive TB skin test. TB commonly presents with unexplained coughing, weight loss, or fever. TB infection normally remains in a latent state and may be dormant throughout life, with the first 1 to 2 years after infection the most crucial for developing the disease. TB is often manifested during periods of stress, decreased immunity, old age, pregnancy, and with other diseases. In immunocompromised individuals, symptoms often appear soon after exposure.

Etiology: Caused by the tubercle bacillus *Mycobacterium tuberculosis*. It is an airborne infection, mostly transmitted by inhalation of droplet nuclei. Incubation period is 2 to 10 weeks. PPD becomes positive in about 12 weeks.

Occurrence: Over the past decade, there had been a resurgence of TB. People with HIV infection are highly susceptible to TB. The incidence and prevalence in the United States varies greatly by region; it may be as high as 32 to 100 per 100,000.

Age: Occurs in all age groups. Except for the group of patients with HIV, adults older than age 65 have the highest case rate of TB. Children up to the age of 14 have increased vulnerability to TB. In recent years, there has been an increased incidence in the age range of 25 to 44 years.

Ethnicity: More than two thirds of reported cases occurred among non-white populations.

Gender: Occurs more often in men than in women.

Contributing factors: Groups at high risk for TB include the homeless, minorities, older adults, immigrants from other countries with higher prevalence of TB, prisoners, alcoholics, those with malnutrition, residents and staff of long-term care facilities. Groups at high risk for progression from TB infection to disease include children younger than 5 years of age, those who have acquired the infection within the last 2 years, those with fibrotic lesions on CXR, those with disabling conditions such as HIV, silicosis, recent gastrointestinal (GI) surgery, chronic renal disease, diabetes, and those who are immunosuppressed. Those who are pregnant, and those on chronic high-dose steroids.

Signs and symptoms: The history is important in determining whether to treat the patient for TB infection or disease. Obtain information regarding previous skin tests, CXRs, and possible exposure. Common symptoms of active disease include cough lasting over 3 weeks, purulent mucous, fatigue, diaphoresis, night sweats, low-grade fever, anorexia, weight loss, flulike symptoms, pleuritic chest pain, swollen lymph nodes, headache, and pain.

The physical exam may reveal pallor, generalized wasting (late sign), adenopathy, dullness of lung fields, crackles near the apex of the lungs, whispered pectoriloquy, bronchial breath sounds, and hepatosplenomegaly.

Diagnostic tests

Test	Result Indicating Disorder	CPT Code
PPD*	Determined by the diameter of the induration, not by erythema: induration of greater then 15 mm is considered positive in all populations. Induration of 10 mm or greater is considered positive in a high-risk population; induration of 5 mm or greater is considered positive in those with compromised immunity or with old x-ray studies suggestive of previous disease.	86580-86585
CXR	Presence cavitary lesion, air space consolidation in middle and lower lobes, patch or nodular consolidation in upper lobes. May see pleural effusion, hilar and mediastinal lymphadenopathy.	71010 (PA), 71020 (PA & LAT)
Sputum C&S/ gram stain	Positive in 50% of patients for *Mycobacterium*. Acid fast bacilli on Gram stain. Culture will confirm diagnosis. A series of three morning sputum samples is recommended for culture.	87116-7

* PPD testing is **not contraindicated** for person's who have been vaccinated with bacille Calmette-Guérin BCG. However, no method can reliably distinguish tuberculin reaction caused by BCG from those caused by natural mycobacterial infection. Therefore, a positive PPD in BCG-vaccinated persons indicates infection when the person is at increased risk or has comorbidities that increase risk.

Differential diagnosis:

- Pneumoconiosis (chronic cough)
- Pneumonia (cough, fever)
- Sarcoidosis (cough, DOE)
- Neoplasm (cough, hemoptysis)
- Lung abscess(cough, fever, consolidation)
- Fungal infection

Treatment: It is important to note that before starting therapy, baseline laboratory tests must be obtained. These should include: CBC, BUN and creatinine, liver function tests (LFTs), uric acid (if pyrazinamide is used). Baseline visual acuity should also be tested with attention to red-green color perception (if ethambutol is used). LFTs should be monitored monthly during treatment—if LFT's become elevated by 3 to 5 times the baseline, consider discontinuing isoniazid. If there is suspected noncompliance to therapy by the patient, consider directly observed therapy (DOT) – treatment given in the office, clinic, or patient's home).

Initial Treatment

Option 1: Isoniazid, rifampin, and pyrazinamide daily for 8 weeks, followed by isoniazid and rifampin daily for two to three times per week for 16 weeks. If isoniazid resistance is not documented or < 4%, add ethambutol or streptomycin to the initial regimen.

Option 2: Isoniazid, rifampin, pyrazinamide, and streptomycin or ethambutol daily for 2 weeks, followed by administration of same drugs two times weekly for 6 weeks; subsequently, isoniazid and rifampin two times weekly for 16 weeks.

Option 3: Isoniazid, rifampin, pyrazinamide, and ethambutol or streptomycin three times weekly for 6 months. Dosage recommendations depend on the number of times per week the patient is taking the medication.

Daily dosage: Isoniazid 5 mg/kg (maximum 300 mg); rifampin 10 mg/kg (maximum 600 mg); pyrazinamide 15 to 30 mg/kg (maximum 2 g); ethambutol 15 to 25 mg/kg; streptomycin 15 mg/kg (maximum 1 g).

Two times per week dosage: Isoniazid 15 mg/kg (maximum 900 mg); rifampin 10 mg/kg (maximum 600 mg); pyrazinamide 50 to 70 mg/kg (maximum 4 g); ethambutol 50 mg/kg (maximum 2.5 g); streptomycin 25 to 30 mg/kg (maximum 1 g).

Three times per week dosage: Isoniazid 15 mg/kg (maximum 900 mg); rifampin 10 mg/kg (maximum 600 mg); pyrazinamide 50 to 70 mg/kg (maximum 3 g); ethambutol 25 to 30 mg/kg (maximum 2.5 g); streptomycin 25 to 30 mg/kg (maximum 1 g).

For the patent who cannot take pyrazinamide: isoniazid and rifampin for 9 months. If isoniazid resistance is demonstrated, continue rifampin and ethambutol for at least 12 months.

For the patient with infection resistant to isoniazid use rifampin: for pregnant patient with TB use isoniazid and rifampin.

Follow-up: See the patient at least once a month for repeat sputum cultures; continue until sputum cultures are negative. Continue treatment for at least 3 months after sputum is negative. Re-evaluate in 6 months. If findings on x-ray studies fail to improve after 3 months of therapy, this suggests the abnormality is the result of either previous TB or another disease process.

Sequelae: Secondary infections, drug resistance, death.

Prevention/prophylaxis: Education about mode of transmission and disease process. Education on how to prevent transmission. Preventive therapy for adult is 300 mg isoniazid daily for 6 to 12 months; for the patient with HIV isoniazid for 12 months (Table 5-5).

Referral: Refer to TB expert for consultation. Report all incidences of TB to the health department.

Education: Explain the disease process, signs and symptoms. Explain medications and treatments used; foster compliance to treatment. Educational resource materials available from American Lung Association.

UPPER RESPIRATORY TRACT INFECTION

SIGNAL SYMPTOMS▶ Rhinitis and myalgias

Upper respiratory tract infection   ICD-9-CM: 460

Description: An upper respiratory tract infection (URI), also known as

Table 5–5   Criteria for Preventive Therapy

The CDC has recommended using the following criteria to determine the need for preventive TB therapy for persons with a positivie Mantoux reaction to 5 tuberculin units (TU) of purified protein derivative (PPD).

Category	Age 35 and Younger	Age 35 and Older
With risk factors	Treat if PPD reaction is 5–10 mm. Treat if PPD reaction is 5 mm *and* patient is recent TB contact, is HIV-infected, or has radiographic evidence of old TB.	Treat if PPD reaction is 5-10 mm. Treat if PPD reaction is 5 mm *and* patient is recent TB contact, is HIV-infected, or has radiographic evidence of old TB.
Without risk factors; high-incidence group	Treat if PPD reaction is 10 mm or greater.	No treatment indicated.
Without risk factors; low-incidence group	Treat if PPD reaction is 15 mm or greater.	No treatment indicated.

Adapted from the CDC: The use of preventive therapy for tuberculoses infection in the US. Recommendations of the Advisory Committee for Elimination of TB MMWR 39(RR-8): 9–12;1990.

the common cold, is usually caused by a virus and results in inflammation of the nasal passages. Most URIs are self-limiting and accompanied only by minor somatic complaints.

Etiology: Usually caused by a virus such as rhinovirus; influenza A, B, and C viruses; parainfluenza viruses; respiratory syncytial viruses; coronaviruses; adenoviruses; and ECHO viruses. In 40% of cases, no agent can be identified. The usual mode of transmission is hand to hand from contaminated nasal secretions. The usual URI lasts 5 to 14 days.

Occurrence: URIs are the most common cause of short-term disability in the United States, with episodes reported in 31/100 people per year.

Age: Occurs more frequently in children than in adults.

Ethnicity: Native Americans and Eskimos are at higher risk than other ethnic groups, and may suffer more frequent complications of colds.

Gender: Occurs equally in men and in women.

Contributing factors: Exposure to infected individuals, contact between nose or conjunctiva and contaminated fingers.

Signs and symptoms: Most common signs and symptoms include rhinorrhea, cough, fever (temperature never > 102°F), malaise, myalgias.

Physical examination may reveal mucopurulent nasal drainage, nasopharyngeal mucosal swelling, and lymphadenopathy. (Pharyngeal exudates are unusual in viral infections and more common in bacterial infections.)

Diagnostic tests

Test	Result Indicating Disorder	CPT Code
CBC, if symptoms persist over 10 days or patient has a temperature above 100°F	Leukocytosis over 10,000 indicates bacterial infection	85027
Nasal smear for eosinophils, if allergic rhinitis is suspected	Will be positive if etiology is allergic rhinitis	87205
Throat cultures, if streptococcal pharyngitis is suspected	Will be positive if etiology is strep; will document any other organism	87060
Monospot test to rule out mononucleosis	Positive if due to Epstein-Barr virus (EBV)	86403
Skin testing may be performed in patients with rhinitis when the diagnosis is not clear	Will be positive for allergy if chronic rhinitis is due to allergy rather than infection	86580-86585

Differential diagnosis:

- Influenza
- Chronic rhinitis
- Sinusitis
- Epstein-Barr virus (sore throat, adenopathy, fatigue, fever)
- Use of medications such as: nasal sprays, antihypertensives, hormones, ASA, NSAIDS, psychotropic drugs

Treatment: Usually managed on an outpatient basis.

Physical

Rest, increased fluid intake, and symptom relief measures such as humidified air.

Pharmacologic

OTC medications for pain, fever, congestion, or cough relief. When a cough is nonproductive or prevents normal rest and activities, it may be treated with a cough suppressant containing DM or codeine. Mouthwashes, lozenges, hard candy, gargling with warm saline, and products with local anesthetics such as benzocaine or phenol may provide subjective relief of sore throat pain. The use of antihistamines, vitamin C (ascorbic acid), and expectorants is controversial. Avoid medications with pseudoephedrine in patients with history of HTN and cardiac dysrhythmias.

Follow-up: See the patient if symptoms last longer than 14 days; or if the patient develops a fever associated with systemic symptoms; SOB, or cough and nasal drainage with purulent sputum.

 Clinical Pearl: In patients who have more than four episodes per year, look for underlying chronic sinus/allergy problems.

Sequelae: Possible complications include lower respiratory tract infection, sinusitis, and aggravation of asthma symptoms.

Prevention/prophylaxis: Prevention strategies include advising the patient to perform frequent, proper hand washing, avoid touching the face, and avoid contact with infected people.

Referral: Referral or consultation is usually not necessary if the patient has an uncomplicated URI.

Education: Explain disease process, signs and symptoms, and treatment (including side effects of medications). Discuss prevention strategies and when to contact health-care provider.

VALVULAR HEART DISEASE (MITRAL STENOSIS, MITRAL REGURGITATION, AORTIC STENOSIS, AORTIC REGURGITATION, TRICUSPID STENOSIS, TRICUSPID REGURGITATION)

SIGNAL SYMPTOMS▶ Varies depending on the severity of the stenosis or insufficiency. Severe aortic stenosis causes frequent presyncope and syncope: may be chest pain with mitral insufficiency. May be asymptomatic if not severe.

Mitral and aortic stenosis	ICD-9-CM: 396.0
Mital and aortic insufficiency	ICD-9-CM: 396.3

Description: Valvular heart disease describes cardiac dysfunction that results from structural or functional abnormalities of one or more valves. There are two major types of diseased valves: valvular stenosis, in which the flow of blood from one chamber to the next is impeded, and valvular insufficiency or regurgitation, in which blood leaks back (regurgitates) into the chamber from which blood is being pumped. Valvular heart disease includes mitral stenosis, mitral regurgitation (insufficiency), mitral valve prolapse, aortic stenosis, aortic regurgitation (insufficiency), tricuspid stenosis, and tricuspid regurgitation (insufficiency). (For information on mitral valve prolapse, see the section Mitral Valve Prolapse on page 250.)

Etiology: With valvular stenosis, the valve orifice's opening narrows and the valve leaflets (cusps) become fused together in such a way that the valve cannot open freely. As a result, the chamber behind the affected valve must build up more pressure to overcome the resistance and push the blood through the narrowed opening. Gradually, the muscle hypertrophies in response to the added workload.

With valvular regurgitation (insufficiency), the valve cannot close completely, resulting in blood flowing backward through the opening. The incomplete closure usually results from scarring and retraction of the valve leaflets. Hypertrophy and dilation are compensatory mechanisms that occur. When stenosis and regurgitation occur simultaneously, the defect is called a mixed lesion. It is usually seen in advanced disease.

Occurrence: Common; mitral stenosis is the most common valvular disorder in people with rheumatic heart disease (40% of all valvular disease).

Age: Occurs at any age.

Ethnicity: No significant ethnic predisposition.

Gender: Mitral stenosis and mitral regurgitation: Occur more often in women than in men. Aortic stenosis and aortic regurgitation: Occur more often in men than in women.

Contributing Factors: Acute rheumatic fever, rheumatic valve disease, CAD.

Signs and symptoms:

Mitral Stenosis

Mild: usually asymptomatic; diastolic murmur.

If severe, may cause CHF with the following symptoms: DOE, SOB, orthopnea PND, fatigue. Physical examination may reveal ruddy cheeks; bloody, productive cough; peripheral edema; right ventricular tap along left sternal border (increased RV size); displaced point of maximal pulse (PMI), enlarged liver; decreased arterial pulse volume; thrill over apical area; crackles; irregular pulse if atrial fibrillation present; diastolic murmur; accentuated S_1 with opening snap.

Mitral Regurgitation

Mild: usually asymptomatic; may have palpitations; systolic murmur radiating from left sternal border to the left axilla

If severe, may cause CHF with the following signs and symptoms: weakness, fatigue, orthopnea, PND, and DOE.

Physical examination may reveal dyspnea, diaphoresis, JVD, peripheral edema, regular pulse with sharp upstroke or irregular pulse if patient has atrial fibrillation, systolic thrill at apex, enlarged liver, laterally displaced PMI, and crackles.

Auscultation may reveal a soft S_1, systolic murmur, holosystolic murmur radiating from left sternal border to left axilla, split S_2; severe MR may hear S_3.

Aortic Stenosis

Signs and symptoms may include chest pain, palpitations, presyncope, DOE; if severe may have heart failure; fatigue, vertigo, syncope, ventricular tachycardia, and bradycardia. If severe, physical examination may reveal altered mental status; peripheral edema; hair loss; shiny skin over shins; forceful, sustained apical impulse; delayed carotid upstroke; cool extremities; pulsus alternans; decreased systolic blood pressure; inferiorly and laterally displaced PMI; systolic thrill in aortic area at jugular notch and along carotid arteries; CHF to pulmonary edema; and narrowed pulse pressure. Auscultation reveals S_3 or S_4, mid ejection murmur in the aortic area that radiates to the carotids; split S_2.

Aortic Regurgitation

Signs and symptoms may include palpitations, dyspnea; if severe: orthopnea, PND, fatigue, weakness, and presyncope, and syncope. If the condition is severe, physical examination may reveal altered mental status; symptoms of left ventricular failure; peripheral edema; de Musset's sign (nodding head); flushed skin; forceful, diffuse apical impulse; widened aortic pulse pressure; abrupt rise and fall of carotid and other peripheral pulses; water-hammer pulse (bounding); Quincke's sign (capillaries in nail base pulsate on pressing of the fingertips); Hill's sign (popliteal blood pressure is about 40 mm Hg > brachial blood pressure). Auscultation reveals early to mid-diastolic murmur over the aortic area; as the condition worsens, it may become a holodiastolic murmur, which may have S_3.

Tricuspid Stenosis and Tricuspid Regurgitation

Signs and symptoms include those of right ventricular failure (neck vein distention, peripheral edema, RUQ pain).

Auscultation reveals a diastolic, rumbling murmur in the left sternal border that increases with inspiration.

Diagnostic tests:

Mitral Stenosis

Test	Result Indicating Disorder	CPT Code
Chest x-ray	WNL unless advanced MS and then may have CHF with cardiomegaly and pulmonary venous congestion.	71010 (PA), 71020 (PA & LAT)
ECG	May show left atrial and right ventricular hypertrophy; P mitrale: prolonged, notched P waves, atrial fibrillation	93000
Echocardiogram	Shows thickened mitral valve with diminished movement of leaflets, left atrial and right ventricular enlargement.	93307, 93320, 93325
Cardiac catheterization	Reveals increased pressure gradient across mitral valve, increased left atrial pressure and pulmonary vascular resistance, increased left ventricular end-diastolic pressure (LVEDP) and pulmonary artery wedge pressure (PAWP), decreased cardiac output	93510, 93543, 93545, 93555, 93556

CHF, congestive heart failure; ECG, electrocardiogram; LAT, lateral; MS, mitral stenosis; PA, posteroanterior; WNL, within normal limits.

Mitral Regurgitation

Test	Result Indicating Disorder	CPT Code
Chest x-ray	May be WNL unless advanced MR and then may have CHF with cardiomegaly and pulmonary vascular congestion	71010 (PA), 71020 (PA & LAT)
ECG	May show left atrial and ventricular hypertrophy, P mitrale, atrial fibrillation	93000
Echocardiogram	Shows bizarre motion of mitral leaflets, hyperdynamic left ventricle, enlarged left atrium and ventricle	93307, 93320, 93325
Cardiac catheterization	Reveals increased left atrial pressure, increased amount of regurgitant flow; rules out prolapse and congenital disorders, increased VEDP and PAWP, decreased cardiac output	93510, 93543, 93545, 93555, 93556

CHF, congestive heart failure; ECG, electrocardiogram; LAT, lateral; VEDP, ventricular end-diastolic pressure; MS, mitral stenosis; PA, posteroanterior; PAWP, pulmonary artery wedge pressure; WNL, within normal limits..

Aortic Stenosis

Test	Result Indicating Disorder	CPT Code
Chest x-ray	WNL unless advanced; then may show calcification of aortic valve, left ventricular enlargement, prominent ascending aorta	71010 (PA), 71020 (PA & LAT)
ECG	Shows left ventricular hypertrophy, sinus tachycardia, atrial fibrillation, AV conduction delay, left and right bundle branch block	93000
Echocardiogram	Shows limited aortic valve movement, thickened left ventricular wall	93307, 93320, 93325
Cardiac catheterization	Reveals increased pressure gradient in systole across aortic valve, decreased size of aortic orifice, increased VEDP	93510, 93543, 93545, 93555, 93556

AV, atrioventricular; ECG, electrocardiogram; VEDP, ventricular end-diastolic pressure; PA, posteroanterior.

Aortic Regurgitation

Test	Results Indicating Disorder	CPT Code
Chest x-ray	WNL unless advanced, then may show calcification of aortic valve, left ventricular enlargement, dilation of ascending aorta	71010 (PA), 71020 (PA & LAT)
ECG	Shows left ventricular hypertrophy, sinus tachycardia, PVCs	93000
Echocardiogram	Shows dilated and hyperdynamic left ventricle, enlargement of aortic root and left atrium, early closure of mitral valve, diastolic fluttering of aortic valve	93307, 93320, 93325
Cardiac catheterization	Reveals decreased aortic diastolic pressure, increased VEDP, decreased regurgitant flow, reflux through aortic valve	93510, 93543, 93545, 93555, 93556

ECG, electrocardiogram; LAT, lateral; VEDP, ventricular end-diastolic pressure; PA, posteroanterior; PVCs, premature ventricular contractions..

Tricuspid Stenosis

Test	Results Indicating Disorder	CPT Code
Chest x-ray	Shows right atrial enlargement	71010 (PA), 71020 (PA & LAT)
ECG	Shows tall, peaked P waves, right atrial hypertrophy, and atrial arrhythmias	93000
Echocardiogram	Shows thickening and abnormal motion of tricuspid valve	93307, 93320, 93325
Cardiac catheterization	Reveals increased pressure across the tricuspid valve	93510, 93543, 93545, 93555, 93556

ECG, electrocardiogram; LAT, lateral; PA, posteroanterior.

Tricuspid Regurgitation

Test	Result Indicating Disorder	CPT Code
Chest x-ray	Shows right atrial and ventricular enlargement	71010 (PA), 71020 (PA & LAT)
ECG	Shows tall, peaked P wave and right ventricular hypertrophy	93000
Echocardiogram	Shows right ventricular dilation, paradoxic septal motion, and tricuspid valvular thickening and abnormal motion	93307, 93320, 93325

ECG, electrocardiogram; LAT, lateral; PA, posteroanterior.

Differential diagnosis:

Mitral stenosis: Atrial myxoma or vegetation caused by endocarditis, anemia, thyrotoxicosis.

Mitral regurgitation: Rheumatic or ischemic heart disease, mitral valve prolapse, infective endocarditis, mitral annular dilation or calcification, congenital valve deformities (parachute mitral valve, endocardial cushion defects, endocardial fibroelastosis, and transposition of the great arteries), cardiac trauma, prosthetic mitral valve malfunction.

Treatment: For the asymptomatic patient, no treatment is indicated, except for prophylactic antibiotic therapy before any dental or surgical procedure to protect against bacterial endocarditis.

Mitral stenosis: For symptomatic patient, cardiac glycosides (digitalis); beta blockers; diuretics, and sodium restriction to reduce blood volume and pulmonary and systemic venous pressures; anticoagulation therapy with warfarin if patient has a history of systemic embolism, atrial fibrillation, or a large left atrium; or surgical interventions, including mitral commissurotomy, balloon valvuloplasty, and mitral valve replacement.

Mitral regurgitation: For symptomatic patient, vasodilators to reduce ventricular filling volume and decrease systemic vascular resistance; administration of digitalis and anticoagulants to control ventricular rate and decrease embolic complications if patient has atrial fibrillation; management of CHF if indicated (see CHF).

Aortic stenosis: For symptomatic patient, surgical interventions, such as aortic commissurotomy or aortic valve replacement, may be indicated.

Aortic regurgitation: For symptomatic patient, treatment may include digitalis and diuretics to treat symptoms of heart failure and arterial vasodilators to reduce left ventricular afterload, or aortic valve replacement.

Tricuspid stenosis and tricuspid regurgitation: For symptomatic patient, sodium restriction, digitalis, or diuretics to relieve or treat the symptoms of CHF.

Follow-up: See the patient at regular intervals for close monitoring of the progression of symptoms.

Sequelae: Possible complications include cardiac arrhythmias; CHF, which may progress to pulmonary edema and respiratory failure; sudden death; TIAs; brain attack (stroke).

Prevention/prophylaxis: Prevention strategies include advising the patient to maintain compliance with therapy; take measures to reduce stress, including using stress relaxation techniques; maintain diet and fluid intake as prescribed; obtain appropriate rest and physical activity; and avoid sodium and caffeine. Advise patients to inform other healthcare providers of their condition. Provide the patient considering pregnancy with information about the associated risks.

Referral: Refer to, or consult with a physician/cardiologist in order to make the diagnosis and guide treatment.

Education: Explain the disease process, signs and symptoms, and treatment (including side effects of medications). Discuss prevention strategies. Advise patient when to seek medical attention.

REFERENCES

General

Dambro, M: Griffith's 5 Minute Clinical Consult. Williams & Wilkins, Baltimore, 2002.

Dunphy, L, and Winland-Brown, J: Primary Care: The Art and Science of Advanced Practice Nursing. F.A. Davis Company, Philadelphia, 2001.

Fauci, A, et al (eds): Harrison's Principles of Internal Medicine, ed. 14. McGraw-Hill, New York, NY, 1998.

Goroll, A, et al: Primary Care Medicine. Lippincott-Raven, Philadelphia, 2000.

Grubb, N, and Newby, D: Churchill's Pocketbook of Cardiology. Harcourt Publishers Limited, New York, 2000.

Hurst, JW (ed): Medicine for the Practicing Physician, ed. 5. Appleton & Lange, Norwalk, Conn, 2001.

Noble, J (ed): Primary Care Medicine, ed. 3. Mosby, St Louis, 2001.

Rakel, R: Textbook of Family Practice. WB Saunders, Philadelphia, 2000.

Sellers, R: Differential Diagnosis of Common Complaints, ed. 3. WB Saunders, Philadelphia, 1996.

Swartz, M: Textbook of Physical Diagnosis. WB Saunders, Philadelphia, 2000.

Uphold, C, and Graham, MV: Clinical Guidelines in Family Practice, ed. 3. Barmarrae Books, Gainesville, Fla, 1998.

US Preventive Service Task Force: Guide to Clinical Prevention Services, ed. 2. Williams & Wilkins, Baltimore, 1998.

Wachtel, R, and Stein, M: The Care of the Ambulatory Patient. Mosby, St Louis, 2000.

Woolf, J, et al (eds): Health Promotion and Disease Prevention in Clinical Practice. Williams & Wilkins, Baltimore, 2000.

Angina

ACC/AHA Task Force on Practice Guidelines: ACC/AHA/ACP-ASIM Pocket Guidelines for Management of Patients With Chronic Stable Angina. March, 2000.

Braunwald, E, et al: Unstable angina: Diagnosis and management. Clinical Practice Guideline, number 10. AHCPR Publication No. 94-0602. Agency for Health Care Policy and Research and the National Heart, Lung, and Blood Institute, Public Health Service, US Department of Health and Human Services, Rockville, Md, 1994.

Julian, DG, et al: Management of stable angina pectoris. Eur. Heart J 18(3):394, 1997.

U.S. Preventive Services Task Force: Aspirin for the primary prevention of cardiovascular events: Recommendations and rationale. Ann Intern Med 136:2, 2002.

Wenger, NK, et al: Cardiac Rehabilitation as Secondary Prevention: Quick Reference Guidelines for Clinicians, No. 17, AHCPR Publication No. 96-0673. U.S. Department of Health and Human Services, Rockville, Md.

Asthma

Bethesda (MD) : U. S. Dept. of Health and Human Services, Public Health Service, National Institutes of Health, National Heart, Lung and Blood Institute: Expert Panel Report 2: Guidelines for the Diagnosis and Management of Asthma. Jul. 1997 (update Mar. 1999).

Bloomington (MN): Institute for Clinical Systems Improvement (ICSI): Diagnosis and management of asthma. June, 2000.

Carroll, P: How to Intervene Before Asthma Turns Deadly. RN 64(5), 2001.

Janson, S: Practical Issues in asthma management. Advance for Nurse Practitioners, 1999.

National Asthma Education and Prevention Program, Expert Panel II: Guidelines for the Diagnosis and Management of Asthma. National Heart, Lung, and Blood Institute of NIH (NHLBI), Washington, DC, 1997.

Spector, S, et al (ed): Practice Parameters for the diagnosis and treatment of asthma. J Allergy Clin Immunol 96(5 pt 2):707–870, 1995 (reviewed 1998).

Chronic Obstructive Pulmonary Disease

Bethesda (MD): Global Initiative for Chronic Obstructive Lung Disease, World Health Organization, National Heart, Lung and Blood Institute: Global Strategy for the Diagnosis, Management, and Prevention of Chronic Obstructive Pulmonary Disease, 2001.

Chapman, K: The diagnosis of COPD: Does it differ by gender? The Journal of COPD Management 3:1, 2002.

Friedman, M: Formulating a pharmacologic management plan for COPD. The Journal of COPD Management 3:1, 2002.

Hafner, J, and Ferro, T: Acute bronchitis in adults: A modern approach to management. Hospital Management 34:8, 1998.

Niederman, M: Antibiotic therapy of acute exacerbations of chronic bronchitis. The Clinical Advisor (Suppl), 2001.

Congestive Heart Failure

ACC/AHA Task Force Heart Failure Guidelines: Guidelines for the Evaluation and Management of Chronic Heart Failure in the Adult—A Report of the American College of Cardiology/American Heart Association Task Force on Practice Guidelines (Committee to Revise the 1995 Guidelines for the Evaluation and Management of Heart Failure). 2001.

Adams, K: Beta-Blockers across the cardiovascular continuum. Cardiology 8:1, 2002.

Burns, D, Goldenberg, I, and Pritzker, M: Strategies for the management of congestive heart failure. Cardiology 7:2, 2001.

Connolly, K: New directions in heart failure management. The Nurse Practitioner 25:7, 2000.

Klapholz, M: Emerging therapies in heart failure. Cardiology 7:1, 2001.

Konstam, M, et al: Heart Failure: Management of Patients with Left Ventricular Dysfunction. AHCPR Publication No. 94-0613. US Department of Health and Human Services, Rockville, Md, June 1994.

Miller, J: Congestive heart failure: Clinical assessment and pharmacologic management. Advance for Nurse Practitioners 5(6):17, 1997.

Packer, M, and Cohn, J: Consensus recommendations for the management of chronic heart failure. Am J Cardiol 1999.

Young, J, and Mills, R: Clinical Management of Heart Failure, ed. 1. Professional Communications, Inc., Caddo, OK, 2001.

Hypertension

Fitzgerald, MA: Hypertensive update: Highlights from the sixth report of the Joint National Committee on Prevention, Detection, Evaluation, and Treatment of High Blood Pressure. Clinical Excellence 2(4):197–201, 1998.

Grimm, R: Cardiovascular risk factor management—the role of hypertension treatment. Supplement to Clinician Reviews (Suppl) 2001.

Guidelines Subcommittee. 1999 World Health Organization—International Society of Hypertension guidelines for the management of hypertension. Journal of Hypertension 17, 1999.

Moser, M: Clinical Management of Hypertension, ed. 4. Professional Communications, Inc., Caddo, OK, 1999.

National Heart, Lung, and Blood Institute: Seventh Report of the Joint National Committee on Prevention, Detection, Evaluation, and Treatment of High

Blood Pressure. US Department of Health and Human Services, National Institutes of Health, Bethesda, Md, 2003.

The Medical Letter: Drugs for hypertension. The Medical Letter 41:1048, 1999.

Pneumonia

Bartlett, J, et al: Practice Guidelines for the management of community-acquired pneumonia in adults. Clin Infect Dis 31:2, 2000.

Fitzgerald, M: Community acquired pneumonia —the Captain of Death can be controlled. Advance for Nurse Practitioners , 2000 .

Green, D, and Pedro, G: Making sense of guidelines for CAP. The Clinical Advisor.

Meredith, P: Community acquired pneumonia. The American Journal for Nurse Practitioners 5:6, 2001.

The Medical Letter: The choice of antibacterial drugs. The Medical Letter 43:1111–1112), 2001.

Sleep Apnea

Chesson, A, et al: Practice parameters for the indications for polysomnography and related procedures. Sleep 20:6. 1997.

Tuberculosis

Centers for Disease Control and Prevention: Targeted tuberculin testing and treatment of latent tuberculosis infection. MMWR 50(34), 2001.

Horsburgh, R, et al: Practice guidelines for the treatment of tuberculosis. Clin Infect Dis 31:3, 2000.

Upper Respiratory Infection

Bloomington (MN): Institute for Clinical Systems Improvement (ICSI) Health Care Guidelines no. GRD07. Viral Upper Respiratory Infection (VURI) in Children and Adults, 1999.

Casiano, R: A rational approach to treating rhinosinusitis. The Clinical Advisor, 2001.

Valvular Heart Disease

Grubb, N, and Newby, D: Churchill's Pocketbook of Cardiology. Harcourt Publishers Limited, New York, 2000.

Hines, S: Update on mitral valve prolapse. Patient Care for the Nurse Practitioner, 2000.

PATIENT EDUCATION WEBSITES

American Academy of Family Physicians (AAFP): Health Information for the Whole Family. Self-care flowcharts covering symptoms, diagnosis, self-care; Herbal and alternative drugs and drug interactions. *http://familydoctor.org*

DiscoveryHealth.com From the producers of the Discovery Channel – offers consumer health information for all age groups. *http://health.discovery.com/*

MayoClinic.com Answers to patient questions, site search engines for health information and prescription drug information; A-to-Z index of diseases and conditions. *http://www.mayohealth.org/home*

MDAdvice.com Patient fact sheets covering symptoms, conditions, medical tests. Support groups, expert advice and live chats. *http://www.mdadvice.com*

MEDLINEplus A service of the National Library of Medicine; offers information on a wide variety of health topics; directories, organizations, and publications. Hundreds of diseases and disorders with a direct link to MEDLINE database. *http://www.medlineplus.gov*

Chapter 6

ABDOMINAL DISORDERS

ANAL FISSURE

SIGNAL SYMPTOMS▶ Rectal pain exacerbated by defecation often associated with fresh blood loss from the anus and perianal itching

| Anal fissure | ICD-9-CM: 565.0 |

Description: An anal fissure is an acute or chronic ulcer on the margin of the anus. It may occur anteriorly or posteriorly.

Etiology: Posterior fissures (90%) are believed to result from traumatic passage of hard stools; anterior fissures from strain on the perineum during childbirth or some other type of trauma, such as anal intercourse. May be acute or chronic.

Occurrence: Common cause of rectal bleeding.

Age: Posterior fissures may occur at any age, with increasing prevalence among older adults. Anterior fissures are associated with childbearing age in women.

Ethnicity: No significant ethnic predisposition.

Gender: Posterior fissures occur equally in men and in women. Anterior fissures are 10 times more common in women. 11% of women develop after childbirth.

Contributing Factors: Low intake of dietary fiber. Constipation, diarrhea, childbirth (anterior fissures), anal intercourse, insertion of objects into the anal canal, irritable bowel disease, tuberculosis, syphilis, cancer, inflammatory bowel diseases, acquired immunodeficiency syndrome (AIDS).

Signs and symptoms: Knifelike pain and bright red rectal bleeding associated with bowel movements, commonly after a recent bout of constipation. Pain may persist for several hours following each bowel movement. Bleeding is usually minor and seen mainly on the toilet paper. May also present with perianal itching.

Physical examination may be difficult because of fear and tenderness. Digital examination is very painful and usually unnecessary.

 Clinical Pearl: Use 2% lidocaine.

Acute fissures: Acute anal fissures have sharply demarcated, fresh, mucosal edges, often with granulation tissue at the base. Often, gentle eversion of the anoderm in the posterior midline is all that is required. Physical findings include an approximately 1-cm split in the anoderm in the posterior midline just distal to the dentate line. Mucosal tears are demonstrable usually at 6 o'clock or 12 o'clock.

Chronic fissures: Classic triad (hypertrophy of the anal papilla, anal fissure, and sentinel skin tag) may be present. Margins are indurated, there is less granulation tissue, and muscle fibers of the internal sphincter may be seen at the base. Fissures persisting for more than 6 weeks are generally classified as chronic.

Diagnostic tests: Diagnosed by visual examination. Not seen on colonoscopy. Anoscopy may be used.

Differential Diagnosis:

- Hemorrhoids (bleeding associated with passage of stool; pruritus)
- Anorectal abscess (discharge may be associated; odor)
- If multiple fissures or fissures occurring away from the anterior or posterior midline are present, suspicion should be raised for other problems such as inflammatory bowel disease, AIDS, tuberculosis, leukemia, or syphilis.

Treatment:

Pharmacologic

- Topical analgesic, such as glyceryl trinitrate (GTN), benzocaine, dibucaine, or pramoxine hydrochloride, applied as needed
- Stool softener
- Avoid suppositories because they are painful and rest in the rectum rather than the anal canal
- Topical nitroglycerine or injection with botulinum A toxin-HC, or botulinum A toxin-HC followed by three times daily application of topical isosorbide dinitrate

Physical

- Warm sitz baths for 15 to 20 minutes several times a day
- High-fiber diet including bran cereal, fresh fruits, and vegetables
- Fiber supplements, such as Metamucil or FiberCon
- Encourage liberal water intake (six to eight 8-ounce glasses daily).

Surgical

- Chronic, recalcitrant cases may require sphincterotomy or fissurectomy.

Follow-up: May require 6 to 8 weeks to heal. Advise patient to contact practitioner if pain is not relieved by recommended treatment, bleeding is excessive (more than trace or streak on toilet paper, dripping into the toilet bowel), or occurring between bowel movements, or if constipation persists.

Sequelae: Possible complications include bleeding, anemia (rare), secondary infection, pain, and constipation.

Prevention/prophylaxis: Prevention strategies include avoiding constipation.

Referral: Refer to, or consult with, physician if patient presents with persistent pain, bleeding, or poor healing of fissure.

Education: Explain disease process, signs and symptoms, and treatment (including side effects of medications). Discuss the relationship between diet, fluid intake, exercise and bowel regularity, the physiology of defecation, and importance of establishing a routine. Advise avoiding straining and prolonged sitting on the toilet; recommend putting feet on a low footstool and removing reading material from the bathroom. Advise using soap and water for cleanup after bowel movement. Explain that external application of creams and ointments is better than suppositories.

APPENDICITIS

SIGNAL SYMPTOMS ▶ Periumbilical pain of recent onset; localizes to right lower quadrant (RLQ) within 24 hours; Rebound tenderness

Appendicitis, without mention of peritonitis	ICD-9-CM: 540.9
Appendicitis with generalized peritonitis	ICD-9-CM: 541.0

Description: Appendicitis is an inflammation of the vermiform appendix caused by infection or obstruction.

Etiology: Caused by hardened fecal occlusion of the lumen (a fecalith); fibrous disease affecting the bowel wall; an adhesion externally occluding the lumen; invasion of the appendix by bacteria such as *Escherichia coli* or *Klebsiella*; hypertrophy of lymphoid tissue; an inspissate of barium from a previous contrast study; foreign-body occlusion of the lumen (such as by vegetable or fruit seeds); and intestinal worms (ascarids). Once infected, the appendix becomes swollen, inflamed, and pus filled.

Occurrence: Accounts for the majority of acute abdominal pain and acute abdominal surgical conditions in the United States; 1 in 15 people (8%) will be affected at some point in their lifetime. The incidence of acute appendicitis is falling for unknown reasons. **Appendicitis is the most common surgical emergency requiring operation.**

Age: Occurs most commonly in people age 10 to 30 years; peak incidence between age 15 to 24 years. (May be difficult to assess in older patients, only about one third have classic symptoms.)

Ethnicity: No significant ethnic predisposition.

Gender: Occurs more in men age 10 to 30 years; occurs equally in men and in women older than age 30 years.

Contributing Factors: Intra-abdominal tumors, family history, recent illness (especially roundworm infestation or viral infection of the gastrointestinal [GI] tract).

Signs and symptoms:

- Epigastric or periumbilical pain accompanied by anorexia (almost 100%), nausea (90%), and vomiting (75%), with pain shifting to right lower quadrant within 6 to 24 hours of the onset of symptoms. Pain is continuous and dull in character; may intensify with moving, coughing, sneezing, walking, riding over bumps in a car, or with touch; usually increases with percussion; may be located posteriorly (occasionally flank tenderness, RLQ), in the suprapubic region (pain on rectal examination), or on the right side of the rectum. Diffuse pain and non-localized tenderness is more common in older patient.

 Clinical Pearl: Anorexia, then abdominal pain, then vomiting. Urge to defecate, but no relief of pain on defecation.

- Other common complaints include malaise related to indigestion, change in bowel habits (constipation or diarrhea), inability to pass gas
- Low-grade fever (may present after onset of other symptoms); slight tachycardia
- Physical examination may reveal patient lying in a fetal position, flexing the knees and pulling them up to the chest; diminished bowel sounds on auscultation; and rebound tenderness, McBurney's sign, obturator sign, iliopsoas or psoas sign, or Aaron's sign on palpation.

 Clinical Pearl: Cutaneous hyperesthesia. Pain lessened with flexion of thigh.

Diagnostic tests:

Test	Result Indicating Disorder	CPT Code
Complete blood count (CBC)	May show moderate leukocytosis (10,000–18,000/mm³) with a shift to the left. **Above 18,000, suspect perforation**	85025
Erythrocyte sedimentation rate (ESR)	May be elevated (above 20)	85651
Human chorionic gonadotropin (hCG)	Rules out ectopic pregnancy	80414, 84702-3
Urinalysis	Detects elevated specific gravity, occasional presence of red blood cells (RBCs), pyuria, and albuminuria; also rules out pregnancy in women	81001
Flat plate and upright abdominal films	Identify fecaliths, rule out other pathology	74020

(Continued)

Test	Result Indicating Disorder	CPT Code
Pelvic ultrasound	Determines appendiceal inflammation, rules out other abdominal pathology, identifies free fluid or abscess	76856
Computerized tomography (CT) scan of the abdomen	Shows periappendiceal abscess or cecal inflammation	74170 without and with contrast 74160 with contrast 74150 without contrast
Diagnostic laparoscopy	May be considered for young adult female patients; rules out ectopic pregnancy, tubo-ovarian process, and pelvic inflammatory disease (PID)	49320

Differential diagnosis: 75% of erroneous diagnoses accounted for by acute mesenteric adenitis, no organic pathology, acute PID, acute gastroenteritis, ruptured graafian follicle

- Gastritis (no RLQ localization of pain, burning epigastric pain usually associated with food intake)
- Gastroenteritis (crampy, diffuse abdominal pain usually relieved by vomiting or defecation)
- Colitis (no localization of pain; more diffuse pain pattern)
- Diverticulitis (lower left quadrant [LLQ] pain, intermittent cramping)
- Mesenteric adenitis (may be detected on ultrasound)
- PID, ruptured ectopic pregnancy, ovarian cyst– (female patients; pregnancy test, history, pelvic examination)
- Cholelithiasis (RUQ pain, radiates to back and shoulder, occurs 1 to 6 hours after meals)
- Renal calculi (back pain, hematuria, fever, costovertebral angle (CVA) tenderness)
- Pancreatitis (epigastric abdominal pain which may radiate to back, elevated amylase, nausea, vomiting)
- Peptic ulcer disease (gnawing, burning epigastric pain 1 to 3 hours after meals)

Treatment:

Red Flag: Patient should not take anything by mouth (NPO), intravenous (IV) should be started for fluid replacement, and immediate surgical consult if highly suspicious of appendicitis. Intensive in-house observation.

Pharmacologic
Medications may include analgesics, antipyretics, antibiotics.

Clinical Pearl: Uncomplicated acute appendicitis, one preoperative dose of broad-spectrum antibiotic; in a nonsurgical candidate, antibiotic therapy may be used also. Spontaneous resolution has been reported in approximately 8% of cases

IV fluids or electrolyte replacement therapy.

Physical

Bed rest, limited activities, and NPO status until diagnosis is confirmed.

Surgical

Open or laparoscopic appendectomy within 24 to 48 hours after onset of symptoms. **The mortality from acute appendicitis is < 0.3%, rising to 1.7% following perforation.**

Sequelae: Possible complications include rupture of the appendix and peritonitis (especially if diagnosis is delayed or missed, or in very young or old patients); wound infections (5% to 33%). Abscess occurs < 2% of the time after appendectomy.

Prevention/prophylaxis: None.

Referral: Immediate referral to surgeon.

Education: Explain disease process, signs and symptoms, and treatment (including side effects of medications).

Refer to Figure 6–1 for the steps in the differential diagnosis of abdominal pain.

BLADDER CANCER

SIGNAL SYMPTOMS▶ Painless hematuria (primary presenting symptom of 75% of patients)

Neoplasm bladder, primary	ICD-9-CM: 188.9

Description: Second most common urologic malignancy, after prostate cancer. Approximately 90% are transitional cell carcinomas, 6% to 7% are squamous cell carcinomas, and 1% to 2% are adenocarcinomas. The most important prognostic indicator is the depth of bladder wall penetration. The overall 5-year cure rate for superficial bladder tumors that have been completely resected is about 70%.

Etiology: The majority of tumors arise from transitional epithelial tissue that lines the bladder; 70% are characterized by papillary lesions (papillomas), which are generally superficial and noninvasive, although they tend to recur. Nonpapillary tumors that lie flat are less common but more invasive. Carcinogens in the urine and chronic inflammation or irritation of the bladder mucosa are implicated in the development of bladder cancer.

Occurrence: Accounts for about 4% to 5% of all reported cancers in the United States. Approximately 50,000 new cases per year are diagnosed and about 10,000 deaths reported. Incidence is higher in industrialized areas. It is the second most common genitourinary (GU) cancer after prostate cancer.

Age: Occurs primarily in persons older than age 50 years; median age at diagnosis is 67 to 70 years.

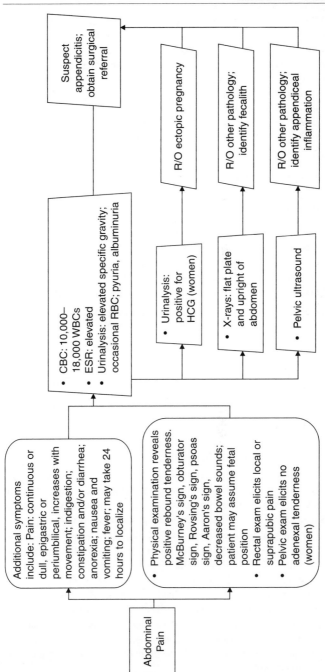

Figure 6–1. Differential diagnosis: abdominal pain.

Ethnicity: Occurs more frequently in white men than in black men.

Gender: Occurs in men four times more often than in women.

Contributing Factors: Cigarette smoking (one third of all cases); occupational exposure, such as working with textile dyes, leather, rubber, paint, and metal; long-term use of analgesics with phenacetin; long-term use of cyclophosphamide.

Signs and Symptoms: Painless hematuria (primary presenting symptom of 75% of patients), dysuria, frequency, urgency, bladder irritability. Weight loss and abdominal or bone pain in advanced disease. Physical examination is usually unremarkable.

 Clinical Pearl: Often asymptomatic

Diagnostic Tests:

Test	Result Indicating Disorder	CPT Code
Urinalysis	Reveals gross or microscopic hematuria	81002
Urine cytology	Evidence of malignant cells	88104
Flow cytometry	Examines DNA content of urine cells	88180, 88182
Intravenous pyelogram	Unilateral or bilateral ureteral obstruction; hydronephrosis; filling defects or lack of bladder distensibility suggest bladder cancer. Renal ultrasound reveals presence of tumors	74400
CT scan	Detects variations in tissue density	72194 without and with contrast
Cystoscopy or urethroscopy	Allows direct visualization, assessment, and biopsy of lesions	52224

Differential diagnosis:

- Urinary tract infection (resolves with treatment)
- Nephrolithiasis (usually painful)

Treatment: Treatment depends on stage. The staging system used is the Jewett-Strong and TNM combined, evaluating tumor penetration with size and presence of spread or metastases. Serum chemistries, chest x-ray study, and CT scan of the abdomen and pelvis are needed for staging.

Superficial tumors: Endoscopic resection. Local recurrence occurs within 3 years in 50% to 70% of patients. Recurrences are usually managed with intravesical therapy (instillation of chemotherapy directly into the bladder).

Invasive disease: Radical or simple cystectomy. For men, this involves removal of the prostate and seminal vesicles; for women this involves removal of the uterus, fallopian tubes, ovaries, and part of the vaginal vault. Radiation therapy and/or chemotherapy are also recommended in some patients; the 5-year survival rate is 40% to 50%.

Metastatic disease: Various chemotherapeutic options. Initial response rate is usually < 6 months of remission in 30% to 70% of patients; most die within 2 years.

Follow-up: Follow-up is managed by the urologist using periodic cystoscopy, usually every 3 months for 2 years, then every 6 months for 2 years. Patients with advanced disease are followed more frequently.

Sequelae: Complications include impotence (from surgical intervention); altered quality of life (from radical cystectomy); urinary tract hemorrhage, inflammation, tissue necrosis, and hemorrhage; urinary tract fistulas; invasion, inflammation, and destruction of adjacent tissue; and obstruction leading to renal failure.

Prevention/prophylaxis: Prevention strategies include smoking cessation (key component) and monitoring occupational hazards.

Referral: Once urinary tract infection is ruled out, refer to, or consult with, a urologist for a urological workup. Depending on the stage of disease, consultation with radiation oncology and medical oncology is indicated. Referral to a hospice program may be made for patients with advanced disease.

Education: Explain disease process, signs and symptoms, and treatment (including side effects of medications). Discuss treatment options. If the patient undergoes cystoscopy, or radical cystectomy, address questions or issues regarding sexual changes and possible complications. Provide patient with telephone number of the Cancer Information Services (1-800-4CANCER). Educational resources are available from the United Ostomy Association, Inc., 19772 MacArthur Blvd., Suite 200, Irvine, CA 92612 (714-660-8624) or (800-826-0826). Website: *www.voa.org*

CHOLECYSTITIS

SIGNAL SYMPTOMS▶   Severe upper right quadrant pain; Rebound tenderness

Cholecystitis, acute	ICD-9-CM: 575.0

Description: Cholecystitis is an inflammation of the gallbladder occurring acutely or chronically, often secondary to previously occurring gallstones. Acute inflammation of the gallbladder usually follows obstruction of the cystic duct by a stone. Chronic inflammation is almost always associated with the presence of gallstones and is believed to be a result of repeated bouts of subacute or acute inflammation or persistent mechanical irritation of the gallbladder.

Etiology: Caused by gallstones (90% to 95% of cases), mechanical inflammation (especially in patients with diabetes), bacterial inflammation (commonly *Escherichia coli, Klebsiella,* group D *Streptococcus, Staphylococcus,* and *Clostridium*), and chemical inflammation (such as from the release of lysolecithin and other local tissue factors). Cholesterol stones account for 80% of the biliary stones in developed Western nations. Pigment stones (20%) often secondary to cirrhosis or hemolytic anemia.

Occurrence: Most western countries; occurs in an estimated 16 to 20 million people in the United States, approximately 1 million new cases develop each year.

Age: Occurs primarily in middle age (fifth to sixth decades) and older.

Ethnicity: Increased prevalence in Northern European or Native American ancestry. Occurs in 30% of whites by age 60; 20% of blacks by age 60; 30% of Native Americans by age 30 and 80% by age 60.

Gender: Occurs twice as often in women than in men.

Contributing factors: Gallstones, acalculous, secondary to stressful situations, such as cardiac surgery, multiple trauma; bacteria; neoplasms; ischemia; torsion. Female gender, history of estrogen therapy, obesity, Northern European or Native American ancestry are all risk factors for development of gallstones. Factors that increase bile stasis such as weight reduction, and prolonged bowel rest, may also be contributing factors.

Signs and symptoms: Often asymptomatic.

> *Acute*: Abdominal pain (sudden onset, severe in epigastrium or right upper quadrant, radiates to the shoulder or back); nausea and vomiting; low-grade fever, may have shaking chills; positive Murphy's sign; recurrent attacks after meals for 1 to 6 hours, lasting more than 12 hours until relieved, usually < 2 to 3 days.
>
> With common bile duct calculi: Jaundice, biliary colic, fever, chills, pruritus, loose bowels (light in color), hepatomegaly, abdominal distention.
>
> With empyema: Phlegmon of obstructed gallbladder, weight loss, infectious signs, fever, anorexia, palpable mass, tenderness absent.
>
> *Chronic:* Usually asymptomatic; may have mild dyspepsia following fatty meals.

Diagnostic tests:

Tests	Result Indicating Disorder	CPT Code
CBC	Shows leukocytosis	85025
LFTs—obtain CBC first; if leukocytosis, then do LFTs	Show increased ALT, AST, and alkaline phosphatase; elevated GGPT with duct obstruction	80076 82977 GGT
Serum amylase and lipase	May be elevated with concomitant pancreatitis	82150 (amylase) 83690 (lipase)
Serum bilirubin, alkaline phosphatase and-glutamyltransferase(GGT)	Elevated with common duct occlusion	82247 (bilirubin included in LFT) 84075 alk Phos, (included in LFT) 82977 GGT
Abdominal upright	20% of gallstones are radiopaque	74240

(Continued)

Tests	Result Indicating Disorder	CPT Code
Ultrasound (HBUS).	Best technique (high sensitivity–95% and specificity–98%) Ultrasound will reveal gallbladder stones; not reliable for common bile duct stones but may reveal ductal dilatation > 75% of the time	78223
99m iminodiacetic acid (HIDA) scan Most effective when client is experiencing pain.	97% sensitive for diagnosis of acute cholecystitis–use if ultasound is negative–assesses gallbladder functioning (ejection fraction < 35% with reproduction of pain a positive result)	56342
Endoscopic retrograde cholangiopancreatography (ERCP).	Will visualize the common bile duct and other portions of the gastrointestinal tract and will allow for papillotomy plus stone extraction in the majority of cases	74330
Percutaneous transhepatic cholangiography (PTC).	Gives additional information about intrahepatic biliary system; use if retained common bile duct stone	74320

ALT, alanine aminotransferase; AST, aspartate aminotransferase; CBC, complete blood count; GGPT, γ-glutamyl transpeptide; LFTs, liver function tests.

Differential diagnosis:

- Perforated peptic ulcer (tachycardia, tachypnea, abdomen diffusely tender, signs and symptoms of peritonitis)
- Thoracic disease (cough, shortness of breath [SOB], dyspnea, stabbing pain)
- Hepatitis (fever, nausea, vomiting, > liver function tests)
- Pancreatitis (acute pain through to back and vomiting)
- Appendicitis (RLQ pain)
- Ectopic pregnancy (pelvic pain, amenorrhea followed by irregular vaginal bleeding; abdominal tenderness, referred pain pattern [shoulder pain])
- Bowel obstruction (decreased bowel sounds; vomiting)
- Pneumonia (fever, coughing, SOB)
- Angina (radiating pain, relieved with rest, nitroglycerine)
- Perforated colon (diffuse abdominal tenderness, pneumoperitoneum)

Treatment: Laparoscopic cholecystectomy is the procedure of choice for uncomplicated acute cholecystitis. Inpatient treatment suggested in patients with biliary colic lasting longer than 6 hours, jaundice, rigors, or requiring narcotics for pain. Give nothing by mouth; start intravenous fluid replacement.

 Clinical Pearl: use meperidine, not morphine.

Intravenous antibiotics with activity against gram-negative, gram-positive, and anaerobic bacteria are usually indicated. One regiman is gentamycin 3.5 mg/kg/day and clindamycin 1.8–2.7 gm/day. Diclofenac 75 mg IV may abort early attack. Cholecystectomy should be performed in 24–72 hours.

Follow-up: See patient who has had surgery for routine postoperative care. See the patient in 3 to 6 months if patient has symptomatic gallstones with recurrent symptoms.

Sequelae: Possible complications include perforation, abscess formation, fistula formation, gangrene, empyema, cholangitis, hepatitis, pancreatitis, gallstone ileus, and carcinoma.

Prevention/Prophylaxis: Prevention strategies include advising the patient to avoid risk factors when possible, and to eat small, frequent meals of nongaseous, low-fat foods. During rapid weight loss, ursodeoxycholic acid 10 mg/kg/day.

Referral: Refer to, or consult with, surgeon (acute cases).

Education: Explain disease process, signs and symptoms, and treatment. Explain that even after cholecystectomy gallstones may recur in common bile duct. Educational resource materials available from National Digestive Diseases Information Clearinghouse, PO Box NDDIC, Bethesda, MD 20892 (301-468-6344).

CHOLELITHIASIS

SIGNAL SYMPTOMS▶ May be asymptomatic

| Calculus of gallbladder with acute cholelithiasis | ICD-9-CM: 574.0 |

Description: Cholelithiasis refers to the formation of calculi (gallstones). Gallstones are classified by chemical composition and include cholesterol stones (most common), pigment stones (calcium bilirubinate), or mixed stones. Once stones have developed, the gallbladder has the tendency to continue production of more stones, with two thirds of all patients developing chronic pain and one third of patients developing other acute problems such as cholecystitis.

Etiology: Caused by changes in the composition of bile or in the absorptive ability of the gallbladder epithelium. Bile supersaturated with cholesterol causes crystal formation or microstones, which continue to build up to macrostones. Pigmented stones are associated with biliary infection and are formed by increased unconjugated bilirubin in the bile. Mixed stones are produced by a combination of the preceding factors.

Occurrence: Eight to ten percent of the U.S. population (about 20 million) have gallstones; this increases to 20% in people older than age 40 years.

Age: Increases with age; peaks in the sixth decade.

Ethnicity: Increased occurrence in people of Native American, Hispanic, and Northern European heritage.

Gender: Occurs two times more frequently in women than in men.

Contributing factors: Short gut syndrome, inflammatory bowel disease, disorders of the small intestine, biliary parasites, cirrhosis (pigmented stones), obesity or rapid weight loss, prosthetic heart valves, coronary artery disease (CAD), hereditary hemolytic disorders, childhood malignancy, diabetes mellitus, long-term total parenteral nutrition, increased alcohol use; high-fat, low-fiber diets; family history of gallstones; medications that increase cholesterol saturation, such as oral contraceptives, estrogen, estrogen-progestin therapy, and clofibrate.

Signs and symptoms: Many patients are asymptomatic, with the gallstones found during assessment of other complaints.

If patient has symptoms, most common is abdominal pain occurring in the right upper quadrant or epigastrium and radiating to the right shoulder, scapula, or between the shoulder blades. Pain may be aching or sharp and lancing and last for 15 to 60 minutes; may progress to a chronic, steady pain lasting several hours; and usually has a diurnal variation, peaking at midnight.

Physical examination may reveal tenderness to palpation of the right upper quadrant, Murphy's sign, and occasionally, jaundice.

Diagnostic tests: No laboratory test is diagnostic; however, the following may be performed. Imaging studies are diagnostic of gallstones.

Tests	Result Indicating Disorder	CPT Code
WBC	Count greater than 15,000 occurs with biliary infection	85032
Serum bilirubin and alkaline phosphatase	Elevated in one third of patients	84075, 82247
Serum amylase and lipase	Elevated with pancreatic duct obstruction	82150, 83690
Ultrasound (CT scan has no advantage over ultrasound)	Best technique to diagnose gallstones	76700
HIDA scan	Shows stones in biliary tree	
Oral cholecystography	Visualized gallbladder; only useful if cystic duct is patent	74290
X-ray study of the gallbladder	Shows stones only if enough calcium is present	74240
ERCP	Shows obstruction in hepatobiliary tree and pancreatic ducts	74330

CT, complete blood count; ERCP, endoscopic retrograde cholangiopancreatoscopy; HIDA, hepato-iminodiacetic acid; WBC, white blood cell.

Differential diagnosis:

- Peptic ulcer disease (burning pain, epigastric tenderness)
- Pancreatitis (acute pain through to back, vomiting, tenderness and > amylase)
- Appendicitis (RLQ pain)
- Hepatitis (fever, nausea, jaundice, RUQ tenderness, > LFTs)
- Gallbladder cancer (diagnosed on biopsy)
- Gallbladder polyps (biopsy)

- Biliary sludge (episodic, low-grade symptomatology)
- Stricture (check imaging)
- CAD (radiating chest pain, diaphoresis, SOB)
- Pneumonia (Fever, cough, SOB)
- Renal stones (severe pain, diaphoresis, vomiting)
- Blood clots (SOB, anxiety, panic)

Treatment:

Pharmacologic

- For mild attacks: Analgesics, such as nonsteroidal anti-inflammatory drugs (NSAIDs) or acetaminophen for symptomatic relief.
- For oral dissolution of cholesterol stones, when surgery is not an option: Ursodiol, 8 to 10 mg/kg twice or three times a day, or chenodeoxycholic acid, 250 mg twice a day for 2 weeks, then increase by 250-mg increments until a dose of 13 to 16 mg/kg daily or intolerance develops. Oral dissolution may take up to 2 years. Lifetime maintenance therapy is usually required because gallstones recur 10% a year and then plateau at 50% to 60% after 5 years.
- For direct contact dissolution of cholesterol stones: Instillation of methyl *tert*-butyl directly into the gallbladder. A high recurrence rate occurs with all dissolution medications.

Physical

- Therapies include the application of heat to the area of pain and a low-fat, high-fiber diet. During attacks, encourage rest and sipping water frequently, but no eating.

Surgical

- For patients with severe attacks or pain lasting longer than 6 hours. Procedures include laparoscopic cholecystectomy (preferred for most patients) and open cholecystectomy. After cholecystotomy, stones may recur in the bile duct.

Other

- Noninvasive procedures that may be used to break up the gallstones include extracorporeal shock-wave therapy and lithotripsy. For lithotripsy, stones may recur by 30% in 5 years.

Follow-up: See the patient receiving outpatient therapy as needed for management of symptoms. See the patient receiving oral dissolution agents as follows: See the patient monthly for the first 3 months, then every 3 months to monitor liver enzymes. Monitor serum cholesterol every 6 months, and perform serial imaging studies every 6 to 9 months to evaluate response and monitor for recurrence. See the patient who has undergone surgery or other procedures for routine postoperative or postprocedure care.

Sequelae: Fewer than half of patients with cholelithiasis become symptomatic. Possible complications include acute cholecystitis (90% to 95% of patients), gallstone pancreatitis, acute cholangitis, common bile duct stones with obstructive jaundice, gallstone ileus, liver abscess, biliary-enteric fistula, peritonitis, gallbladder cancer, and infection or rupture of the gallbladder.

Prevention/Prophylaxis: Prevention strategies include advising the patient to eat a high-fiber, low-fat diet and to avoid or reduce risk factors (obesity, excess alcohol consumption, oral contraceptives, rapid weight loss). Use of ursodiol (Actigall) during rapid weight loss may prevent stone formation.

Referral: Refer to, or consult with, a surgeon if the patient has a severe case or has pain lasting longer than 6 hours; to a physician if patient is a candidate for lithotripsy or direct contact dissolution.

Education: Explain disease process, signs and symptoms, and treatment (including side effects of medications). Discuss prevention strategies, especially dietary strategies, the importance of rest during painful episodes, the importance of follow-up medical care and tests, and when to seek medical attention (for example, if pain lasts longer than 3 hours). Additional information is available from the National Digestive Diseases Information Clearinghouse, PO Box NDDIC, Bethesda, MD 20892 (301-468-6344); http://www. niddk.nih.gov/; e-mail: nddic@aerie.com.

CIRRHOSIS

SIGNAL SYMPTOMS ▶ *Early:* May be asymptomatic or have a condition such as infertility, impotence, or decreased libido, or have minimal abnormalities on routine liver function tests.

Late: Signs and symptoms may include severe anorexia and weight loss; occasional vomiting; lethargy; low-grade fevers; general body pruritus, resulting in scratching causing bruising and bleeding; an increase in bruising tendency; frequent nosebleeds; and menstrual abnormalities (usually amenorrhea).

Cirrhosis	ICD-9-CM: 571.5

Description: Cirrhosis is a chronic, irreversible inflammatory disease of the liver that causes disruption of the organ's structure and function. Types of cirrhosis include alcoholic, biliary, and postnecrotic cirrhosis.

Etiology: Many forms of liver disease are the consequence of alcohol consumption. Use of alcohol is responsible for most cases of liver disease in the western hemisphere, whereas hepatitis B and C are the leading causes of the disease worldwide.

Alcoholic, early and late: Results primarily from alcohol abuse but may also be a result of obesity, postsurgical jejunoileal bypass, exposure to toxic chemicals, chronic cholestatic diseases (such as primary biliary cirrhosis and sclerosing cholangitis), peripheral hepatic thrombosis, and malignancies of the liver and gallbladder.

Primary biliary: The exact cause is unknown, but it is thought to be the result of an autoimmune response because it frequently accompanies collagen disease disorders.

Secondary biliary: Results from prolonged, partial, or complete mechanical obstruction of the bile ducts, either internal or external to the liver, for a period of 1 year or more. Chronic bile duct obstruction is usually caused by postoperative strictures of gallstones often associated with infectious cholangitis and, rarely, pancreatic, biliary duct, and gallbladder tumors.

Postnecrotic: Results from many types of chronic severe liver disease or liver injury that causes the liver to regenerate lost hepatic mass with nodules.

Occurrence: One of the 10 leading causes of death in the United States; about 40% from alcoholic cirrhosis; 0.6% to 2% from primary biliary. Postnecrotic cirrhosis occurs in about 25% of patients with hepatitis C.

Age: Varies, but age at onset is usually between 35 and 45 for alcoholic and primary biliary cirrhosis.

Ethnicity:

Alcoholic: In the United States, the incidence is lower in whites and higher in cultures that favor the ongoing practice of wine drinking.

Postnecrotic: Incidence higher in areas where hepatitis B is endemic, such as in Southeast Asia.

Gender: Alcoholic cirrhosis occurs more often in men than in women; primary biliary occurs more frequently (90% to 95%) in women than in men.

Contributing factors:

Alcoholic: Alcohol consumption; exposure to toxins such as carbon tetrachloride or trichloroethylene; use of hepatic toxic medicines such as acetaminophen, alpha-methyldopa, methotrexate, isoniazid, nitrofurantoin, and amitriptyline; metabolic disorders such as hemochromatosis, Wilson's disease, $alpha_1$-antitrypsin deficiency, and glycogen storage disease.

Primary biliary: Collagen diseases.

Secondary biliary: Gallstones, chronic pancreatitis, biliary atresia, cystic fibrosis, neoplasms, history of ascending cholangitis.

Postnecrotic: Hepatitis C, hepatitis B, metabolic disorders, advanced alcoholic cirrhosis, primary biliary cirrhosis.

Signs and symptoms:

Alcoholic, early: May be asymptomatic or have a condition such as infertility, impotence, or decreased libido, or have minimal abnormalities on routine liver function tests. Signs and symptoms include transient nausea, occasional vomiting, fatigue, weight loss, or occasional right upper quadrant pain. Physical examination may reveal slight jaundice, palmar erythema, enlarged and tender liver, and hepatosplenomegaly. The liver may palpate as large and smooth in contour, with a sharply defined border 5 cm or more below the right costal margin. Pain secondary to hepatic enlargement may be elicited when the patient is asked to lean forward from the waist. Percussion often elicits an increased vertical span of liver dullness in the right upper quadrant.

Alcoholic, late: Signs and symptoms may include severe anorexia and weight loss; occasional vomiting; lethargy; low-grade fevers; general body pruritus, resulting in scratching causing bruising and bleeding; an increase in bruising tendency; frequent nosebleeds; and menstrual abnormalities (usually amenorrhea). Physical examination may reveal a patient who appears chronically ill and confused or possibly even in a comatose state; slurred speech; musty smelling breath; a beefy red tongue; bleeding gums; jaundice; spider angiomas on the face, neck, arms, or trunk; gynecomastia and testicular atrophy (men); upper body wasting; enlarged, prominent parotid glands; palmar erythema; Dupuytren's contracture of palmar fascia; asterixis (flapping tremor of the hands when arms are extended with palms upward); "milk maid's grip" (a pulselike sensation when patient's hands grip the examiner's fingers); white nailbeds with a loss of nail lunulae; and clubbed fingers. Palpation may reveal a small, hard liver, with a nodular, irregular surface; ascites; a positive abdominal fluid wave; and possibly splenomegaly. Abdominal pain may be elicited with palpation. Percussion may reveal extended dullness, both horizontally and vertically, along the right upper quadrant.

Primary biliary: May be asymptomatic (15% of patients), or patient may complain of a general deterioration of health that is difficult to describe. Signs and symptoms may include generalized pruritus, an insidious onset of easy fatigability, clay-colored stools, dark urine, general malaise, fatigue, anorexia, and weight loss. Physical examination may reveal slightly jaundiced color; dry eyes; dry oral mucous membranes; deep skin excoriation (secondary to pruritus); xanthomas in periorbital areas or on elbows, knees, and palmar surfaces; peripheral neuropathies; hepatosplenomegaly; and ascites.

Secondary biliary: Signs and symptoms of primary biliary cirrhosis accompanied by right upper quadrant pain (from gallstones).

Postnecrotic: Signs and symptoms as listed above.

Diagnostic tests:
Alcoholic

Tests	Result Indicating Disorder	CPT Code
Mean corpuscular volume (MCV)	Elevated	85032
GGPT	Elevated	82977
Uric acid	Elevated	84550
Immunoglobulin G (IgG) and immunoglobulin A (IgA)	Both elevated	86332
Fine-needle biopsy	Confirms diagnosis	47000 (88170-73)

GGPT, γ-glutamyl transpeptidase.

Laboratory test findings may also include bone marrow suppression, thrombocytopenia, leukopenia, hypoalbuminemia, hypoprothrombinemia, and hyperbilirubinemia. Ultrasound may be performed.

Primary Biliary

Tests	Result Indicating Disorder	CPT Code
Alkaline phosphatase	Elevated	84075
GGPT	Elevated	82977
Serum bilirubin	Initially normal or minimally elevated	82247
IgG and IgM	Elevated	82784 (for each test)
Antimitochondrial antibody (AMA) test	Positive	86038-86039 (for AMA)
Liver biopsy	Confirms diagnosis	47000

GGPT, γ-glutamyl transpeptidase; IgG, immunoglobulin G; IgM, immunoglobulin M.

Ultrasound or CT scan may be performed.
Secondary Biliary

Tests	Result Indicating Disorder	CPT Code
Alkaline phosphatase	Elevated	84075
Bilirubin	Elevated	82247
WBC	Shows leukocytosis	85007

WBC, white blood cell.

Impaired coagulation, anemia, thrombocytopenia, and folic acid deficiency may also be present. Cholangiography provides the most definitive diagnosis; however, liver biopsy and endoscopy may be performed.

Postnecrotic

Test	Result Indicating Disorder	CPT Code
Needle biopsy	Confirms diagnosis	47000

Laboratory findings mimic those mentioned for the other types of cirrhosis.

Differential diagnosis:

Alcoholic: Alcoholic fatty liver, alcoholic hepatitis.

Primary biliary: Pruritus, hypothyroidism, sarcoidosis, chronic active hepatitis, sclerosing cholangitis, secondary biliary cirrhosis, drug-induced cholestasis, biliary obstruction.

Secondary biliary: Cholecystitis, cholelithiasis.

Postnecrotic: Alcoholic cirrhosis, primary biliary cirrhosis.

Treatment:

Alcoholic: The only treatment for alcoholic cirrhosis is complete abstinence from alcohol. Patients who comply with abstinence may be able to enjoy clinical improvement and reduce their rate of hepatic mass loss. Referral to an alcohol rehabilitation program is suggested. Additional treatment includes rest, nutritional therapy (with amino acid supplements, a daily multivitamin, and a well-balanced diet that includes 1 g protein per kilogram per day and 2000 to 3000 cal/day); colchicine, 0.6 mg orally twice a day; spironolactone, 100 to 400 mg orally each day, or furosemide, 40 to 80 mg/day (to reduce fluid retention); stool softeners; and antibiotics such as neomycin (to reduce ammonia level buildup). Management of late disease includes symptom management, medical management, and control of complications, such as propranolol at a dose to lower resting pulse when esophageal varices seen on endoscopy. Possible surgical procedures for portal hypertension include splenorenal or portocaval anastomosis or transjugular hepatic portal systemic shunt. Possible liver transplant.

Primary biliary: No standard treatment recommendations. Symptom control includes ursodiol 13 to 15 mg/kg in four divided doses/day; colchicine, 0.6 mg orally twice a day; cholestyramine, 8 to 12 g daily; phenobarbital or antihistamines (for pruritus); vitamin K and D injections (for vitamin deficiency); low-fat diet; and administration of estrogen, sodium fluoride, calcitonin, biphosphates, or ursodeoxycholic acid (UDCA) (for osteopenia). For end-stage primary biliary cirrhosis: liver transplant (treatment of choice).

Secondary biliary: Treatment includes surgical or endoscopic evacuation of bile duct stones, correction of bile duct strictures, dilation and stenting of strictures.

Postnecrotic: Only treatment is symptom management and control of complications.

Sequelae: Major complications include portal hypertension and associated esophageal varices, hemorrhage, disabling edema and ascites, and death caused by hepatic encephalopathy and coma.

Prevention/prophylaxis: Prevention strategies include advising the patient to decrease or abstain from alcohol intake; to obtain early detection and treatment of alcoholism; to diligently monitor liver function in patients with known risk for liver damage related to medications or environmental exposure to hepatotoxic substances; and to maintain a balanced nutritional diet and good general health.

Referral: Refer to, or consult with, radiologist for liver ultrasound studies; with a surgeon for fine-needle or laparoscopic liver biopsy or visceral angiography; nutritionist or dietitian for nutritional and dietary considerations; gastroenterologist for esophagogastroduodenoscopy if varices are suspected; to support groups such as Alcoholics Anonymous as indicated.

Education: Explain disease process, signs and symptoms, and treatment (including side effects of medications). Educational resources are available from the National Digestive Diseases Information Clearinghouse, PO Box NDDIC, Bethesda, MD 20892 (301-468-6344) and the American Liver Foundation, 1425 Pompton Ave., Cedar Grove, NC 07009 (201-256-2550).

COLORECTAL CANCER

SIGNAL SYMPTOMS Rectal bleeding; Change in bowel habits

Colorectal cancer ICD-9-CM: 154.0

Description: Colorectal cancer is cancer of the large intestine, arising from the mucosal lining, including all sections of the colon (70% of cases) and rectum (30% of cases); 95% of all colorectal cancers are adenocarcinomas. After involving the regional lymph nodes, colorectal cancers metastasize primarily to the liver via the portal venous circulation. Overall survival rate remains about 50% and has not changed over the past 40 years, although disease-specific mortality is decreasing.

Etiology: Majority are believed to begin as adenomatous polyps. Etiologic factors include consumption of high levels of animal fats and protein and genetics (25% of patients have a positive family history).

Occurrence: Prevalence of adenomatous polyps increases with age at a rate of more than 25% in patients older than age 50 years. Colorectal cancer second only to lung cancer in regard to number of new cases and reported deaths; 155,000 new cases per year, and approximately 60,000 deaths each year in the United States. Although the mortality rate has remained relatively constant, overall occurrence is falling for unknown reasons.

Age: Most frequently occurs in patient older than age 50 years; peak incidence is in the seventh decade.

Ethnicity: Higher incidence in highly industrialized countries and African Americans.

Gender: Occurs equally in men and in women.

Contributing factors: Inflammatory bowel disease, adenomatous polyps, previous history of colon cancer, diet (including insufficient calcium in the diet, diet high in animal fats and proteins), genetics.

Signs and symptoms: Signs and symptoms vary with location and size of lesion, and because of the elasticity of the bowel, may often reach advanced stages without symptoms.

Signs and symptoms include vague abdominal pain; peptic ulcer-like symptoms; weight loss; anorexia; crampy, colicky pain; change in bowel habits; constipation alternating with diarrhea; weakness; iron deficiency anemia.

Right-sided: May present with pain or mass in the right lower quadrant, anemia, and occult blood in the stool.

Left-sided: May present with changes in bowel habits such as constipation or diarrhea, changes in the shape of the stool such as decreased caliber, or hematochezia (red blood mixed in stool).

Rectal: May present with gross rectal bleeding, tenesmus, urinary frequency, pain in the sacrum or sciatic pain.

Later presentations: May present with abdominal pain and cramping secondary to intestinal obstruction. Presenting symptoms may be systemic and include fatigue, weight loss, anemia, and fever (occasionally) associated with hepatic metastasis.

Physical examination may reveal rectal mass on digital rectal examination, possible occult blood in the stool, abdominal asymmetry, and possible acute abdomen or bowel obstruction. Digital rectal examination (DRE) (detects rectal mass; identifies 15% of rectal cancer [approximately 30% of colorectal lesions arise in the rectosigmoid area]).

Diagnostic tests:

Tests	Result Indicating Disorder	CPT Code
Colonoscopy with biopsy	Confirms diagnosis; rules out other causes of symptoms	45380
Anoscopy and possibly flexible proctoscopy	Especially for patients over age 40 with change in stool caliber or nonspecific abdominal pain and family history of colorectal cancer; helps rule out other causes	46615

(Continued)

Tests	Result Indicating Disorder	CPT Code
Carcinoembryonic antigen (CEA)	Helps define prognosis; is necessary for follow-up surveillance; not recommended for screening or diagnosis because many things can cause an elevated CEA	82378
Stool for guaiac	Positive stool warrants follow-up and evaluation; however, many agents, such as aspirin-containing products, anti-inflammatory agents, animal proteins and dietary irons, may cause false-positive results	82270

Differential diagnosis:

- Rectal polyps (differentiate on biopsy and pathologic examination)
- Hemorrhoids (bright, red bleeding associated with defecation, itching, burning rectal pain)
- Diverticulosis (acute localized pain, fever, changes in bowel habits)
- Rectal fissures (acute pain, bleeding)
- Inflammatory bowel disease (chronic, recurrent pain, fever, rectal bleeding, weight loss, variable abdominal exam, > WBCs and >ESR)
- Colorectal strictures (seen on imaging)
- Other neoplasms (determined on biopsy and pathologic examination)
- Extrinsic masses (abscesses or cysts)
- Colorectal infectious or inflammatory lesions (pathology reports)

Treatment: Treatment will depend on tumor type (classified according to histologic characteristics: well-differentiated, moderately differentiated, or poorly differentiated); staging (based on TNM or Duke's classification systems); and overall prognosis (best for well-differentiated tumor).

Surgical: Treatment of choice. Even if metastatic disease precludes bowel resection for cure, it may be done for palliative reasons. Before surgery, a metastatic workup, which includes liver function tests, CEA level, colonoscopy, and chest film, is usually performed.

Chemotherapy: Usually palliative; drug of choice is 5-fluorouracil; addition of levamisole reduces rate of tumor recurrence.

Radiation therapy: May be used in conjunction with surgical excision for stages B2 and C rectal tumors which tend to metastasize early because of extensive lymphatic drainage.

Follow-up: Following resection, see patient semiannually for physical examination, including history, physical, CEA levels, stools for guaiac, chest films, and liver function tests. Patient should have colonoscopy annually for the first 2 years, then every 2 to 3 years, depending on symptom status. If an adenomatous polyp is excised, colonoscopy should be performed within 6 months.

Sequelae: Possible complications include metastatic disease; complications following resection (mortality rate, 5% to 10%; wound infections, as

high as 15%; pneumonia, 5% to 10%), complications from chemotherapy and/or radiation therapy, stoma after bowel resection, and colostomy.
Prevention/Prophylaxis: Prevention strategies include screening for early detection (although 5-year survival is about 55% and has not changed in spite of screening programs). Yearly digital rectal examinations are recommended for patients over age 40; the American Cancer Society and the National Cancer Institute recommend annual stool checks for guaiac. The American Cancer Society also recommends an initial flexible sigmoidoscopy at age 50 with follow-ups every 3 to 5 years. In addition, all colonic polyps should be removed and identified. Recent studies have supported use of colonoscopy as the gold-standard for screening, with baseline exam at age 50 and repeated every 5 years (every 3 years for patients with adenomatous polyps).

Changes in dietary habits, including consumption of more fiber, fruits, and vegetables and less animal fats and proteins, appear to hold the most promise for decreasing colorectal cancer. Some studies have suggested that daily aspirin intake may lower the risk of this cancer; likewise, adequate calcium intake is thought to provide protection (although this is unsubstantiated).

Referral: Refer to, or consult with, physician or surgeon for colonoscopy if polyps are suspected. On diagnosis, refer to surgeon, and, depending on staging, to an oncologist.

Education: Explain disease process, signs and symptoms, and treatment (including side effects of medications). Discuss treatment options. If patient has colostomy, discuss management and care of colostomy, including avoiding gas-producing foods, such as cabbage, onions, beans, and alcoholic beverages. Educational resource materials are available from the American Cancer Society (Facts on Colorectal Cancer) and from

Table 6–1   Colorectal Screening Guidlines

History	
Identify risk factors	• Family history of colorectal cancer or polyposis. • History of inflammatory bowel disease • History of cancer (colon, ovarian, breast, endometrial) and/or adenomatous polyps • High-fat, low-fiber diet

Screening Recommendations		
Age	*Appropriate Population*	*Recommended Examinations*
Beginning at age 35	• Patients with 2 or more identified risk factors	• Yearly digital rectal examination • Serial stool specimens for guaiac • Baseline colonoscopy with follow-up as appropriate
Beginning of age 40 Beginning of age 50	• All Patients • All Patients	• Yearly digital rectal examination • Yearly digital rectal examination • Serial stool specimens for guaiac • Flexible sigmoidoscopy, barium enema, or colonoscopy every three years

the National Cancer Institute, Department of Health and Human Services, Public Inquiries Section, Office of Cancer Communications, Building 31, Room 101-18, 9000 Rockville Pike, Bethesda, MD 20892 (301-496-5583).

Refer to Table 6-1 for colorectal cancer screening guidelines.

DIVERTICULA DISEASE (DIVERTICULOSIS, DIVERTICULITIS)

SIGNAL SYMPTOMS▶ LLQ pain; Intermittent cramping; may be asymptomatic

Diverticulosis	ICD-9-CM: 562.10
Diverticulitis	ICD-9-CM:562.11

Description: Diverticula disease consists of diverticulosis, in which bulging pouches (diverticula) in the wall of the gastrointestinal tract push the mucosa lining through the surrounding muscle, and diverticulitis, in which inflamed diverticula cause obstruction, infection, hemorrhage, and stagnation of feces. Diverticula are most common in the sigmoid colon, but may develop anywhere from the proximal end of the pharynx to the anus.

Etiology: Diverticula probably result from high intraluminal pressure on weak areas in the GI wall. Diverticulosis commonly results from habitual consumption of low-fiber diet that reduces fecal bulk, thus reducing the diameter of the colon. Diverticulitis commonly results when undigested food mixes with bacteria and accumulates in the diverticular sac, forming a hard mass (fecalith). This mass cuts off the blood supply to the thin walls of the sac, making them more susceptible to the attack of bacteria.

Age: Most common in older adults. About 5% affected during fifth decade; as high as 50% by ninth decade.

Occurrence: Affects up to 20% of the general population; incidence increases with age. Recurrent diverticulitis is observed in approximately 33% of cases, about half within 1 year and the remainder within the next 5 years. Almost unknown in rural Africa and Asia. Most common in developed countries, although a lower prevalence in western vegetarians consuming a diet high in roughage.

Gender: Gender distribution varies with age.

Contributing factors: Habitual consumption of foods low in fiber or those with small seeds; increased age; sedentary lifestyle; obesity.

Signs and symptoms: Symptoms may be vague or absent; only 10% to 25% of patients present with symptoms.

Common symptoms: Cramping pain that localizes to the left lower abdomen or midabdominal pain radiating to the back, increased flatus, constipation alternating with diarrhea, rectal bleeding; pain usually worse after eating, with relief after defecation. Recent change in bowel habits not uncommon

With inflamed or abscessed diverticulitis: Localized left lower abdominal pain with rebound tenderness, mild nausea, flatus, irregular bowel movements, fever, leukocytosis. Rectal examination may reveal a mass from a pelvic abscess.

With ruptured diverticulitis: Left lower abdominal pain, tenderness, and rigidity; fever, chills, leukocytosis, hypoactive bowel sounds, signs and symptoms of peritonitis.

Diagnostic tests:

Tests	Result Indicating Disorder	CPT Code
WBC	Normal with diverticulosis; increased with diverticulitis	85007
ESR	May be increased	85652
Stool for guaiac	May be positive	82270
Barium enema	Diagnoses diverticulosis best; less useful for diverticulitis	74270
CT scan with or without contrast	Diagnoses size and location of mass, abscess, or fistula	74183
Flat and upright x-ray studies of abdomen	Can evaluate for an intestinal obstruction or perforated viscus	74250
Colonoscopy and flexible sigmoidoscopy	Diagnoses diverticulosis; rules out malignancy	45380

ESR, erythrocyte sedimentation rate; WBC, white blood cell.

Differential diagnosis:

- Intestinal ischemia (sharp, excruciating pain)
- Meckel's diverticulitis (painless rectal bleeding, anemia, lower abdominal pain)
- Ulcerative colitis (diarrhea, rectal bleeding)
- Appendicitis (RLQ pain)
- Crohn's disease (chronic, abdominal pain, anorexia, non-bloody diarrhea, weight loss)
- Irritable bowel syndrome (chronic pain, varying bowel habits, relief after bowel movement, normal examination)
- Malignancy (biopsy and pathological examination)
- Lactose intolerance (associated with ingestion of dairy products)

Treatment:

Diverticulosis: Treat pain with antispasmodics, such as hyoscyamine, 0.125 mg every 4 hours or dicyclomine hcl 10 to 20 mg every 6 hours. Encourage a high-fiber diet (15 to 20 g/day, including fruits, vegetables, coarse cereals, and bran) and increased fluids to increase bowel motility (although two small randomly controlled studies found no consistent effect of bran or ispaghula husk versus placebo on symptoms after 6 to 12 weeks).

Bed rest and clear liquid diet may be recommended during acute attack.

Diverticulitis: Treat as noted earlier. Add antibiotic therapy. For mild attack, antibiotics, such as metronidazole, 250 to 500 mg orally every 8 hours; amoxicillin with clavulanic acid, 500 mg orally every 8 hours; ciprofloxacin, 500 mg orally twice a day; or levofloxacin 500 mg each day. Expect a response in 3 days; continue treatment for 1 week.

Signs of toxicity, peritonitis, septicemia, or failure to resolve: Hospitalize patient; treat with parenteral antibiotics, IV fluids, analgesia. Surgery may be indicated.

Rupture: Severe complications, such as an abscess, rupture, or perforation, is a surgical emergency requiring resection of the bowel with a temporary colostomy.

Follow-up: Follow-up will depend on the severity of the patient's condition.

Sequelae: Sixty-seven percent of patients have only one attack; 33% will have a recurrence. Possible complications include hemorrhage, perforation, bowel obstruction, abscess, peritonitis, rebleeding.

Prevention/prophylaxis: Prevention strategies include high-fiber diet, and use of bulk-forming medications such as Metamucil, FiberCon, and psyllium.

Referral: Refer to, or consult with, physician if patient does not respond to antibiotic therapy and bed rest.

Education: Explain disease process, signs and symptoms, and treatment (including side effects of medications). Discuss prevention strategies. Encourage patient to keep a diary of foods eaten before symptoms started and to report changes or symptoms. Encourage family and/or group support. Educational resource materials available from the National Digestive Diseases Information Clearinghouse, PO Box NDDIC, Bethesda, MD 20892 (301-654-3810). Website: *www.niddk.nih.gov/health/digest/nddic.htm*

GASTRITIS

SIGNAL SYMPTOMS▶ *Erosive gastritis:* ranges from asymptomatic to anorexia, nausea, vomiting, and epigastric distress to upper GI bleeding (pallor, tachycardia, hypotension).
Nonerosive, nonspecific gastritis: From no symptoms to nausea, and/or abdominal pain of several days' duration.

Gastritis	ICD-9-CM: 535

Description: Gastritis is mucosal inflammation of the stomach. Mucosal erosions are present, but ulcerations are not.

Etiology: Gastritis is commonly classified according to three categories: erosive or hemorrhagic acute gastritis, caused by medications (such as aspirin or NSAIDs), stress (such as severe trauma, major surgery, hepatic, renal, or respiratory failure, massive burns, and infections with septicemia), and alcohol; *Helicobacter pylori* gastritis, caused by inflammatory changes along the greater curvature of the stomach (fundal gland or type A) or in the antrum of the stomach (antral or type B), with the gram-negative bacterium *Helicobacter pylori* possibly an opportunistic cause; and, occasionally, viral infection, usually as a component of systemic infection.

Occurrence: Common; approximately 60% of patients over age 60 harbor *H. pylori*.

Age: Occurs in all ages; increases with age. Adult prevalence is believed to represent the persistence of a historically high rates of infection acquired in childhood rather than increasing acquisitions of infection during life.

Ethnicity: Occurs more in nonwhite people than in whites.

Gender: Occurs equally in men and in women.

Contributing factors: Peptic ulcer disease; chronic *H. pylori* infection; smoking; ingestion of alcohol, caffeine, or caustic acids; radiation therapy; use of NSAIDs and aspirin; emotional stress; pernicious anemia; sequelae of physiologic stressors such as hypoxia, hypovolemia.

Signs and symptoms:

> *Erosive gastritis:* Signs and symptoms range from asymptomatic to anorexia, nausea, vomiting, and epigastric distress to upper GI bleeding (pallor, tachycardia, hypotension).
>
> *Nonerosive, nonspecific gastritis:* Signs and symptoms include no symptoms, nausea, and/or abdominal pain of several days' duration.

Diagnostic tests:

Tests	Result Indicating Disorder	CPT Code
Upper GI endoscopy	Provides definitive diagnosis	43235
Gastroscopy	Reveals mucosal hemorrhages, friable and congested mucosa, and presence of erosions in the fundus or body of the stomach	43234
Gastric biopsy	Permits extraction of cultures for *H. pylori*	43239
Serologic test for *H. pylori*; ELISA for anti-*H. pylori* immunoglobulin G.	Positive	86317, 86318

ELISA, enzyme-linked immunosorbent assay.

Differential diagnosis:

- Peptic ulcer disease (gnawing pains after eating, epigastric region)

- Gastroesophageal reflux (persistent burning sensation after meals, relieved with antacids; postprandial regurgitation precipitated by bending over or recumbency)
- Gastric cancer (imaging; biopsy)
- Biliary tract disease (ERCP)
- Pancreatitis (pale, frothy stools; elevated lipase, amylase; low-grade temperature; may have mucous or blood in vomitus; paroxsyms of deep-seated epigastric pain)
- Food poisoning (usually accompanied with nausea, vomiting, sometimes fever)
- Atypical angina pectoris (more common presentation in older adults)

Treatment:

Physical

   For mild cases: Nonpharmacologic actions include removing the offending agents, stopping smoking, reducing alcohol and caffeine consumption, stopping the use of NSAIDs and aspirin, and reducing emotional physiologic stress. In cases of physiologic stressors of acute illness, treat prophylactically IV with H_2 blockers.

Pharmacologic

Treatment includes antacid therapy with over-the-counter (OTC) antacids and H_2 blockers and proton pump inhibitors. Sucralfate 1 g orally four times a day is effective in healing peptic ulcers.

- Antacids: OTC antacid 2 tablespoons orally four times a day 1 hour after meals and at bedtime (hs).
- H_2 blockers: cimetidine, 300 mg orally four times a day or 400 mg three times a day (highest incidence of side effects and drug interactions); famotidine, 20 mg orally three times a day; or ranitidine, 150 mg orally twice a day.
- Proton pump inhibitors such as omeprazole 20 g daily, iantoprazole (prevacid) 15 mg daily, pantoprazole (protonix) 40 mg daily are more potent than the H_2 blockers.
- For treatment of *H. pylori*: The following "triple therapy" may be prescribed: bismuth subsalicylate (Pepto-Bismol), 2 tablespoons or two tablets orally four times a day; and metronidazole, 250 mg orally three times a day; and tetracycline, 500 mg orally four times a day for 14 days. (Warn patient of occurrence of black stools with bismuth use.); or esomeprazole 40 PO each day or lansoprazole 30 orally each day or omeprazole 20 PO bid and amoxicillin 1 gm PO bid and clarithromycin 500 mg bid for 10 to 14 days.
- Anxiolytics or antidepressants as appropriate if emotional stress is a major contributor to gastritis.

Follow-up: See the patient for recurrence of symptoms as indicated.
Sequelae: Most cases resolve with proper treatment. Possible complications include reinfection with *H. pylori*.

Prevention/prophylaxis: Prevention strategies include advising the patient to avoid known offending agents, stop smoking, decrease alcohol and caffeine intake, reduce ingestion of NSAIDs and aspirin, and learn techniques to reduce emotional stress.

Referral: Refer to, or consult with, gastroenterologist.

Education: Explain disease process, signs and symptoms, and treatment (including side effects of medications). Discuss prevention strategies. Provide reassurance.

GASTROENTERITIS

SIGNAL SYMPTOMS Crampy, diffuse abdominal pain relieved by vomiting or defecation

Viral gastroenteritis	ICD-9-CM: 008.8
Gastroenteritis, other and unspecified	ICD-9-CM: 558.9

Description: Gastroenteritis is an inflammation of the gastric and mucous membrane. It is commonly caused by ingestion of contaminated food or water or by fecal-oral transmission. Largely self-limiting.

Etiology: Commonly caused by infection by viruses, bacteria, and protozoa. It may also be caused by toxic agents in food, as well as allergic or chemical reactions and enzyme deficiencies. Recent travel to underdeveloped countries and not exercising proper precautions is the most common cause for nonindigenous gastroenteritis. Travelers from developed countries are frequently susceptible to endemically caused gastroenteritis ("traveler's diarrhea"). May also be caused by *Clostridium difficile* infection secondary to recent antibiotic therapy.

Occurrence: Common (second to the common cold as the cause of lost work time). Viral enteritis occurs more often in winter (winter vomiting disease).

Age: Occurs in all ages.

Ethnicity: No significant ethnic predisposition.

Gender: Occurs equally in men and in women.

Contributing factors: History of ingestion of contaminated food, untreated water, and known GI irritants; age (infants and elderly at most risk); institutionalized, debilitated, or immunocompromised patient; workers in health-care facilities, institutions, or day-care centers.

Signs and symptoms: Symptoms vary depending on the level of GI tract involvement and infecting pathogen. It is important to obtain an accurate history concerning recent food and water intake, travel, or GI illness with close contacts.

> *Diarrhea (classic symptom),* varying in amount and consistency. In mild diarrhea, there may be 2 to 10 stools per day with increased fluid content; with severe diarrhea, the frequency and fluidity increase and may contain mucus or blood. May be flatulence and

explosive diarrhea. Other signs and symptoms may include nausea or vomiting; abdominal pain, discomfort, or cramping; fever (with some pathogens); anorexia; malaise; myalgia; and headache.

Severe gastroenteritis: Signs and symptoms of dehydration, fluid loss, and electrolyte imbalance, such as weight loss, dry and flushed skin, dry mucous membranes and lips, poor skin turgor, decreased urinary output, and rapid pulse. Presence of neurologic symptoms may indicate botulism. Refer to emergency department immediately.

Physical examination may reveal hyperactive bowel sounds, diffuse abdominal tenderness, and abdominal distention. Fever may be present and may accelerate dehydration.

Diagnostic Tests: Because most cases of gastroenteritis are short lived and symptoms rapidly resolve with appropriate supportive therapy, diagnostic tests are frequently not necessary but may include

Test	Result Indicating Disorder	CPT Code
BUN, creatinine	Assess in young and elderly patients	84520, 82565
Stool cultures, ova and parasites, *C. difficile*	Helps identify causative organism	87045, 87177, 87324
Gram stains	Identify WBCs and RBCs for diagnosing organisms	87205
Serum electrolytes, hemoglobin, and hematocrit	Evaluate for dehydration	80051, 85018, 85014
CBC	Shows leukocytosis in bacterial infection	85025
Blood cultures	Identify causative organism; provide sensitivity testing for antibiotic therapy	87072, 87075
ESR	Risk of irritable bowel	85652
Stool for occult blood	Should be negative except in cases of gastroenteritis	82270

CBC, complete blood count; ESR, erythrocyte sedimentation rate; RBCs, red blood cells; WBCs, white blood cells.

Differential diagnosis:

- Ingestion of toxins such as food-borne, pharmacologic, heavy metal, poisonous plant, or household products (history)
- Food intolerance (related to ingestion of certain foods)
- Drug allergies (history)
- Obstructive diseases of the GI tract (anorexia, vomiting, abdominal pain, decreased bowel sounds)
- Acute presentations of systemic disorders (check associated diagnostic tests to evaluate)
- Acute appendicitis (RLQ pain)
- Cholecystitis (RUQ pain)
- Fecal impaction with overflow (history of constipation)
- PID (pelvic examination, history)

Treatment: Intervention and treatment is determined by the severity of the condition.

Physical

In most cases, treatment is supportive with bed rest and replacing fluid and electrolytes. Fluid replacement therapy consists of providing the patient with adequate fluid and electrolyte content. Gatorade is the cheapest and most readily available fluid containing electrolytes. Carefully monitor intake and output, and progress diet as tolerated. Cracked ice chips may be used if patient has nausea and vomiting; then progress to clear liquids for 24 hours. Rice, applesauce, ripe bananas may be tried next.

Other supportive care includes using enteric precautions, developing good hand-washing techniques, and maintaining good skin integrity. Maintain skin integrity by careful washing and drying, using hydrocortisone cream or Desitin ointment to anus if irritated, taking sitz baths for 10 minutes three times a day, or applying witch hazel compresses to relieve anal irritation.

Pharmacologic

Use of antidiarrheal agents is controversial, because infective agents need to be eliminated from the body. For relief of mild, nondysentery symptoms, consider loperamide, 4 mg after the first loose stool and 2 mg after each subsequent stool, up to 16 mg in 24 hours, or diphenoxylate with atropine, 5 mg four times a day for loose stools. If antiemetics are required, consider prochlorperazine or trimethobenzamide. If antimicrobial therapy is indicated, administer therapy for the specific causative agent, such as ciprofloxacin, 500 mg twice a day for 7 days; norfloxacin, 400 mg twice a day for 7 days; trimethoprim-sulfamethoxazole, double strength, one tablet twice a day for 7 days or metronidazole 250-500 mg four times a day for 7 days.

Follow-up: See the patient if symptoms persist for more than 72 hours or if symptoms worsen.

Sequelae: Possible complications include prostration, irritability, convulsions, dehydration, protracted diarrhea, acquired lactase deficiency, protein-losing enteropathy, and metabolic acidosis.

Referral: Refer to, or consult with, physician if patient has severe dehydration or is a very young or old patient, debilitated, or immunocompromised. Hospitalization may be necessary for IV fluid or electrolyte replacement, IV antimicrobial therapy, severe abdominal pain, rebound tenderness, or neurologic symptoms. The local health department must be notified of identified individual cases of salmonellosis, shigellosis, cholera, campylobacteriosis, and yersiniosis; of epidemics; and of outbreaks of *E. coli, Rotavirus,* Norwalk virus, *S. aureus,* and *Clostridium perfringens,* cryptosporidiosis, and *Giardia.*

Prevention/prophylaxis: Prevention strategies include advising the patient to maintain good personal hygiene, to perform good hand-washing techniques, to take care when handling animals and pets, to maintain good sanitation, to treat other family members with gastroenteritis, and to follow the World Health Organization (WHO) guidelines for safe food preparation: choose food processed for safety; cook food thoroughly; eat cooked food immediately; store cooked food carefully; reheat cooked food thoroughly; avoid contact between raw and cooked food; wash hands repeatedly; keep all kitchen surfaces meticulously clean; protect food from insects, rodents, and other animals; and use safe water. Routine antibiotic prophylaxis is usually not recommended, however, antibiotics such as ciprofloxacin, 500 mg/day; norfloxacin, 400 mg/day; or trimethoprim-sulfamethoxazole DS, 1 tablet per day) and antidiarrheal prophylaxis (such as with bismuth subsalicylate [Pepto-Bismol], 2 tablets four times a day) may help prevent "traveler's diarrhea" when traveling to underdeveloped countries. Caution patient to avoid tap water, ice, unpasteurized milk, raw or rare meats, and raw fruits or vegetables that have not been peeled by the patient.

Education: Explain disease process, signs and symptoms, and treatment (including side effects of medications). Discuss prevention strategies and when to seek medical attention. Explain the self-limiting nature of the disease (up to 48 hours, but may persist up to 2 weeks).

GASTROESOPHAGEAL REFLUX

SIGNAL SYMPTOMS▶   Heartburn, regurgitation, dysphagia

| Gastroesophageal reflux disease | ICD-9-CM: 530.81 |

Description: Gastroesophageal reflux disease (GERD) is a chronic condition in which gastric contents, usually acidic, reflux into the esophagus, causing symptoms and tissue damage.

Etiology: Complex multifactor process. There may be acid hypersecretion or structural etiology, such as lower esophageal sphincter (LES) relaxation related to food, drugs, or idiopathic causes.

Occurrence: Very common; 65% of all adults have heartburn at some time during their lives.

Age: Occurs at all ages.

Ethnicity: Common in whites. Not common in African Americans.

Gender: Two to three times more common in men than women.

Contributing factors: Lower esophageal sphincter dysfunction; esophageal peristaltic dysfunction; delayed gastric emptying; sliding hiatal hernia; supine position for sleep; lying down immediately after eating; obesity; cigarette smoking; diet high in fatty, acidic, and spicy foods; caffeine and alcohol ingestion.

Signs and Symptoms:

 Red Flag: Any patient presenting with dysphagia, weight loss, and blood in the stool must be referred for definitive diagnostic testing such as endoscopy.

Heartburn occurring 30 to 60 minutes after meals and on reclining (most common); substernal pain, often radiating upward; regurgitation of a sour or bitter taste into the mouth; and cough. Atypical symptoms, such as dysphagia, asthma, chronic laryngitis, and noncardiac chest pain, have also been associated with GERD.

Diagnostic tests: Heartburn and regurgitation may be treated without the need for diagnostic tests; stool for occult blood may be performed. Atypical symptoms, such as dysphagia, hematemesis, guaiac-positive stools, weight loss, and anemia, and symptoms that persist despite treatment may warrant tests such as

Test	Result Indicating Disorder	CPT Code
Upper endoscopy	Reveals esophageal tissue damage, presence of Barrett's esophagus or peptic stricture	43202
Bernstein's test	Replicates and confirms symptoms	82926-82928
Ambulatory esophageal pH monitoring	Acid reflux	91032-91033
Barium swallow	Reveals sliding hiatal hernia; a predictor of reflux esophagitis	74230

Differential diagnosis:

- Esophageal motility disorders (check diagnostic test results, i.e. hiatal hernia)
- Peptic ulcers (gnawing epigastric pain associated with eating)
- Cholelithiasis (RUQ pain)
- Esophageal tumor (imaging; biopsy)
- Angina pectoris (Relieved with nitroglycerin [NTG], rest; electrocardiogrram [ECG])
- Pill- and radiation-induced esophagitis (history)
- Infections such as with cytomegalovirus (CMV; appropriate cultures, history)
- Herpes (appropriate cultures, history, immune status)
- *Candida* (drug history, i.e., antibiotics; check immune status)

Treatment:

Phase I (mild disease): Lifestyle changes: Avoid eating within 3 to 4 hours of bedtime; elevate head of bed 6 inches or use wedge under pillow; lose weight if overweight; stop smoking; eat small, frequent meals; avoid overeating; avoid foods that provoke symptoms such as high-fat, spicy, acidic foods, chocolate, citrus fruits, mints, caffeine, and alcohol. Medications: OTC antacids and OTC histamine 2 (H_2) blockers.

Phase II (moderate disease): H_2 blockers: Cimetidine, 800 mg orally hs or 400 mg orally twice a day; ranitidine, 150 mg orally twice a day; famotidine, 20 mg orally twice a day; nizatidine, 150 mg twice a day. Thirty to 50 percent of patients respond to therapy in 6 weeks; 50% to 80% in 12 weeks.

Phase III (erosive disease): Esomeprazole 40 mg each day; lansoprazole, 30 mg each day; omeprazole, 20 mg each day; pantoprazole 40 mg each day; or rabeprazole 20 mg each day; or increase dosage of H_2 blockers.

Phase IV (surgical): Surgical interventions (Nissen fundoplication, Hill posterior gastropexy, Belsey Mark IV operation) may be appropriate for patients who are noncompliant with medical treatment or in whom medical treatment fails.

Follow-up: See the patient 2 weeks after beginning treatment for reevaluation. If treatment is effective, have patient continue it for 6 to 8 weeks. Maintenance therapy (H_2 receptor antagonists: or esomeprazole 40 mg each day; lansoprazole, 30 mg each day; omeprazole, 20 mg each day; pantoprazole 40 mg each day; or rabeprazole 20 mg each day; should be considered to prevent relapse (80% relapse within 6 months).

Sequelae: Possible complications include hemorrhage (3%), noncardiac chest pain, and peptic stricture (10% to 15%).

Prevention/prophylaxis: Although GERD is a chronic, lifelong condition in most patients, prevention strategies include lifestyle changes (such as those listed previously), and maintenance with H_2 blockers.

Referral: Refer to, or consult with, physician or specialist (gastroenterologist) if patient does not respond to therapy, or has dysphagia, weight loss, anemia, or blood loss.

Education: Explain disease process, signs and symptoms, and treatment (including side effects of medications). Discuss the chronic nature, importance of compliance with lifestyle changes and drug therapy, need for re-evaluation if symptoms intensify or nature of the pain changes, and how to monitor stools for signs of bleeding. Educational resource materials available from the National Digestive Diseases Information Clearinghouse, PO Box NDDIC, Bethesda, MD 20892 (301-654-3810). Website: *www.niddk.nih.gov/health/digest/nddic.htm*

Refer to Figure 6-2 for the differential diagnosis and treatment of epigastric pain.

HEMORRHOIDS

SIGNAL SYMPTOMS ▶ Painless bleeding, anal discomfort, rectal itching, pain, burning

| Hemorrhoids | ICD-9-CM: 455.6 |

Description: Hemorrhoids (piles) are dilated varicosities of the hemorrhoidal venous plexus that may be internal or external, thrombosed or prolapsed. Hemorrhoids are classified as follows: first degree, no pro-

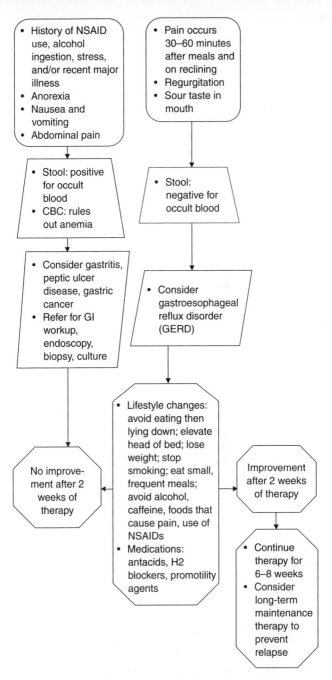

Figure 6–2. Differential diagnosis and treatment: epigastric pain.

lapse; second degree, prolapses but reduces spontaneously; third degree, prolapses but reduces with manual reduction; and fourth degree, permanently prolapsed, will not reduce.

Etiology: The primary cause is straining at stool with resultant increased intra-abdominal and hemorrhoidal venous pressures. Hemorrhoids probably result from venous congestion caused by interference with venous return from the hemorrhoidal veins and increased intravenous pressure in the hemorrhoidal plexus.

Occurrence: Common; about half of the population have hemorrhoids by age 50 years.

Age: Occurs most often in people older than age 50; uncommon under age 25, except for women who have been pregnant.

Ethnicity: No significant ethnic predisposition.

Gender: Occurs equally in men and women.

Contributing factors: Constipation, pregnancy, episiotomy, congestive heart failure (CHF), prolonged sitting or standing, obesity, anal intercourse, loss of muscle tone, rectal surgery, liver disease, colon cancer, portal hypertension.

Signs and symptoms: Physical examination reveals inflammation, appearance of hemorrhoid, flabby skin sac, dilated hemorrhoidal veins, anal protrusion, hemorrhoidal prolapse, hemorrhoidal thrombosis (tense, tender, bluish purple mass covered with skin), or anal fissure. Digital rectal examination is often negative. Internal hemorrhoids above the anorectal junction are not palpable unless thrombosed.

Diagnostic tests:

> *External hemorrhoids:* Visualize on physical examination if external hemorrhoids.
>
> *Internal hemorrhoids*: Diagnosed by digital palpation and visualization through an anoscope. Asking the patient to strain will cause the veins to enlarge, aiding in diagnosis.
>
> Additional tests may include sigmoidoscopy or colonoscopy (rules out other causes of GI bleeding), and hemoglobin and hematocrit (if anemia is suspected).

Differential diagnosis:

- Crohn's disease (chronic, abdominal pain, anorexia, non-bloody diarrhea, weight-loss)
- Anal tags (visible in physical examination)
- Prolapse of the rectal mucosa
- Colon cancer (colonoscopy, biopsy)
- Anal fissure (rectal pain exacerbated by defecation)
- Colorectal neoplasm or adenoma (firm painless nodule)
- Anorectal abscess (pain, possible drainage, foul smelling)
- Anorectal fistula (communication between epithelialized viscera, periodic discharge occasionally filled with blood)

- Pilonidal disease (hair containing cyst or sinus located in midline over coccyx or lower sacrum)
- Thrombosed hemorrhoid (hemorrhoid containing clotted blood that becomes painful, shiny and blue, itchy and bleed on defecation)
- Pruritus ani (rectal itching, symptom of hemorrhoids, fissures, condylomata)

Treatment:

Pharmacologic

Stool softener. Topical steroids (for severe inflammation and itching). Local analgesic sprays or ointments such as benzocaine or dibucaine (avoid suppositories because they deliver medication to the rectum not the anus). Witch hazel pads (may help itching and burning). For pruritus, use hydrocortisone ointment. For bleeding, use an astringent suppository such as Preparation H.

Physical

Warm sitz baths for 15 to 20 minutes several times a day, ice packs, and witch hazel compresses for symptomatic relief. Bed rest to reduce pain and swelling, especially if thrombosed. High-fiber diet including bran cereal, fresh fruits and vegetables. Fiber supplements. Encourage liberal water intake (six to eight 8-ounce glasses daily).

Surgical

Excision under local anesthesia (for thrombosed hemorrhoids). Hemorrhoidectomy (for severe cases with prolonged, intolerable pain, recurrent thrombosis, and prolonged bleeding).

Nonsurgical

(Most effective with first- and second-degree hemorrhoids.) Rubber band ligation (for very large, prolapsing lesions). Sclerotherapy (for large lesions). Infrared photocoagulation. Cryosurgery. Laser coagulation.

Follow-up: See the patient if pain is not relieved by recommended treatment, if rectal bleeding is excessive (more than a trace or streak on toilet paper or stool), or if constipation persists.

Sequelae: Spontaneous resolution often occurs; however, recurrence may be frequent. Possible complications include bleeding, thrombosis, hemorrhoidal strangulation, secondary infection, ulceration, anemia (rare), and incontinence.

Prevention/prophylaxis: Prevention strategies include avoiding constipation, prolonged sitting on the toilet, and prolonged sitting at work. Weight loss, if overweight, is also recommended. Regular daily exercise such as walking. High-fiber diet.

Referral: Refer to, or consult with, physician if patient presents with persistent bleeding, extensive mucosal erosion, severe pain, thrombosis, or rectal prolapse.

Education: Explain the disease process, signs and symptoms, and treatment (including side effects of medications). Discuss the relationship between diet, fluid intake, exercise, and bowel regularity; the physiology of defecation; and importance of establishing a routine. Advise to avoid straining and prolonged sitting on the toilet; respond only to the urge to defecate. Recommend putting feet on a low footstool to aid bowel movement and removing reading material from the bathroom. Advise cleaning the anal area gently with soft, moist paper and using soap and water for cleanup after bowel movement. Explain that creams and ointments are better than suppositories.

HEPATITIS, VIRAL

SIGNAL SYMPTOMS▶ Jaundice, tender hepatomegaly, malaise and nausea

Hepatitis, Viral	ICD-9-CM: 070.0

Description: Viral hepatitis is a viral infection of the liver. There are six commonly accepted forms of viral hepatitis: A, B, C, D, E, and, recently, hepatitis G. Viral hepatitis may also be classified as acute, which lasts < 6 months and is common with hepatitis A virus (HAV) and hepatitis E virus (HEV); or chronic, which lasts longer than 6 months and is common with hepatitis B virus (HBV), hepatitis C virus (HCV), and hepatitis D virus (HDV). HDV is usually identified only with a concurrent HBV infection. Examples are Epstein Barr virus and cytomegalovirus. Additionally, nonhepatotropic viruses may also cause hepatitis, although typically they infect many organs as well as the liver.

Etiology: Caused by the hepatitis virus, HAV and HEV may be contracted by fecal-oral transmission and transmitted enterically; whereas hepatitis B, C, D, and G may be contracted by blood, parenteral, perinatal, or sexual transmission.

Occurrence: HAV antibodies have been found in > 50% of adults older than age 49 years in the United States; account for about 25% of the cases of acute hepatitis.

HBV: Occurs in about 200,000 adults each year; with about another 500,000 being carriers.

   HDV: Occurs concurrently in about 1% of all HBV infections.
   HCV: The most common cause of acute hepatitis, it accounts for about 150,000 infections each year.
   HEV: Occurs primarily in underdeveloped countries.
   HGV: About 2% of non-A, non-B chronic hepatitis. In chronic HDV, 20% coinfection with HGV (Japan).

Age: Occurs in all ages; rare in infants.

Ethnicity:

HAV: Highest incidence in American Indians and native Alaskans.

HEV: Occurs primarily in people from underdeveloped and third-world nations, transmitted enterically by fecal-oral route.

HBV, HCV, and HDV: No significant ethnic predisposition.

Gender: HBV: Occurs two times more in men than in women. HAV, HCV, HDV, HEV: Unknown. HDV: Identified only with HBV infection.

Contributing factors: Occupational risk of exposure to blood and/or body fluids (such as with health-care workers); patients undergoing hemodialysis; recipients of blood or blood products; people with hemophilia; IV drug users; sexually active homosexual men; people with household exposure to an infected person; adopted children from areas of high exposure; people who have experienced a positive needle stick; those with high-risk sexual behavior or regular sexual contact with an infected partner; day-care center workers exposed to the diaper contents of infected children; and anyone exposed to an HAV-infected food handler.

Signs and symptoms: Signs and symptoms for all six types are similar; however, the severity of the symptoms varies with the infecting agent. The signs and symptoms are categorized according to disease progression: phase 1, prodromal or pre-icteric phase; phase 2,-icteric or active phase; and phase 3, posticteric or recovery phase. The most common patient complaints include fatigue (HAV); malaise; nausea; anorexia; jaundice; dark urine; abdominal pain (primarily right upper quadrant); headache; low-grade fever (unusual with HBV and HCV); tender, enlarged liver; vomiting; hepatomegaly; and other hepatic symptoms such as urticaria, rash, arthritis, photophobia, pharyngitis, and diarrhea.

Physical examination may reveal jaundice of the skin, mucous membranes, and sclera; spider angiomas; dark urine; clay-colored stools; fever; a mildly to generally debilitated appearance; postcervical adenopathy; and a possibly enlarged tender spleen.

Diagnostic tests:

Test	Result Indicating Disorder	CPT Code
AST and ALT	Increase during prodromal phase of acute hepatitis	80053 (panel: includes bilirubin, alkaline phosphatase, and CBC)
Serum bilirubin	Elevated	With above panel
CBC	May show that atypical lymphocytosis is acute hepatitis	With above panel
Prothrombin time (PT)	May be prolonged	85610-11
Serum alkaline phosphatase	May be normal or mildly elevated	With above panel

(Continued)

Test	Result Indicating Disorder	CPT Code
Urinalysis	May reveal protein and/or bilirubin	81001
Hepatitis panel	Elevated in acute phase, decreased in posticteric phase	80074
Ultrasound	May show ascites or exclude obstruction	76700
Liver biopsy	Shows type and extent of liver damage	47100

ALT, alanine aminotransferase, AST, aspartate aminotransferase CBC, complete blood count,

Laboratory:

Tests for acute viral hepatitis include HBsAg, anti-HAV, IgM anti-HBc, and anti-HCV. Tests for chronic hepatitis include HBsAg and anti-HCV.

HAV is confirmed by detecting an IgM antibody to HAV (IgM anti-HAV); HBV by HBsAg and IgM anti-HBC (when HBeAg is detected, the patient is highly infectious); HCV by ELISA-2 and RIBA-2; and HDV by anti-HDV and serologic markers for HBV. For HEV, only research-based tests are available at this time.

Differential diagnosis:

- Viral disorders such as CMV, herpes simplex, coxsackievirus, infectious mononucleosis, and toxoplasmosis (mono-spot, viral testing, history)
- Malignancy (liver biopsy)
- Use of medications such as acetaminophen and anesthetic agents such as halothane (history)
- Alcoholic hepatitis (history)
- Acute cholecystitis (RUQ pain)
- Common duct stone (seen on ERCP)
- Wilson's disease (accumulation of copper in various organs including liver; check copper levels in blood; pigmented ring [Kayser-Fleischer ring] at the outer margins of the cornea is pathognomonic)
- Cirrhosis (Liver biopsy)
- Rheumatoid disorders such as rheumatoid arthritis and systemic lupus erythematosus (SLE; ESR elevated; positive rheumatoid factor)

Treatment: All newly diagnosed cases must be reported to the local health department.

Physical

Supportive measures are generally advocated in uncomplicated cases that resolve spontaneously in 4 to 8 weeks. Measures include frequent rest periods because too much activity may cause liver and/or spleen trauma; a fluid intake of 3 to 4 liters per day; a diet with adequate protein, carbohydrate, and green leafy vegetables or other foods high in vitamin K (consider vitamin K therapy for patients with prolonged prothrombin time PT levels); an antiemetic to control symptoms of nausea and vomiting if needed; and colloid baths, soaps, and lotions to lessen the symptoms of pruritus.

Pharmacologic

HBV: Pegylated interferon SC once weekly with ribavirin orally each day for 16 to 26 weeks; reduce dosage if granulocyte or platelet count is decreased.

HCV: Pegylated interferon SC once weekly for 24 weeks; if no response in 16 weeks, re-evaluate effectiveness of current therapy. Nonresponder may respond to a second course of therapy, with remission in 40-50% of patients treated with a 6-month course.

Follow-up: See the patient regularly to perform and monitor appropriate diagnostic tests (including liver biopsies for patient with chronic hepatitis) and to evaluate effectiveness of treatment. Serial measurements of serum AST/ALT.

Sequelae: Possible complications include acute or subacute necrosis, chronic active or chronic hepatitis, cirrhosis, hepatic failure, and hepatocellular cancer.

HAV: May cause mild disease; usually does not result in chronic liver disease.

HBV: May proceed to a chronic state, and those infected may become HBsAg carriers; fulminant liver failure occurs with about 5% of patients.

HCV: About 50% develop chronic hepatitis; about 20% develop cirrhosis.

HDV: About 70% develop cirrhosis.

HEV: Does not result in chronic disease.

HGV: Same as for HCV

Prevention/prophylaxis: Prevention strategies include advising the patient to use standard (universal) precautions when in contact with body fluids, including blood; to use safe sex practices; to use proper hygiene and hand-washing techniques (especially for food handlers); and to abstain from IV drug use or properly dispose of needles. Specific prevention strategies for HAV include administering immunoglobulin, 0.02 mL/kg IM 1 to 2 weeks after exposure (prevents illness in 80% to 90% of those exposed), or for high-risk individuals, administering HAV vaccine, 1 mL IM with a booster dose in 1-6 months. Specific prevention strategies for HBV include screening all pregnant women for HBV, vaccinating all infants at birth, and, for high-risk individuals, administering HBV vaccine (1 mL IM Heptavax) repeated 1 month and 6 months after initial vaccination. Screening of all blood products and possible disposal of needles.

Referral: Because of the high incidence for development of chronic hepatitis, refer to, or consult with, physician as soon as possible if patient has HBV, HCV, HDV, and HGV; to physician, if patient has HAV or HEV, for development of treatment plan.

Education: Explain disease process, signs and symptoms, and treatment (including side effects of medications). Discuss prevention strategies. Advise the patient to abstain from alcohol intake and to avoid other medications that are detoxified by the liver. For women, advise the patient that use of birth control pills may increase bilirubin levels.

HERNIAS, ABDOMINAL

Inguinal (direct, indirect) hernia	ICD-9-CM: 550.9
Femoral (unilateral) hernia	ICD-9-CM: 533
Umbilical hernia	ICD-9-CM: 553.1
Incisional hernia	ICD-9-CM: 553.4

Description: A hernia, often called a "rupture," is a protrusion of a viscus through the wall of the cavity in which it is normally contained. Types of hernias include direct or indirect, ventral or incisional, hiatal, traumatic, irreducible or incarcerated (contents cannot be replaced into the abdomen), and strangulated (irreducible hernia in which the blood supply to the entrapped bowel loop is compromised). Hernias are also classified according to location, for example, inguinal, femoral, or umbilical.

Etiology: Caused by congenital or acquired weakness of the abdominal wall; tends to increase in size and occurrence with increase in intra-abdominal pressure from coughing, straining, prostatitis, or a tumor.

Occurrence: Umbilical hernias occur more frequently in obese women, children, and patients with cirrhosis and ascites. Femoral hernias occur most often in women. Ventral or incisional hernias occur most often after surgery. Incidence increases if patient has a family history of hernia, if child has a premature or undescended testicle, or if patient has a congenital connective tissue disorder such as Ehlers-Danlos syndrome. Groin hernias (inguinal, direct, indirect) account for 75% of all cases; ventral, 10%; umbilical, 3%; and others, 3%.

Ethnicity: No significant ethnic predisposition.

Age: Occurs in all ages. Hernias in children are usually indirect; in adults, usually direct.

Gender: Indirect inguinal hernias occur 8 to 10 times more often in men than in women. Femoral hernias occur three to five times more often in women than in men.

Contributing factors: Underlying illnesses that cause an increase in intraabdominal pressure, such as chronic coughing, constipation, prostatism, emphysema, bronchitis, obstructing intestinal neoplasm, bronchogenic carcinoma, uterine fibroid, obesity, and excessive weight loss.

Signs and symptoms:

Uncomplicated or reducible external hernias: Protrusion of viscus through the wall of the cavity in which it is normally contained;

signs and symptoms are related to the degree of pressure on its content.

Irreducible or incarcerated hernia: Bulge or lump in herniated area; slight burning sensation on the hernia.

Strangulated hernia: Colicky abdominal pain, nausea and vomiting, abdominal distention, abdominal tympany, hyperperistalsis.

Diagnostic tests:

Inguinal, femoral, umbilical, ventral, and incisional hernias: Diagnosed by history and physical examination; also abdominal ultrasonography and CT scan

Hiatal and Traumatic Hernias: Diagnosed by chest and abdominal x-ray or barium swallow.

Differential diagnosis:

- Inguinal adenopathy (enlarged, palpable inguinal lymph nodes)
- Incarcerated hernia (hernia that cannot be reduced)
- Hydrocele (imaging)
- Varicocele (imaging)
- Undescended testicle (imaging)
- Strangulated hernia (blood supply of incarcerated contents is interrupted; gangrene may quickly ensue)
- Groin abscess (palpable, painful, fever)

Treatment:

Physical

(For reducible hernia only) Abdominal truss (prevents abdominal contents from entering hernial orifice; may be used in treatment of hernia in adults when, because of disease or age, it is inadvisable to perform surgery).

Surgical

Primary treatment. Hernia repair (herniorrhaphy) is recommended to correct the hernia before strangulation occurs, which then becomes an emergency situation. Strangulated hernia requires resection of ischemic bowel in addition to hernia repair.

Follow-up: See patient as needed for symptomatic evaluation.

Sequelae: Possible complications include small bowel obstruction and/or infarction (with strangulated hernia).

Prevention/prophylaxis: Prevention strategies include advising the patient to lose weight, if overweight, and to use support devices such as trusses, as indicated.

Referral: Refer to, or consult with, surgeon if surgery is indicated.

Education: Explain disease process, signs and symptoms, and treatment (including side effects of medications). Discuss prevention strategies and provide reassurance.

INFLAMMATORY BOWEL DISEASE
(ULCERATIVE COLITIS, CROHN'S DISEASE)

SIGNAL SYMPTOMS▶ Bloody stools, tender colon, abdominal pain, RLQ pain, diarrhea, weight loss, anorexia

| Ulcerative colitis (idiopathic proctocolitis) | ICD-9-CM: 556 |
| Crohn's disease (regional enteritis) | ICD-9-CM: 555.9 |

Description: Inflammatory bowel disease (IBD) is a general term for a chronic, episodic, inflammatory disorder of various portions of the bowel. IBD is divided into two major categories: ulcerative colitis (also known as idiopathic proctocolitis) and Crohn's disease (also known as regional enteritis). Both conditions are characterized by periods of acute exacerbations, alternating with periods of remission.

Etiology: Exact mechanism unknown; however, infectious and autoimmune immunologic mechanisms are thought to play a part.

Occurrence: Ulcerative colitis is more common (70-150/100,000) compared with Crohn's disease (20-100/100,000).

Age: Peak age of onset for both diseases is between the ages 15 and 30 years, with a second smaller peak around age 60.

Ethnicity: More common in whites than in blacks and Asians; greater incidence in people of Jewish heritage (three to six times) than in people of non-Jewish heritage.

Gender: Occurs slightly more often in women than in men.

Contributing factors: Several factors have been proposed, but none have been proved. Genetic factors (first-degree relative with disease) and immunologic dysregulation have been found significant. Emotions may exacerbate symptoms.

Signs and symptoms:

Ulcerative colitis: Primary feature is frequent, watery stools with blood and mucus. Associated signs and symptoms include intermittent, mild cramping, abdominal pain, abdominal tenderness (often lower bowel), anorexia, malaise, weight loss, fatigue, rectal tenesmus, intolerance to dairy products and arthritis.

Crohn's disease: Primary features are intermittent diarrhea, abdominal pain (usually right lower quadrant or periumbilical) and weight loss. Associated signs and symptoms include anorexia, malaise, low-grade fever and chills, flatulence, perianal disease and fistula, apthous ulcers in the mouth, and arthritis. Ingestion of coarse foods and dairy products may exacerbate symptoms (Table 6-2).

Diagnostic tests: Diagnostic tests are often nonspecific and reflect degree of bleeding and inflammation.

Test	Result Indicating Disorder	CPT Code
Colonoscopy	Needed to diagnose	45378 45380 with biopsy

Differential diagnosis:

- Other causes of rectal bleeding such as hemorrhoids, neoplasm, and diverticula
- Causes of diarrhea, such as infection, lactose intolerance, and antibiotic-associated diarrhea.

Treatment

Ulcerative colitis: For mild flare-ups and chronic treatment, the treatment of choice is sulfasalazine, 0.5 g twice a day to 1 g four times a day (increase dose gradually), to a total dosage of 1 to 4 g/day, as tolerated. Other medications may include antidiarrheal agents and topical (enemas and suppositories) and/or systemic corticosteroids. Severe symptoms usually require hospitalization, IV fluids, nasogastric (NG) suction, and parenteral corticosteroids, and infusions of tumor necrosis factor. Symptomatic treatment includes advising the patient to avoid dairy products, if they are irritating; applying heat to the abdomen to decrease cramping; and taking warm baths. Also important in treatment is a close supportive relationship between the patient and health-care provider. Surgical interventions may include proctocolectomy with ileostomy to help prevent recurrences. Disease limited to the rectum (proctitis) or to the left side of the colon may be treated topically with steroid enemas or mesalamine (5-aminosalicylic acid [5-ASA]) enemas or suppositories.

Crohn's disease: For maintenance, 5-ASA, methotrexate, or azathioprine. Prednisolone or mesalamine enemas for rectal symptoms. For exacerbations, prednisone 20 to 40 mg/day.

Table 6–2 Compairing Ulcerative Colitis And Crohn's Disease

Features	Ulcerative Colitis	Crohn's Disease
Signs and Symbols		
Rectal bleeding	+++	+
Malaise, fever	+	+++
Abdominal pain	+	+++
Abdominal mass or fistulas	0	++/+++
Rectal tenesmus	+++	+
Diagnostic Tests		
Anemia	Microcytic	Macrocytic
Nutritional deficiencies (vitamin B_{12}, folate, fat-soluble vitamins)	0	++
Rectal occult blood	+++	+

Response in 1 to 3 weeks. Taper after 4 to 6 weeks. Sulfasalazine (2 to 8 g/day) or 5-ASA preparation, enteric coated, 800 mg orally three times a day. Begin sulfasalazine therapy in higher doses (2 to 8 g/day). Corticosteroids may also be indicated. For acute symptoms, antibiotics, such as metronidazole, 15 mg/kg per day; ampicillin, 2 to 4 g/day; or tetracycline, 1 to 2 g/day, may be indicated. (Newer 5-ASA compounds are now available for both disorders.) Infusions of tumor necrosis factor may also be considered. Symptomatic treatment includes advising the patient to eat a well-balanced diet high in protein and vitamins, using vitamin supplements as needed, avoiding raw fruits and vegetables, and applying heat to the abdomen to decrease pain or take warm baths. Also important in treatment is a close supportive relationship between the patient and health-care provider. Surgical interventions may be needed; 60% of patients undergo surgery within first 5 years, usually for intra-abdominal strictures or fistulas.

Complementary Therapy

Yoga

Relaxation therapy

Meditation

Biofeedback

Aromatherapy: Lavender for relaxation—put 5 drops of essential oil in warm bath water or use an aromatherapy lamp with a few drops of lavender oil in the water, heat, let lovely fragrance fill the room.

Peppermint tea—soothes stomachache

Camomile tea

Valerian: the drug Valium named for the substance. Chemically, the drug and herbs are not related but the end result is the same— both soothes frazzled, jangled nerves. Take one capsule three times a day or make a cup of tea by mixing 2 teaspoons of dried herb with boiling water, then steep for 15 minutes and drink.

Follow-up: See the patient frequently to provide psychological support, to evaluate effectiveness of therapy, and to monitor for disease exacerbation.

Sequelae:

Ulcerative colitis: The mortality rate in severe cases may be as high as 10% to 25%. Seventy-five to eighty percent of patients relapse after first attack; ultimately, about 20% of patients require surgery. Colon cancer is the single most important risk factor affecting long-term prognosis. Possible complications include sepsis and perforation.

Crohn's disease: The mortality rate is lower than with ulcerative colitis; however, recurrence and progression of disease are common. Average patient has surgery every 7 years. After four surgeries, expect short bowel syndrome. Life span usually shortened. Possible complications include fistula (15% of patients), abscess, perforation, and malnutrition.

Prevention/prophylaxis:

Ulcerative colitis: Prevention strategies include advising the patient to undergo colonoscopy and biopsy of tissue every 1 to 2 years after disease has been present for 7-8 years because of increased risk for colon cancer.

Crohn's disease: Prevention strategies include advising the patient to maintain good nutritional status.

Referral: Refer to, or consult with, gastroenterologist as needed.

Education: Explain disease process, signs and symptoms, and treatment (including side effects of medications). Discuss prevention strategies and importance of compliance with therapy. Advise patient and family about support groups. Educational resource materials available from the Crohn's and Colitis Foundation, 444 Park Avenue South, 11th Floor, New York, NY 10016 (800-343-3637).

IRRITABLE BOWEL SYNDROME

SIGNAL SYMPTOMS Recurrent, intermittent dull crampy, abdominal pain relieved with bowel movement; may be characterized by episodes of diarrhea and/or constipation; abdominal bloating

Irritable colon	ICD-9-CM: 564

Description: Irritable bowel syndrome (IBS) is a chronic, noninfectious disease with altered bowel habits, abdominal pain, and gaseousness in the absence of organic pathology. There are four types of altered bowel habits: combination diarrhea and constipation, predominantly diarrhea, predominantly constipation, and upper abdominal bloating and discomfort. IBS is also known as mucous colitis, spastic colon, and irritable colon.

Etiology: The cause is unknown but is believed to relate to a gut motility abnormality (thought to be associated with response to stress or stimulants) or lower pain threshold in response to gut distention. The increase or decrease in motility or changes in smooth-muscle contraction result in nonpropulsive colonic contractions, leading to constipation or increased contractions in the small bowel and proximal colon with diminished activity in the distal colon, leading to diarrhea. Other causes include specific food intolerances and malabsorption of bile acids. Also, about three fourths of all patients with IBS have psychological problems, such as depression, personality disorder, hysteria, anxiety, and somatization, that predate their treatment.

Occurrence: Occurs in 15% to 20% of the population. Comprises 20% to 50% of all visits to gastroenterologists and 12% of all visits to primary care physicians; second only to the common cold in lost work and school days.

Age: Occurs in all ages; most common between ages of 20 to 40 years.

Ethnicity: Occurs in all ethnic groups; most common in whites.

Gender: Occurs two times more often in women than in men in the United States; in other parts of the world, occurs more in men than in women.

Contributing factors: Familial history; anxiety or tenseness; emotional stressors, such as marital tension, fear of loss, and obsessively worrying about everyday concerns; physical stressors, such as overwork, improper diet, alcohol use, and poor physical fitness; abuse, including history of childhood sexual abuse and/or sexual domestic abuse.

Signs and symptoms: Patient must have recurrent symptoms of disturbed defecation and abdominal pain for 3 to 6 months to be diagnosed with IBS; however, each does not need to be present every time. Symptoms are often precipitated by stress and abate while asleep.

> Disturbed defecation: Stools may be described as constipation alternating with irregular passage of small, hard stools; small, dry pellets; pasty colored stools; or straining for normal-consistency stools. Diarrhea (common in the morning; four to six movements per day) may be described as ribbonlike, pencil thin, small, watery, or with clear mucus in the stool. Feelings of incomplete evacuation or urgency may also be reported.

> *Abdominal pain:* May be described as aching or cramping in the lower quadrant or periumbilical area, may radiate to the chest or arm, and is relieved by defecation; may be worse 1 to 2 hours after eating.

Other symptoms include backache or rectal pain, bloating or flatulence after eating, headache, loss of appetite, nausea and vomiting (rare); anxiety, fatigue, depression, difficulty concentrating, or low self-esteem; and exaggerated response to, or preoccupation with, the bowels.

Physical examination may reveal distention or guarding over the upper or lower abdomen; abdominal rigidity; tenderness over the ascending or descending colon (more common) (a tender cord [the "sigmoid cord"] indicates presence of stool in the sigmoid colon); abdominal tympany if air trapping occurs; and normal or mildly hyperactive bowel sounds.

Positive Carnett's test: Palpate abdomen to discern minimal pressure needed to elicit pain. Then ask patient to cross arms and assume a partially sitting position (tightens abdominal muscles). Palpate abdomen again using the same amount of pressure. If pain is more severe with muscles taut and less pressure, then this is a positive test that indicates diagnoses such as abdominal wall hernias or costochondritis.

Diagnostic tests:

Test	Result Indicating Disorder	CPT Code
CBC with differential	Usually normal	85025
ESR	Usually normal	85651
Stool for ova and parasites and occult blood	Usually negative	87177, 82270
24-hour stool collection	Weight is atypical if greater than 300 g/day; may indicate inflammatory bowel disease	82705-82715
Endoscopy, small bowel series, colonoscopy, sigmoidoscopy, and barium enema	All usually normal	43200, 74249 45378, 45330 74270
Bowel scintiscan	Shows areas in bowel where spasm occurs	78290
Lactose deficiency breath test	May be positive	91065
Endoscopic biopsies		43260–72 (check area for specific code)

CBC, complete blood count; ESR, erythrocyte sedimentation rate.

Differential diagnosis:

- Inflammatory bowel disease (diarrhea, rectal bleeding; diagnosed on biopsy)
- Lactose intolerance (symptoms related to intake of food/fluid with lactose)
- Infections such as *Giardia lamblia, Entamoeba histolytica, Salmonella, Campylobacter, Yersinia, Clostridium difficile* (rule out with appropriate laboratory tests)
- Diverticula (LLQ pain, not relieved with defecation)
- Adenocarcinoma of the colon (colonoscopy, biopsy)
- Villous adenoma (colonoscopy, biopsy)
- Use of medications (or their side effects) that alter bowel motility (medication history)
- Psychologic disorders such as depression, anxiety, and somatization (psychological evaluation, history)

Treatment: Treatment usually begins with a 2-week trial of diet, education, reassurance, and bulk agents, because more than two thirds of all patients respond to these techniques alone. Medication is reserved for more severe cases.

Diet: Diet can be a major factor in controlling symptoms. Encourage a high-fiber, low-fat diet with small, frequent meals. Increase dietary fiber gradually (may cause gas and bloating) up to 30 to 40 g/day; include fresh fruits, vegetables, bran, and whole grains. Increase water or fluids to 8 glasses or more per day. Limit dairy products if they cause cramping and diarrhea. Include a calcium supplement if limited dairy products are eaten; a multivitamin if a significant number of foods are limited. Encourage patient to keep a food diary to identify problem-causing foods; eliminate those foods from the diet. Have patient eat regularly scheduled meals to encourage regular bowel function.

Education/reassurance: Successful treatment relies on a strong practitioner-patient relationship. Use a nonjudgmental, attentive attitude, provide emotional support, and emphasize that all symptoms are real. Discuss ways to decrease stress such as biofeedback, meditation, self-hypnosis, and behavioral modification. Have patient keep a stress diary to be aware of symptoms. Lifestyle changes include stopping smoking. Physical therapies may include application of heat to relieve pain, physical activity and exercise to decrease stress and improve bowel function.

Pharmacologic

Bulk agents or psyllium (helps diarrhea and constipation): 1 tablespoon twice or three times a day or Fibercon tablets.

Antidiarrheals (for significant diarrhea): Loperamide, 4 mg initially, then 2 mg after each unformed stool to a maximum of 16 mg/day; or diphenoxylate, 2.5 to 5 mg after each loose stool.

Antiflatulents (for bloating and gas pain): Simethicone, 2 to 4 tablets after meals and at bedtime.

For milk intolerance: Lactase, 1 to 2 tablets before milk product ingestion.

Antispasmodics and anticholinergics (for pain and spasm after a trial of diet and bulking agents prove ineffective): Dicyclomine, 10 to 20 mg twice or four times a day; hyoscyamine sulfate, 0.125 to 0.25 mg. Chlordiazepoxide-clidinium (Librax, an antispasmodic with a mild tranquilizer), 1 to 2 tablets before meals and at bedtime.

For chronic, unremitting abdominal pain, antidepressants in lower-than-usual doses may be effective: Amitriptyline, 25 to 50 mg at bedtime.

For anxiety: Buspirone, 5 mg three times a day, increase by 2.5 mg/day at 2- to 3-day intervals up to 60 mg/day, or diazepam, 2 mg twice a day. Alprazolam (Xanax), 0.25 to 0.5 mg three times a day as needed.

Complementary Therapies:

- Apples relieve constipation and diarrhea
- Bayberry—boil 1 tsp of powdered root bark for 10 to 15 minutes. Sweeten and drink two cups per day
- Tea - both green and black contain tannins which exert a drying or astringent effect that can be helpful in relieving diarrhea
- Cascara sagrada contains compounds called anthraquinones that stimulate intestinal contractions. Boil a teaspoon of dried bark in 3 cups of water for 30 minutes. Let it cool, and drink 1 or 2 cups before bed. Also found in aloe vara, buckthorn, and rhubarb, but these are more harsh.

- Olive oil—1 to 2 oz a day for constipation
- Alfalfa—take 6 tablets daily for constipation; add alfalfa to salads

Follow-up: See the patient initially every 2 weeks until condition improves, then every month, then every 6 months.

Sequelae: IBS is a chronic disorder controlled by recognition and adaptation of the precipitating factors; one third of patients progress to becoming symptom free; however, a small minority progress to daily symptoms. A possible complication involves fixation on bowel functions, leading to psychological disability.

Prevention/prophylaxis: Prevention strategies include advising the patient to avoid stress or adapt to stressful situations by learning stress-relieving techniques, such as relaxation and guided imagery, and by allowing time for regular exercise and recreation. Also advise the patient to follow a healthy lifestyle with consistent, adequate sleep and scheduled times for elimination; to follow a high-fiber, low-fat diet; to avoid foods that cause gastric problems (such as fried, fatty, and spicy foods; concentrated fruit juices; dietetic sweeteners that include sorbitol, mannitol, raffinose, or fructose); to avoid medications that cause diarrhea (magnesium antacids and lactulose) and constipation (sucralfate and calcium channel blockers); and to avoid tobacco, alcohol, and caffeine. Daily walking or regular exercise.

Referral: Refer to, or consult with, a gastroenterologist for further workup and management if diet, bulk agents, and antispasmodics fail, or if patient has more than six episodes per year; to a psychologist for counseling in stress relief if indicated.

Education: Explain the disease process, signs and symptoms, and treatment (including side effects of medications). Discuss prevention strategies. Explain need for annual rectal examinations and sigmoidoscopy after age 40 years; have patient call if fever, black tarry stools, vomiting, unexplained weight loss, or a change in symptoms occurs, or if there is no improvement in symptoms. Discuss the chronic nature of the disease, with frequent recurrences, exacerbations, and quiescent periods; expect recurrences when under stress throughout life. However, as age increases, bouts of diarrhea and constipation usually lessen. Explain that treatment depends on coping with the disease, not curing it. Help patient understand that there is an organic basis to the disease, not just a psychosocial one. Educational resource materials are available from the International Foundation for Functional Gastrointestinal Disorders (414-964-1799). Website: *www.IFFgd.org*

LACTOSE INTOLERANCE

SIGNAL SYMPTOMS▶   Bloating, cramping, abdominal discomfort, diarrhea or loose stools, flatulence, rumbling.

Intolerance or malabsorption of lactose	ICD-9-CM: 271.3

Description: Lactose intolerance is the inability to digest lactose (the primary sugar in milk) into its constituents, glucose and galactose, because of low levels of the lactase enzyme in the brush border of the duodenum. It may be classified as primary or secondary.

Etiology: Primary lactose intolerance is caused by the normal decline in the lactase activity in the intestinal mucosa after weaning, which is genetically controlled and permanent. Secondary lactose intolerance, caused by any condition injuring the intestinal mucosa, such as diarrhea, is usually transient.

Occurrence: Primary lactose intolerance is common. Secondary lactose intolerance is common in people with giardiasis and ascariasis, inflammatory bowel disease, and AIDS malabsorptive syndrome.

Age: Primary lactose intolerance occurs from teenagers to adults. Age for secondary lactose intolerance depends on the underlying condition.

Ethnicity: Primary lactose intolerance occurs in 100% of Native Americans; 80% to 90% of blacks, and people of Asian, Mediterranean, and Jewish heritage; and < 5% of people of northern and central European heritage.

Gender: Occurs equally in men and women; however, 44% of lactose-intolerant women will regain the ability to digest lactose during pregnancy.

Contributing factors: Race, age, nontropical and tropical sprue, regional enteritis, abetalipoproteinemia, cystic fibrosis, ulcerative colitis, immunoglobulin deficiency.

Signs and symptoms: Symptoms often do not appear until 1-2 hours after ingestion of milk or milk products or up to 12 hours after ingestion of lactose. Degree of symptoms varies with lactose load and with other foods consumed at the same time. Only about 20% to 33% of patients will develop symptoms. Symptoms include bloating, cramping, abdominal discomfort, diarrhea or loose stools, flatulence, rumbling.

Diagnostic tests:

Test	Result Indicating Disorder	CPT Code
Low fecal pH and reducing substances	Only valid when stools are collected fresh and assayed immediately	83986
Lactase breath hydrogen test	Usually used in children	91065
Lactose absorption test	Used as an alternative to lactose breath hydrogen test in adults	83633-83634 (urine) 82951-2 (tolerance)
Small bowel biopsy for assay of lactase activity	May be normal if deficiency is focal or patchy	44361

Differential Diagnosis: IBS.

Treatment:

Pharmacologic

Recommend commercially available "lactase" preparations, such as LactAid or Dairy Ease, to help control or reduce symptoms. These products contain the lactose enzyme, which will help digest the lactose in food so patients will not experience discomfort after eating. Some tablets can be added to milk before drinking.

Physical

To control symptoms, reduce or restrict dietary lactose by using lactose-reduced and lactose-free dairy products or by eating lactose-rich foods in small amounts or in combination with low-lactose or lactose-free foods. Eat fermented dairy products such as aged or hard cheeses and cultured yogurt, because they are easier to digest and contain less lactose than other dairy products. Supplement calcium in the form of calcium carbonate. Prehydrolyzed milk is available and effective.

Follow-up: See patient as needed for education and observation for complications.

Sequelae: Possible complications include calcium deficiency, malnutrition, and dehydration.

Prevention/prophylaxis: Prevention strategies include avoiding large quantities of lactose. Encourage patients to learn what levels of lactose are tolerable in their diets.

Referral: Refer to, or consult with, physician if the patient has malnutrition or dehydration. Refer to surgeon for biopsy if needed.

Education: Explain disease process, signs and symptoms, and treatment (including side effects of medications). Reassure patient. Explain how to carefully read food labels because not all sources of lactose are obvious, such as whey, which is a lactose-rich ingredient, and to carefully read medication labels because some OTC and prescription medications also contain lactose. Educational resource materials, coupons, and free samples are available from LactAid (800-522-8243; Website: *www.Lactaid. com*) and Dairy Ease (800-331-4536; Website: *www.dairyease.com/ products*).

LIVER CANCER (HEPATOMA)

SIGNAL SYMPTOMS▶   Dull, localized ache in the right upper quadrant abdomen (80% of patients); may radiate to right scapula.

Malignant neoplasm of the liver, primary	ICD-9-CM: 155.0

Description: Liver cancer, or hepatocellular carcinoma, is a malignancy of the liver. Malignant liver tumors (hepatomas) may be classified as primary (arising from the liver parenchyma and almost always associated with an underlying disease of the liver) or secondary (resulting from metastasis from other primary sites). Metastatic disease is far more common than primary liver cancer.

Etiology: The etiology is only partially understood. Chronic liver injury, in association with alcohol-induced, nutritional, or posthepatic state, results in inflammation, which may precipitate the development of cancer cells. Alcoholic cirrhosis accounts for 60% to 80% of cases in the western world; endemic hepatitis accounts for a higher incidence of primary liver cancer in Africa and Asia. The majority of primary malignant hepatomas are adenocarcinomas; about 85% to 95% arise from malignant epithelium. Secondary liver cancer results from metastasis from other primary sites, frequently the lung, breast, kidney, gallbladder, pancreas, stomach, colon, or rectum. Primary liver cancer may not affect liver function until the tumor has grown to massive proportions; however, with coexisting cirrhosis, symptoms may occur earlier or precipitate liver failure or portal hypertension. Secondary liver cancer usually does not cause liver dysfunction or failure.

Occurrence: The incidence of primary liver cancer in the United States is 1 to 5/100,000 per year; among patients with cirrhosis, 2 to 5/100 per year.

Age: Average age of onset is between age 50 to 60.

Ethnicity: More common in African and Asian people.

Gender: Occurs four times more in men than in women.

Contributing factors: Chronic liver injury associated with alcohol, nutrition, or following hepatitis; cirrhosis; chronic hepatitis B infection; malnutrition; hemochromatosis; long-term use of oral contraceptives; underlying carcinomas.

Signs and symptoms: Onset may be insidious or sudden. Dull, localized ache in the right upper quadrant abdomen (80% of patients); may radiate to right scapula.

Other symptoms may include fatigue, weakness, loss of appetite, weight loss (30% of patients), epigastric fullness after eating, nausea, emesis (with or without hematemesis), diarrhea, constipation, severe pruritus, low-grade fevers (10% to 50% of patients), irregular menstrual cycles (female patient), and symptoms of thrombophlebitis.

Physical examination may reveal hepatomegaly (80% to 90% of patients; irregular, nodular, firm to hard, and tender liver) and hepaticarterial bruit (20% of patients).

Diagnostic tests

Test	Results indicating disorder	CPT code
Liver function tests (LFTs)	Usually demonstrate abnormalities	80076
Alpha-fetoprotein (AFP)	Most important test for screening and diagnosis; level above 500 ng/mL is diagnostic for disorder	82105

(Continued)

nitis (abdomen rigid, pain, increased WBC, fever, toxic)

(RLQ pain)

use abdominal pain, relieved with defecation)

is (LLQ pain)

examination)

s (RUQ pain)

(rectal examination)

nless the condition is associated with infection, excessive miting, hypertension, or uncontrolled pain, patients with r less in diameter can be managed as outpatients (90% of ny stones are < 5 mm in diameter and pass in the urine quence or any additional treatment. Struvite, uric acid, and dissolve more readily than calcium stones. Goals of treat- relief and aggressive fluid management.

gic

cs such as NSAIDs (ibuprofen, 600 to 800 mg three times a narcotics such as hydrocodone-acetaminophen (Vicodin) tablets every 4 hours as needed. Occasionally may need rcotic such as Demerol for relief. For calcium stones caused uria: Hydrochlorothiazide, 50 mg orally twice a day. For cal- e stones with hyperuricosuria: Allopurinol, 100 mg orally day.

y patient with a single stone visible on IVP or abdominal flat ormal laboratory results: Have patient strain all urine for report if stone has passed. Needs to be brought in for analy- ical composition. Increase fluids to more than 3 liters/day low of urine and reduces the concentration of stone-forming . Take measures to avoid new stone formation, such as avoid- gh in purines and fats and increasing fiber in diet. Soak in hot relaxes the ureteral muscles and can provide relief).

nt with relentless pain, obstruction, or infection: Surgical hotripsy (fragments stones, allowing the smaller particles to eously). Extracorporal shock using lithotripsy (ESWL) for

ee the patient weekly to monitor creatinine level and re' 1 to 2 weeks, have plain film of abdomen perform ession of stone. Have patient continue to strain a equired.

eriod of diuresis lasting several days gene struction. Possible complications include failure, bladder cancer, and compl

Test	Results indicating disorder	CPT code
Chest x-ray study of two views: frontal and lateral	May reveal abnormally raised right diaphragm	71020
Ultrasound of liver; CT scan of abdomen, with and without contrast; and MRI*	Differentiates primary liver tumor from metastatic and confirmed versus diffuse tumor	76700, 74170, 74185
Liver biopsy	Positive pathology report	47000
Liver ultrasound	Helps identify hepatocellular cancer when lesion is smaller than 2 cm	76700

*Ultrasound is the primary screening for hepatic lesions, especially for focal lesions rather than parenchymal disease. CT scanning is superior for parenchymal disease. MRI has sensitivity to CT scanning for mass lesion.

CT, computed tomography; MRI, magnetic resonance imaging.

Differential diagnosis:
- Hepatitis (elevated liver enzymes)
- Cirrhosis (history, biopsy)
- Gastritis (symptoms relieved with treatment)

Treatment: Once pathologic diagnosis has been made, evaluate the extent of disease using the Union International Centre Le Cancer Staging System (ICC) to classify primary liver cancer. Selection of treatment and subsequent survival is based on extent of tumor involvement and functional status of the patient. Prognostic indicators include the stage of disease and size of tumor; involvement of nodes; site of metastasis; performance and functional status; liver function and degree of cirrhosis; degree of symptom distress; presence of comorbid disease; and support systems.

Surgical
Lobectomy, liver segmentectomy, or liver transplant (2-year survival rate is 15% to 20%).

Radiotherapy
For patient with primary liver cancer: Provides palliative therapy and relief of symptoms.

Chemotherapy
For the patient who is not a surgical candidate: Provides palliative therapy. Agents administered systemically or intrahepatically (via hepatic artery or portal vein).

Physical
Supportive care for problems such as pain, nutrition, nausea, emesis, bowel problems, metabolic disorders, and bleeding is crucial. Refer to supportive care agencies such as hospice care.

Follow-up: See patient as indicated by disease progression. Obtain AFPs every 3 months and ultrasound every 4 to 6 months.

Sequelae: For patient with primary liver cancer, the prognosis is poor; most die within 6 months. The 5-year survival rate is < 2%. Most patients are diagnosed with advanced disease; about 80% have symptoms before seeking medical care. Sequelae may include hepatic failure, severe ascites, infection, bleeding, diathesis, pain, weight loss, weakness, and pneumonia. For the patient with metastatic liver cancer, prognosis is based on primary tumor site.

Prevention/prophylaxis: Prevention strategies include, in areas where hepatitis B is endemic, administration of hepatitis B vaccine to help reduce risk of later developing the disease (especially for high-risk individuals such as health-care workers). Also advise the patient to abstain from alcohol or IV drug use.

Referral: After initial diagnosis, refer to medical oncologist for management. Patient may also be referred to radiation-oncologist and to a supportive agency such as hospice.

Education: Explain the disease process, signs and symptoms, and treatment (including side effects of medications). Discuss hospice and supportive care; reassure patient that efforts will be made to provide comfort and relief of symptoms. Advise patient of the telephone number of the National Cancer Institute Hotline (1-800-FOR-CANCER) to inquire about treatments, clinical trials, and educational resource materials and the telephone number of the local branch of the American Cancer Society.

NEPHROLITHIASIS (RENAL CALCULI, KIDNEY STONES)

SIGNAL SYMPTOMS▶   sudden, severe pain

Calculus of kidney	ICD-9-CM: 592.0

Description: Nephrolithiasis, also called renal calculi or kidney stones, involves masses of crystals and proteins, which can cause obstruction in the urinary tract.

Etiology: Caused by masses of crystals and protein, which form in the presence of high urinary concentration; major types include calcium oxalate, struvite, and uric acid stones.

Occurrence: Occurs in approximately 1% of the U.S. population. More common in warm climates, where people become dehydrated more quickly and in geographic areas where there is a high mineral content in the water.

Age: 30 to 50 years; third decade most common.

Ethnicity: No significant ethnic predisposition.

Gender: Calcium stones are more common in men; struvite stones more common in women.

Contributing factors: High urinary concentration of stone-forming substances and an alkaline urine. Calcium stones: High levels of calcium and uric acid in the urine, diet high in calcium, vitamin D, and purines,

---

bone demineralization caused
Struvite stones: Infections such
duce an alkaline urine. Uric aci
often resulting from high-purine
roidism. Low water intake. Geneti

Signs and symptoms:

Stones above the ureters: Usu
obstruction occurs.

Stones below the ureters: Often
severe agonizing flank pain (h
angle (CVA) pain; or pain radia
urinary retention. Pain may be
tachycardia, tachypnea, chills, a
as nausea, vomiting, diarrhea, a
possible.

Diagnostic tests:

Test	Result Indicating Di
Routine urinalysis	May reveal an alkalin and gross or micro (80% of cases)
Urine pH	Acidic urine: uric acid alkaline urine: stru
24-hour urinalysis	Evaluates for uric acid oxalate, total volum clearance, calcium
Glomerular filtration rate (GFR)	Decreases with even a obstruction
Urine culture and sensitivity	Indicates infection
CBC with differential	Indicates infection
BUN; and creatinine calcium phosphorus protein electrolytes uric acid	Evaluates renal functio
Abdominal x-ray study, IVP, or renal ultra-sound	Reveals presence of stones are not rar
ncontrast h cal puted tom g (CT) BUN,	Superior to IVP or Level of obstru can be assess

Pe   nitrogen; CBC, complete blood
and oth
Differe tion may be ne
• Gastic problems)

ous

• Acute perit
• Appendiciti
• Colitis (dif
• Diverticuli
• PID (pelvi
• Pancreati
• Prostatiti

Treatment: U
nausea and v
stones 6 mm
the time). Ma
without conse
cystine stones
ment are pai

Pharmacol
Oral analgesi
day) or oral
one or two
injectable na
by hypercal
cium oxala
three times

Physical
For a heal
plate and
stones an
sis of che
(increase
substance
ing foods
water bat

Surgical
For the pa
removal or
pass sponta
certain ston

Follow-up:
function. Eve
monitor prog
Stone analysis

Sequelae: A
relief of the o
infection, rena

Usually resolves within 4 weeks but recurrences are common (50% within 5 years).

Prevention/prophylaxis: Prevention strategies include avoiding dehydration by maintaining an adequate fluid intake and increasing activity level; diet low in animal fats and increased fiber (especially bran) is recommended. Daily fluid intake of 3–4 L/day with avoidance of nonsoftened and mineral water. Specific dietary and pharmacologic recommendations relate to stone type.

Referral: Refer to, or consult with, a urologist if patient has evidence of obstruction, if symptoms last more than 2 weeks, or if patient is unresponsive to conservative treatment.

Education: Explain the disease process, signs and symptoms, and treatment (including side effects of medications). Discuss prevention strategies. Provide reassurance.

PEPTIC ULCER DISEASE

SIGNAL SYMPTOMS Gnawing, burning epigastric pain 1 to 3 hours after meals, relieved with food and/or antacids.

Peptic ulcer disease	ICD-9-CM: 536.8
Duodenal ulcer	ICD-9-CM: 532.9
Gastric ulcer	ICD-9-CM: 531.9

Description: Peptic ulcer disease (PUD) is a chronic erosion of the gastric or duodenal mucosa, usually over 5 mm in diameter or with multiple sites of erosion. Duodenal ulcers occur five times more frequently than gastric ulcers do.

Etiology: Causes include *Helicobacter pylori* (*H. pylori*) infection (present in > 90% of peptic ulcers and > 75% of gastric ulcers); use of nonsteroidal anti-inflammatory drugs (NSAIDs); and pathologically high acid-secreting states, such as Zollinger-Ellison syndrome. Alcohol use and dietary factors do not appear to cause ulcers, and the role of stress on ulcer formation is uncertain.

Occurrence: Approximately 500,000 new cases and recurrence of 4 million cases annually in the United States, with a 10% prevalence rate.

Age: Occurs in any age group. Duodenal ulcers occur most frequently between ages 30 and 55 years. Gastric ulcers occur most frequently between ages 55 to 70.

Ethnicity: No significant ethnic predisposition.

Gender: Duodenal ulcers occur more often in men than in women. Gastric ulcers occur equally in men and women.

Contributing factors: Use of aspirin, NSAIDs, and corticosteroids; smoking; familial history of ulcers (50% of patients with duodenal ulcers).

Signs and symptoms:

Red Flag: Any patient presenting with anemia, GI bleeding, weight loss, early satiety, and new onset of symptoms after age 50 must be referred for definitive diagnostic testing such as endoscopy.

Gnawing, burning, or "hunger-like" epigastric pain, which may radiate to the back (80% to 90% of patients); usually fluctuates in intensity throughout the day and night and is relieved with antacids or by eating. Duodenal ulcer pain classically occurs 1 to 3 hours after eating or after taking an antacid; gastric ulcer pain is more variable and may worsen with food ingestion. Nocturnal pain that awakens the patient from sleep may also occur (one third of patients with gastric ulcers; two thirds of patients with duodenal ulcers).

Dyspepsia or a variety of nonspecific dyspeptic complaints.

Anorexia and nausea may occur with gastric ulcers.

Physical examination may reveal mild, localized epigastric tenderness on deep palpation.

Diagnostic tests:

Test	Result Indicating Disorder	CPT Code
Stool for occult blood	Positive in one third of patients	82270
CBC	Rules out anemia from blood loss	85025
WBC	Elevated (may suggest that an ulcer has perforated),	Included in CBC
Fasting serum gastrin levels	Screens for Zollinger-Ellison syndrome	82938-82941
Serology or a carbon isotope urea breath test	Reveals presence of *H. pylori;* tests have a 5-15% false-negative rate	83013
Serologic test for *H. pylori.*	Positive	86677
Upper GI endoscopy	Diagnoses peptic and gastric ulcers; obtains biopsies for malignancy and *H. pylori* infection	43239 with biopsy

CBC, complete blood count; WBC, white blood cell.)

Differential diagnosis:

- GERD (acid regurgitation, heartburn, occasional hoarseness, asthma, chronic cough)
- Gastric neoplasms (verify by imaging, biopsy, vague epigastric discomfort, anorexia, weight loss, iron deficiency anemia)
- Cholecystitis and biliary tract disease (acute: RUQ pain, nausea and vomiting, eructation. Chronic: pain at night after a fatty meal)
- Cardiovascular disease (chest pain, dyspnea)

Treatment: The goals of therapy are to heal the ulcer, relieve symptoms, and prevent complications and recurrences. For new-onset dyspepsia not associated with taking NSAIDs, the following are options:

Option 1: Short-term trial of antiulcer therapy. If symptoms do not respond in about 2 weeks, a further workup should be pursued.

Treatment should be continued for 6 to 8 weeks if a good response is obtained. If symptoms reoccur, a further workup will be required. Recommended medications include the following: ranitidine, 150 mg twice a day or 300 mg hs , cimetidine, 400 mg twice a day or 800 mg hs; famotidine, 20 mg twice a day or 40 mg hs; nizatidine, 150 mg twice a day or 300 mg hs; esomeprazole 40 mg each day; lansoprazole 30 mg each day; omeprazole 20 mg each day; pantoprazole 40 mg each day; or rabeprazole 20 mg. Other initial alternative treatments include use of mucosal protective agents including antacids pc and hs (to prevent changes in absorption, separate from other medications by 2 hours), as well as sucralfate, 1 g ac and hs, or bismuth subsalicylate, two tablets qid.

Option 2: Useful in the presence of other complications such as anemia, anorexia, weight loss, GI bleeding, and in patients over age 50 where there is concern for neoplasms. Perform endoscopy. Treatment based on clinical findings. Patients with duodenal or gastric ulcers are generally treated with at least 8-12 weeks of acid suppression, sometimes longer, depending on the size of the ulcer. Patients with gastric ulcers need follow-up endoscopy at 2 to 3 months to assess healing and to rule out gastric carcinoma; duodenal ulcer may be assessed by alleviation of symptoms.

Option 3: (Involves noninvasive detection of *H. pylori* and treatment.) Treatment is controversial because of growing concern for the development of resistant strains and adverse effects of antimicrobial therapy. However, the National Institutes of Health (NIH) recommends that all patients with ulcers who are infected with *H. pylori* receive antimicrobial therapy. For *H. pylori* infection: Treat active ulcer disease with H_2 receptor antagonists for 6 to 8 weeks. Concomitant use of various regimens (these therapies have an eradication rate greater than 90%): 14-day triple therapy: tetracycline, 500 mg four times a day, metronidazole, 250 mg three times per day, and bismuth subsalicylate, two tablets four times a day; *or* tetracycline, 500 mg four times a day, clarithromycin, 500 mg three times a day; and bismuth subsalicylate, two tablets four times a day; *or* amoxicillin, 500 mg four times a day, clarithromycin, 500 mg three times a day, and bismuth subsalicylate, two tablets four times a day; *or* amoxicillin, 500 mg four times a day, metronidazole, 250 mg three times a day, and bismuth subsalicylate, two tablets four times a day. Ten 14-day triple therapy: amoxicillin, 1 g twice a day, clarithromycin, 500 mg twice a day, and lansoprazole 30 mg each day or esomeprazole 40 mg each day or omeprazole 20 mg each day taken with meals; or clarithromycin, 500 mg twice a day, metronidazole, 500 mg twice a day, and lansoprazole 30 mg each day or esomeprazole 40 mg each day or omeprazole 20 mg each day taken with meals. These regimens change frequently; check current sources.

For NSAID-associated ulcers, begin with discontinuing or reducing NSAID dose or substituting a nonacetylated NSAID. Follow option 1 for initial drug therapy. Screen and treat for *H. pylori* if detected.

Follow-up: See patient within 2 weeks to evaluate effectiveness of treatment and relief of symptoms; eradication of *H. pylori* in about 80% to 90% of patients. If treatment is not effective, try a different antimicrobial regimen. If the patient remains symptomatic, further testing is needed to rule out malignancy or *H. pylori* infection. For the patient with gastric ulcers, a follow-up endoscopy 12 weeks after the beginning of therapy is needed to document complete healing; nonhealing ulcers are suspicious for malignancy.

Sequelae: Possible complications include hemorrhage and perforation.

Prevention/prophylaxis: Prevention strategies include advising the patient taking NSAIDs and who has a high risk of developing NSAID-induced complications or who has serious medical problems, such as prior GI complications or on chronic corticosteroid therapy, to consider the administration of misoprostol, 100 to 200 mcg four times a day or 400 mcg twice a day or consider a COX-2 inhibitor NSAID to help reduce or prevent the occurrence of PUD. For the patient with recurrent *H. pylori*–negative ulcers not attributed to NSAIDs, with recurrent ulcers in whom *H. pylori* cannot be successfully eradicated, and with a prior history of ulcer bleeding, consider administration of a daily maintenance therapy of half of the dosage of an H_2 receptor antagonist at bedtime.

Referral: Refer to, or consult with, physician or gastroenterologist for endoscopic evaluation if patient has symptoms such as sustained and progressive weight loss, dysphagia, persistent vomiting, hematemesis, melena, or GI bleeding; or if patient fails to respond to H_2 receptor antagonists within several weeks or has relapsing symptoms after discontinuation of treatment.

Education: Explain the disease process, signs and symptoms, and treatment (including side effects of medications). Discuss the importance of reporting symptoms. Encourage the patient who smokes to stop smoking; offer assistance with smoking cessation programs. Advise patient who is on high-dose aspirin or other NSAIDs not to take OTC H_2 receptor antagonists since these drugs may mask the symptoms of ulcers.

RENAL FAILURE, ACUTE

SIGNAL SYMPTOMS▶ Fatigue, weakness, low urine output

Renal failure, acute	ICD-9-CM: 548.9

Description: Acute renal failure (ARF) is the sudden decline of kidney function, resulting in failure to clear metabolic wastes, rendering the body incapable of maintaining fluid and electrolyte balance, eliminating wastes, and safeguarding acid-base balance. The process is often reversible, but prolonged episodes may lead to irreversible renal failure.

Etiology: Causes are divided into three categories.

Prerenal: Conditions that originate outside the kidney, such as from events that result in a decrease in the amount of blood supplied to the kidneys (for example, hypovolemia, hypoperfusion, or hypotension).

Intrarenal: Damage to renal tissue itself such as from acute tubular necrosis, glomerulopathies, malignant hypertension, vascular diseases such as polyarteritis nodosa, nephrotoxicities, or SLE. Prolonged prerenal and postrenal conditions can also result in intrarenal damage.

Postrenal: Conditions such as obstructive uropathies, ureteral destruction, or bladder neck obstruction, which block the flow of urine, resulting in a greater pressure in the collecting tubules affecting filtration and reabsorption.

Occurrence: Occurs in 5% of patients admitted to hospitals (half of which are iatrogenic); 10 to 15% of intensive care unit (ICU) patients; 2% to 7% of open heart surgery patients. The mortality rate as high as 50%.

Age: Occurs in all ages; incidence higher in older adults after surgery.

Ethnicity: No significant ethnic predisposition.

Gender: No significant gender differentiation.

Contributing factors: History of surgery, trauma, cardiovascular disorder, exposure to nephrotoxins (such as radiocontrast materials, insecticides, or heavy metals), volume depletion (as seen in diabetes), use of nephrotoxic drugs (such as ACE inhibitors, aminoglycoside, NSAIDs), upper or lower urinary tract obstruction.

Signs and symptoms: Oliguria ($<$ 500 mL/day); anuria (less common); nausea, vomiting, pruritus, and fatigue (from electrolyte imbalance); edema (dependent on pulmonary function; from fluid retention); symptoms of CHF in patients with cardiovascular disease. Assess skin turgor and jugular veins. Signs of fluid depletion can, in turn, indicate prerenal disease; fluid overload can indicate the degree of renal dysfunction. A rectal or pelvic exam may reveal a cause of obstruction, such as a mass. The presence of abdominal bruits indicates renovascular disease.

Diagnostic tests:

Test	Results indicating disorder	CPT code
BUN and creatinine	Elevated with BUN to creatinine ratio normal or greater than normal	84520 BUN 82565 Creatinine included in complete history

(Continued)

Test	Results indicating disorder	CPT code
Serum chemistries including potassium, magnesium, phosphorus	Usually elevated	80053, 83735, 84100
pH (blood)	Usually increased	82803
Sodium, total calcium, and carbon dioxide	Usually decreased	Included in complete chemistry above
Urinalysis	Usual findings include proteinuria, muddy brown or tubular cell casts, high osmolality, high specific gravity, low urine sodium concentration).	81001
Renal ultrasonography	Helps detect malignancy, urolithiasis or bladder outlet obstruction	76770

BUN, blood urea nitrogen.

Differential diagnosis: Diagnosis is one of exclusion.

Treatment:

Physical

Fluid management: Fluid replacement should equal insensible loss (about 500 mL/day) plus urinary losses. Weigh patient daily; each pound of weight gain may represent 500 mL of retained fluid. Carefully regulate fluid and sodium balance to avoid volume overload. Restrict sodium intake to 2 to 4 g daily. Monitor fluid intake and output. If urine output decreases, fluid-challenge patient who is not volume overloaded with 500 to 1000 mL normal saline IV over 30 to 60 minutes; urine output generally follows. If no response, administer furosemide, 100 to 400 mg IV. If effective, continue furosemide at the lowest effective dose to maintain fluid balance.

Dietary modification: Limit protein intake to approximately 0.5 g/kg per day (decreases nitrogenous waste production). Malnourished or highly catabolic patient may require higher protein intake and should be considered for early institution of dialysis. Restrict potassium intake to 40 mEq/day; phosphorus intake to 800 mg/day.

Pharmacologic

Closely monitor drug dosages of renally excreted drugs (narcotic and nonnarcotic analgesics; narcotic sedative; antihypertensives; antiarrhythmics; diuretics; anticoagulants; hypoglycemic agents; antibiotics, especially aminoglycosides [gentamicin, tobramycin, vancomycin]); readjust as necessary.

Renal Replacement Therapies

Dialysis (indicated when hyperkalemia, acidosis, or volume overload cannot be controlled by conservative measures; BUN above 100 mg/dL and serum creatinine above 10 mg/dL).

Follow-up: Watch patient closely during the recovery phase (commonly occurs within 6 weeks; may take up to 1 year) for monitoring of serum electrolytes and volume status, clinical assessment, and assessment of patient and family coping mechanisms.

Sequelae: Possible complications include infection, gastrointestinal bleeding, uremia, anemia, permanent kidney damage, and chronic renal failure. High mortality rate; at 1 month from onset, about 50% of patients die from a number of causes; 20% continue dialysis; and 30% recover.

Prevention/prophylaxis: Prevention strategies include early detection of impending renal failure and timely interventions (such as maintaining fluid volume before and after surgery, avoidance of nephrotoxic medications) to reverse the process, and to prevent or minimize serious and permanent kidney damage.

Referral: Refer to a nephrologist for diagnosis and management.

Education: Explain disease process, signs and symptoms, and treatment (including side effects of medications). Discuss importance of diet, fluid restrictions, avoidance of infection, daily weights, and intake and output. Educational resource materials are available from the National Kidney and Urologic Diseases Information Clearinghouse, PO Box NKUDIC, Bethesda, MD 20893 (301-654-4415; Website: *www.niddk.nih.gov/ health/kidney/nkudic.htm*) and the National Kidney Foundation, Inc., 30 East 33rd St., New York, NY 10016 (800-622-9010; Website: *www. kidney.org*).

RENAL FAILURE, CHRONIC

SIGNAL SYMPTOMS Generally, none until < 25% function

Renal failure, chronic	ICD-9-CM: 585

Description: Chronic renal failure (CRF) is the progressive, irreversible decline in kidney function manifested by the kidney's inability to rid the body of wastes and maintain homeostasis.

Etiology: Occurs with a decrease in glomerular filtration rate and a reduction in the clearance of solutes excreted by the kidneys (chronic elevation of creatinine greater than 2.0 mg/dL) as a result of damage to the kidneys from a variety of disease processes.

Occurrence: Occurs in 2.8/100,000; an estimated 160,000 people per year are treated for end-stage renal disease (ESRD).

Age: Occurs in all ages; more common in adults.

Ethnicity: No significant ethnic predisposition.

Gender: No significant gender differentiation.

Contributing factors: Diseases that damage the kidneys, such as nephrosclerosis, glomerulonephritis, diabetic nephropathy, interstitial nephritis, polycystic kidney disease, connective tissue disease, hypertension, and diabetes; volume depletion; urinary tract obstruction; analgesic abuse; nephrotoxic substances.

Signs and symptoms: Because of the compensatory ability of the remaining nephrons to filter wastes, patients with declining renal function do not manifest symptoms until renal function declines to < 25% of normal.

Initial symptoms may be those of contributing diseases.

Characteristic signs and symptoms include hypertension, anorexia, nausea, vomiting, diarrhea, metallic taste in the mouth, tremors, weight loss, yellow-brown pigmentation, pruritus, and signs and symptoms of uremia (anemia, acidosis, azotemia).

Late-stage symptoms include general malaise, lassitude, forgetfulness, loss of libido, weight loss, altered mental status, and severe peripheral nerve deterioration.

Uremic syndrome.

Diagnostic tests:

Test	Result Indicating Disorder	CPT Code
Serum chemistries	Reveals hyperkalemia, hyponatremia, hypocalcemia, hyperphosphatemia, metabolic acidosis, and electrolyte imbalance	80053 complete 80049 Basic
BUN and serum creatinine levels and relationship to each other*	As disease progresses, serum creatinine will rise proportionately	Basic/complete metabolic panel includes BUN/CR
CBC	Shows profound anemia (normochromic, normocytic).	85025
Urinalysis	Commonly shows proteinuria and casts in the urine	81001
24-hour urine	Quantifies proteinuria and calculates creatinine clearance	81050
Renal ultrasound	Provides information on kidney size and presence of obstruction	76770
Renal biopsy	confirms the diagnosis	50555

*If the BUN-creatinine ratio is greater than 20:1 (normal), consider an extrarenal cause. A ratio of 10:1 is indicative of acute and/or chronic renal failure.
BUN, blood urea nitrogen; CBC, complete blood count.

Differential diagnosis: One of exclusion

Treatment: Slowing the progression of the renal failure is extremely important.

Pharmacologic

Recombinant human erythropoietin, 50 U/kg, subcutaneous (SQ) tid (starting dose). Calcium supplements (200–400 mg with meals) (for renal osteodystrophy).

Physical

Conservative treatment with dietary restrictions of protein, potassium, phosphorus, and sodium (for patients with slow deterioration and minor symptoms). Fluid intake should equal daily urine output plus an additional 500 to 1000 mL.

Because it may accelerate the disease, hypertension should be treated aggressively. Careful monitoring of diuretics is essential. Acidosis is treated with oral sodium bicarbonate, 300-600 mg PO tid. Azotemia does not require treatment until the BUN exceeds 100-125 mg/dL, when dialysis should be considered.

Renal Replacement Therapies

Hemodialysis or continuous ambulatory peritoneal dialysis (for uncontrolled hypertension, uncontrollable uremia, and when neuropathies are present). Renal transplant (when conservative treatment and dialysis have failed).

Follow-up: See patient closely to monitor serum chemistries (determines progression of disease) and hematocrit levels (monitors for anemia), and to assess clinical status.

Sequelae: Renal disease causes pathologic changes in almost all body systems. When $< 10\%$ of renal function remains, end-stage renal failure results. Mortality rate is estimated at 50%.

Prevention/Prophylaxis: Deceleration of the disease can be accomplished by conservative medical treatment and avoidance of factors known to exacerbate an acute decline in renal function, such as volume depletion, hypertension, hypotension, infection, urinary tract obstruction, and nephrotoxic drugs (for example, aminoglycosides or NSAIDs).

Referral: Refer to nephrologist for diagnosis and management.

Education: Explain the disease process, signs and symptoms, and treatment (including side effects of medications). Discuss importance of diet, fluid restrictions, avoidance of infection, daily weights, and intake and output. Educational materials are available from the National Kidney and Urologic Diseases Information Clearinghouse, PO Box NKUDIC, Bethesda, MD 20893 (301-654-4415; Website: *www.niddk.nih.gov/health/kidney/nkudic.htm*) and the National Kidney Foundation, Inc., 30 East 33rd St., New York, NY 10016 (800-622-9010; Website: *www.kidney.org*).

STOMACH CANCER (GASTRIC CANCER)

SIGNAL SYMPTOMS▶ Weight loss, dysphagia, nausea/vomiting

Malignant neoplasm of stomach ICD-9-CM: 151

Description: Stomach (gastric) cancer refers to a malignancy that occurs anywhere in the stomach. Infiltration of the lymph nodes, omentum, lungs, and liver may be rapid. Ninety percent of these cancers are adenocarcinomas.

Etiology: Unknown cause; thought to be associated with food preservatives such as nitrates and sulfites; probably arises from nonspecific mucosal injury; some sources suggest association with untreated *H. pylori* infection. It is two to four times more common in first-degree relatives, suggesting a genetic link.

Occurrence: Occurs in 10/100,000; accounts for approximately 14,000 deaths. Overall 5-year survival rate is 12% to 14%.

Age: Incidence increases with age; two thirds of all cases occur older than age 65.

Ethnicity: More common in people from Japan and Iceland (possibly because of a diet high in smoked fish); also a high incidence in people from Peru and Costa Rica (possibly also diet-related).

Gender: More common in men than in women.

Contributing factors: Diet low in fruits and vegetables and high in foods with additives such as smoked, pickled, or salted foods, or highly spiced Oriental foods (primary contributing factor); pernicious anemia; atrophic gastritis; *H. pylori* infection; prior gastric resection; polyps or dysplasia in the GI tract; smoking; alcohol abuse; lower socioeconomic status.

Signs and symptoms: Most patients are diagnosed with advanced disease and have had vague symptoms for a while. Common signs and symptoms include the following: Persistent abdominal pain and weight loss; anorexia; nausea; vomiting, with or without hematemesis; change in bowel habits, with or without melena; weakness; and fatigue.

Physical examination may reveal an abdominal or epigastric mass (50% of patients), firm hepatomegaly, enlarged lymph nodes, spider angiomas, palmar erythema (hepatic failure), distended firm abdomen, hyperactive or hypoactive bowel sounds, and dullness on percussion (may or may not be present). Jaundice, ascites, a periumbilical metastatic node, and positive Virchow's node are poor prognostic signs.

Diagnostic tests:

Test	Result Indicating Disorder	CPT Code
Hematology	Anemias are common in ulcerated lesions; eosinophilia and polycythemia may be seen	85025
Chemistry with liver function	Rules out liver involvement; elevated liver function enzymes and elevated bilirubin may be seen	80053 80076
Nutritional assessment including albumin	Often decreased	82040
Electrolytes		Included in complete chemistry above
Serum protein		Included in complete chemistry above
Stools for guaiac	Often positive	82770

(Continued)

Test	Result Indicating Disorder	CPT Code
Barium studies, including a barium swallow with follow-through		72426
Endoscopy and biopsy	Endoscopy may reveal esophageal varices; biopsy is definitive for diagnosis	43200, 43202
CT scan of the abdomen; chest x-ray study	May reveal elevation or displacement of the diaphragm	74170, 71010

CT, computed tomography.

Differential diagnosis:

- Colon cancer (imaging, biopsy, weight loss, anorexia, blood in stools)
- Peptic ulcer (abdominal pain, weight loss, nausea and vomiting, food intolerance, bloating, belching)
- Functional dyspepsia (abdominal cramping, relief with defecation)
- Pancreatic cancer (vague abdominal complaints, needle biopsy to differentiate)
- Crohn's disease (diarrhea)

Treatment:

Surgical

Surgical excision with resection of lymph nodes (only chance of cure).

Procedures include a radical subtotal gastrectomy or total gastrectomy. Local excision may be performed for palliation. Radiation therapy is of little benefit because of the radioresistance of gastric tumors. Chemotherapy also has little effect; however, the effect it may have is improved after surgical resection.

Follow-up: See patient for routine, frequent follow-up to monitor disease progression, assess nutritional status, and provide palliative care. (Serious problems with pain, nutrition, nausea, emesis, bowel elimination, metabolic imbalances, and bleeding commonly occur.) Because prognosis is poor, supportive care is crucial; therefore, referral to a supportive program or agency such as a hospice is appropriate, even if palliative radiotherapy or chemotherapy is administered.

Sequelae: Possible complications include anemias, metastatic disease (especially hepatic, cerebral, pulmonary), and pyloric stenosis. Overall 5-year survival rate is 18% (local disease, 57%; regional spread, 19%; distant spread, 2%).

Prevention/prophylaxis: Prevention strategies include advising patient not to ignore symptoms of indigestion that last more than a few days; to eat a well-balanced, nutritious diet; to decrease alcohol consumption to < one to two drinks per day; and to have stools examined yearly for blood. In geographic areas where occurrence is high, routine screening is advocated. Early gastric cancers that are successfully resected are usually accidentally discovered by endoscopy done for another reason.

Referral: Refer to, or consult with, surgeon or oncologist for definitive diagnosis of cancer. Refer to hospice program for palliative care.

Education: Explain disease process, signs and symptoms, and treatment (including side effects of medications). Discuss treatment options and importance of nutritional status. Educational and resource materials are available from the American Cancer Society or the Cancer Research Institute, 681 Fifth Ave., New York, NY 10022 (1-800-99 Cancer). Website: *www.cancerresearch.org*

URINARY TRACT INFECTION

SIGNAL SYMPTOMS ▶ *Cystitis:* Dysuria, frequency, urinary urgency
Pyelonephritis: UTI symptoms, back pain, fever

Urinary tract infection in adults, acute	ICD-9-CM: 599.0
Pyelonephritis, acute	ICD-9-CM: 590.1
Pyelonephritis, chronic	ICD-9-CM: 590.0
Cystitis	ICD-9-CM: 595
Acute cystitis	ICD-9-CM: 595.1
Chronic cystitis	ICD-9-CM: 595.2

Description: A urinary tract infection (UTI) is an inflammation of some portion of the urinary tract. A descending UTI, or cystitis, typically affects the urinary bladder or ureters. An ascending UTI, or pyelonephritis, is an inflammation of the renal parenchyma and collecting system.

Etiology: Most commonly caused by bacterial infection, typically a gram-negative organism such as *Escherichia coli* (70 to 80% of all cases). Anatomic or functional pathology may also predispose toward infection.

Occurrence: Three to eight percent of all women have bacteriuria at any given time; 43% of women age 14 to 61 have had at least one UTI. Uncommon in men. Hospital-acquired pyelonephritis, 7.3/10,000 hospitalized patients; community-acquired, 7/100,000.

Age: Occurs in all age groups, especially in women.

Ethnicity: No significant ethnic predisposition.

Gender: Much more common in women than in men; after age 65, tends to occur equally in men and in women.

Contributing factors: Ascending urethral infection caused by contaminated urologic instruments, fecal contamination, indwelling catheters, more frequent and vigorous sexual activity, use of spermicides or diaphragm; shortness of urethra (in women); secondary to infected prostate, epididymitis, or bladder stones (in men); pregnancy, diabetes, ascending infection from bladder, history of UTIs.

Signs and symptoms:

Cystitis: Urgency, frequency, painful urination, perineal and suprapubic pain, hematuria, chills, and fever. Occasionally, gross hematuria, low back pain. No flank or costovertebral pain.

Pyelonephritis: Fever, lower back pain, chills, malaise, frequency, burning urination, nausea and vomiting, flank pain, shaking chills, dysuria, frequency urgency. Patient generally has systemic illness and appears sick.

Diagnostic Tests:

Cystitis

Urinalysis (microscopic exam, culture and sensitivity).

Pyelonephritis

Urinalysis (RBC, WBC, penteururia), cystoscopy, retrograde pyelography.

Differential diagnosis:

Cystitis: Vaginitis, sexually transmitted diseases (STDs), urethritis, cervicitis, pyelonephritis, abdominal disease.

Pyelonephritis: Cystitis, PID, prostatitis, ectopic pregnancy, toxic shock syndrome.

Treatment:

Cystitis: Treatment includes antibiotics as indicated by sensitivities of causative organisms and increased fluid intake. A 3-day treatment may be used if the patient's symptoms last < 3 days; if vaginitis or an overt upper UTI is not present; and if the patient can be relied on for follow-up visits; and should include the use of antibiotics, such as ampicillin, trimethoprim-sulfameth oxazole (Bactrim os/Jeptra) one tablet 3 times per day or ciprofloxacin 500 g/day × 3 day. For other cases, treat with same medications for 7–10 days. In young men may be trusted with same drugs but for 7 days.

Pyelonephritis: Outpatient treatment includes antibiotics trimethoprim, 160 mg, and sulfamethoxazole, 800 mg one tablet orally every 12 hours for 10 to 14 days, or floxacin (Floxin) 400 g BID or levofloxacin (Levaquin) for 7–10 days is as efffective as a standard two-drug parenteral regimen in a patient who can retain oral fluids. May need analgesics, increased fluid intake, bed rest, and hospitalization for administration of parenteral medication (usually ampicillin and gentamicin). Postcoital treatment may be recommended: one dose of trimethoprim/sulfamethoxazole or cephalexin may reduce frequency of UTIs in sexually active women.

Follow-up: See the patient as needed to evaluate effectiveness of treatment and for follow-up urine cultures.

Sequelae: For cystitis, possible complications include chronic cystitis and pyelonephritis. For pyelonephritis, possible complications include chronic pyelonephritis and septicemia.

Prevention/prophylaxis: Prevention strategies include advising the patient to avoid a full bladder; to increase fluid intake to 2000 to 3000 mL/day to flush out bacteria; to avoid alcohol and caffeinated beverages

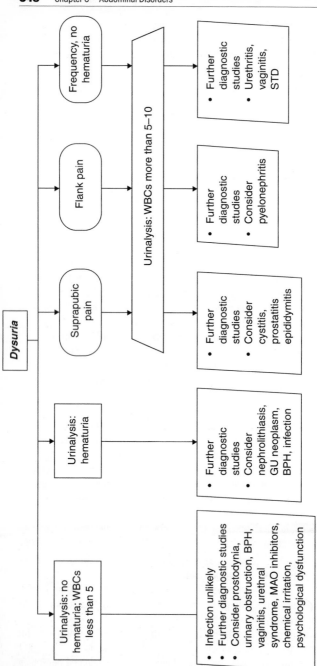

Figure 6–3. Differential diagnosis: dysuria.

if bladder spasms are present; and, for women, to void after sexual intercourse and to consider other birth control methods if using a diaphragm.
Referral: Refer to, or consult with, physician if patient is male, because UTI may indicate a more serious underlying abnormality; if patient is female with recurrent infections; if patient fails to improve in 3 to 4 days; if patient has diabetes or known kidney stones; or if growth of original pathogens is found on follow-up examination.

Education: Explain disease process, signs and symptoms, and treatment (including side effects of medications). Discuss prevention strategies. Advise patient to complete entire regimen of medication even though symptoms may be alleviated within 72 hours. Refer to Figure 6-3 for the differential diagnosis of dysuria.

REFERENCES

Dambro, M: Griffith's 5 Minute Clinical Consult. Williams & Wilkins, Baltimore, 2003.

Dunphy, LM and Winland-Brown, E: Primary Care: The Art & Science of Advanced Practice Nursing. FA Davis, Philadelphia, 2001.

Goroll, A, et al (eds): Primary Care Medicine, ed. 4. Lippincott-Williams & Wilkins, Philadelphia, 2000.

Graber, MA. and Lanternier, ML (eds): University of Iowa The Family Practice Handbook, ed. 4. Mosby, St. Louis, 2001.

Koda-Kimble, MA, et al: The Handbook of Applied Therapeutics, ed 7. Lippincott Williams & Wilkins, 2002.

Lin, TL, and Rypkema, SW (eds). The Washington Manual of Ambulatory Therapeutics. Lippincott Williams and Wilkins, Philadelphia, 2002.

NIH Consensus Development Panel on *Helicobacter pylori* in Peptic Ulcer Disease. JAMA 272:65, 1994.

Noble, J (ed): Primary Care Medicine, ed. 2. Mosby, St Louis, 2002.

Rakel, R: Textbook of Family Practice, ed. 6. WB Saunders, Philadelphia, 2002.

Rippe, JM (ed): Lifestyle Medicine. Blackwell Science, Malden, MA, 1999.

Running, A, and Berndt, A: Management Guidelines for Nurse Practitioners Working in Family Practice. FA Davis, Philadelphia, 2003.

Sellers, R: Differential Diagnosis of Common Complaints, ed. 4. WB Saunders, Philadelphia, 2002.

Taylor, R (ed): Manual of Family Practice, ed. 2. Lippincott Williams & Wilkins, Philadelphia:2002.

Tierney, LM et al (eds): Current Medical Diagnosis and Treatment, 2003, ed. 43. Lange Medical Books/McGraw-Hill, New York, 2003.

US Preventive Service Task Force: Guide to Clinical Prevention Services, ed. 2. Williams & Wilkins, Baltimore, 1998.

Wachtel, R, and Stein, M: The Care of the Ambulatory Patient. Mosby, St Louis, 2001.

Woolf, J, et al (eds): Health Promotion and Disease Prevention in Clinical Practice, ed. 2. Lippincott Williams & Wilkins, Philadelphia, 2001.

Chapter 7

MALE GENITALIA DISORDERS

CHANCHROID

SIGNAL SYMPTOMS Acutely painful penile or rectal ulcer; regional adenopathy

Chanchroid	ICD-9-CM: 099.0

Description: An acute sexually transmitted, gram-negative bacillus infection manifested as painful penile or rectal lesion and often accompanied by regional adenopathy. Associated with increased risk for human immunodeficiency (HIV) infections.

Etiology: Source is by direct contact with lesions or exudates, *Haemophilus ducreyi*, the Ducrey bacillus. The incubation period is 1 to 21 days, with an average of 7 days. The infection is spread through sexual contact and autoinoculation.

Occurrence: Most often found in tropical and sub-tropical regions of the world. May be as few as 1000 new cases in the United States annually as regional outbreaks but likely under-reported.

Age: If the condition is found in children, it is highly suggestive of sexual abuse.

Ethnicity: In the United States, it has been found primarily in Hispanic and Black heterosexual men who patronize sex workers.

Gender: More often in men than women.

Contributing factors: Unprotected intercourse, especially with sex workers. Uncircumcised men. Sexual activity in tropical, subtropical, and endemic areas.

Signs and symptoms: Red tender papule that becomes a painful, deep, friable, necrotizing ulcer with undetermined borders. The ulcer quickly becomes pustular, and multiple lesions may erupt. Found on the glans, shaft of the penis, urinary meatus, or rectal area. Regional lymphadenitis occurs in one third of the cases. May be accompanied by fever, anorexia, and malaise.

Diagnostic tests: Up to 25% of patients will have a false-negative culture. Diagnosis is presumptive by exclusion.

Test	Result Indicating Infection	CPT Code
Culture only means of confirmation but results variable	Isolation of *H. ducreyi,* however may be indistinguishable from other *Haemophilus* bacilli	87082–87085
RPR/VDRL and darkfield	If negative for *T. pallidum* and clinically negative for HSV, then diagnosis is presumptive but probably high rate of false positive results	86592–86593

HSV, herpes simplex virus; RPR, rapid plasma reagin; VDRL, Venereal Disease Research Laboratory.

Differential diagnosis:

- Syphilis (nontender, nonpustular lesion)
- Genital herpes (appearance of lesion, but may be difficult to differentiate)
- Lymphogranuloma venereum (small, painless, solitary lesion)

Treatment: The finding of true chancroid is unusual in the United States and should include consultation with an infectious disease specialist. *H. ducreyi* bacteria in the United States have become resistant. Antibiotics to attempt include ceftriaxone, 250 mg intramuscular (IM) single dose or azithromycin 1.0 g oral single dose; alternately use erythromycin, 500 mg orally every 6 hours for 7 days or ciprofloxacin, 500 mg orally every 12 hours for 3 days. Sex partners should be treated if there has been contact within 10 days of the patient's eruption.

Follow-up: Patient should expect to have improvement in symptoms in 3 days. If no improvement in 7 days, then the diagnosis must be questioned and consideration of co-infection or resistance. Baseline testing for syphilis, HIV, and hepatitis B with retest in 3 months is recommended.

Sequelae: A small number of treated persons relapse. Failure to treat infection may result in destruction of the affected tissue.

Prevention/prophylaxis: Safe sex practices, increased surveillance when visiting in endemic areas. Avoid exchange of, or purchase of, sex.

Referral: Consultation with an infectious disease specialist is recommended as noted above. Usually a reportable condition, check with local health department.

Education: Patient must prevent contact between lesion and others or other body parts while lesions are present. Need to treat sex partners. Instruction in wound care and techniques to prevent further inoculation. Patient is at high risk for concurrent HIV, syphilis, and HSV.

CONDYLOMA ACUMINATA

SIGNAL SYMPTOMS ▶ Flesh-colored protuberance on the genitals

Condyloma acuminata	ICD-9-CM: 078.11
Warts, condyloma	ICD-9-CM: 078.1

Description: Condyloma acuminata is a highly contagious human papillomavirus (HPV), which is sexually transmitted. It manifests as a soft, skin-colored, villous growths, which protrude from the skin and can become ulcerated if moist. They may appear singly or in a conglomerate and found most often on the frenulum, corona, glans, prepuce, meatus, shaft, scrotum or in the anal region. Commonly known as venereal warts.

Etiology: Of the more than 60 types of HPV identified in humans, more than 10 (including types 6, 11, 16, 18, 31, and 33, which have been associated with condyloma acuminata) infect the lower genital tract. The virus enters the body through an epithelial defect and infects the stratified squamous epithelium of the lower genital tract.

Occurrence: One of the fastest increasing sexually transmitted diseases (STDs) in men and women. A minimum of 10% to 20% of sexually active young adults may be infected with HPV; an estimated 500,000 cases of genital warts occur annually. The incubation time is 1 to 6 months.

Age: Occurs in men primarily aged 15 to 30 years who are at the peak of their sexual activity.

Ethnicity: More in whites than in nonwhites.

Gender: Occurs equally in men and women.

Contributing factors: Unprotected sexual activities, poor hygiene, cigarette smoking.

Signs and symptoms: In many cases, the appearance of the condyloma is subclinical. They most often are completely asymptomatic other than their appearance. The individual or his intimate partner or partners may notice the lesion on observation. Bleeding at the site may occur as a result of mechanical trauma to the lesion.

Diagnostic tests:

Test	Result Indicating Disorder	CPT Code
Acetic acid: 5% solution on a towel to wrap the area. Leave on for 5 minutes and attempt to visualize with a 10× hand lens.	Appearance of typical whitish papules	Part of usual E & M code
Biopsy	Positive path report for HPV	55700–55705

HPV, human papillomavirus.

Differential diagnosis:
- Condyloma lata (initial flat appearance)
- Squamous cell carcinoma (if ulcerated may be unable to differentiate without biopsy)

Treatment: Although no therapy has been shown to eradicate HPV infection completely, it may become dormant even without intervention. Owing to the appearance and location of the lesions, patient may prefer cosmetic removal. This can be done with simple cryotherapy for smaller lesions and laser or electrocoagulation for larger lesions. Alternately, the lesions can be treated chemically with any of the following:

Pharmacologic Agent	Directions for Use	Frequency
Imiquimod 5% cream	Apply three times a week before sleep and remove after 6 to 10 hours	Repeat for maximum of 16 weeks if needed
Podofilox, 0.5% solution or gel	Apply every 12 hours for 3 days, no treatment for 4 days	May repeat sequence 4-6 times
Podophyllin, 10% to 25% (provider applied)	Apply, leave on for 1 to 4 hours, then wash off	Repeat every 7 days as needed

Follow-up: Consider evaluation for other STDs, HIV infection, and hepatitis B infection.

Sequelae: Possible complications include secondary infection and bleeding in untreated, extensive, or refractory disease; and recurrence. Leading risk factor for cervical cancer in infected woman. Asymptomatic infection persists indefinitely.

Prevention/prophylaxis: Only prevention is to avoid exposure, encourage use of protective barriers during sexual activity; circumcision may prevent recurrences in some cases.

Referral: Refer to, or consult with, urologist if patient has extensive or refractory disease or urethral meatus warts; to dermatologist or proctologist if patient has rectal mucosal warts.

Education: Explain the chronicity of HPV and the association with other STDs. Teach self-treatment as indicated and danger of exposing female sexual partner.

EPIDIDYMITIS

SIGNAL SYMPTOMS ▶ Acute pain in testes; presence of Prehn's sign (relief with elevation)

Epididymitis	ICD-9-CM: 604.90

Description: Epididymitis is an acute bacterial infection and inflammation of the epididymis, which is the result of trauma or an infection of the other structures of the genitourinary (GU) tract.

Etiology: In men younger than 35 years of age, the usual causative agents are sexually transmitted, that is, *Chlamydia trachomatis* or *Neisseria gonorrhoeae*. In men older than 35 years of age, or the insertive partners in anal intercourse, the usual causative agents are enteric; that is *Pseudomonas aeruginosa,* and *Escherichia coli.*

Transmission of pathogens can occur through a urinary tract infection (UTI), prostatitis, anal intercourse, trauma, urethral instrumentation or prostate surgery.

Occurrence: Common.

Age: Occurs at any age; however, it is most often associated with STDs in men younger than 35 years. Immunocompromised or immunosuppressed men are especially susceptible.

Ethnicity: None.

Gender: Men only.

Contributing factors: Unprotected anal intercourse, voiding dysfunction, neurogenic bladder, prostatic enlargement, presence of indwelling urinary catheter, UTI, and immunocompromised states.

Signs and symptoms: Symptoms are associated with inflammation, including scrotal pain with radiation into spermatic cord or flank, rapid scrotal swelling (may double in size in a matter of hours), epididymal tenderness, and urethral discharge. Elevation of the scrotum decreases pain (Prehn's sign).

Signs are an enlarged scrotum; overlying skin may be reddened. If an abscess is present, skin may appear dry and flaky. Palpation of the spermatic cord reveals thickening (from edema); a reactive hydrocele secondary to inflammation may develop.

Diagnostic tests: Diagnosis is usually through a combination of laboratory tests and the clinical exam. Causative agent must be determined for appropriate treatment.

Test	Result Indicating Infection	CPT Code
Gram stain for gonorrhea	Identification of gonorrhea	87082–87085
Culture of drainage	Identification of causative pathogen.	87082–87085
Urine analysis with culture and sensitivity as indicated (mid-stream collection)	Identification of causative pathogen.	81000–81099 87086–87088

Differential diagnosis:

- Testicular torsion (unable to differentiate the epididymis from the teste).
- Incarcerated inguinal hernia (may be visible on transillumination).
- Tumor (nodular).

Treatment: Treatment includes both comfort measures and antibiotics. There are no associated herbal preparations. Comfort measures include bed rest and scrotal elevation, ice, analgesics and antipyretics. No sexual or physical activities during acute phase. Antimicrobial drugs based on culture and sensitivity. *Antibiotics:* For empiric treatment of men younger than 35 years of age, presume *Chlamydia trachomatis* or *Neisseria gonorrhoeae:* ceftriaxone 250 mg IM single dose plus doxycycline 100 mg orally twice a day for 10 days. Alternately: ofloxacin 300 mg orally twice a day for 10 days. For empiric treatment of men older than 35 years of age and anal insertive partners presume *Pseudomonas aeruginosa or E. coli:* ciprofloxacin (Cipro) 500 mg orally twice a day or olfaction 200 mg twice a day for 10 to 14 days. Alternately, Floxin 300 mg twice a day for 10 days.

Follow-up: A follow-up culture to ensure resolution should be considered at the conclusion of the course of antibiotics.

Sequelae: Untreated or chronic epididymis can lead to orchitis and potential infertility. Adequately treated infection should resolve without sequelae.

Prevention/prophylaxis: If infection is acquired sexually, using a condom may prevent its recurrence. Prompt treatment of UTIs will also decrease the likelihood of epididymitis.

Referral: Refer to, or consult with, urologist if symptoms recur with treatment or do not improve within 2 weeks, or if further diagnostic studies or surgical exploration is indicated. Causative agent may be reportable.

Education: Explain the disease process, signs and symptoms, and treatment (including side effects of medications). Discuss safe sex practices, use of condoms, prevention of UTI, and need for hydration. If infection from gonorrhea or *Chlamydia,* it is essential that partner be treated as well.

ERECTILE DYSFUNCTION (IMPOTENCE)

SIGNAL SYMPTOMS▶   Inability to obtain or maintain an erection

Erectile dysfunction	ICD-9-CM: 302.72

Description: Erectile dysfunction is the persistent inability to obtain or maintain a penile erection adequate for sexual activity.

Etiology: Often multifactorial in nature. There are generally two types of causes, psychogenic causes, such as performance anxiety or depression, and organic causes including vasculogenic problems (the most common single cause) resulting in poor inflow or arterial insufficiency, or enhanced outflow from venous leak. Other causes include diabetes, hypogonadism, hyperthyroidism, hyperprolactinemia, Cushing's disease, and mechanical trauma. Neurogenic causes include disease or dysfunction of the brain, spinal cord, cavernous and pudendal nerves. Pharmacologic causes include the use of certain medications, such as antihypertensive drugs, antidepressants, tranquilizers, hypnotics, estrogen, antiandrogens (cimetidine, ketoconazole), marijuana, alcohol and narcotics.

Occurrence: Occurs in approximately 20 million men in the United States.

Age: Incidence progressively increases with age; in men younger than age 35, psychogenic erectile dysfunction is more common than organic; in men older than age 50, organic erectile dysfunction is more likely than psychogenic.

Ethnicity: None.

Gender: Men only.

Contributing factors: See etiology. Cigarette smoking also increases the likelihood of vascular disturbances. Psychological problems such as depression, anxiety, and psychosis may contribute to psychogenic erectile dysfunction, as do interpersonal conflict and personal beliefs about sexual activity.

Signs and symptoms: Persistent inability to obtain or maintain a penile erection during sexual activity.

Diagnostic tests: The initial approach is most often the differentiation of psychogenic from organic causes. Determine whether any erections occur during sleep. Inability to achieve erection with stimulation despite erections during sleep is highly suggestive of psychogenic etiology. This information may be available from the patient or the patient's sleeping partner.

If this information is not available or, in the absence of nocturnal penile tumescence, a compete history and physical must be performed to determine the etiology of the dysfunction. If no abnormalities are apparent in vascular, endocrine, or neurological function, and other potential causes are ruled out, patient must be referred to a urologist for further testing.

Laboratory tests to consider include:

Test	Result Indicating Problem	CPT Code
Serum-free testosterone (if older than 50 years or with s/s of hypogonadism)	≤9 ng/mL	84402–84403
Serum prolactin (test only if low testosterone)	Elevated	80418, 80440, 84146
UA	Positive for infection	81000–81099
Chemistry panel	Abnormalities associated with chronic diseases and elevated glucose	80054
TSH	Low levels suggestive of hyperthyroidism	80418, 80438–440, 80443

TSH, thyroid-stimulating hormone; UA, urinalysis.

Differential diagnosis: Differential will relate to the determination of the cause of the erectile dysfunction.

Treatment: For psychogenic erectile dysfunction,psychotherapy or sex therapy is recommended. *General health care*, such as decreasing alcohol and smoking, performing regular exercise, and reducing weight (if indicated), may also help reverse erectile dysfunction. Yohimbine, 5.4 mg (1 tablet) three times a day, may be prescribed. For organic erectile dysfunction, treat or control the underlying cause. Psychotherapy or sex therapy may also be of benefit both for possible psychogenic component and, if limited treatment is available, for adjustment to this change in life and sexual activity.

Additional pharmacologic therapies may be considered after a complete physical examination. These include sildenafil (Viagra): start with 25 to 50 mg orally 0.5 to 4 hours before intercourse. Contraindicated with nitrate use—fatalities have been reported. Alprostadil injectable (Caverject): Intracavernous injections (5-4 0 micrograms, start with 2.5) may be prescribed; however, careful supervision required. Alprostadil suppositories (MUSE): 125-500 micrograms into urethra. Testosterone cypionate, IM or transdermal: 200 mg IM every 2 weeks or patches (increases risk for prostate cancer, only with documented testosterone deficit).

Other approaches include vacuum erection devices: The penis is inserted into an acrylic chamber with an attached vacuum pump (pump creates a vacuum, resulting in an erection-like state). A constriction ring is transferred from the outside of the device to the base of the penis to maintain the erection. Alternatively, there are two types of penile prostheses (devices implanted into the corpora produce an erection-like state). The nonhydraulic penile prostheses are paired, nodelike devices implanted into the corpora cavernosa to create permanent penile rigidity. The hydraulic (inflatable) penile prostheses, consists of paired penile cylinders, a pump, and a fluid reservoir. Pumping fluid from the reservoir to the cylinders creates an erection.

Follow-up: See the patient as indicated by patient's satisfaction with chosen therapeutic modality.

Sequelae: Possible complications include those related to the underlying disease process or treatment modality.

Prevention/prophylaxis: Counsel regarding drug and alcohol use or abuse. Evaluate for depression.

Referral: Refer to, or consult with, a urologist if patient requires more than general education or medication adjustments. Psychologists, social workers, sex therapists, and other counselors can provide psychotherapy and/or sex therapy. Verify health-care provider's knowledge of erectile dysfunction management before referral.

Education: Explain disease process (especially multifactorial nature), signs and symptoms, and treatment (including side effects of medications). Discuss treatment options. Provide support. Educational resources: *The New Male Sexuality*, by Bernie Zibergeld, PhD, 1992; and problem-specific handouts. See also the websites for the American Urologic Association *(www.auanet.org)* and the American foundation for Urologic Disease *(www.afud.org)*

GONORRHEA

| Gonorrhea | ICD-9-CM: 098 |

Description: Gonorrhea is a sexually transmitted infection of the mucous membranes. In men, the infection can result in urethritis, epididymitis, or prostatitis. Up to 60% of the patients with gonorrhea are co-infected with *Chlamydia*.

Etiology: Causative agent is *Neisseria gonorrhoeae*, a gram-negative diplococcus. The incubation period is 2 to 7 days.

Occurrence: Occurs in an estimated 1.3 million people per year.

Age: Can occur at any age; most often (60%) found in sexually active young men aged 15 to 24.

Ethnicity: Although there is no ethnic predisposition, gonorrhea is seen most often in African American men.

Gender: Occurs more often in men than in women; more men manifest symptomatic disease than women. A single episode of unprotected sexual intercourse with an infected woman carries a transmission risk of 17% to 20% for the man; conversely, unprotected sexual intercourse with an infected man carries a transmission risk of 80% for the woman.

Contributing factors: Highest incidence in the southeastern states in the United States. Unprotected sexual activity with an infected partner, multiple sex partners, sex in exchange for drugs or money, purchased sex, autoinoculation (finger to eye).

Signs and symptoms: Men infected with gonorrhea usually become symptomatic and seek treatment; however, symptoms may not appear until 45 days after exposure. Purulent, yellowish urethral discharge with dysuria most common. May have bilateral lymph nodes enlargement. Urethra most common site of infection in men, however receptive partner in anal intercourse may have rectal discharge, tenesmus, burning or itching. Without treatment, urethritis will persist for 3 to 7 weeks; after 3 months, 95% of men become asymptomatic but are still contagious.

Diagnostic tests:

Test	Result Indicating Infection	CPT Code
Urethral swab on Thayer-Martin culture plate	Presence of bacteria	Call lab
Gram stain of discharge (not useful for rectal discharge)	Presence of bacteria	Call lab
DNA probes and enzyme immunoassays of urine (EIA)	Presence of infection	87797–99 86317–18

Differential diagnosis:

- Nongonococcal urethritis (serous discharge)
- Chlamydial infection (may be indistinguishable except with culture)

Treatment: No sexual intercourse until cure is established. Owing to the high rate of co-infection with Chlamydia treatment should cover both organisms. There has been an increasing incidence of treatment resistance in various parts of the United States and other countries. Refer to web site *www.cdc.gov/ncidod* for the latest recommendations for treatment in your local area.

Antibiotics for uncomplicated urethral or rectal infection: Ceftriaxone, 125 mg IM single dose; ciprofloxacin, 500 mg oral single dose; *or* ofloxacin 400 mg oral single dose plus azithromycin 1.0 g Orally for one dose, or doxycycline 100 mg orally every 12 hours for 7 days.

Follow-up: See the patient 1 week after completing treatment for reculture of mucosal sites. If infection persists, consider resistance or reinfection. Partner or partners require treatment.

Sequelae: If the condition is not treated or is treated inadequately, possible complications include abscess formation, urethral fibrosis and urethral strictures (from periurethritis); prostatitis; epididymitis; testicular atrophy or infertility; disseminated infection (seen as petechiae or small, tender papules or pustules on the arms and legs); arthritis and tenosynovitis (knees are the most common joint involved); hepatitis; myocarditis; endocarditis; and meningitis (rarely).

Prevention/prophylaxis: Prevention strategies include the use of condoms. The spermicidal nonoxynol-9 had been thought to have protective qualities, but this feature has not been supported by research and is not recommended. Whether they are symptomatic or not, those who have been in contact with infected partners should be examined, cultured, and treated. There should be no sexual activity until the infected partner is treated and recultured. Avoid sold, purchased, or exchanged sex.

Referral: Refer to, or consult with, a urologist if patient has complicated or disseminated disease or fails to respond to treatment. Report to local public health unit.

Education: Explain disease process, signs and symptoms, and treatment (including side effects of medications). Discuss prevention strategies and methods for preventing STDs, including HIV infection. Emphasize need for partner or partners to be treated.

LYMPHOGRANULOMA VENEREM

SIGNAL SYMPTOMS Small painless lesion; flocculent lymph nodes with surrounding edema and erythema

| Lymphogranuloma venereum | ICD-9-CM: 099.1 |

Description: Lymphogranuloma venereum (LGV) is a sexually transmitted *Chlamydial* infection manifested primarily in the lymphatic system. It begins as a tiny, painless ulcer on the penis or the perianal area that may resolve unnoticed and followed by unilateral regional adenopathy. The incubation time is 3 to 21 days.

Etiology: LGV is caused by one of the three most virulent strains of *Chlamydia trachomatis* (L1, L2, and L3), the same organisms responsible for *Chlamydial* urethritis.

Occurrence: Approximately 300 cases are reported annually to the CDC. Although LGV has been rare in the United States, it is occurring with increased frequency, especially in homosexual men who engage in anal intercourse. May be endemic in tropical countries including especially Africa, the Caribbean (Haiti, Jamaica), South America, East Asia, and Indonesia.

Age: Occurs most often during the peak of sexual activity, between the ages of 15 and 35.

Ethnicity: None

Gender: Occurs 10 times more often in men than in women.

Contributing factors: Unprotected sexual activity, multiple sex partners, anal intercourse (especially receptive partner), and sexual activity in tropical or developing countries where LGV is prevalent.

Signs and symptoms: Initially a small (1-mm), painless papule, pustule, or vesicle and may appear on the penis at the sight of inoculation 3 to 21 days after exposure. The lesion usually heals spontaneously and rapidly, and may be unnoticed. One to two weeks later, tender, matted lymph nodes (called buboes) appear with characteristic overlying erythema and edema. Constitutional symptoms of fever, headache, malaise, and myalgias are prominent. In 60% of the cases, the adenopathy is unilateral. If the condition is left untreated, the buboes become flocculent and rupture in 1 to 2 weeks, with creamy purulent or serosanguinous exudate. If the infection has been introduced anally, the patient may experience anal pruritus, rectal discharge, pain, and tenesmus.

Diagnostic tests

Test	Result Indicating Infection	CPT Code
Culture of lesion or buboes aspirant	*Chlamydia trachomatis*	87110
Serology of antibody titers to L1, L2, L3 serovars	Four fold rise in the MIF titer to LGV antigen (only available in specialized labs) or complement fixation titer > 1:64 probable diagnosis; > 1:128 confirmatory	86631, 86632

Differential diagnosis:

- Syphilis (no edema or erythema at nodes)
- Herpes simplex (painful lesion)
- Chancroid (extensive ulcer)

Treatment: There is no known herbal treatment. If rectal LGV it may require re-treatment.

Antibiotics: Doxycycline, 100 mg orally every 12 hours for 21 days; alternately, use erythromycin, 500 mg orally every 6 hours for 21 days.

Follow-up: Symptoms should begin to resolve 24 to 48 hours after onset of antibiotic therapy. Monitor for constitutional symptoms and for responsiveness to treatment. Testing for co-existing STDs, including HIV and hepatitis B, is highly recommended. All sexual contacts in the previous 30 days require treatment.

Sequelae: If they are left untreated, the buboes may develop fistulas. Other possible complications include proctitis, rectal strictures, and fistulas involving the rectum and bladder, and elephantiasis of the genitalia.

Prevention/prophylaxis: Prevention strategies include advising patients to use protective safe sex. Monitor for other STDs.

Referral: Refer to, or consult with, surgeon if patient has infected or fluctuant nodes requiring aspiration, draining sinuses requiring excision, or rectal stenosis requiring surgical measures. Refer to an infectious disease specialist if patient does not quickly respond to antibiotics. LGV is a reportable infection in many states, check with local health department.

Education: Explain disease process, signs and symptoms, and treatment (including side effects of medications). Discuss prevention strategies and advise patient of HIV risk factors for transmission, prevention, and detection.

PROSTATE CANCER

SIGNAL SYMPTOMS▶   Urinary frequency; urinary retention

Prostate Cancer	ICD-9-CM: 185

Description: Prostate adenocarcinoma is the most common noncutaneous cancer in men in the United States.. The 10-year disease-specific survival for disease localized to the prostate is 75%; this percentage decreases to 55% for local disseminated disease and 15% for those persons with widespread metastases.

Etiology: The exact etiology of prostate cancer is unknown. A genetic predisposition has been postulated, because it appears that men with one first-degree relative with prostate cancer have a twofold-increased risk and a ninefold increased risk if two first-degree relatives have or have had prostate cancer. It occurs only in the presence of testosterone. Dietary factors (especially high-fat diets), environmental conditions, and contagion such as viruses and bacteria are currently under consideration as causative agents.

Occurrence: The exact number of men with prostate cancer is unknown. However approximately 35,000 to 40,000 men die every year with prostate cancer, or 70 out of 100,000. The American man has a 3.4% risk of death from prostate cancer.

Age: Rarely occurs in men younger than age 50; approximately 30% of men older than age 50 have histologic evidence of prostate cancer; the percentage rises with age.

Ethnicity: Prostate cancer is the most common of all malignant disorders seen in African American men. Compared with whites, blacks have both a 50% higher incidence and a higher mortality rate, and are usually at a more advanced stage of the disease at the time of diagnosis. There is a very low incidence of prostate cancer in men of Asian descent.

Gender: Men only.

Contributing factors: Persons with a positive family history, are older than 50 years old, or who are African-American are at greater risk. Other possible contributing factors may be vasectomy, high-fat diet, alcohol use, and exposure to certain chemical carcinogens such as cadmium, pesticides, and rubber.

Signs and symptoms: Prostate cancer is most often asymptomatic until it is established and may not be detected until it is advanced. If there are any early symptoms, they are similar to those of benign prostatic hyperplasia, such as weak urinary stream, urgency, and nocturia. Later symptoms are associated with enlarged prostate and the effects of metastases such as skeletal pain, weight loss, anemia, shortness of breath, or lymphadenopathy. Hematuria, obstructive uropathy, neurologic signs from cord compression, or pathologic fractures are uncommon signs of cancer that may occur in advanced disease. The most significant (but possibly misleading) sign is the palpation of an asymmetrical discrete, rock-hard nodule on the posterior lobe of the prostate. With more advanced disease, the entire prostate may be involved and the median furrow may become obliterated.

Diagnostic tests: If prostate cancer is suspected, a transrectal ultrasound is recommended. Only a biopsy is confirmatory of prostate cancer; other screening measures are used to determine the level of suspicion, including annual prostate-specific antigen (PSA) levels and digital rectal exam (DRE).

Test	Results Indicating Disorder	CPT code
Serum prostate-specific antigen (PSA)	Observe rate of change from 1 year to another. Increases of > 0.75 ng/mL are highly predictive. 70% of men with PSA > 10 ng/mL will have cancer. False-positives can occur with benign prostatic hyperplasia (BPH), infection, and inflammation.	84153, 86316
Digital rectal exam (DRE)	Palpation of hard nodular prostate indicates need for further evaluation	Visit code

Differential diagnosis:

- BPH (not significantly elevated PSA, boggy texture to prostate)
- Inflammation (prostate pain)

Treatment: For asymptomatic men with no evidence of disease outside of the prostate, a course of "watchful waiting" is often selected. The type of treatment will depend on the age, life expectancy, and the extent of disease spread. In most cases, aggressive treatment is confined to men younger than 70 years old and those with > 10-year life expectancy. Possible treatments include prostatectomy, radiotherapy, or either chemical or surgical (bilateral orchiectomy) hormonal ablation.

Follow-up: The level of follow-up depends on stage and treatment approach and is done in conjunction with the treating urologist or oncologist. Regardless of treatment approach, follow for changes in urination and complaints of pain in genitourinary area or bone.

Sequelae: Possible complications of uncontrolled prostate cancer are long term and include urinary outflow obstruction, causing hematuria and pelvic pain. With metastases, the patient may have painful bony lesions, pathologic fractures, spinal cord compression, weight loss, anemia, shortness of breath, lymphedema, lymphadenopathy, and death.

Prevention/prophylaxis: Although some groups recommend them, there is no statistical evidence that screenings (e.g., DRE and PSA) will reduce morbidity or mortality rates. There are no prevention strategies.

Referral: If the patient has an elevated PSA or abnormal DRE, refer to, or consult with, urologist for further evaluation and possible ultrasound-guided biopsy for diagnosis.

Education: Because treatment and watching is in conjunction with a urologist, the nurse practitioner (NP) plays in active role in ensuring that the patient has the information he needs to make informed choices about treatment. Advanced planning is also recommended, for example, pre-paring a living will, durable power of attorney for health care, and so on. Resources for support and further information should be offered: American Cancer Society and Help for Incontinent People are valuable. Additional educational resources are available from the National Kidney and Urologic Disease Information Clearinghouse, PO Box NKUDIC, Bethesda, MD 20893 (301-654-4415); the American Institute for Cancer Research, 1759 R Street, NW, Washington, DC 20069 (800-843-8114 or 202-328-7744), "Reducing Your Risk of Prostate Cancer" (Brochure E42-BHP); the American Urologic Association, Baltimore, MD (410-727-1100): and the American Cancer Society (800-ACS-2345). Other sites of excellent patient education are at the American Urologic Association(www.auanet.org) and the American Foundation for Urologic Disease (*www.afud.org*).

PROSTATIC HYPERPLASIA, BENIGN

SIGNAL SYMPTOMS Urinary hesitancy; weak stream

Prostatic hyperplasia, benign	ICD-9-CM: 600
See also code for presenting symptom	ICD-9-CM: variable

Description: BPH is an adenomatous enlargement of the prostate gland that may result in bladder outlet obstruction.

Etiology: The etiology is unknown. It is suspected that BPH is the result of hormonal alterations that stimulate growth. This may or may not be associated with growth factors. Dietary factors and genetics may play a role.

Occurrence: Up to 50% of men 51 to 60 and 90% of men older than 80 have prostatic enlargement to some extent.

Age: Rare in men younger than 40 years. Increases with age.

Ethnicity: None.

Gender: Men only.

Contributing factors: Increasing age and intact testes in the presence of testosterone. High-fat diet and family history of BPH may increase risk.

Signs and symptoms: Palpable prostate size does not necessarily correlate with symptoms. See the American Urological Association Symptom Index for quantification of symptoms into mild (0 to 7), moderate (8 to 19), or severe (20 to 35) (Table 7–1). Many symptoms are associated with obstruction: weak or split stream, decreased urine force, hesitancy, postvoid dribble, double or incomplete void, urinary retention, increased postvoid residual, distended bladder, and overflow incontinence. Other symptoms are irritative: dysuria, frequency, urgency, nocturia or hematuria. An enlarged prostate may be palpable. The symmetrically enlarged lateral lobes of the prostate will feel smooth with elastic to rubbery to firm consistency, but it is usually described as "boggy." The rectal mucosa is freely movable over the prostate. If the hyperplasia is of the median lobe, no enlargement may be palpable as growth is anterior. Focal neurologic examination will be negative.

Diagnostic tests: Laboratory data are for the diagnosis of potentially associated conditions and are only suggestive of BPH. Computed tomography (CT) scan, magnetic resonance imaging (MRI), or transrectal ultrasound provides volumetric estimate of gland and indicate need for biopsy. Only a biopsy is confirmatory.

Table 7–1 American Urological Association Symptom Index for Evaluating Benign Prostatic Hyperplasia

Circle frequency for each question and enter the score in last column

Questions	Not at All	Less than 1 time in 5	Less than half the time	About half the time	More than half the time	Almost always	Score
Over the past month, how often have you had a sensation of not empty-ing your bladder completely after you finished urinating?	0	1	2	3	4	5	
Over the past month, how often have you had to urinate again less than 2 hours after you finished urinating?	0	1	2	3	4	5	
Over the past month, how often have you found you stopped and started again several times when you urinated?	0	1	2	3	4	5	
Over the past month, how often have you found it difficult to postpone urination?	0	1	2	3	4	5	
Over the past month, how often have you had a weak urinary stream?	0	1	2	3	4	5	
Over the past month, how often have you had to push or strain to begin uri-nation?	0	1	2	3	4	5	
Over the past month, how many times did you most typically get up to urinate from the time you went to bed at night until the time you got up in the morning?	None 0	1 time 1	2 times 2	3 times 3	4 times 4	5 or more times 5	
						TOTAL SCORE:	

Mild symptoms 0–7 points, moderate symptoms 8–19 points, severe symptoms 20–35 points.

Source: Barry, M.J, et al H. (1992). The American Urological Association symptom index for benign prostatic hyperplasia. *J Urol 148(5)*, 1549–1557.

Test	Result Indicating Disorder	CPT Code
Urinanalysis, culture as indicated to rule out infection	If positive, does not rule out BPH but indicates need for treatment that may resolve the presenting symptoms.	81000–81099 (ua) 87086–87088 (culture)
Serum creatinine	If elevated, further evaluation for extent of renal impairment and for more aggressive evaluation of BPH.	82565
Biopsy, resection, or aspiration	Will provide definitive diagnosis and information about the type of tissue involved (stromal, fibromuscular, muscular, fibroadenoma, or fibromyoadenoma)	55700–55705
PSA (optional)	Increased in 25% but rarely over 10 ng/mL. Not specific for BPH.	84153, 86316

BPH, benign prostate hyperplasia, PSA, prostate-specific hormone.

Differential diagnosis:

- Strictures (no prostatic enlargement)
- Neurogenic bladder (large post void residual without obstruction)
- Medication side effect (presence of anticholinergic medications)
- Infectious / inflammatory processes (positive urine culture, tender prostate)
- Cancer (nodular prostate)

Treatment: Watchful waiting is the recommended treatment for asymptomatic men.

For symptomatic men: Alpha blockers may be used with caution in persons with cardiac disease but are especially helpful for use in persons with hypertension because all lower blood pressure. For example, terazosin (Hytrin), begin with 1 mg/day, may increase to 10 mg; doxazosin (Cardura), 0.5 to 8 mg/day; or tamsulosin (Flomax), 0.4 to 0.8 mg/day. The 5-alpha inhibitor finasteride (Proscar), 5 mg/day may also be used.

Phytotherapy: These include saw palmetto (in studies of self-report especially effective in reducing nocturia), beta-sitosterol plant extract, *Serena repens,* and rye grass pollen extract. As with all nonregulated preparations, exact ingredients and dosages are unknown. Sexual side effects have occurred in some men.

Surgery is commonly recommended for severe symptoms. All forms of surgery are initially highly effective but with high complication rates, especially ejaculatory abnormalities. Procedures include the less invasive transurethral balloon dilation (TUDP), transurethral microwave thermotherapy (TUMT), and transurethral needle ablation (TUNA), and the more invasive transurethral resection (TURP) and prostatectomy.

Follow-up: Monitor AUA symptom index every 1 to 6 months. Perform or refer for urodynamic testing if concerned about obstruction. Annual

DRE for men older than 50 years of age. In 70% to 80% of patients, symptoms will improve or stabilize over time.

Sequelae: Detrusor instability, bladder diverticuli, recurrent UTIs, prostatitis, bladder stones, urinary retention, and subsequent renal failure are all possible.

Prevention /prophylaxis: None. Some men are taking phytotherapy in hope of preventing BPH but there are no clinical trials related to this factor at this time.

Referral: Refer to a urologist if the patient has moderate or severe symptoms, when a definitive diagnosis is necessary, or the patient has recurrent infections.

Education: Explain the disease process, signs and symptoms, and treatment (including side effects of medications). For the patient with mild symptoms, discuss behavioral techniques to improve symptoms, including reducing fluid intake after dinner; and avoiding caffeine, alcohol, artificial sweeteners, decongestants, anticholinergics, tranquilizers, and antidepressants. For the patient with moderate to severe symptoms, offer information on all management options. Encourage patient to view and search for the latest information, see especially *www.healthfinder.gov*

PROSTATITIS

SIGNAL SYMPTOMS ▶ Perineal or suprapubic pain; hematuria

Prostatitis, acute	ICD-9-CM: 601.0
Prostatitis, chronic	ICD-9-CM: 601.1

Description: Prostatitis is an infection of the prostate gland. It is classified as acute bacterial, chronic bacterial, or nonbacterial and is one of the most common and important results of UTI in men. Acute bacterial prostatitis is fairly uncommon, painful, and potentially serious in nature. The chronic nonbacterial form is more common and may cause persistent, frustrating symptoms.

Etiology: Both acute and chronic prostatitis originate from an ascending urethral infection, reflux of infected urine due to nonrelaxation of the internal sphincter and pelvic floor muscles, direct extension or lymphatic spread from the rectum. Acute and chronic bacterial infections are most often caused by *Escherichia coli, Klebsiella, Proteus, Chlamydia, Pseudomonas,* and *gonorrhea,* or a number of other organisms. The source for the nonbacterial prostatitis is either undetermined or caused by *Ureaplasm* or *Mycoplasma.*

Occurrence: Common; may account for 25% of all office visits.

Age: When occurring in a younger man. it is most often from an STD. When occurs in an older man, it is often after the placement of a Foley catheter. Chronic prostatitis is rarely seen in men younger than 50 years.

Ethnicity: None.

Gender: Men only.

Contributing factors: Exposure to STDs, recurrent UTI, age older than 50 years, anal receptive or insertive partner in anal intercourse.

Signs and symptoms: In acute prostatitis, the patient may present with chills, fever, low back and perineal pain, urinary urgency and frequency, nocturia, dysuria, and difficulty starting to urinate or urinating at all. Gentle rectal palpation typically discloses an exquisitely tender, swollen prostate gland that is firm to boggy, and warm to the touch. In chronic bacterial prostatitis, symptoms may be absent or include voiding dysfunction, such as urgency, frequency, and dysuria, or pain in the perineal, scrotal, or penile areas, or the lower back. Hematospermia and decreased potency may be seen. Similar symptoms are seen in nonbacterial cases but they may be intermittent.

Diagnostic tests

Test	Results Indicating Infection	CPT Code
Routine UA	Bacteriuria with large mucus threads	81000–81099
Segmented urine analyses	> 20 WBCs / HPF in third specimen suggestive of acute infection 10 to 15 WBCs / HPF with a negative culture indicative of nonbacterial infection	81000–81099
Segmented urine and prostatic secretion cultures (Including specialized cultures for *Chlamydia* or gonorrhea if indicated)	= 1 logarithmic increase in the bacterial count from the first and second cultures in the third and fourth cultures is confirmatory.	87086–87088
Digital rectal exam	Acute tenderness is suggestive	Visit code

UA, urinalysis; WBCs, white blood cells, HPF, high-powered field.

Differential diagnosis

- BPH (non-tender prostate)
- Prostate cancer (nodular, non-tender prostate)

Treatment: Hospitalization is required for men with suspected abscess or urosepsis and for those who are immunocompromised. Outpatient treatment includes antibiotics; comfort measures, including sitz baths lasting 20 to 30 minutes two to three times daily; bed rest; stool softener; analgesics. Alpha- blockers, especially terazosin and doxazosin, may be helpful for prostatodynia. Final treatment depends on the isolated causative agent. For immediate empiric *antibiotic* treatment of bacterial infections when STD is suspected: ofloxacin 400 mg orally for first dose, then 300 mg every 12 hours for 10 days. For non-STD infections: fluoro-quinolones (e.g., ciprofloxacin [Cipro] 500 mg orally twice a day) for10 to 14 days for acute infection and 4 weeks for chronic infection. Alternately, use trimethoprim-sulfamethoxazole 1 tablet orally every 12 hours for 10 to 14 days for acute infection and 1to 3 months for chronic infection. For non-bacterial prostatitis, a 2- to 4-week trial of antimicro-bial therapy may be helpful to relieve symptoms: minocycline, 100 mg orally every 12 hours; erythromycin, 500 mg orally every 6 hours; *or* ofloxacin, 300 to 400 mg orally every 12 hours. However, if no response to therapy is noted, do not continue therapy. If suppression therapy is necessary for chronic conditions, prescribe trimethoprim/sul-famethokazole (Bactrim DS), 1 tablet orally every night or nitrofurantoin (Macrodantin), 100 mg orally every night.

Follow-up: No unprotected intercourse while undergoing treatment. For acute bacterial prostatitis, repeat urinalysis and cultures 30 days after ini-tiating treatment. For chronic bacterial prostatitis, repeat urinalysis and cultures every 30 days. To control symptoms: Anti-inflammatory agents, such as ibuprofen (for symptomatic flare-ups); alpha-blocking agents, such as prazosin (for urinary symptoms). Frequent prostatic ejaculations may be helpful; therefore, prostatic massage may be useful.

Sequelae: Prostatitis is often prolonged and difficult to cure. Possible complications of acute infections include abscess, sepsis, urinary reten-tion, and chronic prostatitis.

Prevention/prophylaxis: Suppression therapy may benefit the patient with chronic prostatitis. Avoid exposure to causative agents through safe sexual practices. If using a Foley catheter, the patient can be taught to maintain the sterility of the drainage system.

Referral: Refer to, or consult with, urologist if the patient fails to respond to treatment. May be reportable depending on infectious agent.

Education: Advise patient to discontinue all over-the-counter (OTC) drugs with anticholinergic properties, such as antihistamines and decon-gestants; and to avoid caffeine (colas, coffee, tea), alcohol, and foods that cause irritative urinary outlet symptoms

SYPHILIS

SIGNAL SYMPTOMS Painless anal, penile or oral lesion after unpro-tected sexual contact

Syphilis	ICD-9-CM: 090.0-097

Description: An STD with three sequential stages. If the condition is left untreated, the disease evolves through the following course: the infec-tious stage (with primary and secondary symptoms), the noninfectious latent stage, and the third or tertiary stage. The secondary and tertiary stages may be asymptomatic. Neurosyphilis may develop at any stage.

Etiology: Caused by the spirochete bacteria *Treponema pallidum* and transmitted through contact with lesions or rash.

Occurrence: Third most common reported infectious disease in the United States, with about 100,000 new cases annually. Highest incidence is in select metropolitan areas and in the south eastern United States.

Age: May be seen at any age; however, it is most common in men 20 to 35 years old.

Ethnicity: Those at greatest risk are African American men and women, and men who have sex with men. There has been an increasing rate among Hispanic men.

Gender: Occurs more frequently in men than in women.

Contributing factors: Unprotected sexual activity, sex in exchange for drugs or money. Often found simultaneously with other STDs.

Signs and symptoms: Signs and symptoms are specific to the stage of the disease. In primary syphilis, the patient presents with an ulcer that appears from 1 to 5 weeks after exposure. The punched-out ulcer is usually painless, with indurated borders and a clean base. It may be accompanied by regional lymphadenopathy (firm and bilateral). Without treatment, the lesion and adenopathy will resolve in about 6 weeks. Anywhere from 6 weeks to 2 years, later the patient develops constitutional flu-like symptoms, lymphadenopathy, and a generalized rash. The rashes may be macular, papular, papulosquamous, pustular, or nonspecific and involve only the palms and soles. This secondary phase of the first stage of syphilis is the most contagious state, but the signs and symptoms resolve spontaneously in 3 to 12 weeks. Any infection that has been untreated for more than 1 year is considered "latent." About one third of people with latent syphilis are little inconvenienced by the disease. Latent syphilis is usually only detectible by serology. Tertiary syphilis is a widely disseminated disease that may affect one or any number of organs, resulting in uveitis, gummatous, aortitis, or neurologic impairments including dementia. Owing the high rate of antibiotic use in the United States, it is unlikely that a patient would present with tertiary syphilis.

Diagnostic tests:

Test	Results Indicating Infection	CPT Code
Darkfield examination of scrapings of active lesions (gold standard)	Presence of organism	87164–87166

(Continued)

Test	Results Indicating Infection	CPT Code
Serology: VDRL or RPR (more sensitive)	Positive within 7 days of exposure but decreases with time or treatment. Titer of 1:64 probably positive. Successful treatment indicated with a fourfold decrease in serum RPR at 6 months for primary syphilis and an eightfold decline within 12 months for secondary syphilis. High rate of false-positive and false-negative findings.	86592–86593
VDRL on CSF for all patients with syphilis of > 1 year or in presence of neurologic symptoms	Positive	86592–86593

CSF, cerebrospinal fluid, RPR, repeat plasma reagin test;

Differential diagnosis:

- Chancroid (painful lesions and concurrent adenopathy)
- LGV (self-limited lesion, extensive lymph involvement)
- HSV (prodromal, first case may have systemic manifestations of acute viral infection)

Treatment: The treatment of choice in all cases is parenteral penicillin G. The preparation, dosage, and duration are dependent on the stage and clinical manifestations. For infections of < 1 year, the usual treatment is penicillin G benzathine, 2.4 million units IM in one dose. For infections of an unknown duration or more than 1 year, the usual treatment is penicillin G benzathine, 2.4 million units IM weekly for 3 weeks. Alternatives should be used only when allergy is conclusively documented. Either a neurologist or infectious disease specialist should treat all cases of suspected neurosyphilis. Confirm choice of treatment with current infectious disease guide or CDC at *www.cdc.gov/*. Treatment of all sexual contacts is presumptive regardless of serology.

Follow-up: See the patient 6 months, 12 months, and 24 months after initial diagnosis and treatment for clinical and serologic examination and to confirm eradication. If at any time there is a fourfold increase in serum RPR, the treatment has failed or the patient has become reinfected and retreatment is necessary. Lumbar puncture should then be considered. All persons treated for syphilis should also be screened for HIV and hepatitis. All sexual contacts require empiric treatment.

Sequelae: Primary and secondary syphilis is highly curable, and sequelae are uncommon. However, when the condition is left untreated or inadequately treated, multiple organs can become affected.

Prevention/prophylaxis: Avoid unprotected sexual contact, and the avoidance of sex in exchange for drugs or money or purchased sex. Syphilis screening should be performed on individuals at high risk for developing syphilis, sexual partners of known cases, and individuals with multiple sex partners, especially those in areas with a high prevalence.

Referral: Consult with infectious disease and public health specialists as needed. This is a reportable infection in all jurisdictions.

Education: Explain the disease process, signs and symptoms, and treatment (including side effects of medications). Discuss prevention strategies, including abstaining from sexual activity until the conclusion of treatment and all contacts are treated as well. Inform the patient of the high rate of false negative and false-positive findings. Discuss with the patient the very high rates of infection in selected areas of the country and the need for increased caution when engaging in sexual activity in these areas. Refer the patient to CDC web sites and hotlines. Watch for Jarisch-Herxheimer reaction, that is, rash, fever, headache, which occurs 6 to 8 hours after penicillin injections and is a reaction to the proteins released by the dead treponemas, not the penicillin.

TORSION OF TESTIS

SIGNAL SYMPTOMS▶ Acute scrotal pain; edematous mass in scrotum

Torsion of Testis	ICD-9-CM: 608.2

Description: Torsion of the spermatic cord or testicular torsion is an acute urologic emergency that results when the spermatic cord becomes twisted, the arterial blood supply to the testis is interrupted, and the venous and lymphatic drainage are blocked. It is frequently confused with a strangulated scrotal hernia or acute epididymitis and must be differentiated from varicocele and hydrocele. Figure 7–1 provides a comparison.

Etiology: Usually spontaneous and idiopathic; may be stimulated by trauma, exercise, cold, and sexual stimulation; initiating factor appears to be spasm of the cremaster muscle; occurs during sleep in about half of patients. Testis may have inadequate, incomplete, or absent fixation within scrotum.

Occurrence: Seen in about 1:160 men.

Age: Most common in adolescents.

Ethnicity: None

Gender: Men only.

Contributing factors: Congenital abnormality of tunica vaginalis or spermatic cord, winter months (possibly because of cold), paraplegia.

Signs and symptoms: The patient complains of acute pain. On examination, the testis of the affected side lies higher than usual, the testis and the epididymitis are indistinguishable, leg on the affected side is often flexed, and elevation does not provide relief (Prehn's sign).

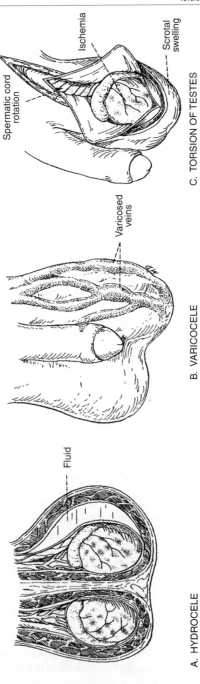

Figure 7–1. Comparing hydrocele, varicocele, and testicular torsion.

A. HYDROCELE

B. VARICOCELE

C. TORSION OF TESTES

Diagnostic tests: If the physical examination suggests torsion, the patient is urgently referred to a surgeon for diagnostic surgery and correction. If correction is delayed, the affected tissue will die.

Differential diagnosis:

- Acute epididymis (epididymis can be differentiated in examination, relief with elevation).
- Strangulated scrotal hernia (unable to differentiate without visualization during surgery).

Treatment: Surgeon may attempt manual detorsion before surgery. Detorsion within 12 hours of onset has good results; within 12 to 24 hours, recovery is possible; after 24 hours, preservation is doubtful. Beyond 48 hours, orchiectomy is advised.

Follow-up: As needed in cooperation with surgeon.

Sequelae: Testicular recovery is directly related to duration of torsion.

Prevention/prophylaxis: Surgical orchiopexy is performed bilaterally to prevent recurrence.

Referral: Urgent referral to urologist or surgeon.

Education: Explain need for urgency in obtaining treatment. If orchiectomy is performed, address physiologic, emotional, and psychological aspects in follow-up.

VARICOCELE

SIGNAL SYMPTOMS▶ Infertility; heaviness or dull ache in groin

Varicocele	ICD-9-CM: 456.4

Description: A varicocele is an abnormal degree of venous dilation of the pampiniform plexus above the testis. It is clearly distinguishable owing to its characteristic feel of a "bag of worms" above the testis. The left side is most commonly affected although may be bilateral. See Figure 7–1 for comparison of varicocele with hydrocele (very unusual in adults) and torsion.

Etiology: Results from a backflow of blood secondary to incompetent or absent valves in spermatic veins. The sudden development of a varicocele in older men is sometimes a late sign of a renal tumor.

Occurrence: The incidence is between 10% and 15%; in individuals evaluated for infertility problems, the incidence is approximately 21% to 41%.

Age: May occur at any age but most often in the 10- to 20-year-old person.

Ethnicity: None.

Gender: Males only.

Signs and symptoms: May be completely asymptomatic and only found during an evaluation for infertility. Patient also may report "heaviness" or a dull ache in the groin. Physical examination reveals (with patient standing) a mass of dilated, tortuous veins lying posterior to and above the testis; may extend up to the external inguinal ring; often tender. The Valsalva maneuver can increase degree of dilation; in the recumbent position, venous distention abates. Testicular atrophy may be present. On palpation, a varicocele often feels like a "bag of worms." Grade I varicocele: palpable only when patient performs Valsalva's maneuver; grade II varicocele: palpable when patient is standing; grade III varicocele: visual inspection reveals varicocele.

Diagnostic tests: Diagnosis is made primarily by physical examination.

Test	Results Indicating Disorder	CPT Code
Ultrasound	Can confirm the diagnosis	Pelvic: 76856-57 Retroperitoneal: 76770–76775 Scrotum: 76870

Differential diagnosis:
- Indirect inguinal hernia (place finger over the inguinal ring while patient lying, when stands, veins refill, whereas hernia would be held back)

Treatment: The only treatment, if necessary, is surgical ligation of the internal spermatic vein.

Follow-up: In asymptomatic patients with no history of infertility, a yearly physical examination is prudent. Have patient return if he experiences pain or any other changes.

Sequelae: Possible complications include testicular atrophy and infertility (if condition is not corrected).

Prevention/prophylaxis: Scrotal support for pain.

Referral: Refer to, or consult with, physician or surgeon if the patient has a right-sided varicocele of new onset, infertility, pain, or testicular atrophy.

Education: Explain that varicoceles are usually not problematic but could cause infertility.

REFERENCES

General
Goroll, A, et al: Primary Care Medicine. Lippincott-Raven, Philadelphia, 2000.

Hurst, JW (ed.): Medicine for the Practicing Physician, ed. 4. Appleton & Lange, Norwalk, Conn, 2001.

Noble, J (ed.): Primary Care Medicine, ed. 2. Mosby, St. Louis, 2000.

Rakel, R: Textbook of Family Practice, ed. 8. W. B. Saunders, Philadelphia, 2001

Resnick, MI, and Novick, AC: Urology Secrets. Hanley & Belfus, Philadelphia, 2001.

Sellers, R: Differential Diagnosis of Common Complaints, ed. 4. Saunders, Philadelphia, and 2000.

Swartz, M: Textbook of Physical Diagnosis, ed. 4. Saunders, Philadelphia, 2001.

Tierney, LM, et al: Current Medical Diagnosis and Treatment, ed. 42. Appleton & Lange, Norwalk, Conn, 2003.

Uphold, C, and Graham, MV Clinical Guidelines in Family Practice, ed. 2. Barmarrae Books, Gainesville, Fla, 1999.

US Preventive Service Task Force: Guide to Clinical Prevention Services, ed. 2. Williams & Wilkins, Baltimore, 1998.

Wachtel, R, and Stein, M: The Care of the Ambulatory Patient. Mosby, St Louis, 2001.

Woolf, J, et al (eds): Health Promotion and Disease Prevention in Clinical Practice, ed. 2. Williams & Wilkins, Baltimore, 2001.

Chanchroid

Benenson, A (ed): Control of Communicable Disease Manual. American Public Health Association, Washington, DC, 2001.

Centers for Disease Control and Prevention: Sexually transmitted diseases treatment guidelines. MMWR 51(RR-6), 2002.

Gilbert, DN, et al: The Sanford Guide to Antimicrobial Therapy 2001. Pfizer, Hyde Park, Vt, 2002.

Isada, CM, et al (eds.): Infectious Disease Handbook, ed. 4. Lexi-Corp, Hudson, Oh, 2001.

Tierney, LM, et al: Current medical diagnosis and treatment, ed. 42. Appleton & Lange, Norwalk, Conn, 2003.

Workowski, KA, and Levine, WC: Sexually transmitted diseases guidelines 2002. MMWR 51(RR-6):1–78, 1992.

Condyloma Acuminata

Benenson, A (ed): (2001). Control of Communicable Disease Manual. American Public Health Association, Washington, DC, 2001.

Isada, CM, et al (eds.): Infectious Disease Handbook, ed. 4. Lexi-Corp, Hudson, Oh, 2001.

Pfenninger, JL, and Fowler, GC: Procedures for Primary Care Physicians. Mosby, St Louis, 2000.

Workowski, KA, and Levine, WC: Sexually transmitted diseases guidelines 2002. MMWR 51(RR-6):1–78, 2002..

Epididymitis

Centers for Disease Control and Prevention: Sexually transmitted diseases treatment guidelines. MMWR 51(RR-6), 2002.

Dambro, M: Griffith's 5-minute Clinical Consult. Williams & Wilkins, Baltimore, 2001.

DeGowin, RL: DeGowin and DeGowin's Diagnostic Examination, ed. 6. McGraw-Hill, New York, 2001.

Gilbert, DN, et al: The Sanford Guide to Antimicrobial Therapy 2001. Pfizer, Hyde Park, Vt, 2002.

Nelson, JB: Prostate diseases. Clin Geriatr 8(12):60, 63–66, 2000.

Workowski, KA, and Levine, WC: Sexually transmitted diseases guidelines 2002. MMWR 51(RR-6):1–78, 2002.

Erectile Dysfunction

Chan, PD, and Johnson, MT: Treatment Guidelines for Medicine and Primary Care. Current Clinical Strategies Publishers, Laguna Hills, Cal, 2002.

Olsson, AM, and Persson, C: Efficacy and safety of sildenafil citrate for the treatment of erectile dysfunction in the man with cardiovascular disease. Intern J Clin Pract 55(3):171–176, 2001.

Tierney, LM, Current Medical Diagnosis and Treatment, ed. 42. Appleton & Lange, Norwalk, CN, 2003.

Gonorrhea

Centers for Disease Control and Prevention: Sexually transmitted diseases treatment guidelines. MMWR 51(RR-6), 2002.

Benenson, A(ed.): Control of Communicable Disease Manual. American Public Health Association, Washington, DC, 2001.

Gilbert, DN, et al: The Sanford Guide To Antimicrobial Therapy 2001. Pfizer, Hyde Park, Vt, 2002.

Isada, CM, et al (eds.): Infectious Disease Handbook, ed. 4. Lexi-Corp, Hudson, Oh, 2001.

Workowski, KA, and Levine, WC: Sexually Transmitted Diseases Guidelines 2002. MMWR 51(RR-6):1–78, 2002.

Lymphogranuloma Venerem

Benenson, A (ed): Control of Communicable Disease Manual. American Public Health Association, Washington, DC, 2001.

Isada, CM, et al (eds.): Infectious Disease Handbook, ed. 4. Lexi-Corp, Hudson, OH, 2001.

Workowski, KA, and Levine, WC: Sexually transmitted diseases guidelines 2002. MMWR 51(RR-6):1–78, 2002.

Prostate Cancer

Chan, PD, and Johnson, MT: Treatment guidelines for medicine and primary care. Current Clinical Strategies Publishers, Laguna Hills, Cal, 2002.

Cotter, VT, and Strumpf, NE (eds.): Advanced Practice Nursing with Older Adults: Clinical Guidelines. McGraw Hill, New York, 2002.

Fracchia, J, et al: Scrotal lesions: Cystic, benign or serious? Consultant 42(9):1097–1100, 1102–1103, 2002.

Nelson, JB: Prostate diseases. Clinical Geriatrics 8(12):60, 63–66, 2000.

Tierney, LM, et al: Current Medical Diagnosis and Treatment, ed. 42. Appleton & Lange, Norwalk, Conn, 2003.

Prostatic Hyperplasia, Benign

Chan, PD, and Johnson, MT: Treatment Guidelines for Medicine and Primary Care. Current Clinical Strategies Publishers, Laguna Hills, Cal, 2002.

Cotter, VT, and Strumpf NE (eds.): Advanced Practice Nursing with Older Adults: Clinical Guidelines. McGraw Hill, New York, 2002.

McConnell JD: Epidemiology, etiology, pathophysiology and diagnosis of benign prostatic hyperplasia. In Walsh, P, et al (eds): Campbell's Urology, Vol 2, ed. 7. W.B. Saunders, Philadelphia, 1998, pp. 1429–1452.

Nelson, JB: Prostate diseases. Clinical Geriatrics 8(12):60, 63–66, 2000.

Tierney, LM, et al: Current Medical Diagnosis and Treatment, ed. 42. Appleton & Lange, Norwalk, Conn, 2003.

Tunuguntla, H: Medical management of benign prostatic hypertrophy. Clinical Geriatrics 10(5):20–22, 24–25, 2002.

Wilt, T, et al: Serenoa Repens for Benign Prostatic Hypertrophy. The Cochrane Library, 2003, (3), CD 001423.

Prostatitis

Centers for Disease Control and Prevention: Sexually transmitted diseases treatment guidelines. MMWR 51(RR-6), 2002.

Chan, PD, and Johnson, MT: Treatment Guidelines for Medicine and Primary Care. Current Clinical Strategies Publishers, Laguna Hills, Cal, 2002.

Collins, MM, et al: Diagnosis and treatment of chronic abacterial prostates: A systematic review. Ann Intern Med 133(5):367–381, 2000.

Gilbert, DN, et al: The Sanford Guide to Antimicrobial Therapy 2001. Pfizer, Hyde Park, Vt, 2002.

Isada, CM, et al (eds.): Infectious Disease Handbook, ed. 4. Lexi-Corp, Hudson, OH, 2001.

Stevermer, JJ, and Easley, SK: Treatment of prostatitis. Am Fam Physician 61(10):3015–3022, 3025–3026, 3061–3064, 2000.

Tierney, LM, et al: Current Medical Diagnosis and Treatment, ed. 42. Appleton & Lange, Norwalk, Conn, 2003.

Workowski, KA, and Levine, WC: Sexually transmitted diseases guidelines 2002. MMWR 51(RR-6):1-78, 2002.

Syphilis

Benenson, A (ed.): Control of Communicable Disease Manual. American Public Health Association, Washington, DC, 2001.

Centers for Disease Control and Prevention: Sexually transmitted diseases treatment guidelines. MMWR 51(RR-6), 2002.

Isada, CM, et al (eds.): Infectious Disease Handbook, ed. 4. Lexi-Corp, Hudson, OH, 2001.

Velasquez, BJ: When is a rash more than a rash? Sexually transmitted diseases: A dermatological perspective. Athletic Therapy Today 7(3):16–23, 38–39, 64, 2000.

Workowski, KA, and Levine, WC: Sexually transmitted diseases guidelines 2002. MMWR 51(RR-6):1—78, 2002.

Torsion of Testis

Dambro, M: Griffith's 5-minute Clinical Consult. Williams & Wilkins, Baltimore, 2001.

DeGowin, RL: DeGowin and DeGowin's Diagnostic Examination, ed. 6. McGraw-Hill, New York, 2001.

Nelson, JB: Prostate diseases. Clinical Geriatrics 8(12):60, 63–66, 2000.

Varicocele

Dambro, M: Griffith's 5-minute Clinical Consult. Williams & Wilkins, Baltimore, 2001.

DeGowin, RL: DeGowin and DeGowin's Diagnostic Examination, ed. 6. McGraw-Hill, New York, 2001.

Kass, EJ, and Stok, BR: Mitigating the effects of pediatric varicole. Contemporary Urology 13(4):33, 36, 38, 2001.

Tierney, LM, et al: Current medical diagnosis and treatment, ed. 42. Appleton & Lange, Norwalk, Conn, 2003.

Chapter *8*
MUSCULOSKELETAL DISORDERS

BURSITIS

SIGNAL SYMPTOMS▶ Abrupt onset of pain with increasing intolerance to motion

Bursitis	ICD-9-CM: 727.3

Description: Bursitis is inflammation of the bursa (soft, fluid-filled sacs that serve as a cushion between tendons and bones. There are more than 70 bursae on each side of the body, which are either superficial (in subcutaneous tissue) or deep (beneath the fibrous fascia). The bursae commonly affected are those near the shoulder (swimmers; football, baseball, and tennis players), elbows (tennis and golf players), knees ("housemaid's knee"), pelvis and hips, and Achilles tendons. Bursitis frequently occurs with tendinitis.

Etiology: The inflammatory process set in motion by trauma (overuse), infection, autoimmune disease (rheumatoid arthritis), or gout.

Occurrence: Common.

Age: Commonly occurs between ages of 15 and 75 years.

Ethnicity: No significant ethnic predisposition.

Gender: Occurs in men more than in women.

Contributing factors: Improper, overzealous stretching, and sudden increases in exercise by out-of-shape individuals; underlying degenerative joint disease; trauma; previous episode of bursitis; family history of arthritis.

Signs and symptoms:

Usually presents with an abrupt onset of pain with increasing intolerance to motion, local tenderness and erythema in superficial cases. Pain is exacerbated by activity and relieved with rest.

Physical examination may reveal a classic sign: Tenderness to palpation over the joint; occasionally with redness and swelling (most com-

Table 8–1 Bursitis: Comparing Signs and Symptoms

Musculoskeletal Disorder	Signs and Symptoms
Bursitis 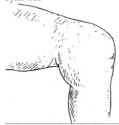	Pain: Localized to area of bursa. Heat and swelling: Minimal. ROM: Pain on isometric contraction with or without ROM.
Synovitis 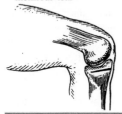	Pain: Entire joint. Heat and Swelling: Entire joint. ROM: Pain and stiffness on ROM.
Trauma to joint from medial meniscus tear	Pain: Localized to joint line adjacent to the medical meniscus. Hemarthrosis may be present. Loose body or tear may cause "locking" of joint.

mon over the knee and elbow joints). There is usually some decrease in range of motion. In early inflammation, bursa may be distended with watery or mucoid fluid; later the bursal wall may feel thickened with gritty, calcific precipitations (Table 8–1).

Diagnostic tests:

Test	Result Indicating Disorder	CPT Code
Complete blood count (CBC)	WBCs increased. Neutrophils increased (rheumatic disease) but decreased in connective tissue disease. Eosinophils increased in autoimmune disease, chronic inflammatory disease, and systemic lupus erythematosus Monocytes increased in collagen diseases and systemic lupus erythematosus May be essentially normal in soft tissue injury. All may help distinguish soft tissue injury from rheumatic and connective tissue diseases	85025
Rheumatoid factor (RF),	Present in rheumatic in connective tissue diseases, but not in soft tissue injury	86430 (qual.) 86431 (quant.)
Erythrocyte sedimentation rate (ESR),	Increased in connective tissue and rheumatic diseases. Decreased in degenerative joint disease Normal with soft tissue injury	85652
Serum uric acid	Increased in acute tissue destruction and with medications	84550
Venereal Disease Research Laboratory test (VDRL),	False-positive results can be seen in autoimmune diseases.	80080 (TORCH panel)
Joint fluid analysis	Includes RBC, WBC, WBC differential and morphology, microscopy for crystals, Gram stain and culture and sensitivity in order to classify cause of joint pain into five categories (non-inflammatory, inflammatory, septic, crystal-induced, or hemorrhagic)	27330 Knee 23066 Shoulder 24100 Elbow 27620 Ankle 21920 Back 26100 Finger/Foot 27050 Sacroiliac 25065 Wrist 87205 Gram stain
Culture and sensitivity (if septic bursitis is suspected). Aspiration with Gram stain	Shows causative organism	87070 culture 87184 sensitivity

(Continued)

Test	Result Indicating Disorder	CPT Code
Computed tomography (CT) scan, magnetic resonance imaging (MRI) scan, or plain x-ray	Shows calcific deposits	Upper extremity: 73200 CT without contrast 73201 CT with contrast 73221 MRI without contrast 73222 MRI with contrast Lower extremity 73700 CT without contrast 73701 CT with contrast 73721 MRI without contrast 73722 MRI with contrast 73000 series for X-ray specific to area

RBC, red blood cell; TORCH, toxoplasmosis, other infections, rubella, cytomegalovirus infection, and herpes simplex; WBC, white blood cell.

Differential diagnosis: Definitive diagnosis may be difficult because there may be an associated tendinitis. You must also rule out

- Rheumatoid arthritis (bilateral morning stiffness, + rheumatoid factor, redness, swelling in hands, wrists, symmetrical involvement, multiple joints.)
- Osteoarthritis (insidious, slow onset; peak intensity with use/relieved with no use; affects only one or a few)
- Cellulitis (red, warm streaking)
- Gonococcal septic arthritis (fever, chills, migratory polyarthralgia, polytendinitis, rash)
- Gout or pseudogout (abrupt onset, usually monoarticular pain, usually large toe; red, swollen, tender joint, synovial fluid, + leukocytes, - birefrin, birefringent crystals)
- Septic arthritis (nongonococcal) (acute onset of joint pain and swelling with limited ROM and fever)

Treatment: Conservative management is usually effective. Goals are to decrease pain and increase function. May include local heat for 30 minutes, immobilization of affected part by splint or sling, and range of motion (ROM) to prevent chronic loss. Encouraging a patient to decrease certain activity will speed up recovery. In the acute phase, the injured part should be treated with rest, ice, and elevation.

Pharmacologic

Full-dose regimen of nonsteroidal anti-inflammatory drugs (NSAIDs), such as ibuprofen, 600-800 mg orally three times a day, or indomethacin, 25 to 50 mg orally three times a day. Injection with corticosteroid or Xylocaine may be necessary, as well as stronger pain medication. For septic bursitis, empiric antibiotic therapy with a penicillinase-resistant agent or a first-generation cephalosporin antibiotic initially, along with bursal drainage is appropriate. Remember: The choice of antibiotic therapy should be based on bursal fluid analysis.

Physical

Modify activity and use site-specific stretching exercises. Rest and immobilization during acute phase (48 to 72 hours), followed by active mobilization and exercise as soon as acute signs subside. Ice to affected part three times a day for 10 to 15 minutes may be helpful in acute phase, then use heat. Do not use heat until pain and edema resolved. Application of local analgesic balm such as capsaicin cream.

Complementary Therapy

See Table 8–4 Summary of Complementary Therapies for Musculoskeletal Disorders at the end of this chapter.

Follow-up: See the patient in 3 to 5 days; discontinue NSAIDs as soon as possible to decrease side effects.

Sequelae: Usually resolves in 7 to 10 days. Possible complications include chronic bursitis, which may require surgical removal of calcification and, occasionally, permanent decrease in ROM.

Prevention/prophylaxis: Prevention strategies include advising the patient to avoid overuse, have adequate rest between workouts, have adequate warm-ups and cool downs, perform ROM exercises, and apply ice to area and begin NSAIDs if symptoms flare or before exercise.

Referral: Refer to, or consult with, physician or orthopedic specialist if patient has severe pain and loss of function or condition does not improve with rest.

Education: Explain the disease process, signs and symptoms, and treatment (including side effects of medications). Discuss prevention strategies.

CARPAL TUNNEL SYNDROME

SIGNAL SYMPTOMS▶ Tingling and numbness in the fingers (typically first three digits) that is relieved by shaking or rubbing the hands.

| Carpal Tunnel Syndrome | ICD-9-CM: 354.0 (first) |

Description: Carpal tunnel syndrome (CTS) is an entrapment neuropathy caused by compression of the median nerve as it passes the transverse carpal ligament.

Etiology: Caused by compression of the median nerve as it passes the transverse carpal ligament. This may be related to underlying inflammation of the tendon sheaths. It can also restrict motor function as well as sensation along the median nerve distribution of the hand.

Occurrence: Common.

Age: Occurs commonly in adults age 40 to 60 years of age.

Ethnicity: No significant ethnic predisposition.

Gender: Occurs in women more than in men.

Contributing factors: Repetitive activity involving the upper extremities, such as gardening, computer work; synovitis of the wrist; pregnancy (common in the third trimester, but usually resolves after delivery); local trauma; local constrictions; prolonged, improper positioning; hypothyroidism, diabetes, rheumatoid arthritis; degenerative joint disease; ganglion cyst.

Signs and symptoms:
Tingling and numbness in the fingers, which are relieved by shaking or rubbing the hands. A classic symptom is acroparesthesia (awaking at night with numbness and burning pain in the fingers). During waking hours, symptoms occur with repetitive activity; there may be a loss of manual dexterity, weakness, and pain that radiates proximally up the forearm.

Physical examination reveals a the presence of Tinel's sign (percussion of median nerve produces distally radiating paresthesia), the presence of Phalen's sign (flexion of wrist produces numbness and tingling after 1 minute), difficulty with pinch and grasp, thenar eminence atrophy (advanced disease).

Diagnostic tests: Usually diagnosed by history and physical examination.

Test	Results indicating disorder	CPT code
EMG and nerve conduction studies	Confirms median neuropathy at the wrist but unable to exclude the diagnosis of CTS	95904
Radiographic or magnetic imaging (wrist)	Shows local structural disease	73115 X-ray study of wrist 73221 MRI without contrast 73222 MRI with contrast
Carpal tunnel pressure measurements	Indicated narrowing and pressure on the nerve	Included in EMG
MRI quantitation of the carpal tunnel, ultrasound of the carpal tunnel	Visualize narrowing of tunnel area and absence of tumors, growths, or masses	76880 Ultrasound (other 73218 (MRI without contrast) 73219 (MRI with contrast)
Sensory quantification, current perception threshold, and grip strength	Numbness or decreased sensation to feel of hot or cold, sharp or dull, weakness noted.	Included in examination, not separate CPT code

CTS, carpal tunnel syndrome; EMG, electromyography; MRI, magnetic resonance imaging.

Differential diagnosis:
- Rheumatoid arthritis (rheumatoid arthritis [bilateral morning stiffness, + rheumatoid factor, redness, swelling in hands, wrists, symmetrical involvement, multiple joints.])
- Osteoarthritis (insidious, slow onset; peak intensity with use but relieved with no use; affects only one or a few)
- Diabetes (blood glucose)
- Tumors (imaging, biopsy)

- Multiple myeloma (bone marrow biopsy)
- Osteoarthritis (x-ray study consistent with changes of osteoarthritis [insidious, slow onset; peak intensity with use/relieved with no use; affects only one or a few])
- Vascular occlusion (cool or mottled skin)
- Myxedema (waxy appearance to skin, hypothyroid and symptoms of same)
- Acromegaly (increased growth hormone level, imaging of pituitary gland)
- Previous wrist fracture (x-ray study)
- Cervical radiculopathy (sensory changes, usually more pronounced than motor changes, paresthesias radiating from neck to arm, weakness is primary symptom, paresthesia over dermatome supplied by involved nerve)
- Soft-tissue injury (history of trauma)

Treatment: If symptoms are interfering with activities of daily living (ADLs), noninvasive treatment should be tried, unless there is progressing motor or severe sensory deficit or severe electrodiagnostic abnormality. Occupational splints or braces.

Pharmacologic
NSAIDs, 400 mg orally three or four times a day. Diuretics (for limb swelling). Pyridoxine (controversial).
Local steroid injection into carpal tunnel; repeated up to three times at 3- to 6-week intervals (if noninvasive treatment is not effective, or if there is progressing motor deficit, severe sensory deficit, or more severe electrodiagnostic abnormality).

Physical
Splinting of the wrist in extension may provide significant relief of symptoms; patient must wear splint during the day and at night. Modification of activities.

Surgical
Surgical therapy (decompression of the carpal tunnel) provides relief in 90% to 95% of patients; reoccurrence is rare after surgery.

Complementary Therapy
See Table 8–4 Summary of Complementary Therapies for Musculoskeletal Disorders at the end of this chapter.

Follow-up: See the patient every 2 to 3 weeks for 4 to 12 weeks when treating patient with splints (brace), NSAIDs, or steroid injections.

Sequelae: Possible complications include failure to respond to surgery (may indicate coexistent cervical spine involvement; reoperation rate is 7%).

Prevention/prophylaxis: Prevention strategies include advising the patient to avoid trauma and repetitive motions; to take a break at least once an hour when doing repetitive work; to wear a brace while doing repetitive work; and to make sure work area, such as desk, chair, and keyboard, are at proper height and position.

Referral: Refer to, or consult with, surgeon if patient does not respond to conservative measures.

Education: Explain disease process, signs and symptoms, and treatment (including side effects of medications). Discuss prevention strategies.

FIBROMYALGIA (MYOFASCIAL PAIN SYNDROME)

SIGNAL SYMPTOMS ▶ History of widespread pain
Tender nodules and trigger points

Myofascial Syndromes	ICD-9-CM: 729.1

Description: Fibromyalgia, also known as myofascial pain syndrome, is a chronic pain syndrome characterized by a dull, constant ache localized to the soft tissues of the neck, shoulders, gluteal area, knees, or upper back. It may also be accompanied by local tenderness of the jaw muscles and difficulty opening the mouth.

Etiology: The pathophysiologic cause unknown; however, some cases may be associated with a primary fibromyalgic disorder. Clenching and grinding of the teeth (bruxism) may play a causative role. Localized inflammation of fibromyalgia usually results from tension and strain associated with repetitive motions of the head and neck or prolonged awkward postures, such as using a poorly positioned keyboard; sitting at a computer terminal for long periods of time; or carrying a heavy backpack, purse, or briefcase consistently on one side of the body. Pain may also be referred from any strained muscle in the back, shoulder or neck.

Occurrence: The incidence is unknown; however, it is one of the most common diagnoses of patients seen at pain treatment centers.

Age: Occurs in all age groups. Peak onset appears to be from 30 to 40 years of age, but younger and elderly patients can also be affected.

Ethnicity: No significant ethnic predisposition.

Gender: More common in women

Contributing factors: Desk jobs involving extended computer work or telephone use, poor posture, a sedentary or routine lifestyle, excessive stress or tension.

Signs and symptoms:

- History of widespread pain. Must be above and below the waist, on both sides of body, and along axial skeleton.

- Associated non-musculoskeletal symptoms include fatigue, sleep disturbance, headache, irritable bowel syndrome (IBS), dysmenorrhea and parathesis as well as anxiety and depression.
- Physical examination usually reveals tender nodules or cords in the posterior musculature; palpation of these focal trigger points produces local pain that radiates to surrounding structures (points are sites of local muscle inflammation).
- Pain on palpation in at least 11 of 18 defined points throughout the body.

Diagnostic tests:

Tests	Result Indicating Disorder	CPT Code
Active range of motion	Decreased range of motion to full extension of ability	95851
MRI	Localizes soft tissue lesions such as the trigger points	70547 without contrast 70548 with contrast
Cervical x-ray studies	Evaluate alignment of cervical spine due to the muscle tension. Expected to be out of alignment toward the more tense muscle area, also to have a flattened cervical spine.	70360

magnetic resonance imaging.

Usually diagnosed by history and physical examination. Diagnostic tests are used primarily to rule out differential diagnoses or to determine whether symptoms continue past the point of expected improvement. Tests may include MRI (localizes soft tissue lesions such as the trigger points) and cervical x-ray studies (evaluate neck pain). On polysomnogram there is a characteristic alpha wave intrusion on delta rhythm sleep.

Differential diagnosis:

- Migraine or tension headache (most common type of headache, symmetric, posterior, sensation of pressure and squeezing, nausea and vomiting. photosensitivity)
- Cervical strain (neck pain)
- Trauma-related causes of neck pain and history of trauma of the back such as acceleration injuries (whiplash), assess activities that precede the pain.
- Osteoarthritis (insidious, slow onset; peak intensity with use/relieved with no use; affects only one or a few)
- Rheumatoid arthritis (bilateral morning stiffness, + rheumatoid factor, redness, swelling in hands, wrists, symmetrical involvement, multiple joints.)
- Hyperthyroidism (thyroid levels)
- Diabetes mellitus and various autoimmune disorders such as systemic lupus erythematosus.

- Depression (no relief from analgesics may need to add antidepressant treatment/therapy)

Treatment:

Pharmacologic

NSAIDs such as ibuprofen, 600 mg orally every 4 to 6 hours, or aspirin, 600 mg orally every 4 to 6 hours. If pain persists, stronger analgesics such as codeine, 30 mg orally every 6 hours, may be prescribed. Steroid injection (0.5 mL triamcinolone acetonide with 2% lidocaine) into muscular trigger points.

Try low dose SSRIs such as fluoxetine (Prozac) 10–20 mg/day or paroxetine (Paxil) 125 mg controlled release or low-dose heterocyclics such as Elavil 10–15 mg/day or cyclobenzaphine (Flexoril) 10–30 mg/day. Tramadol may also be useful for pain.

Physical

Initially, ergonomic management may relieve the pain, although the patient may need to remain recumbent for days to weeks. Rest should be encouraged and any behavioral patterns suspected of contributing to the syndrome discontinued. Local application of ice (30 minutes on; 60 minutes off) during the acute pain phase may also be palliative. If neck or back pain fails to subside after 3 days, heat and massage therapy may ameliorate symptoms. Physical therapy such as passive muscle stretching (helps relieve pain and establish proper bodily mechanics and posture).

Complementary Therapy

See Table 8–4 Summary of Complementary Therapies for Musculoskeletal Disorders at the end of this chapter.

Chamomile tea: relieves stress, calms a nervous stomach; used for four centuries in Europe as a remedy for neuralgia, arthritis, and insomnia. Drink three cups per day.

Follow-up: See the patient as needed to assess the efficacy of initial treatment modalities and need to alter treatment plan.

Sequelae: A possible complication includes temporomandibular joint (TMJ) syndrome.

Prevention/prophylaxis: Prevention strategies include advising the patient to maintain proper posture; to exercise regularly (promotes good muscle tone); to change position frequently if required to sit, stand, or carry heavy objects for long periods of time; and to avoid consistent tasks or behaviors that contribute to the pain.

There is also a relationship between fibromyalgia and sleep disorders demonstrating that deprivation of stage IV sleep can produce symptoms of fibromyalgia in the average person.

Referral: Refer to, or consult with, a physician if the patient requires local steroid injection; to pain treatment center or physical therapist if the patient does not respond to treatment.

Education: Explain disease process, signs and symptoms, and treatment (including side effects of medications). Discuss prevention strategies.

GOUT

SIGNAL SYMPTOMS ▶ Sudden, excruciating pain, frequently monoarticular, classically affecting the first metatarsophalangeal joint, or "big toe." Fever.

Gout	ICD-9-CM: 274.9

Description: Gout is a metabolic disorder with higher than normal accumulations of urates in the joints, bones, and subcutaneous structures. It is characterized by an acute, inflammatory arthritic reaction to these accumulations. The classic gouty attack is podagra, involving the big toe.

Etiology: Hyperuricemia results from overproduction (10%) or underexcretion (90%) of urates. Primary gout results from inborn errors in the metabolism of purines or inherited defects in the renal tubular secretion of urate. Secondary gout occurs because of a variety of acquired diseases such as the myeloproliferative diseases and their treatment; therapeutic regimens producing hyperuricemia; renal insufficiency and renal failure; lymphoproliferative disease; hemolytic anemia; and psoriasis.

Occurrence: Occurs in 2 to 2.6/1000.

Age: Incidence increases with age; initial attack occurs most commonly in the fifth decade.

Ethnicity: Classic Pickwickian picture. Polynesian extraction (Samoan gout).

Gender: Occurs in men more than in women.

Contributing factors: Obesity; alcoholism; hypertension; hyperlipidemia; diabetes mellitus; arteriosclerotic heart disease (ASHD); calcium oxalate urolithiasis; diet high in purines; lead intoxication and ingestion of drugs such as salicylates, diuretics, pyrazinamide, ethambutol, and nicotinic acid for secondary gout; genetics and family history for primary gout.

Signs and symptoms:

- Sudden, excruciating pain, frequently monoarticular, classically affecting the first metatarsophalangeal joint, or "big toe" (other common sites include the instep of the foot, ankle, knee, wrist, or elbow). First attack often begins during the night or early morning and, untreated, peaks in 24 to 36 hours, then subsides in a few days. The joint is reddened, hot, swollen, and exquisitely tender. Condition may become chronic, with asymptomatic intervals becoming shorter and more joints becoming involved.

- Fever
- Tophi (chalky deposits caused by an accumulation of urate crystals) may be found at sites of irritation, such as the joints of hands and feet and pinnae of the ears.

Diagnostic tests:

Test	Result Indicating Disorder	CPT Code
Serum urate level	Above 7.5 mg/dL supports the diagnosis but is not specific	84520
Sedimentation rate and WBC	May be elevated during acute phase	85652 ESR 85021 WBC
Twenty-four hour urinalysis	Assesses urinary acid excretion; levels above 900 mg suggest overproduction of urate	81050
Joint aspiration; fluid sent for smear and culture	Diagnoses disorder; in gout, urate crystals present; rod- or needle-shaped crystals are negatively birefringent (bright yellow) and parallel to the axis of slow vibration (free in synovial fluid or in leukocytes under compensated polarized light.	20600 (small joint) 20605 (intermediate joint) 20610 (large joint) 87205 Gram stain 87070 culture

ESR, erythrocyte sedimentation rate; WBC, white blood cell.

Differential Diagnosis:

- Septic arthritis (nongonococcal) (acute onset of joint pain and swelling with limited ROM and fever)
- Pseudogout (acute onset of joint pain and swelling; joint selling and surrounding warmth; knee and wrists; calcification on x-ray study
- Bursitis related to bunion (bunion present)
- Rheumatoid arthritis (morning stiffness)
- Osteoarthritis (Insidious, slow onset; peak intensity with use/relieved with no use; affects only one or a few)
- Cellulitis (red, warm, streaking)

Treatment:

Acute Therapy

Immediate joint immobilization and decreased weight bearing. Bed rest for 24 hours after the first attack has subsided. Increase fluids, up to daily output of 2000 mL/day. Cold or hot compresses (for comfort). Pharmacologic therapy may include analgesia with NSAIDs, such as indomethacin, 50 mg every 8 hours for 6 to 8 doses, then reduce to 25 mg every 8 hours until attack is resolved; colchicine, 0.6 mg every hour until a total dose of 7.2 mg or 16 doses is reached, symptoms abate, or patient has cramps, diarrhea, nausea, or vomiting. (Aspirin is contraindicated.)

Chronic Therapy

Pharmacologic therapy with uricosuric drugs such as probenecid, 0.5 g/day with gradual increase to 1–2 g/day; avoid use of aspirin. For overexcretion of uric acid, with a history of renal calculi and reduced renal function, drug of choice is allopurinol, 100 mg/day for 1 week, then 200 to 300 mg daily.

Complementary Therapy
See Table 8–4 Summary of Complementary Therapies for Musculoskeletal Disorders at the end of this chapter.

Follow-up: See patient with an acute attack within 24 hours to ensure resolution of acute attack. Follow-up within 4 weeks to discuss maintenance therapy. For patients with chronic gout, obtain yearly uric acid levels.

Sequelae: Possible complications include development of chronic disease, recurrent attacks, tophi (may take up to 10 years to develop), renal stones, and uric acid nephropathy.

Prevention/prophylaxis: Prevention strategies include avoiding provocative factors such as trauma, dietary excess, and alcohol use; advising patient to comply with medication and dietary regimen (usually prevents serious complications), to report attacks promptly, and to not postpone treatment.

Referral: Refer to, or consult with, a physician or an orthopedic specialist as needed.

Education: Explain the disease process, signs and symptoms, and treatment (including side effects of medications). Discuss need for compliance with medication and dietary regimens and lifestyle modifications including gradual weight reduction, reduced alcohol consumption, avoidance of salicylates, and increased fluid intake to approximately 3 liters per day.

MENISCAL TEAR

SIGNAL SYMPTOMS▶ Painful popping or locking of the knee joint. Pain.

| Meniscal tear (knee, unspecified) | ICD-9-CM: 836.2 |

Description: A meniscal tear is a disruption in the medial or lateral surface of the menisci of the knee. This may create an effusion of serosanguineous fluids.

Etiology: Caused by trauma, usually involving rotational stress on a flexed knee, such as that which may occur with sports activities such as roller skating, skiing, football, dancing, motor vehicle accidents, and falls.

Occurrence: The medial meniscus has a higher rate of injury than the lateral.

Age: Occurs primarily in young adults with trauma history and older adults who fall.

Ethnicity: No significant ethnic predisposition.

Gender: Occurs in men more than in women.

Contributing factors: Activities, accidents, muscular weakness related to chronic illnesses.

Signs and symptoms:

- Painful "popping" or locking of joint.
- Most commonly occurs after turning injury.
- Intermittent locking of knee.
- Feeling that leg is "giving way," although the patient may be able to walk after injury.
- Pain.
- Effusion (rapid; postinjury). Ballottement is used to determine if effusion is present, as well as examination for the bulge sign.
- Patellofemoral crepitus may be present.
- McMurray's test: Palpable click and pain in knee when ankle is grasped to turn knee medially and laterally, and while moving knee forward and backward from full flexion to extension. Indicates torn meniscus.
- The Drawer test is used to identify instability of the knee on the mediolateral or anteroposterior plane, more applicable to cruciate ligament injury.
- A positive Apley test also indicates a torn meniscus. Have the patient lie prone and flex the knee to 90 degrees. Place your hand on the heel of the foot and press firmly, opposing the tibia to the femur. Then rotate the lower leg externally and internally cautiously. Any clicks, locking, or pain in the knee indicates a positive Apley sign.

Diagnostic tests:

Test	Result Indicating Disorder	CPT code
X-ray study	Patella may be displaced	73564
Rotatory stress tests	Positive McMurray's test Positive Drawer test Positive Apley test	95851 (ROM studies)
MRI.	Displays meniscal tear	73721 without contrast 73722 with contrast
Arthrocentesis (may perform if effusion is present).	Fluid withdrawn from space	20610
Arthroscopy	Visualize meniscal tear and any other damage	29870

MRI, magnetic resonance imaging; ROM, range of motion.

Differential diagnosis:

- Patellar dislocation (x-ray study)
- Malalignment disorder (x-ray or imaging)
- Acute ligamentous injuries (imaging)
- Osteochondritis dissecans (fragment of cartilage and its underlying bone detached from articular surface)

- Bleeding disorders (prothrombin time [PT]/partial thromboplastin time [PTT])
- Tumors of the knee (imaging; biopsy)
- Tuberculosis (TB) of the knee (positive purified protein derivative [PPD])
- Anterior cruciate ligament tear (positive anterior drawer and Lachman's test)
- Anterior tibial spine fracture (x-ray study)
- Tibial plateau fracture (imaging)
- Osteoarthritis (x-ray study consistent with osteoarthritis, insidious, slow onset; peak intensity with use/relieved with no use; affects only one or a few)

Treatment:

Pharmacologic
NSAIDs (short course of 1 to 2 weeks)

Physical
RICE: Rest, ice, cold, elevation; orthotics, physical therapy for strengthening quadriceps (after healing has occurred) (see Table 8–3 later in the chapter).

Complementary Therapy
See Table 8–4 Summary of Complementary Therapies for Musculoskeletal Disorders at the end of this chapter.

Follow-up: See the patient weekly for reduction of effusion, return of motion, and strengthening exercises (prescribed after healing has occurred).

Sequelae: Possible complications include infection, rupture of meniscus, and loss of ROM.

Prevention/prophylaxis: Prevention strategies include advising patient in use of proper protective equipment for sports activities and prescribing muscle strengthening of quadriceps and biceps femoris.

Referral: Refer to, or consult with, orthopedic surgeon or physical therapist for persistent pain, ligament instability or repetitive knee locking.

Education: Explain disease process, signs and symptoms, and treatment (including side effects of medications). Discuss prevention strategies.

OSTEOARTHRITIS

SIGNAL SYMPTOMS Dull, aching, poorly localized pain of slow, progressive onset in one or a few joints.

Osteoarthritis	ICD-9-CM: 715.9

Description: Osteoarthritis (OA) is a degenerative disorder of the movable joints, characterized by abrasion and deterioration of the articular cartilage, with new bone formation at joint surfaces. It is classified as primary or secondary.

Etiology: Primary, or idiopathic, OA occurs without underlying abnormality or cause, and is considered to be a normal consequence of the aging process. In secondary OA, there is a clearly identifiable cause, such as trauma; an underlying congenital anomaly; a metabolic disturbance, such as gout or acromegaly; or inflammatory processes.

Occurrence: Common. By age 60, more than 80% of the population have some degree of cartilage abnormality in many of their joints, observable on x-ray study. Approximately 40% of this group complain of pain at the affected site. Almost 100,000 total hip replacements, and about as many knee replacements, are performed each year; most of these related to OA. Well over 60 million Americans have pain and limitation of motion as a result of OA.

Age: Predominantly middle-aged and older persons; increases with age.

Ethnicity: Appears to have a lower incidence in northern climates.

Gender: In patients younger than age 55, the condition affects both men and women equally; in patients older than age 55, the condition is more common in women, except in the hips, where more common in men. OA of the distal interphalangeal joints of the hands is 10 times more common in women than in men.

Contributing factors: Age, obesity, repetitive trauma, certain occupational and sports-related stresses, overuse of intraarticular adrenal corticosteroids, familial history.

Signs and symptoms: Commonly affected joints are hips, knees, lumbar and cervical spine, the distal and proximal interphalangeal joints of the hands, and the first carpal-metacarpal and first metatarsophalangeal joint.

- Dull, aching, poorly localized pain of slow, progressive onset in one or a few joints (most common presenting symptom); initially mild and intermittent and brought on by activity and relieved by rest, it progresses to more severe and disabling.
- Heberden's nodes on the dorsal aspect of the distal interphalangeal joints.
- Bouchard's nodes on the dorsal aspect of the proximal interphalangeal joints.
- Other signs and symptoms dependent on affected joint; for example, OA of the spine may also cause neurologic symptoms.
- Physical examination may reveal monoarticular (classically) joint pain and crepitus on passive motion; limitation of motion; localized tenderness. In later stages, there may be subluxation and gross deformity such as a varus knee and contractures.

Diagnostic tests:

Test	Result Indicating Disorder	CPT Code
Sedimentation rate (ESR)	Normal in primary OA, but high in inflammatory process	85652
Rheumatoid factor	Normal in primary OA	86430 (qualitative) 86531 (quantitative)
CBC	Normal in primary OA; but may reflect underlying disorders in secondary OA	85025
X-rays	Normal in early stages; Joint space narrowing, subchondral bone sclerosis, periarticular bone cysts, and osteophytes seen as disease progresses	73000–73225 Upper extremity, chose site 73500–73725 Lower extremity; chose site 720100–72295 Spine and pelvis; chose site

CBC, complete blood count; OA, osteoarthritis.

Differential diagnosis:

- Other types of arthritis (rheumatoid arthritis: bilateral morning stiffness, + rheumatoid factor, redness, swelling in hands, wrists, symmetrical involvement, multiple joints.)
- Osteoporosis (loss of height, kyphosis, back pain, vertebral compression, radiologic evidence)
- Metastatic disease (diffuse bone lesions on x-ray)
- Spinal cord tumors (imaging, biopsy)
- Multiple myeloma (lesions on x-ray, positive Bence Jones protein)
- Bursitis (pain with pressure over affected area)
- Tendonitis (pain with movement in affected joint)

Treatment: Goals are to decrease stress on involved joints, maintain function, and reduce pain.

Pharmacologic

Analgesic therapy with acetaminophen, 650 mg every 8 hours as needed. If pain is not relieved, diclofenac sodium, 50 mg orally twice a day, or ibuprofen, 400 mg orally four times a day (do not exceed 1600 mg/day). May try cyclooxygenase-2 (cox-2) - selective NSAIDS (e.g., celecoxid and rotecoxib). Use regularly for 2 to 3 weeks before switching to another class of NSAIDs. Tailor dosage to maximum benefit within range of tolerance of side effects; may want to start NSAIDs at lower doses for older patients. Concurrent cytoprotective therapy with misoprostol, 200 mcg four times a day with meals and at bedtime (hs), may be needed for patients at risk for peptic ulcer disease (PUD). Capsaicin cream, 0.025% applied topically over affected joint three to four times daily, is sometimes beneficial (most effective in small joints of the hands).

 Clinical Pearl: do not use misoprostol in pregnancy.

Physical

Physical therapies to reduce pain, improve ROM, and maintain patient's ability to function include the following: application of moist heat (decreases muscle spasm and relieves morning stiffness); reduction of weight if patient is overweight; physical therapy (directed at strengthening muscle around affected joint); avoidance of overuse of the involved joint; maintenance of flexibility of the involved joint with stretching exercises (walking, swimming, and bicycle riding are all good for improving muscle tone, also isometric exercises); use of assistive devices and adaptive aids, such as a cane or elastic support, as needed. Occupational therapies to prevent or help decrease functional disability (Table 8–2).

Table 8–2 Prescribing Hot and Cold Physical Therapies

Therapy	Indications	Prescription	
Hot Therapies:	Promote circulation Muscle Relaxation	**Moist Heat** Moist hot packs Contractures	Muscle spasms 20 min three to four times/day
		Whirlpool treatment	Muscle spasms 20 min one to two times/day
		Dry Heat Diathermy Chronic pain	Muscle spasms
		Adhesive capsulitis	20 min, three times/ wk for 1–2 wks
		Infrared therapy Pain	Muscle spasms Buy infrared bulb, keep 20 in from skin; direct it perpendicular to skin for 30 min; may repeat after cooling skin 1 h
		Deep Heat Ultrasound therapy Contractures	Joint pain 10–15 min 3 times/wk
Cold Therapies:	Promote vasoconstriction Reduce swelling and tissue injury	**Direct Application** Cold packs	Acute injury (duration, 72 h or less) Cold pack or ice within a towel, plastic bag, or ice bag. 15 min on; 30 min off. A bag of frozen vegetables (such as peas) works well as a cold pack
		Massage Ice massage	Acute injury (duration, 72 h or less) Freeze water in paper cups; peel away paper at open end; massage affected area with circular movement 5–10 min; may repeat every 30–60 min

Surgical

Surgery, such as arthroscopy with débridement of the joint and removal of free cartilage fragments, osteotomy, and arthroplasty (joint replacement), may be indicated in advanced disease.

Complementary Therapy

- See Table 8–4 Summary of Complementary Therapies for Musculoskeletal Disorders at the end of this chapter.
- Glucosamine sulfate and chondroitin sulfate have been used by many patients with positive results. Research is not definitive.

Follow-up: See patient as needed for exacerbation of pain or dysfunction and to monitor for side effects of medications.

Sequelae: Tends to be a progressive disorder. Possible complications include crippling (generally no systemic complications occur); cervical vertebral lesions can lead to radicular neurologic problems; joint effusions, especially in knees; joint enlargement as disease progresses.

Prevention/prophylaxis: Prevention strategies include advising patient to lose weight if indicated and to maintain physical fitness to help maximize mobility.

Referral: Refer to, or consult with, surgeon, physical therapist, neurologist, or to chronic pain management clinic if patient is unable to achieve symptom management, when function and mobility continue to decline, or for intra-articular injection of corticosteroids during times of acute exacerbations.

Education: Explain disease process, signs and symptoms, and treatment (including side effects of medications). Discuss prevention strategies. Provide support. Explain body mechanics, muscle-strengthening, and ROM exercises. Educational resource materials are available from the American Academy of Family Physicians Foundation, PO Box 8418, Kansas City, MO 64114 (800-274-2237 ext. 4400) and the Arthritis Foundation, PO Box 7669, Atlanta, GA 30357-0669 (1-800-283-7800).

OSTEOPOROSIS

SIGNAL SYMPTOMS▶ Fracture of the hip may be the first sign.

Osteoporosis	ICD-9-CM: 733

Description: Osteoporosis is a heterogenous group of diseases resulting in a reduction in bone mass per unit volume below the level required for adequate mechanical support. It is usually caused by an imbalance between the rates of bone absorption and bone formation. The reduction in bone mass may ultimately lead to fractures, most frequently in the hip, spine, and wrist. Types of osteoporosis include postmenopausal, involutional, idiopathic, juvenile, and secondary.

Etiology: Although in many cases the cause is unknown or unclear, causes include decreased estrogen, excessive corticosteroid therapy, chronic heparin therapy, prolonged immobilization, thyrotoxicosis, Cushing's disease, malabsorption syndromes, renal tubular acidosis, rheumatoid arthritis, chronic liver or kidney disease, systemic mastocytosis, hyperparathyroidism, hyperthyroidism, and a variety of hypogonadal states.

Occurrence: Occurs in 30% to 40% of all women; 5% to 15% of all men.

Age: Incidence increases with age.

Gender: Twice as common in women than in men.

Ethnicity: More common in whites and Asians.

Contributing factors: Risk of osteoporosis increases with age; being female, white, and thin; and with menopause. Other factors include inadequate calcium and excessive phosphate and protein in the diet, immobilization, sedentary lifestyle, alcohol and caffeine use, cigarette smoking, chronic diseases, endocrinopathies, corticosteroids, excessive thyroid replacement, chronic heparin therapy, chemotherapy, loop diuretics, anticonvulsant therapy, tetracyclines, radiation therapy, suboptimal bone mass at maturity (familial fast bone losers).

Signs and symptoms: Most patients are symptomatic because they undergo slow reduction in their bone density.

- Back pain related to vertebral compression fractures (most common symptomatic presentation).
- Fracture of the hip (may be first indication of significant bone disease).

Diagnostic tests:

Test	Result Indicating Disorder	CPT Code
Alkaline phosphatase	May be transiently increased following fractures.	84075
Serum or urine protein electrophoresis	Aid in ruling out Autoimmune diseases	82664
Thyroid function tests	Results corresponding to hyperthyroidism and Cushing's syndrome may be found	84443 (TSH) 84479(T4 uptake) 84480 (T3)
Urinary free cortisol	Increased levels may be found	82530
Urine calcium	Usually normal	82340
Complete blood count	Normal in idiopathic osteoporosis	85025
Serum osteocalcin	Elevation indicates high turnover type	83937
Bone mineral density or dexa scan	Identifies bone mass, decrease bone density.	76075

(Continued)

Test	Result Indicating Disorder	CPT Code
X-ray studies	Show early changes of increased width of intervertebral spaces, relative accentuation of cortical plates, vertical striations of vertebral bodies; late changes of cortical plate fractures, vertebral compression, wedge and crush fractures, peripheral fractures at ends of long bones. Show decreased bone density; but may only be evident after a 40% loss.	70000 series of CPT codes includes x-ray studies. Chose site and then chose number corresponding to site.
Bone scan	May show increased uptake at previous fracture sites, otherwise negative	78102 (limited) 78103 (multiple)

TSH, thyroid-stimulating hormone.

Differential diagnosis:

- Vitamin D deficiency (laboratory results show low levels of vitamin D)
- Metastatic carcinoma (diffuse bone lesions on x-ray study; positive Bence Jones urine)
- Multiple myeloma (diffuse bone lesions on x-ray study; may have systemic symptoms
- Cortisol excess (laboratory studies show increase levels)
- OA (insidious, slow onset; peak intensity with use/relieved with no use; affects only one or a few)
- Primary hyperparathyroidism (muscle weakness, loss of appetite, deafness, weight loss)
- Paget's disease (bone pain, muscle cramps, impaired hearing, loss of height)

Treatment:

Pharmacologic

Calcium intake of 1500 g/day from all sources and vitamin D, 600 to 800 IU/day from all sources.

Hormone replacement therapy, such as estrogen for postmenopausal women (slows bone loss) or testosterone for hypogonadal men. For progressive disease, hormone replacement plus calcium supplementation (increase to 2000 mg/day). For women who are unable to take hormones, salmon calcitonin plus calcium supplementation may be required (prevents movement of calcium from bone to blood; calcitonin can stop bone loss and relieve pain from fractured bones; may also stimulate formation of new bone). Synthetic salmon calcitonin, 100 IU once a day, or synthetic salmon calcitonin nasal spray, 200 IU intranasally, 1 puff per day, alternating nostrils. Additionally, drugs that decrease rate of bone turnover may be used, such as Alendronate (Fosamax), 10 mg once a day or 70 mg once a week on an empty stomach; raloxifene (Eviston) 60 mg daily; or risedronate (Actonel) 5 mg daily.

Physical
Daily exercise, particularly weight-bearing activity such as walking, guided according to age and ability (the minimum to maintain bone strength is to walk for 50 minutes at a 3-mph pace five times a week). Reduce weight if overweight. Avoid high-protein diets.

Complementary Therapy
See Table 8–4 Summary of Complementary Therapies for Musculoskeletal Disorders at the end of this chapter.

Follow-up: See the patient monthly during initial treatment, then every 3 to 4 months thereafter. Perform annual screening such as gynecologic and breast examinations; mammography (for women patients); and annual bone-mineral density using same technique and instrument as for baseline measurement. Repeat x-ray studies of the spine every 3 years, more often when indicated for acute pain or suspected fractures. Perform peripheral bone x-ray studies if patient has acute pain.

Sequelae: In most patients, treatment will lead to skeletal stabilization or increase in bone mass; without treatment, disorder may progress to severe, disabling pain, and limitation of activities.

Prevention/prophylaxis: Prevention strategies include advising the patient of the importance of sufficient dietary intake of calcium. The aim is to achieve a total intake of 1000 mg of calcium by age 40 and total intake of 1500 mg of calcium after menopause (if not on hormone replacement therapy). Good sources of calcium include sardines, green vegetables, cheese, and skim milk. Other strategies include stopping smoking, avoiding excessive alcohol and caffeine intake, and maintaining regular exercise such as walking.

Referral: Refer to, or consult with, physician if patient has symptomatic back pain related to compression fractures or bleeding before the 12th day of progesterone therapy.

Education: Explain disease process, signs and symptoms, and treatment (including side effects of medications). Discuss prevention strategies and importance of regular follow-up, especially if patient is taking estrogen. Educational resource materials available from the National Osteoporosis Foundation, 2100 M Street, Suite 602, Washington, DC 20037 (Website: *www.nof.org*). Refer to Figure 8–1 for strategies to prevent osteoporosis.

SPRAINS, STRAINS

SIGNAL SYMPTOMS Swelling, pain, erythema, ecchymosis, tenderness, gait disturbances

| Sprains and Strains (general, unspecified site) | ICD-9-CM: 848.9 |

Description: A sprain is a complete or partial ligamentous injury, either within the body of the ligament or at the site of attachment to the bone

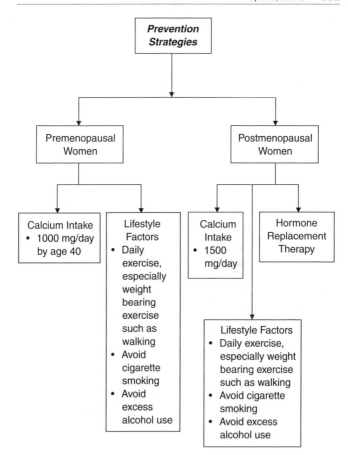

Figure 8–1. Osteoporosis prevention strategies.

such as at the wrist, elbow, and knee joints. Sprains may be classified as first-degree (ligament minimally torn, joint stable, influences physical performance for only few days); second-degree (more severe injury, ligament torn, joint stable, increased swelling and ecchymosis, warrants inactivity or modified activity for several weeks up to 2 months); and third-degree (complete tear of ligament, unstable joint, marked swelling and ecchymosis, pain, prolonged disability and inactivity).

A strain is an injury to the musculotendinous unit such as the hands and feet, knee, upper arm (biceps and triceps), thigh (quadriceps), ankle and the heel (Achilles). Strains may be acute or chronic and classified as first-degree (no gross disruption of the musculotendinous unit), second-degree (partial disruption of the musculotendinous complex), and third-degree (complete tendon or muscle tear).

Etiology:

Sprains: Usually caused by trauma, such as from falls, twisting injury, or motor vehicle accident.

Strains: Usually caused by overuse injuries or unusual activity, excessive exercise, or inadequate warm-up and stretching prior to activity.

Occurrence: Occurs in about 80% of all athletes at one point in their career.

Age: Occurs at any age.

Ethnicity: No significant ethnic predisposition.

Gender: Occurs in men more than in women.

Contributing factors: Improper shoe gear, improper or excessive athletic or physical training, overuse syndromes.

Signs and symptoms: Swelling, pain, erythema, ecchymosis, tenderness, gait disturbances. If severe, decreased ROM of joint and joint instability. In practice, it may be difficult to distinguish between sprains and strains. The following grading system is commonly used for sprains and strains:

- Grade I: Pain or tenderness without loss of motion.
- Grade II: Pain or tenderness; ecchymosis; some limitation in movement.
- Grade III: Pain or tenderness; ecchymosis; complete limitation of movement.

Diagnostic tests:

Test	Result Indicating Disorder	CPT code
X-ray study	For minor injuries; these are not indicated except to rule out fracture.	70000 series (70000–73725) for Musculoskeletal x-ray studies, CT scans, and MRI. Choose site then code specific to area
CT scan	Indicates swelling or tissue damage to area of injury	70000 series (70000–73725) for Musculoskeletal x-ray studies, CT scans, and MRI. Choose site then code specific to area
MRI	Indicates swelling or tissue damage to area of injury. Indicated if injury is severe or not healing.	70000 series (70000–73725) for Musculoskeletal x-rays, CT scans, and MRI. Choose site then code specific to area
Arthroscopy	Visualizes injury to site.	29830 elbow 29860 hip 29870 knee 29900 metacarpophalangeal joint 29805 shoulder 29800 temporomandibular joint 29840 wrist

Test	Result Indicating Disorder	CPT code
Rotary stress tests	Anterior drawer test: may show joint instability in severe cases Talar tilt test: decreased ROM and oain with movement Sequeze test: dull and aching to acute nd sharp when squeezed	95851 (ROM studies)

CT, computed tomography; MRI, magnetic resonance imaging; ROM, range of motion.

Differential diagnosis:

- Tendinitis (pain with movement of involved area)
- Bursitis (pain with pressure on affected area)
- Bony injuries and fractures (confirmed by x-ray, history of trauma)

Treatment:

Pharmacologic
NSAIDs such as ibuprofen, 400 mg orally three times a day as needed, or acetaminophen, 325 mg orally every 4 hours as needed.

Physical
RICE (rest, ice, compression, elevation) (Table 8–3) therapy (decreases swelling). Ice should be applied for 15 to 20 minutes every few hours; after 2 to 3 days, decrease frequency to 3 to 4 times per day. Immobilization or rest of affected area for 2 weeks. Splinting such as with an air cast type device (provides stability and pain relief). Crutches and crutch gait training. Physical therapy and rehabilitation.

Surgical
Surgical repair in cases of complete disruption.

Complementary Therapy
See Table 8–4 Summary of Complementary Therapies for Musculoskeletal Disorders at the end of this chapter.

Follow-up: See the patient in 2 weeks or sooner after injury for re-evaluation if pain and swelling do not decrease.

Sequelae: With appropriate treatment and rest, it may still take 6 to 8 weeks for recovery, depending on the severity of injury. A possible complication is reinjury.

Table 8–3 Rice Therapy

Rest	• Rest affected joint.
	• Reduce or revise exercise of activities of daily living, but do not eliminate them.
Ice	• Ice affected joint by applying cold during the acute phase to help reduce pain and swelling; apply ice 10–15 min every few hours for the first 2–3 days.
Compression	• Compress joint tissue by applying elastic bandages or basket-weave tape to help prevent or reduce swelling; provide support with a brace, tape, or cast.
Elevation	• Elevate the joint above the level of the heart to reduce dependent edema.

Prevention/prophylaxis: Prevention strategies include advising the patient to reduce activity; alter physical training; use arch supports, taping, bracing, or splinting; and perform adequate warm-up and conditioning prior to exercises or activity.

Referral: Refer to, or consult with, orthopedic specialist or surgeon if patient has first- or second-degree injury with little or no improvement or condition worsens in 2 to 3 weeks or immediately if patient has third-degree injury.

Education: Explain disease process, signs and symptoms, and treatment (including side effects of medications). Discuss prevention strategies. Review how to wrap with elastic bandage for compression. Teach crutch walking as necessary.

For First 24 Hours

Immediately after injury, stop all weight bearing; immobilize the affected area. Apply ice to injury as many times as possible a day for 20 minutes. Compression can be accomplished by using an Ace wrap to hold ice in place and after ice application to prevent swelling. Elevate the affected area above the level of heart.

After First 48 Hours (if pain and swelling are resolving normally)

Use hot and cold contrast baths (alternate between hot and cold water four times, ending with cold water; repeat procedure four times per day). Begin exercises, including isometric exercises.

After 2 Weeks (If No Further Problems)

Resistive exercises.

TENDINITIS

SIGNAL SYMPTOMS▶ Swelling and stiffness
Dull and aching pain; becomes acute and sharp when tendon is squeezed

Tendinitis	ICD-9-CM: 726.90

Description: Tendinitis is the inflammation or tear of a tendon, usually occurring at its point of insertion into bone or at the point of muscular origin. Sites frequently affected include the tendons of the rotator cuff around the shoulder, especially the supraspinatus, the elbow, the hand or wrist tendons, and the Achilles tendon.

Etiology: Usually related to repetitive activity or trauma; can occur without obvious cause.

Occurrence: Common. Tendinitis commonly occurs with bursitis.

Age: No significant age differentiation.

Ethnicity: No significant ethnic predisposition.

Gender: Occurs slightly more in men than in women.

Contributing factors: Repetitive activities, mechanical stress, degenerative and attritional changes. Professional athletes and manual laborers are especially prone. May be idiopathic.

Signs and symptoms:

- Swelling and stiffness (may have difficulty dressing, combing hair, reaching up).
- Pain overlying point of inflammation (dull and aching; becomes acute and sharp when tendon is squeezed). With shoulder, pain is initially localized to the area of the greater tuberosity and acromion process (supraspinatus tendon) and worsens with abduction and elevation of shoulder joint; with Achilles tendon, worsens with athletic activity.
- Mild erythema and increased heat of overlying skin, especially if superficial tendon is affected.

Diagnostic tests:

Thorough history and complete physical examination.

Test	Results Indicating Disorder	CPT Code
Metabolic studies	Usually normal	80053
X-ray studies	Plain film may show calcium deposits in the tendon	70000 series (70000-73725) for musculoskeletal x-ray studies, CT scans, and MRI. Choose site then code specific to area
Ultrasound	Shows swelling and inflammation on tendon.	76880 Arm 76880 Leg 76536 Neck 76856 Pelvis 76800 Spine
MRI	Confirms diagnosis; shows extent of injury; demonstrates tear or partial tear	70000 series (70000-73725) for musculoskeletal x-rays, CT scans, and MRI. Choose site then code specific to area
Arthrography	Visualizes extent of injury and may be able to be repaired.	73615 Ankle 73085 Elbow 73525 Hip 73580 Knee 73542 Sacroiliac joint 73040 Shoulder 70328 TMJ 73115 Wrist
Aspiration	Rules out infection, especially in wrist and hand Pathologic findings: Show degenerative changes in the tendon under microscopic examinations with presence of fibrinoid, mucoid, or hyaline degeneration of the connective tissue	20600 (small joint) 20605 (intermediate joint) 20610 (large joint)

CT, computed tomography; MRI, magnetic resonance imaging.

Differential diagnosis:

- Bursitis (frequently coexists) (pain with pressure on affected area)
- Septic arthritis (nongonococcal) (acute onset of joint pain and swelling with limited ROM and fever)
- Avulsion of the tendon (usually complete loss of function)
- Infectious tenosynovitis (fever, increased white blood cells)
- Rheumatoid arthritis (bilateral morning stiffness, + rheumatoid factor, redness, swelling in hands, wrists, symmetrical involvement, multiple joints.)
- Compartment syndrome (limb redness, swelling, pain, overlying skin may feel hard)
- A fracture (history of trauma, confirmed by x-ray study)

Treatment: Goals are to relieve pain, decrease inflammation, and increase flexibility. Rest of the affected joint is important.

Shoulder

Acetaminophen (Tylenol) or NSAIDs such as ibuprofen, 200 to 800 mg orally three or four times a day, not to exceed 2400 mg per day (for short-term use only); you may refer for glucocorticoid injection with 3 to 5 mg of Xylocaine and 40 mg of methylprednisolone (if symptoms are refractory after 10 to 14 days; never inject tendon, only into sheath or surrounding bursa); rest for 2 to 3 days; avoidance of overhead activities; ice packs to area for 15-20 minutes for the first few days (reduces pain and swelling); physical therapy after acute phase to strengthen shoulder muscles (pendulum exercise aids in joint mobility).

Hand and Wrist

NSAIDs, rest, and immobilization (splinting).

Achilles Tendon

Acute phase: NSAIDs, rest, and immobilization (plaster splinting). Chronic phase: NSAIDs, heel lift, ultrasound, heel cord stretching, and orthotics.

Complementary Therapy

See Table 8–4 Summary of Complementary Therapies for Musculoskeletal Disorders at the end of this chapter.

Follow-up: See the patient as needed; follow up with patient on progress during therapy. Patient may need MRI for repeated exacerbations of pain (confirms diagnosis and determines extent of attenuation of the tendon).

Sequelae: Possible complications include rupture or tear of tendon, which may require surgical repair.

Prevention/prophylaxis: Prevention strategies include advising the patient to obtain adequate rest and treatment and to use splints, such as circular bands for forearm extension tendinitis or patella tendinitis. Also, it is important to discontinue the use of NSAIDs as soon as possible.

Referral: Refer to, or consult with, physical therapist once acute episode has resolved to regain muscle and joint strength; to orthopedic specialist if patient has symptoms persisting beyond 2 months in spite of therapy.

Education: Explain disease process, signs and symptoms, and treatment (including side effects of medications). Review how to wrap with Ace bandage; teach crutch walking as necessary. Discuss prevention strategies. Counsel to expect mild discomfort with exercises (trying to stretch the joint capsule), but to do exercises for 5 to 10 minutes three to four times a day. If patient has steroid injection, tell patient that the injection may acutely worsen symptoms after anesthetic wears off, but that the patient will see improvement after 48 hours. Advise patient that injections are limited to every 6 to 12 months if needed.

Table 8–4 Complementary Therapy for Musculoskeletal Disorders

Disorder	Complementary Therapy
Bursitis	Acupuncture Relaxation methods as adjunct for pain relief
Carpel tunnel syndrome	Hatha yoga (controversial) Chamomile tea relieves stress, calms a nervous stomach, used for four centuries in Europe as a remedy for neuralgia, arthritis, insomnia. Drink three cups per day
Chronic pain	Yoga Massage Acupuncture Acupressure Relaxation methods as adjunct for pain relief Biofeedback
Fibromyalgia	Acupuncture Hypnosis Biofeedback Chiropractic medicine Tai chi
Gout	Relaxation methods as adjunct for pain relief Meditation Imagery
Meniscal tear	Relaxation methods as adjunct for pain relief
Osteoarthritis	Acupuncture Acupressure Massage Glucosamine sulfate and chondroitin sulfate have been used by many patients with positive results. Research is not definitive.
Osteoporosis	None recommended. Herbal remedies contain varying amounts of estrogen.

(Continued)

Table 8–4 Complementary Therapy for Musculoskeletal Disorders (Continued)

Disorder	Complementary Therapy
Rheumatoid arthritis	Blueberries, cherries and hawthorn berries are rich sources of flavonoid molecules, particularly proanthocyanidins, which exhibit membrane and collagen stabilizing, antioxidant anti-inflammatory properties. Ginger (eaten or in a tea) has demonstrated the ability to decrease joint pain and swelling in patients with RA. Ginger compresses have also been shown to benefit those with RA inflamed joints. Relaxation methods as adjunct for pain relief Imagery
Sprains, strains	Cold therapy Relaxation methods as adjunct for pain relief
Tendinitis	Acupuncture Relaxation methods as adjunct for pain relief

 Clinical Pearl: Complementary methods for chronic pain may be paid for by medical insurance

REFERENCES

General

Abenhaim, L, et al: The role of activity in the therapeutic management of low back pain: Report of the International Paris Task Force on Back Pain. Spine 15(Suppl 4):1S–33S, 2000.

Bagnell, D, and Gray, G: functional rehabilitation for low back pain: functional restoration and the lower extremity profile. SpineLine 2: 5–10, 2001.

Benson, LS: Orthopaedic Pearls. FA Davis, Philadelphia, 1999

Bigos, SJ, et al: Acute Low Back Problems in Adults. *Clinical Practice Guideline No 14.* Agency for Health Care Policy and Research (AHCPR), Rockville, Md, Pub.#95-0642, 1994.

Bull, CR (ed): Handbook of Sports Injuries. McGraw-Hill, New York, 1999.

Dambro, M (ed): Griffith's 5 Minute Clinical Consult. Lippincottt Williams & Wilkins, Baltimore, 2003.

Dunphy, LM, and Winland-Brown, JE: Primary Care: The Art and Science of Advanced Practice Nursing. FA Davis, Philadelphia, 2001.

Garfin, JM, and Garfin, SR: Low Back Pain: A Quick Guide to Exercise as Acute Therapy. Consultant March 42:350–353, 2002.

Goroll, A, and Mulley, A (eds): Primary Care Medicine, ed. 4. Lippincott Williams & Wilkins, Baltimore, 2000.

Griffin, MR, and Scheiman, JM: Prospects for changing the burden of nonsteroidal anti-inflammatory drug toxicity. American Journal of Medicine 110(Suppl 1A): 488–496, 2000:.

Griffith, HW: Instructions for Patients, ed. 6. W. B. Saunders, Philadelphia, 2000.

Grimsby, O: Evaluation Methods, Soft Tissue Work, Mobilization and Exercises. Ola Grimsby Institute, San Diego, 2000.

Isselbacher, KJ, et al (eds): Harrison's Principles of Internal Medicine, ed. 14. McGraw-Hill, New York, 2001.

Noble, J (ed): Primary Care Medicine, ed. 3. Mosby, St Louis, 2000.

Rakel, R (ed): Textbook of Family Practice, ed. 6. Saunders, Philadelphia, 2002.

Ruoff, G: Strategies to Control Chronic Musculoskeletal pain. Consultant October 39:2773–2781, 1999.

Sellers, R: Differential Diagnosis of Common Complaints, ed. 4. Saunders, Philadelphia, 2000.

Schnare, S: Evaluating and managing acute low back pain. Patient Care for the Nurse Practitioner January 3: 11–17, 1999.

Snyder, RK: Essentials of Musculoskeletal Care. American Academy of Orthopedic Surgeons, Illinois, 2000.

Staley, CA: Oral biphosphonates: Alendronate and risedronate. Women's Health in Primary Care 3(9):662–669, 2002.

Stitik, T, et al: Joint and soft tissue corticosteroid injections: A practical approach. Consultant 40:1469–1475, 2000.

Stitik, T, and Nadler, SF. Sports injuries: When—and how—to apply heat. Consultant 39:144–157, 1999.

Van Tulder, M, et al: Exercise therapy for low back pain: A systemic review within the framework of the cochrane collaboration back review. Spine 25:2784–2796, 2000.

Verst, A: Get in the game: Principles of the preparticipation physical. Advance for Nurse Practitioners August:66–68, 2000.

Wolfe, F, et al: The American College of Rheumatology 1990 Criteria for the Classification of Fibromyalgia: Report of the Multicenter Criteria Committee. Arthritis Rheum 33:160–172, 1990.

Woolf, J, et al (eds): Health Promotion and Disease Prevention in Clinical Practice. Williams & Wilkins, Baltimore, 2000.

Fibromyalgia

Auleciems, LM: Myofacial pain syndrome. Nurse Pract 20:18, 1995.

Clark, S, and Odell, L: Firomyalgia syndrome. Clinician Review 10::57–83.

Consensus Document on Fibromyalgia: The Copenhagen Declaration. Journal of Musculoskeletal Pain 1:295–312, 1993.

Osteoarthritis

Mann, M, and Meehan, N: Counseling seniors about physical activity. Advance for Nurse Practitioners 5(7):36, 1997.

Peck, B: Osteoarthritis treatment. Advance for Nurse Practitioners 4(7):32, 1996.

Ross, C: A comparison of osteoarthritis and rheumatoid arthritis. Nurse Pract 22(9):20, 1995.

Osteoporosis

Bonnick, SL: Intensive healing for brittle bones. Prevention 6:92, 1994.

Brager, R: Alendronate treatment option for osteoporosis. Advance for Nurse Practitioners 5(3):28, 1997.

Kessenich, CR: Breaking the osteoporosis cycle. Advance for Nurse Practitioners 4(8):16, 1996.

Maffie-Lee, J: Osteoporosis: Assessment, prevention and intervention. Clinical Excellence for Nurse Practitioners 1(3):221, 1997.

National Institutes of Health Consensus Development Program. Osteoporosis

Prevention, Diagnosis, and Therapy. Available at: http://odp.nih.gov/consensus/cons/111/111_intro.htm. Accessed, April, 2000.

NIH Consensus Development Panel: Optimum calcium intake. JAMA 272(24):1942, 1994.

Scheiber, LB, and Torregrosa, L: Postmenopausal osteoporosis: When—and how—to measure bone mineral density. Consultant 40: 781–789, 2000.

Rheumatoid Arthritis

Ruoff, G: Rheumatoid arthritis: Emerging treatments. Consultant 42:297–306, 2002.

Sprains and Strains

Onieal, ME: Common wrist and ankle injuries. Advance for Nurse Practitioners 4(8):30, 1996.

Tendinitis

Messer, RS. Bankers, RM. Evaluating and treating common upper extremity nerve compression and tendonitis syndrome...without becoming cumulatively traumatized. Nurse Practitioner Forum 6(3):152-166, 1995.

Chapter 9

PERIPHERAL VASCULAR DISORDERS

PERIPHERAL VASCULAR DISORDERS

SIGNAL SYMPTOMS ▸ Diminished or absent peripheral pulses
Pain, numbness, or tingling of lower extremities

PVD	ICD-9-CM: 443.9

Description: Peripheral vascular disorders (PVD) refer to a group of disorders that affect the blood flow of the arteries, veins, or both. PVD is an independent predictor of increased cardiovascular death. Symptoms of coronary artery disease (CAD) are present in 50% of cases on electrocardiogram, 90% of cases on coronary angiography, and 40% of cases on duplex evidence. Symptomatic PVD reveals a 30% risk of death within 5 years and almost 50% risk of death in 10 years from myocardial infarction (60%) or stroke (12%). The risks are more than doubled with severe disease that requires surgery. Asymptomatic patients with an ankle-brachial pressure index < 0.9 have a twofold to fivefold risk of fatal or nonfatal cardiovascular events.

PVD includes peripheral arterial disease (PAD) and chronic venous insufficiency (CVI). They result from the slow, insidious, and irreversible process of atherosclerosis.

Etiology: PAD results from the accumulation of fatty streaks and fibrous plaques in the arteries, trauma, decreased immune response, and increased coagulability, and it is a progressive, chronic disorder. Acute arterial occlusion results from a thrombosis or embolism regardless of the presence or absence of chronic PAD and is a life-threatening situation. CVI results from congenital absence, genetic defect, or damage to venous valves resulting in valvular incompetence and obstruction.

Occurrence: Incidence of PAD occurs in 20% of the general population; affects 2% of persons aged 40 to 60 years and 20% of persons greater than age 70. Incidence of CVI occurs in 20% of the general population.
Age: Primarily occurs in adults, specifically increased age.

Ethnicity: No significant ethnic predisposition.

Gender: PAD is more common in men than in women with a ratio of 2:1. CVI is more common in men who smoke and obese women; varicosities are more common in women than in men.

Contributing Factors:

PAD: Smoking, advanced age, atherosclerosis, diabetes, hypertension, hyperlipidemia, obesity, sedentary lifestyle, familial history of heart disease, hyperhomocystinemia, hypercoagulable states, and pregnancy.

CVI: Smoking, advanced age, atherosclerosis, diabetes, hypertension, hyperlipidemia, obesity, sedentary lifestyle, familial history of heart disease and deep vein thrombosis, hypercoagulable states, pregnancy, occupations requiring prolonged standing or sitting, varicosities, and oral contraceptives.

Signs and symptoms:

PAD: Symptoms of PAD are staged as: (I) asymptomatic, (II) intermittent claudication with cramping and burning exacerbated by exercise, (III) pain while resting, numbness, and aching in distal portions, and (IV) ulcers with blackened (necrotic) tissue on toes and heels with gangrenous odor. Ten percent of cases are asymptomatic, and 1% of cases present with critical leg ischemia. Five percent of cases present with gradual onset of intermittent claudication, cramping, or aching pain in the calf (most common), thigh, or buttock that increases with walking and relieved by rest along with ischemic rest pain (from tissue hypoxia caused by progressive arteriosclerosis). A comprehensive history determines risk factors and the etiology of leg pain in more than 90% of patients. The determination of walking distance in terms of street blocks before leg pain begins is crucial for diagnosis and therapy. Physical examination includes the 6 Ps (pain, pulselessness, pallor, paresthesia, paralysis, and poikilothermia), decreased or absent peripheral pulses, affected leg smaller in size due to muscular atrophy, thinning of the skin, loss of hair on toes and lower extremities, thickened nails, and possible leg ulcers. Acute arterial occlusion presents with sudden pain, numbness, coldness, tingling, absence of pulses, pallor, and weakness.

CVI: The patient presents with progressive, dependent edema, venous engorgement, localized pain, leg discomforts of pressure, burning, tingling, dull ache, or heaviness, non-healing ankle ulcers, and superficial varicosities. Physical examination reveals normal or diminished peripheral pulses, lipodermatosclerosis (capillary proliferation, fat necrosis, fibrosis of skin, and subcutaneous tissue), hyperpigmentation of reddish brown, brawny edema, and recurrent leg ulcers on the medial malleolus with possible thin scars of fibrotic tissue.

Diagnostic tests:

PAD:

Test	Result Indicating Disorder	CPT Code
Ankle-Brachial Pressure Index (ABPI)	0.6-0.9 = claudication; < 0.5 = severe ischemia (Normal values 0.9-1.1)	93922
Duplex ultrasonography	Degree of ischemia and stenosis of arteries	93922 Single level 93923 Multiple level
Doppler flow study	Severity of ischemia; locates vessel occlusion	93922
Doppler plethysmo-graphic	Changes in leg volume	93922 Single level 93923 Multiple level
Arteriography	Exact location and extent of occlusion	36140
Angiography	Decreased collateral flow and location of occlusion	73225 Upper extremity 73725 Lower extremity
Magnetic resonance imaging	Exact location and extent of arterial occlusion	73225 Upper extremity 73725 Lower extremity

CVI:

Test	Result Indicating Disorder	CPT Code
Duplex Doppler	Locates deep vein thrombosis	93970
Doppler bidirectional flow	Diminished venous flow and presence of thrombus	93970
Doppler flow-velocity	Diminished venous flow and presence of thrombus	93965
Photoplethysnography	Venous reflux of incompetent valves	93965
Outflow plethysmography	Venous reflux	93965

Differential diagnosis:

- Thrombosis (leg pain, tenderness, swelling generally in popliteal area)
- Congestive heart failure (bilateral edema, shortness of breath, more acute cardiac symptoms)
- Phlebitis (asymptomatic or dull ache, tight feeling or frank pain in calf or thigh, edema, fever, tachycardia)
- Polycythemia (increased red blood cell mass associated with smoking and hypertension)
- Anemia (decreased red blood cells associated with chronic infectious diseases)
- Raynaud's disease (small arteries and arterioles of the digits and skin)
- Buerger's disease (more common in men younger than age 30 who are heavy smokers, involves both upper and lower extremities, claudication of arch and calf)
- Aneurysms (common in men older than 50 years, pulsatile extremity mass or acute pain and bleeding)

- Peripheral neuropathy (sensory loss, muscular weakness, falling, unsteadiness)
- Chronic pernio (cold toes commonly seen in women with prior history of cold injury)

Treatment: The therapeutic goal is to improve the blood flow by removing or decreasing the cause of impaired circulation. Treatment focuses on lifestyle modifications and patient education as the conditions are chronic, irreversible processes.

PAD: Treatment focuses on symptomatic management with a daily walking program of 45 to 60 minutes for 6 months to resolve claudication. If the patient lacks motivation for walking, participation in a cardiovascular rehabilitation program for 6 months increases patient adherence. Lifestyle modifications are essential to control contributing factors, such as smoking cessation, reducing blood pressure, controlling diabetes, decreasing cholesterol levels, avoiding trauma to extremities, and maintaining good skin care with prompt treatment of ulcers. Pentoxifylline 400 mg orally three times a day with meals reduces blood viscosity and increases red blood cell flexibility. Aspirin 81 to 325 mg orally each day decreases platelet aggregation. Vasodilators are ineffective.

Complementary Therapy: Alternative therapies include use of antioxidants vitamins E and C to prevent oxidation of low density lipoprotein cholesterol; dietary supplements of fish oil and folic acid reduces homocysteine concentrations; and a diet rich in fish, fruit, vegetables, fiber, and low saturated fats (see the websites listed in Table 9-1 for more information).

CVI: Conservative therapy for CVI alleviates symptoms in approximately 85% of patients. Treatment focuses on lifestyle modifications, such as smoking cessation, low salt diet, losing weight if overweight, controlling edema by wearing below the

Table 9–1 Websites

Agency, Organization, Association	Website
American Heart Association	http://americanheart.org
American Whole Health, Integrative Medicine	http://wholehealthmd.com
Health Finder	http://healthfinder.gov
Mayo Clinic	http://mayoclinic.com
National Center for Complementary and Alternative Therapies	http://nccam.nih.gov
National Health Information Center	http://health.gov/NHIC
National Heart, Lung, and Blood Institute	http://nhlbi.nih.gov/health
Society of Cardiovascular and International Radiology	http://scvir.org
US Preventive Services Task Force	http://hstat.nlm.nih.gov

knees support or compression stockings, elevating extremities, performing light exercise, avoiding constrictive clothing, and avoiding long periods of sitting or standing. Maintaining skin care is essential through daily inspection of feet and extremities for sores or abrasions, avoid being barefoot, wear well-fitting shoes, and use care in trimming nails. Stasis ulcers require bed rest, leg elevation, intermittent moist dressings of saline, and an Unna boot (semirigid boot of calamine, lotion, glycerin, zinc oxide, and gelatin to increase blood flow) that is changed weekly or more frequently depending on the ulcer drainage. Approximately 8% of patients require surgical intervention for discomfort or ulcer refractory.

Follow-up: See the patient every 3 to 6 months to assess effectiveness of walking program on distance and pain, skin care and lifestyle modifications, such as nutrition and smoking. Frequency for follow-up of ulcers depends on stage and status of ulceration and patient adherence to therapeutic regimen.

Sequelae: Potential complications include deep vein thrombosis, leg ulcers, and amputation. Approximately 12.2% of patients with PVD require amputation within 5 years and patients with diabetes have increased risk of 50%. Patients with CVI are at risk for myocardial infarction, stroke, angina, congestive heart failure, and a life-threatening infection. The predicted mortality for patients with claudication at 5, 10, and 15 years are 30%, 50%, and 70%, respectively.

Prevention/prophylaxis: Prevention strategies include lifestyle modification, specifically smoking cessation, walking program, weight loss, reduction of factors that increase atherosclerosis, and tight control of diabetes.

Referral: Refer or consult vascular surgeon immediately for evaluation and treatment of acute arterial occlusion; refer for extensive evaluation of PVD and possible surgical procedures, such as skin grafts for ulcers.

Education: Teach disease process, signs and symptoms of disease especially life-threatening problems, lifestyle modifications, treatment regimen, and side effects of drugs, specifically pentoxifylline, such as dizziness, headache, nausea, vomiting, and upset stomach.

RAYNAUD'S PHENOMENON

SIGNAL SYMPTOMS ▶   Intermittent, bilateral, spontaneous digital vasoconstriction
Triphasic: Pallor (blanching), cyanosis, and rubor or hyperemia (intense redness)

Raynaud's phenomenon	ICD-9-CM: 443.0

Description: Raynaud's disease or primary Raynaud's phenomenon (PRP) is paroxysmal vasoconstriction of the fingers or toes with mild to minimal discomfort. Secondary Raynaud's phenomenon (SRP) presents with more frequent episodes of vasoconstriction of the total digit and sensory symptoms that result in digital ulceration or gangrene.

Etiology: The etiology of PRP is unknown (idiopathic), and a cutaneous ischemia or exaggerated normal physiological response to exposure of cold temperatures or emotional stress. It is a common occurrence, accounts for 50% of all cases, and presents with a familial history in 20% to 30% of cases to suggest a genetic defect. PRP is a vasospastic phenomenon that involves increased sensitivity of the alpha$_2$-adrenergic receptors in the digital vessels that is not disabling. PRP is frequently associated with other vasospastic syndromes, such as migraine headaches and atypical angina.

SRP is generally a manifestation of an underlying systemic process, such as connective tissue disease, trauma, occlusive vascular disease, or abnormal blood flow. It is estimated that 30% of persons with scleroderma or Sjögren's syndrome are more likely to develop SRP. Structural disease is almost always present that creates an ischemic crisis when vasospasm is superimposed. Irreversible obstruction of the vessel lumen may occur with fibrin deposition, platelet activation and aggregation, and clotting. The total obstruction to blood flow causes intense ischemic pain and becomes irreversible in time.

Occurrence: Incidence in the United States is estimated to be 3% to 20% of the population.

Age: PRP primarily occurs in people before the age of 30 and is associated with a teenage onset. SRP usually affects people over age 25.

Ethnicity: No significant ethnic predisposition.

Gender: PRP is more common in women than men, with a ratio of 2:1. SRP occurs equally in men and women.

Contributing factors: The most common factor is smoking, potent vasoconstrictor. Other factors include any existing autoimmune or connective tissue disorder, such as scleroderma, systemic lupus erythematosus (SLE), Sjögren's syndrome, dermatomyositis, mixed connective tissue diseases, rheumatoid arthritis, stress, chronic exposure to extremes in cold temperatures, injury to hands and fingers, vibrating tool use, chronic exposure to repetitive wrist and finger motion, carpal tunnel syndrome, hyperviscosity status, paraproteinemia, cryoglobulinemia, and certain medications, such as nonselective beta blockers, ergotamine preparations, interferon, various chemotherapeutic agents, unopposed estrogen, oral contraceptives, nicotine, caffeine, and various over-the-counter antihistamines and decongestants.

Signs and symptoms:

PRP: Bilateral pallor of fingertips (rarely in thumb) with cold exposure, followed by cyanosis, then redness and pain with warming (white, blue, and red).

SRP: Usually unilateral involvement of total digits with pallor, cyanosis, rubor, intense, throbbing pain, paresthesia, stiffness, diminished sensation, and slight swelling. Attacks terminate spontaneously or with warming and no abnormal findings between attacks. As the disease progresses, the complication sclerodactyly occurs in 10% of all cases and is characterized by tight, white, thick, smooth, and shiny skin over affected digits. Atrophy of terminal fat pads and digital skin with ulceration progresses to autoamputation in severe, prolonged cases (10% of all cases). Physical examination includes pulses, bruits, and signs of ischemia and is generally normal when patient symptoms are not present. Digital pitting scars may be visible.

Diagnostic tests

Diagnosis is largely determined by a history of the three symptoms present with exposure to cold and clinical judgment. A cold challenge test for characteristic color changes is unnecessary and painful. In SRP, a nailfold capillary test shows enlarged, irregular capillary loops under a microscope after placing a drop of oil at the base of the fingernail.

Tests for Secondary Raynaud's Phenomenon	Result Indicating Disorder	CPT Code
Arterial Doppler ultrasonography	Rules out proximal vascular disease, such as occult ulnar artery occlusion	93922
Complete blood count (CBC)	Elevated levels indicate inflammatory process of connective tissue disease	850107
Erythrocyte sedimentation rate (ESR)	Elevated levels indicate inflammatory process of connective tissue diseases	85652
Antinuclear antibodies (ANA)	Presence of autoimmune or connective tissue disease	86038

Differential diagnosis

- Thromboangiitis obliterans (Buerger's disease in younger men who smoke, diminished or absent peripheral pulses, inflammatory occlusion of extremities, intermittent claudication, asymmetric changes, digital foot pale, cold, and rubor)
- Rheumatoid arthritis (palmar erythema, vasculitis, warm, swollen joints)
- Scleroderma (tight, puffy digits, thickened skin, loss of normal folds, telangiectasia pigmentation, fingertip ulceration, subcutaneous calcification)

- SLE ("butterfly" rash, fingertip lesions, periungual erythema, splinter hemorrhages)
- Carpal tunnel syndrome (numbness, burning and pain along median nerve, aching pain radiates to forearm, positive Tinel's sign)
- Thoracic outlet syndrome (pain from brachial plexus compression to hand, paresthesia, weakness, muscle atrophy, pallor of fingers on elevation of limb, sensitivity to cold, edema, cyanosis, engorgement)
- Cryoglobulinemia (palpable purpura on lower extremities)
- Acrocyanosis (persistent, permanent, diffuse coldness and cyanosis regardless of temperatures)
- Polycythemia (generalized pruritus with warm water)
- Frostbite (white or yellow skin, loss of mobility, elasticity)
- Livedo reticularis (purplish, netlike pattern on extremities)
- Effect of certain medications (variety of rashes, pallor, pruritus)

Treatment

Symptomatic

Symptom management or lifestyle modification is the focus of treatment for PRP as 30% to 60% of patients respond positively to smoking cessation, avoid exposure to cold, and practice effective stress management. Follow smoking cessation guidelines and assist the patient to set a stop smoking date. Avoid exposure to cold by dressing warmly in layers, wear socks, shoes, wristlets, gloves, hand warmers, or electric gloves, and use mittens or pot holders in handling foods in a refrigerator or deep freeze. Stress management includes relaxation techniques, deep breathing, visualization, counseling, biofeedback, meditation, and music. Patients need to avoid bruises and trauma to fingertips, aggravating factors, such as repetitive hand and finger motion and use of vibrating tools, and certain medications (beta blockers, amphetamines, ergot preparations, alkaloids, and sumatriptan). Alternative therapies include dietary supplements, such as vitamin E (fruits, vegetables, seeds, and nuts), magnesium (seeds, nuts, fish, beans, and dark green vegetables), and fish oils. Herbs include peony, dong quai, cayenne, ginger, and prickly ash.

Pharmacologic

Nifedipine 30 to 120 mg daily (sustained release form) is first-line treatment, especially during the winter months and offers improvement in 75% of patients with primary disease. However, symptomatic response does not always correlate with objective improvement. Other vasodilators are used with success alone or in combination with calcium blockers, such as nitroglycerin, nitroprusside, hydralazine, papaverine, and phentolamine. In ischemia crisis, vasodilators may have adverse effect by shunting blood away from the ischemic digits and into healthy vessels that easily dilate. Consult with collaborative physician.

Oral prostaglandins are under study because of their potent vasodilatation effect and inhibition of platelet aggregation. Severe SRP and digital ulcers are treated by prostaglandin E_1 (PGE_1), prostacyclin (PGI_2) and iloprost (PGI_2 analog). A referral to specialist is mandatory.

Surgical

Digital sympathectomy provides long-lasting benefits in healing digital ulcers in selected cases. Cervical sympathectomy is considered a "last-ditch option" and not recommended because of high recurrence rate. Dry, gangrenous digits are allowed to autoamputate with surgical amputation reserved for patients with intractable pain or superinfection.

Follow-up: See patient as needed for smoking cessation, stress management, and management of fingertip ulcers, including rapid treatment of infection and application of finger guards over ulcerated fingertips. Observe for signs of associated illnesses as Raynaud's may precede overt development of other conditions by as much as 11 years.

Sequelae: PRP is stable in about 38% of cases, 36% of cases improve, and 16% of cases worsen. Possible complications of SRP include gangrene and autoamputation of the fingertips and worsening of autoimmune or connective tissue diseases.

Prevention/prophylaxis: Prevention strategies include the lifestyle modifications given in symptomatic treatment.

Referral: Refer or consult with a vascular surgeon immediately for a vasospastic event when severe pain or vascular compromise is present.

Education: Teach disease process, signs and symptoms, lifestyle modifications, treatment, and side effects of medications, such as hypotension, dizziness, and headache with use of nifedipine.

THROMBOPHLEBITIS (DEEP VEIN THROMBOSIS)

SIGNAL SYMPTOMS▶ Unilateral swelling, warmth, tenderness, and erythema along the peripheral vein, pain, fever

Thromobophlebitis, phlebitis (superficial vessels, lower extremities)	ICD-9-CM: 451.0
(Deep vessels, lower extremities)	ICD-9-CM: 451.19
Varicose veins	ICD-9-CM:: 454.0

Description: Thrombophlebitis is an inflammation of the vein that usually occurs in the lower extremities. Deep vein thrombosis (DVT) is the development of single or multiple blood clots within the deep veins of the extremities or pelvis.

Etiology: Common cause is primary or secondary hypercoagulability and often complicated by venous stasis or injury to the vessel wall. Septic or suppurative thrombophlebitis results secondary to infection from an iatrogenic cause, such as insertion of an intravenous (IV) catheter.

Occurrence: Common, with more than 2 million cases per year of DVT. Superficial thrombophlebitis accounts for 10% of all nosocomial infections. The incidence of catheter-related thrombophlebitis is 88/100,000.

Age: Incidence increases with age.

Ethnicity: No significant ethnic predisposition.

Gender: Occurs more commonly in women than in men.

Contributing factors: General risk factors include age, immobility, surgery, and advancing age with greater risks after age 40. Inherited risk factors are antithrombin III deficiency and protein culture and sensitivity deficiency. Acquired risk factors include prior DVT, stroke, lupus anticoagulant, cancer, stasis, obesity, varicose veins, pregnancy, postpartum, use of oral contraceptives or estrogen, insertion of IV catheters, infection, long bone trauma, crushing injury, increased blood viscosity due to high altitude, and paroxysmal nocturnal hemoglobinuria. Septic phlebitis occurs secondary to indwelling IV catheter.

Signs and symptoms:

Thrombophlebitis: Swelling, tenderness, induration, pain, erythema along the course of the vein, and fever (70% of patients). In superficial thrombophlebitis, edema and deep calf tenderness are absent.

DVT: Approximately 50% of cases are asymptomatic in the early stages. Usually unilateral, limb swelling, dull ache, tight feeling, or frank pain in calf that worsens with standing and walking and relieved by rest, the presence of Homans' sign (40 % of the time), fever, and tachycardia. Palpable tender cord in affected limb and warmth or redness of skin is less common. Swelling of the affected extremity should be documented by measurement.

Diagnostic tests:

Test	Result Indicating Disorder	CPT Code
Duplex Doppler ultrasonography	Locates thrombosis (high sensitivity, specificity, and repeatability)	93970 Bilateral 93971 Unilateral or limited
Impedence plethysmography	Proximity of thrombosis to calf veins (sensitivity and specificity, 90%)	93965
Prothrombin (PT)	Coagulation factors	85210

Differential diagnosis:

- Lymphedema (unilateral swelling, generally chronic and painless)
- Calf muscle strain or contusion (difficult to differentiate from DVT, use serial duplex Doppler ultrasound)
- Cellulitis (an associated wound, inflammation of skin)
- Arterial occlusion (more painful, absent digital pulses, no swelling, superficial veins in foot fill slowly when emptied)
- Bilateral leg edema (related to heart, kidney, or liver disease)

Treatment: Treatment depends on etiology and includes management of the underlying condition.

Superficial thrombophlebitis: Heat and elevation of the extremity may suffice. Anticoagulation therapy of warfarin (Coumadin) may be necessary with anticoagulation effects beginning 3 to 5 days after initiation. Warfarin dosages are correlated to a therapeutic prothrombin (PT), which is 1.5 to 2 times the control or 15 to 17 seconds. An international normalized ratio (INR) with a target of 2.0 to 3.0 is used. Nonsteroidal anti-inflammatory drugs (NSAIDs) are used for pain. Smoking cessation is critical along with bed rest with bathroom privileges for 3to 5 days.

DVT (except DVT confined to calf): Therapy goals are to restore venous and valvular function and prevent pulmonary embolus. Hospital admission is essential for aggressive IV anticoagulation therapy of heparin and monitoring of signs for further thrombosis or bleeding. Pharmacologic management includes initial IV bolus of heparin (5000 to 10,000 units), followed by a continuous infusion at 1000 units per hour. Dosage adjustment is based on partial thromboplastin time (PTT) with a goal to achieve a PTT that is two times the control value. Begin warfarin (Coumadin) therapy 1 to 5 days after initiation of heparin in a single daily dose beginning at 5 to 10 mg orally daily, titrating to achieve a therapeutic PT, which is 1.5 to 2 times the control or 15 to 17 seconds. An international normalized ratio (INR) with a target of 2.0-3.0 is used. If anticoagulant or thrombolytic therapy is contraindicated, filtering devices such as an "umbrella" may be used to trap emboli before reaching the lungs. Moist heat relieves pain and swelling. Leg elevation with slight flexion of the knees at 15 to 20 degrees is essential with significant leg edema. The duration of bed rest is determined by extent of leg edema.

Septic thrombophlebitis: On hospital admission, initiate antibiotic therapy with a semisynthetic penicillin, such as nafcillin 2 g IV every 4 hours plus an aminoglycoside (gentamicin 2 mg/kg IV every 8 hours), along with anticoagulant therapy.

Follow-up: See the patient in 48 hours because most patients with DVT require hospitalization. For the first episode of DVT, continue warfarin therapy for 3 to 6 months; for subsequent episodes, treat the patient for at least 1 year. For patients on daily warfarin therapy, see the patient until target PT range is achieved, then see patient monthly while on medication.

Sequelae: The more common and serious complication for DVT is pulmonary emboli. About 50% of untreated, proximal (above-the-calf) DVTs progress to pulmonary emboli with 30% mortality. Identified and treated cases of pulmonary emboli result in 2% mortality. Superficial thrombophlebitis may progress to DVT. Treatment may induce hemorrhage or chronic venous insufficiency, a late complication avoided with the thrombolytics used in acute therapy.

Prevention/prophylaxis: Prevention strategies depend on the underlying condition and include identification of risk factors for the development of thrombus. Prevention strategies for patients include

- Avoid prolonged immobility
- Avoid trauma to extremities
- Smoking cessation (especially with oral contraceptive pills)
- Wear elastic stockings
- Avoid constrictive leg wear, such a knee-high hose
- Avoid crossing legs while sitting
- Move legs as much as possible if confined to bed
- Decrease or discontinue estrogen or oral contraceptive pills
- Avoid using any IV medications
- Signs and symptoms of potential complications and when to seek medical care

Provide early interventions, avoid low or extremity cannulation, and for surgical patients, provide active prophylaxis, intermittent mechanical compression therapy, use of support or compression stockings, and early ambulation after surgery. Ensure proper maintenance of IV therapy, including insertion under aseptic conditions, replacement of IV catheter every 48 to 72 hours, and use of a small cannula, such as a scalp vein needle.

Referral: Refer or consult with vascular surgeon for patient with DVT or varicosities.

Education: Teach the disease process, signs and symptoms, treatment, medication side effects, prevention strategies, and when to seek medical care. Advise the patient on anticoagulants to avoid food fads, crash diets, marked changes in eating habits, avoid alcohol consumption, vitamins (especially vitamin E), cold medicines, antibiotics, aspirin, cimetidine, thyroid hormones, mineral oil, or NSAIDs without a healthcare provider's consent.

REFERENCES

General

Barton, S (ed.): Clinical Evidence: The International Source of the Best Available Evidence for Effective Health Care, ed. 5. BMJ Publishing, London, 2001

Collins, KA, and Sumpio, BE   Vascular assessment. *Clin Podiatr Med Surg,* 17:171–189, 2000.

Cotter, VT, and Strumpf, NE (eds): Advanced Practice Nursing with Older Adults. McGraw-Hill, New York, 2002.

Dains, JE, et al: Advanced Health Assessment and Clinical Diagnosis in Primary Care. Mosby, St. Louis, 1998.

Dunphy, LM, and Winland-Brown JE: Primary Care: The Art and Science of Advanced Practice Nursing. F. A. Davis, Philadelphia, 2001.

Samuelson, B, and Norton, VC: Diagnosis and treatment of peripheral vascular disease: The key in evaluating symptomatic patients is determining if acute life-threatening ischemia is present. *Emerg Med* 31:54, 59–60, 63–64, 1999.

Saski, S, et al: Current trends in thromboangiitis obliterans (Burger's disease) in women. *Am J Surg* 177:316–320, 1999.

Stanley, M, and Beare, PG (eds.): Gerontological Nursing: A Health Promotion/Protection Approach, ed. 2. F. A. Davis, Philadelphia, 1999.

Stein, JH (ed.). (1998). Internal Medicine, ed. 5. Mosby, St. Louis, 1998.

Uphold, CR, and Graham, MV: Clinical Guidelines in Family Practice, ed. 3. Barrmarrae Books, Gainesville, Fla., 1998.

US Preventive Services Task Force Screening for asymptomatic coronary artery disease. Guide to Clinical Preventive Services, ed. 2.Washington, DC, U.S. Government Printing Office, 1996. Retrieved December 22, 2001, from http://hstat.nlm.nih.gov/ftrs/pick/collect=cps&dbName=0&cc=1&t=1009200137

US Public Health Service: Put Prevention ito Practice: Clinician's Handbook of Preventive Services, ed. 2. International Medical Publishers, McLean, Vir., 1997.

Zafar, MU, et al: A practical approach to lower-extremity arterial disease. Patient Care 34(10):96–98, 101–104, 109–112.

Peripheral Vascular Disorders

Braum, CM, et al: Components of an optimal exercise program for the treatment of patients with claudication. Journal of Vascular Nursing 17(2):32–36, 1999.

Ciocon, JO, et al: Common and challenging vascular disorders in the elderly. Clin Geriatr 7(3):25–27, 31–32, 1999.

Gibson, JM, and Kenrick, M: Pain and powerlessness: The experience of living with peripheral vascular disease. Journal of Advanced Nursing, 27:737–745, 1998.

Goodall, SG: Peripheral vascular disease. Nursing Standard 14(25):48–54, 2000.

Harvard Medical School Family Health Guide: Peripheral Vascular Disease, 2001. Retrieved December 22, 2001, from http://www.health.haravrd.edu/fhg/doctor/PVD.shtml

Lamaitre Vascular, Inc: Peripheral Vascular Disease: Glossary, Words that Doctors Love to Use, 2001. Retrieved December 22, 2001, from http://lemaitre.com/patient/glossary.html

Lubisch, K: Management of Peripheral Vascular Disease and Pressure Sores. Wild Iris Continuing Education, 2001. Retrieved December 22, 2001, from http://www.nursingceu. com/NCEU/courses/web

Podnos, YD, and Williams, RW: Chronic venous insufficiency. eMedicine Journal 2(11), 2001. Retrieved December 22, 2001, from http:www.emedicine.com/med/topic391.htm

Rowe, VL: Peripheral arterial occlusive disease. eMedicine Journal 2(7), 2001. Retrieved December 22, 2001, from http:www.emedicine.com/med/topic391.htm

Society of Cardiovascular & International Radiology: Peripheral Vascular Disease (PVD). Retrieved December 22, 2001, from http://scvir.org.patient.pcl./page10.htm

Tierney, S, et al: Secondary prevention of peripheral vascular disease. BrMed J 320:1262–1265, 2000.

Virtual FairPeripheral Vascular Disease. Retrieved December 22, 2001, from http://www.vfair.com/conditions.peripheral_vascular_disease.htm

Raynaud's Syndrome

Arthritis Society: Raynaud's Phenomenon. Retrieved December 22, 2001, from http://www.arthritis.ca/types%20of%20arthritis/raynauds%20phenomenon/mode=static

Carson-DeWitt, RS: Raynaud's disease. The PDR Encyclopedia of Medicine, 2001. Retrieved December 22, 2001, from http://www.ahealthyme.com/article/gale/100083960

Fraenkel, L, et al: The associations between plasma levels of von Willebrand Factor and fibrinogen with Raynaud's phenomenon in men and women. Am J Med 108:583–586, 2000.

McGrath, A: Raynaud's syndrome. American Journal of Nursing 97(1):34, 1997.

National Heart, Lung, and Blood Institute: Facts about Raynaud's Phenomenon. Retrieved December 22, 2001, from http://www.nhlbi.gov/health/pubic/blood/other/raynaud.htm.

Raynaud's and Scleroderma Association: Raynaud's. Retrieved December 22, 2001, from http://www.raynaud's.demon.co.uk/raynauds.htm

Surgical-tutor.org.uk: Raynaud's disease. Retrieved December 22, 2001, from http://surgical-turuo.org.uk/system/vascuular/raynauds.htm

Wigley, FM: Raynaud's phenomenon: How to give cold comfort this winter. Consultant 39:540–549, 1999.

Thrombophlebitis

American Heart Association: Thrombolysis, Thrombosis, Thrombus, and Embolus. Retrieved December 22, 2001, from http://www.americanheart.org/presenter.jhtmlidentifer=4745

Brown, CE, et al: Puerperal septic thrombophlebitis: Incidence and response to heparin therapy. Am J Obstet and Gynecol 181(1): 143–148, 1999.

Macklin, D: Removing a PICC. American Journal of Nursing 100(1):52–54, 2000.

Mayo Clinic: Thrombophlebitis. Retrieved December 22, 2001, from http://www.mayoclinic.com/findinformation/diseasesandconditions/invoke.cfmid=DSOO;

Chapter 10
CENTRAL AND PERIPHERAL NERVOUS SYSTEM DISORDERS

BELL'S PALSY

SIGNAL SYMPTOMS ▶ Includes facial paralysis or weakness, mild numbness on affected side, flat nasolabial fold, sagging of eyebrow, inability to close eye, mouth droop, excessive or decreased lacrimation, impairment of taste, loss of ipsilateral blink reflex, and earache. Pain behind the ear may precede paralysis.

Bell's palsy (idiopathic facial paralysis)	ICD-9-CM: 351.0

Description: Bell's palsy is characterized by acute, unilateral facial muscle weakness or paralysis as the result of cranial nerve VII (facial nerve) inflammation and swelling of the nerve within the facial canal. Eighty percent of patients recover within a few weeks to a month. Recovery depends on severity of the lesion.

Etiology: May have viral etiology, such as herpes simplex type I or HIV, or a bacterial etiology, such as syphilis or Lyme disease. Commonly postinfectious (e.g., upper respiratory infection [URI]) secondary to nerve compression from edema. Idiopathic.

Occurrence: Occurs in approximately 23 out of 100,000 people.

Age: Occurs at any age; more common over age 30.

Ethnicity: No significant ethnic predisposition.

Gender: Occurs equally in men and in women.

Contributing factors: Recent upper respiratory viral infection, exposure to cold, familial occurrence, diabetes (fourfold increase in incidence), pregnancy

Signs and symptoms: Onset usually acute (48 hours) but may occur over several days. Symptoms are usually unilateral. If bilateral, consider chronic meningitis or Guillain-Barré syndrome.

Diagnostic tests: None, unless needed to rule out differential diagnosis,

Tests	Result Indicating Disorder	CPT Codes
Lumbar puncture	To rule out Guillain Barré syndrome. A mild increase in lymphocytes and mononuclear clear cells in the cerebrospinal fluid (CSF) may occur in some cases.	62270
Computerized tomo- graphic (CT) scan	To rule out masses, tumors or growths	70450 without contrast 70460 with contrast
Magnetic resonance imaging (MRI)	To rule out masses, tumors or growths	70544 without contrast 70545 with contrast
Chest x-ray (CXR) study	Possible sarcoidosis	71030
Electromyography (EMG)	To determine disease progression and predict prognosis.	95867
Erythrocyte sedi- mentation rate (ESR)	May be elevated	85652
Lyme titer	To rule out Lyme disease	86617
Serum glucose	May be elevated	82947

Differential diagnosis:
- Temporal bone fracture (check x-ray study)
- Tumor (check imaging, biopsy-pathology report)
- Meningitis (fever, stiff neck, lumbar puncture): increased cell count, high globulin, positive culture
- Guillain-Barré syndrome (ascending motor weakness with pain in back and limbs, headache, numbness)
- Otitis media (fever, pain, rhinorrhea, swollen lymphs)
- Multiple sclerosis (ataxia, intention tremor, nystagmus, scanning speech)
- Lyme disease (red macular skin lesions after tick bite)
- Acoustic neuroma (imaging)

Treatment:
Pharmacologic
Methylcellulose eye drops; may need to tape eye shut, especially at night. Steroids such as methylprednisolone (reduces inflammation and edema). Must be started at onset; ineffective if started more than 10 days after onset. Prednisone, 80 mg for 3 days; then 60 mg for 3 days, 40 mg for 3 days, 20 mg for 3 days; then discontinue. May consider acyclovir 400 mg 5 times a day for 10 days.
Mild analgesics.

Nonpharmacologic
Heat and massage therapy for weakened muscles. Facial exercises for 5 minutes three or four times a day after acute phase.

Follow-up: See patient 3 or 4 days after onset, then monthly for 6 to 12 months to assess recovery and presence of corneal abrasion or ulceration. Physical therapy may be initiated after acute phase.

Sequelae: Eighty percent of patients recover in a few weeks to 2 months. Some patients may never recover or may have only partial recovery. May develop corneal abrasion or ulceration. Occasional facial nerve atrophy. Symptoms usually resolve in 3 to 4 weeks.

Prevention/prophylaxis: None. Facial exercises to prevent muscle atrophy. Eye care and protection to prevent corneal abrasion or ulceration.

Referral: Refer to, or consult with, neurologist for steroid use or need for further studies.

Education: Explain disease process, signs and symptoms, and treatment (including side effects of medications). Instruct patient in eye care, comfort measures, necessity of chewing food with unaffected side, and importance of effective oral care and exercise.

BRAIN CANCER

SIGNAL SYMPTOMS Varies with the location and growth rate of the specific neoplasm. Four classic signs and symptoms include early morning headache, nausea, vomiting, and papilledema.

Brain cancer	ICD-9-CM: 191.0

Description: Brain cancer consists of primary neoplasms (originate in the brain) or secondary neoplasms (originate from sites other than the brain) located within the intracranial vault. About half of the primary tumors are gliomas, with astrocytomas grades III and IV (glioblastoma multiform) occurring most frequently. Secondary tumors are commonly metastatic lesions from lung, breast and malignant melanoma. Secondary tumors occur more frequently than primary tumors.

Etiology: Unknown; however, genes and viruses, as well as environmental exposure to ionizing radiation, may be possible causes. Cellular phone use continues to be studied as a possible cause of brain cancer. To date, there is no evidence to support this theory.

Occurrence: Approximately 18,000 primary and 24,000 secondary tumors occur each year.

Age: Can occur at any age; however, some neoplasms occur more often in specific age groups. Children tend to have posterior fossa neoplasms such as astrocytoma grade I or II of the cerebellum. In adults, the most common neoplasm is the highly malignant glioblastoma multiform.

Ethnicity: No significant ethnic predisposition; however, some studies suggest that brain cancer affects whites more than blacks.

Gender: Occurs equally in men and in women; however, meningiomas are found more often in women, and gliomas more often in men.

Contributing factors: None known.

Signs and symptoms: Vary with the location and growth rate of the specific neoplasm. Three classic signs and symptoms are as follows:

Headache: Initially mild and occurs on awakening; tends to dissipate after assuming an upright position. With increased tumor growth, headache becomes more severe and constant; increases with bending, stooping, or coughing; and may awaken patient during sleep.

Nausea and vomiting: Seen more often in children; vomiting may or may not be preceded by nausea and tends to be projectile.

Papilledema: Seen in a small number of patients (about 10%); is more common in children; may cause visual disturbances such as amaurosis fugax (temporary blindness, usually associated with transient ischemic attacks [TIAs]).

Other signs and symptoms may include focal or localized signs and symptoms such as anosmia and diplopia. Approximately 30% of adults with intracranial tumors develop generalized or focal seizure activity.

Diagnostic tests:

Test	Result Indicating Disorder	CPT Code
MRI with/without contrast	Identifies presence and location of neoplasm	70541 without contrast 70542 with contrast
EEG	Detects presence and location of seizure activity	95816
Chest x-ray study	Possible site of primary lesion	71030
Cerebral angiography	Determines vascularity of lesions or proximity to blood vessels; usually performed preoperatively	70496
Positron-emission tomography (PET) and Single proton emission topography (SPECT)	Aids in differentiating tumor recurrence from tissue necrosis	78608/9 (PET) 78803 (SPECT)
Open brain biopsy or a CT- or MRI-directed stereotactic needle biopsy	Provides definitive diagnosis before proceeding with treatment	61140 (Open brain biopsy) 70450 (CT without contrast) 70460 (CT with contrast) 61750 (MRI without contrast) 61751 (MRI with contrast)

EEG, electroencephalography; MRI, magnetic resonance imaging.

Differential diagnosis:

- Pseudotumor cerebri (seen most often in young, overweight men; benign intracranial hypertension; moderate to severe headaches; papilledema on physical examination; no mass on imaging)
- Brain abscess (fever, no mass on imaging)
- Granuloma, or toxic-metabolic disorders

Treatment: Varies with tumor size and location; may include one or more of the following:

Pharmacologic

Chemotherapy (depends on type and stage of tumor); corticosteroids (dexamethasone, 30 to 60 mg, or methylprednisolone, 120 to 200 mg in four to six divided doses to decrease tumor-associated edema); anticonvulsants (phenytoin, 300 mg/day); anticoagulants for deep vein thrombosis (DVT)/pulmonary embolus (PE) prophylaxis (heparin 5000 units subcutaneously twice a day for those with gliomas and associated immobility).

Surgical/Other

Surgery (debulking or removing the tumor); stereotactic radiosurgery or gamma knife surgery; radiation therapy (depends on type of tumor): whole brain or fractionated; interstitial brachytherapy (radioactive beads implanted into tumor) for recurrent tumors.

Follow-up: Varies with the type of neoplasm, treatment method, patient's response to treatment, and residual deficits following therapeutic interventions. Includes follow-up with physical, occupational, or speech therapy, and social worker.

Sequelae: Varies with type of lesion. Possible complications include various neurologic deficits and disabilities, and death (life expectancy after diagnosis with glioblastoma multiform is 8.5 months, for those with astrocytoma, 29 months). Primary tumors rarely metastasize; become symptomatic due to the anatomic confines of the skull.

Prevention/prophylaxis: None known.

Referral: Refer to, or consult with, neurosurgeon for diagnostic workup and treatment. Other referrals and consultants may include neuro-oncologist, physical therapy, occupational therapy, speech therapy, or social worker.

Education: Explain disease process, signs and symptoms, and treatment (including side effects of medications).

CEREBROVASCULAR ACCIDENT

SIGNAL SYMPTOMS▶ Varies with location and severity, and may include altered level of consciousness, disorientation, confusion (40% of patients), aphasia, dysphasia, dysarthria, cortical blindness, disconjugate gaze, visual field defects, diplopia, Horner's syndrome, sluggish pupil, hemiparesis, hemiplegia, ataxia, headache, dysphagia, sensory-perception defects, seizures.

| Cerebrovascular accident (stroke, brain attack) | ICD-9-CM: 436 |

Description: Cerebrovascular accident (CVA) is a syndrome of acute, sustained injury to the central nervous system (CNS) as a result of an arterial or venous disorder of the cerebrovascular system. Types include thrombotic (prognosis difficult), hemorrhagic (prognosis difficult), and embolic (prognosis determined by occurrence of further emboli and gravity of underlying illness).

Etiology: Thrombotic events (50% to 75% of CVAs) are caused by atherosclerotic processes, resulting in endothelial damage, plaques, formation of microemboli composed of platelets and fibrin, and debris that travel to distal arterioles. Hemorrhagic events are usually the result of bleeding within parenchymal tissue (intracerebral) or within spaces (subdural, subarachnoid, ventricular). Embolic events are usually secondary to a cardiac disorder, such as atrial fibrillation, valvular disease, or infectious endocarditis; or follow an acute myocardial infarction (MI) (especially in the anterior wall); or result from a hypercoagulable state from oral contraceptive use or an antiphospholipid antibodies syndrome causing blood vessel occlusion. Refer to Figure 10–1 for steps in the differential diagnosis of CVA.

Occurrence: CVAs, occurring at a rate of approximately 200,000 cases per year, are the third leading cause of death in the United States. The overall incidence is 160/100,000, and the prevalence is 135/100,000.

Age: Incidence increases with age. In patients between the ages of 50 and 65, ht incidence is 1000/100,000; in patients older than 80 years of age, the incidence is 3000/100,000.

Ethnicity: Occurs in blacks two to four times as often as whites.

Gender: Occurs in men three times more than in women.

Contributing factors: Age, race, family history, alcohol abuse, obesity, sedentary lifestyle, diabetes mellitus, smoking, hypertension, hyperlipidemia, atrial fibrillation (usually associated with mitral stenosis), recent myocardial infarction, carotid stenosis, oral contraceptive use after age 35.

Signs and symptoms: Vary with location and severity, and may include altered level of consciousness, disorientation, confusion (40% of patients), aphasia, dysphasia, dysarthria, cortical blindness, disconjugate gaze, visual field defects, diplopia, Horner's syndrome, sluggish pupil, hemiparesis, hemiplegia, ataxia, headache, dysphagia, sensory-perception defects, seizures. If signs and symptoms last less than 24 hours, condition is referred to as TIA.

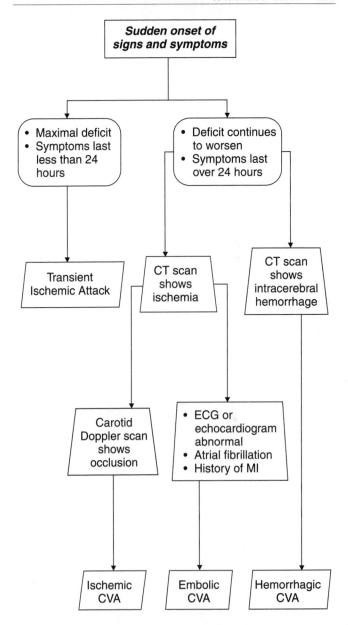

Figure 10–1. Determining types of CVA.

Diagnostic tests:

Tests	Result Indicating Disorder	CPT Code
Serum electrolytes	To rule out other abnormalities that decrease proper function	80051
Serum glucose	Detects hypoglycemia	82947
Complete blood count (CBC)	Look for infection or in flammation	85025
Antithrombin	Decreased	85301
Alanine aminotransferase (ALT)	Moderately elevated in recent CVA (three to five times normal)	84460
Aspartate aminotransferase (AST)	Slightly elevated (two to three times normal)	84450
Lactic dehydrogenase	Elevated	83615
Prothrombin time	May be elevated	85611
Prothrombin time (PT/partial thromboplastin time (PTT)	Done if initiating anticoagulation therapy	85732
ESR	May be elevated	85652
Urinalysis	May show hematuria	81001
Serum glucose, serum electrolytes, ALT, AST, CBC, lactic dehydrogenase	These laboratory tests are incorporated in a general health panel	80050
CT scan	Noncontrast; done first to rule out hemorrhagic CVA when considering thrombolytic therapy	70450
MRI	Shows hemorrhage, focal infarction, size of occluded artery	70544
Carotid duplex scan	Appearance of occlusion of carotid arteries	93880
Cerebral angiography	Rules out carotid occlusion; determines if patient is potential candidate for carotid endarterectomy.	70496
Transcranial Doppler	Assess anterior, middle, posterior and vertebrobasilar artery flow	93875 (extracranial) 93886 (intracranial)
Echocardiogram (ECG)	Determines whether CVA has cardiac etiology.	93320
EEG	Detects presence of seizure activity	95816

CBC, complete blood count; CT, computed tomography; CVA, cerebrovascular accident; EEG, electroencephalography; MRI, magnetic resonance imaging.

Differential diagnosis:
- Seizure disorder with post-ictal Todd's paresis (no resolution or paresis)
- Brain tumor (check imaging, biopsy-pathology report)
- Subacute or chronic subdural hematoma
- Metabolic encephalopathy such as hypoglycemia (blood glucose 50 mg/dL or lower)

- TIA (depends on location; weakness, transient numbness, visual disturbances: symptoms pass)
- Migraine headache (unilateral moderate to severe head pain, pulsating, photosensitivity, nausea, vomiting, phonophobia)

Treatment:

Pharmacologic

Goals for drug therapies for acute CVA include prevention of further thrombotic events (anticoagulation), augmentation of blood flow (reperfusion), and protection of neurons (metabolic adjustment).

Anticoagulation: Heparin (for some thromboembolic events) in prodromal or early phase, IV bolus, 100 units/kg, and drip, 1000 units/hour for 1 to 2 weeks; maintain PTT two times normal. Warfarin therapy initiated to wean drip; maintain PT 1 to 1.5 times normal with International Normalized Ratio (INR) 2 to 3.

Long-term warfarin (maintain PT at 1.5 times normal) for patients with atrial fibrillation with associated congestive heart failure (CHF), hypertension, previous thromboembolism, left ventricular dysfunction, or cardiac valve disease.

Antiplatelet aggregation therapy: Enteric-coated aspirin 325 mg each day (may consider using with dipyridamole), clopidogrel (Plavix) 75 mg each day, or ticlopidine (Ticlid) 250 mg twice a with food for patients who cannot take aspirin.

Hypertension control: monitor carefully to avoid overcontrol.

Thrombolysis: tissue plasminogen activator (tPA) 0.9mg/Kg IV (max. 90 mg)—give 10% of total dose as bolus and the remainder over 60 minutes. Must be given within 3 hours of onset of symptoms and only after meeting very specific criteria.

Surgical

Carotid endarterectomy per recommended guidelines (greater than 70% carotid stenosis).

Follow-up: Dependent on outcome, but usually see the patient every 3 months for the first year, then yearly.

Sequelae: Possible complications vary with location and severity; may range from minimal neurologic deficits and functional loss to catastrophic functional loss and major neurologic deficits, total incapacity, and death.

Prevention/prophylaxis: Prevention strategies include stopping smoking; controlling hypertension and glycemia; maintaining normal serum lipid, cholesterol, and triglyceride levels; maintaining appropriate weight for body type and activity level; avoiding or limiting consumption of alcohol; and performing regular exercise. Aspirin prophylaxis is useful for secondary prevention of ischemic stroke; warfarin (Coumadin) for secondary prevention of cardiogenic emboli.

Referral: Refer to or consult with neurologist for evaluation and treatment. Refer to tertiary care center; physical, occupational, or speech therapist; and social worker.

Education: Explain disease process, signs and symptoms, and treatment (including side effects of medications). After hospitalization and rehabilitation, when optimal functional ability has been achieved, discuss risk-factor control as well as prevention and prophylaxis strategies. Discuss available community services for care management and assessment of home environment, especially for patients with significant functional loss.

ENCEPHALITIS

SIGNAL SYMPTOMS▶ Acute onset of fever, headache, and stiff neck

Encephalitis	ICD-9-CM: 047.9

Description: Encephalitis is a syndrome consisting of an acute febrile illness with evidence of meningeal involvement, in which there is acute inflammation of the brain parenchyma from an infectious agent. Encephalitis is caused by viral invasion or by a viral-mediated inflammatory response in the brain following an acute, systemic infection.

Etiology: Caused by multiple infectious agents, including viral agents (such as herpes simplex virus [HSV] types 1 and 2, Epstein-Barr, varicella-zoster, arthropod-borne [La Crosse virus, California encephalitis, western equine encephalitis, eastern equine encephalitis], enterovirus [Coxsackie B], mumps, cytomegalovirus, HIV, rabies), West Nile virus and nonviral agents (such as TB, tertiary syphilis, *Rickettsia rickettsii, Staphylococcus aureus, Streptococcus pneumoniae, Haemophilus influenzae, Bacteroides fragilis, Brucella* species, *Leptospira* species, and *Cryptococcus neoformans*). May follow vaccination for rabies, measles, rubella, chickenpox, or influenza. Death occurs in 5% to 20%, residual deficits in 20%. With herpes simplex, 50% die or are left with severe impairment. Eastern equine encephalitis is the most serious infectious agent because two thirds of patients die or are left with severe abnormalities.

Occurrence: Not common; approximately 20,000 cases per year; may have seasonal (such as spring and summer) or epidemic (such as a geographic location) occurrences.

Age: Occurs at any age; very young children and older adults are at highest risk.

Ethnicity: No significant ethnic predisposition.

Gender: Occurs equally in men and in women.

Contributing factors: Exposure to vectors such as mosquitoes or ticks; exposure to virus such as HIV.

Signs and symptoms:

- Nonspecific symptoms such as malaise, fever, and rhinorrhea may precede neurologic symptoms.

- Acute onset of fever, headache, and stiff neck.
- Other signs and symptoms include decreased or altered level of consciousness, photophobia, confusion, focal neurologic signs, seizures, aphasia, hemiparesis, and ataxia.
- Physical examination may reveal asymmetry of deep tendon reflexes and the presence of Babinski's sign.

Diagnostic tests:

Test	Result Indicating Disorder	CPT Code
Lumbar puncture for cerebrospinal fluid (CSF) analysis and culture	Reveals elevated white blood cell (WBC) count, normal or moderately increased protein level, normal to subsequently decreased glucose level, presence of HSV antigen.	62270 87070 (culture)
Serum antibody concentrations	Done initially, then 2 to 3 weeks later for comparison of titers	86975
Fluorescent antibody study	Demonstrates antibody	86255
Viral culture of cerebral tissue	Shows positive culture for herpes 1 and herpes 2, Epstein-Barr, varicella-zoster, arthropod-borne, enterovirus or CMV	80090 (TORCH panel) 87531 (herpes culture) 87070 (general culture)
Polymerase chain reaction (PCR)	Positive.	83898
MRI	Focal abnormalities or masses or tumors	70544 without contrast 70550 with contrast
CT scan	Focal abnormalities not observed on scan until 3 days after onset	70450 without contrast 70460 with contrast
EEG	Detects seizure activity	95816
Brain biopsy if CSF PCR ondiagnostic and clinical decline in spite of treatment	Diagnostic	61140

CSF, cerebrospinal fluid; CT, computed tomography; EEG, electroencephalography; MRI, magnetic resonance imaging; TORCH, toxoplasmosis, other infections, rubella cytomegalovirus infection, and herpes simplex virus.

Differential diagnosis:

- Meningitis (fever, stiff neck, lumbar puncture: increased cell count, increased globulin, positive culture)
- Syphilis (painless indurated chancre, malaise, sore throat, positive Venereal Disease Research Laboratory [VDRL] test)
- Lyme disease (red macular skin lesion after tick bite)
- Toxoplasmosis (malaise, headache, myalgia, arthralgia, weakness, fever, transient maculopapular rash)

- Rocky Mountain spotted fever (chills, anorexia, malaise, headache, fever, red or hemorrhagic maculopapules on wrists and ankles)
- Intracranial hemorrhage (lumbar puncture)
- Abscess, or neoplasm (imaging, biopsy)
- Thromboembolism (ultrasound)
- Acute thrombotic thrombocytopenic purpura (pallor, petechiae, bruises, bleeding; lab: microangiopathic hemolytic anemia; elevated LDH and serum creatinine)
- Ingestion of toxic substances (history)
- Sjögren's syndrome (keratoconjunctivitis, Vero stoma, rheumatoid arthritis)
- Protozoal infections (positive identification of organism)

Treatment: Varies with regard to causative agent and based on type of encephalitis in terms of morbidity and mortality expectations. Initially, treat as HSV: acyclovir 30 mg/kg per day IV (shown to decrease the mortality rate by 28%). Aggressive supportive treatment, largely symptomatic. Corticosteroids may be used to reduce cerebral edema.

Follow-up: Depends on outcome; if successfully treated, patient does not need further follow-up; if there is residual deficit or dysfunction; follow-up is individualized based on patient needs.

Sequelae: Possible complications vary with causative agent. For example, with HSV, there is approximately a 70% mortality rate if the patient is not treated before the onset of coma; with eastern equine encephalitis, 80% are left with severe neurologic dysfunction.

Prevention/prophylaxis: Prevention strategies include advising the patient to avoid areas where vectors reside, especially during peak times of the year when the vector populations are increased; to use appropriate insect repellant; and to wear protective clothing.

Referral: Refer to tertiary care center for prompt treatment. Refer to, or consult with, neurologist or infectious disease specialist and physical or occupational therapist as needed.

Education: Explain disease process, signs and symptoms, and treatment (including side effects of medications). Discuss prevention strategies.

MENINGITIS

SIGNAL SYMPTOMS ▶ Sudden, severe, frontal headache
Photophobia
Stiff neck
Nausea and vomiting

Meningitis, bacterial	ICD-9-CM: 320.0
Meningitis, viral	ICD-9-CM: 047.8

Description: Meningitis is the inflammation of the meninges (pia mater and arachnoid) caused by an infectious agent or noninfectious process. It involves the cerebrospinal fluid (CSF) and ventricles. Three types of infectious meningitis are acute bacterial; viral, or aseptic; and subacute, or chronic. Untreated bacterial meningitis is usually fatal; viral meningitis is usually self-limiting; and subacute or chronic meningitis may be infectious or self-limiting.

Etiology: Infectious bacterial meningitis is usually caused by *Streptococcus pneumoniae* (approximately 50%), *Neisseria meningitidis* (Waterhouse-Friderichsen syndrome—approximately 25%), group B streptococci, or *Listeria* species. *Haemophilus influenzae* meningitis has declined since 1987 with the use of the hib vaccine. Viral, or aseptic, meningitis is caused by enteroviruses such as Coxsackie A and B virus and echovirus; mumps; herpes virus (HSV type 2); cytomegalovirus; lymphocytic choriomeningitis; or Epstein-Barr virus. Subacute, or chronic, meningitis is caused by HIV, *Mycobacterium tuberculosis, Cryptococcus neoformans, Coccidioides immitis, Histoplasma capsulatum, Treponema pallidum,* or Lyme disease. Noninfectious meningitis is caused by subarachnoid hemorrhage, sarcoidosis, or cancer.

Occurrence: Bacterial meningitis occurs in approximately >2.5/ 100,000. Viral meningitis has 11/100,000 reported cases per year, but many cases are probably not reported. Viral meningitis also tends to be seasonal, summer to early autumn especially in temperate climates.

Age: Seventy-five percent of bacterial meningitis cases occur in people 15 years old or younger; 70% of viral meningitis cases occur in people 20 years old or younger; pneumococcal meningitis predominates in the very young and people over 40 years old.

Ethnicity: Some people of Native American heritage, such as Navajos, and American Eskimo heritage may be more vulnerable.

Gender: Occurs equally in men and in women.

Contributing factors: Exposure to causative agents or to someone infected with a causative agent; immunosuppression; disruption of meninges, such as head injury and neurosurgical procedures.

Signs and symptoms: Classic onset is a sudden, severe, frontal headache; photophobia; stiff neck; and nausea and vomiting. Key signs to establish the diagnosis are nuchal rigidity, a positive Kernig's sign (have patient lie supine and flex knees and hips, then extend knee; if pain occurs with extension, consider this a positive sign), and the presence of Brudzinski's sign (have patient lie supine, then bend patient's neck forward; if knees flex spontaneously, consider this a positive sign). May progress rapidly to confusion, lethargy, loss of consciousness.

> *Bacterial:* Approximately 25% have acute onset, whereas in others, it develops over 1 to 7 days; may follow 1 to 3 weeks after an URI. Fever; severe headache; drowsiness; confusion; meningismus (stiff neck); irritability; maculopapular erythematous rash (*Neisseria* meningitidis); generalized seizures; focal neurologic signs.
>
> *Viral:* History should include immunizations, family outbreaks, insect bites, contact with animals, and recent travel. Fever, headache

(retro-orbital to frontal), nausea and vomiting, photophobia, generalized aches. Nuchal rigidity is usually mild, and Kernig's and Brudzinski's signs are usually absent.

Subacute to chronic: Develops over several days to weeks; may be infectious, depending on organism or seeding in other body areas. Headache, fever, meningismus, confusion, irritability, hydrocephalus

Noninfectious: Photophobia, meningismus.

Diagnostic tests:

Test	Result Indicating Disorder	CPT Code
Lumbar puncture with CSF cell count, glucose, protein, and culture	*Bacterial meningitis:* turbid, markedly increased WBC count (mostly neutrophils), decreased glucose, elevated protein (usually 150 to 400 mg/dL), and positive Gram stain and culture *Viral meningitis:* pleocytosis (elevated WBC count), normal glucose, normal or less than 100 mg/dL protein, normal or mildly elevated opening pressure, negative Gram's stain, positive PCR and positive serum antiviral antibody	62270
EEG	R/O seizure activity	95816
Meningeal biopsy	Pathology Report	61140
MRI with/without contrast	Diagnostic for meniscal tears or meningioma	70541 with contrast 70542 without contrast 70543 with contrast initially then without contrast
General health panel (CBC with diff, glucose, electrolytes, BUN, creatinine, amylase), ESR, and lipase, CPK.	Viral/bacterial infection, increased glucose	80050 85652 83690 82550
Coxsackie B virus	Positive (viral)	86658
Fungal antibody tests	Positive for cryptococcal meningitis	86671
Throat and blood cultures	Detect suspected organism	87071 (throat) 87040 (blood)
Nasopharyngeal swab	May be positive in bacterial meningitis	42999 (other nasopharynx)

BUN, blood urea nitrogen; CPK, creatine phosphokinase; EEG, electroencephalography; ESR, erythrocyte sedimentation rate; MRI, magnetic resonance imaging; WBC, white blood cell.

Differential diagnosis:

For bacterial meningitis

- Brain abscess (often associated with fever or other signs of infection, confirmed by MRI or CT scan)
- Nonbacterial meningitis especially HSV (positive culture for HSV)

- Bacteremia (blood culture)
- Sepsis (associated fever and other signs of infection)
- Seizures (convulsions, confirmed by EEG)

For viral meningitis

- Bacterial meningitis (lumbar puncture)
- Encephalitis (nuchal rigidity, changes in consciousness level)
- Subacute meningitis (lumbar puncture)
- Migraine headache (unilateral moderate to severe head pain, pulsating, photosensitivity, nausea, vomiting, phonophobia)
- Subdural empyema
- Neoplastic meningitis or noninfectious meningitis such as sarcoidosis.

Treatment

Bacterial: Immediate hospitalization (medical emergency, septic shock must be counteracted). Begin aggressive treatment while waiting for laboratory results. Any circumstance that prolongs bacterial meningitis increases the risk of damage to the unaffected areas and structures.

Antimicrobial agents include the following: Vancomycin (because of emergence of PCN and cephalosporin resistant strains of *S. pneumoniae*), penicillin G (drug of choice for *N. meningitidis*), and third-generation cephalosporin (cefotaxime or ceftriaxone). Corticosteroids (decrease morbidity and mortality): dexamethasone, 0.15 mg/kg every 6 hours for 4 days (start 15 minutes before antibiotics).

Viral: A prudent course is to administer empiric antibiotic therapy while awaiting culture results. Depends on causative agent; if herpes simplex virus, treat with acyclovir.

Subacute and chronic: Depends on causative agent; refer to neurologist.

Noninfectious: Treat to relieve symptoms.

Follow-up: See patient as needed depending on patient outcome.

Sequelae: Possible complications vary with causative agent and virulence. Patient with bacterial meningitis may have residual focal neurologic deficits, obstructive hydrocephalus, deafness, death (approximately 30%). Patient with viral meningitis usually has complete recovery within 1 to 2 weeks. Patient with chronic meningitis may have pronounced neurological deficits. Death can occur if the condition is left untreated.

Prevention/prophylaxis: Prevention strategies include advising patient to seek medical attention promptly for infections, to wear appropriate protective clothing when outdoors, and to avoid direct contact with infected individuals; if exposed to respiratory secretions, take rifampin, 600 mg every 12 hours for 2 days to help prevent meningococcal meningitis. Consider meningococcal polysaccharide vaccine especially for college students residing in dormitory. Advise parents that a vaccine

Haemophilus influenzae type B is available for children. Health-care workers should maintain strict aseptic technique when treating patients with head wounds or skull fractures.

Referral: Refer to, or consult with, physician, neurologist, tertiary care center (for in-patient management), and physical or occupational therapist as indicated.

Education: Explain the disease process, signs and symptoms, and treatment (including side effects of medications). Discuss prevention strategies.

MULTIPLE SCLEROSIS

SIGNAL SYMPTOMS▶ Acute (approximately 85%) or subacute onset with combinations of the following: unilateral vision loss or diplopia, nystagmus, optic neuritis, or ocular paralysis; motor weakness; dysarthria; ataxia; paresthesias; vertigo; fatigue; incontinence or bladder dysfunction; hyperreflexia; the presence of Babinski's reflex; intention tremor; emotional lability; depression; Lhermitte's sign (with neck flexion, patient experiences electric shocklike sensations radiating down spine to lower extremities); decreased or absent vibration and position sense; heat sensitivity.

Multiple sclerosis   ICD-9-CM: 340

Description: Multiple sclerosis (MS) is a disorder in which there is chronic, progressive inflammatory demyelination of the brain and spinal cord nerve fibers. It is characterized by multiple areas of white matter inflammation, demyelination, and glial scarring. The clinical course varies from a benign, largely symptom free-disease to a rapidly progressing, disabling disorder. Periods of relapse and remission during the clinical course vary according to the following typical patterns: relapsing-remitting (acute exacerbations with recovery; stable between exacerbations); primary progressive (gradual neurological decline); secondary progressive (seen in those with relapsing-remitting pattern–progressive neurologic decline with or without exacerbations) and progressive relapsing (gradual neurological decline with exacerbations).

Etiology: The cause of MS is unknown, but it may be related to epidemiologic factors, autoimmune mechanisms (evidence strongly suggestive for this), genetic susceptibility, viral infections.

Occurrence: It is estimated that there are 350,000 persons affected in United States; with approximately 25,000 new cases per year. It is the second leading cause of neurologic dysfunction in the early to middle-aged adult.

Age: Onset of symptoms is usually between age 16 to 40 years but may occur in all age groups.

Ethnicity: Occurs more in people of northern European descent.

Gender: Occurs more in women than in men.

Contributing factors: Living in colder climates or having lived in one as a child (age 15 or younger), familial tendency; 15% have an affected relative.

Signs and symptoms:

- History may include vague symptoms such as lack of energy, weight loss, vague muscle and joint pains.
- Specific symptoms usually start unilaterally and focally, but progress to a bilateral and disseminated pattern.
- Acute (approximately 85%) or subacute onset with combinations of the following: unilateral vision loss or diplopia, nystagmus, optic neuritis, or ocular paralysis; motor weakness; dysarthria; ataxia; paresthesias; vertigo; fatigue; incontinence or bladder dysfunction; hyperreflexia; positive Babinski's reflex; intention tremor; emotional lability; depression; Lhermitte's sign (with neck flexion, patient experiences electric shock-like sensations radiating down spine to lower extremities); decreased or absent vibration and position sense; heat sensitivity.

Diagnostic tests:

Test	Result Indicating Disorder	CPT Code
Lumbar puncture with CSF analysis	Shows increased gamma globulin IgG, elevated protein, and more than two oligoclonal bands	62270
Visual evoked responses—evoked potentials are quantitative, neurophysio-logic means of demon-strating the interruption of the message-carrying capacity of axons whose myelin is inflamed—pathways tested raw either visual, auditory, or poste-rior columns of the spinal cord	Shows a slowing transmission—although abnormalities are specific for location they are not specific for pathophysiologic process More than 75% have abnormal results; may show clinically unsus-pected lesions Supporting data for MRI results	95930
Somatosensory evoked potentials	Slowing transmission—more than 72% have abnormal results—supporting data for MRI	95925
Brain stem auditory evoked responses	Slowing transmission—55% to 65% have abnormal results Supporting data for MRI results	92585 (brain stem) 92585 (auditory)
*MRI (more sensitive than CT scan)—most sensitive diag-nostic tool but suffers from lack of specificity with a large number of other dis-eases having similar changes	Shows presence of demyelinating plaques in 90% of patients with MS; however, interpret MRI cau-tiously and in context of total clini-cal picture. Changes also found in other conditions such as normal elderly patients, chronic uncon-trolled hypertension, advanced Lyme disease, CNS vasculitis	70544 without contrast 70545 with contrast

CNS, central nervous system; CSF, cerebrospinal fluid; IgG, immunoglobulin G; MRI, magnetic resonance imaging.

Differential diagnosis: No diagnostic test is specific for MS; diagnosis should be based on history, physical examination, CSF analysis, MRI, evoked potential studies, and repeated observations over a period of time. A diagnosis of exclusion.

- CNS neoplasms (imaging)
- Small cerebral infarctions from arteriovenous malformations (imaging)
- Friedreich's ataxia
- Neurosyphilis (positive VDRL)
- Lyme disease (red, macular skin lesions after tick bite)
- HIV-associated myelopathy (positive for HIV)

Treatment:

Pharmacologic

Interferon-beta 1a(Avonex), Interferon-beta 1b(Betaseron) or Glatiramer acetate (Copaxone) for specific patients with relapsing-remitting MS.

Methotrexate 7.5 mg by mouth weekly for those with secondary progressive MS.

Methylprednisolone, 1 g IV each day for 7 to 10 days; then oral prednisone, tapered, such as follows: prednisone, 80 mg each day for 4 days; then 60 mg, 40 mg, 20 mg, 10 mg, and 5 mg, each for 4 days; then four doses of 5 mg once a day (for patients with severe symptoms and acute exacerbation).

Baclofen, 40 to 80 mg/day in divided doses (to control spasticity).

Physical

Support and treat symptoms.

Follow-up: See the patient as needed depending on type and effects on patient.

Sequelae: Possible complications vary but may include permanent disability, coma, and death. Of MS patients, 70% have prolonged remissions, 30% relapse within 1 year, 20% relapse within 5 to 9 years, and 10% do not have a relapse for 10 to 30 years. Many patients can lead full, productive lives for many years; 60% are fully functional 10 years after onset; and 28% are fully functional 25 to 30 years after onset. Thirty to forty percent of patients with optic neuritis alone eventually develop other signs. Approximately 60% experience depression and are at risk for suicide.

Prevention/prophylaxis: There is no known prevention; however, adequate nutrition, hydration, and rest; regular elimination; avoidance of stress and temperature extremes (especially hot); scheduling activities to promote rest; maintaining regular exercise to promote optimal functioning; and discussion of pregnancy with neurologist before conception can assist in preventing relapses or exacerbation of condition.

Referral: Refer to, or consult with, neurologist for complete workup and evaluation; refer to MS specialty clinic, national MS society, or social services agencies as needed. A multidisciplinary approach is most effective.

Education: Explain the disease process, signs and symptoms, and treatment (including side effects of medications). Discuss prevention strategies. Encourage participation in local support groups. National Multiple Sclerosis Society, 733 Third Ave., NY, NY 10017-3288; phone: 212-986-3240 or 800-FIGHT MS; Web site: http://www.nmss.org

PARKINSON'S DISEASE

SIGNAL SYMPTOMS ▶ Resting tremors

Parkinson's disease	ICD-9-CM: 332.0

Description: Parkinson's disease, or paralysis agitans, is a chronic, degenerative CNS disease affecting the extrapyramidal system and resulting from an alteration in the dopaminergic pathway and loss of dopaminergic neurons in the substantia nigra. The disease may begin slowly and remain unnoticed until symptoms appear. It continues to progress at an individual pace, with some patients becoming totally incapacitated. Parkinsonism is a symptom complex manifested by any combination of the following six clinical features: tremor at rest, rigidity, bradykinesia, flexed posture, loss of postural reflexes, and masklike facies. For a positive diagnosis, at least two of these clinical features, including either tremor at rest or bradykinesia, must be present.

Etiology: Cause unknown in Parkinson's disease. Parkinsonism may be caused by postviral encephalitis; exposure to toxic agents such as 1-methyl-4-phenyl-1,2,5,6-tetra-hydropyridine (MPTP); or medications such as chronic use of high-dose antipsychotic agents (phenothiazines, butyrophenones).

Occurrence: At present, 0.5 million are affected with Parkinson's disease, with approximately 50,000 new cases each year.

Age: Occurs primarily in people age 40 to 70, with peak incidence at age 60.

Ethnicity: No significant ethnic predisposition.

Gender: Occurs more in men than in women at a ratio of 3:2.

Contributing factors: Parkinson's disease: unknown. Parkinsonism: Use of MPTP.

Signs and symptoms:

- Cardinal early symptoms are resting tremors (approximately 70%), often involving a hand, relieved with activity or complete rest.
- Other symptoms include muscle weakness; slow, difficult-to-initiate movements; bradykinesia; stooped posture; gait disturbances (no arm

swing; small, shuffling steps); rigidity ("lead pipe," "cogwheeling" with passive movement of limbs); slow, slurred speech with monotone voice; masklike face.
- As the disease progresses, symptoms include slowed mental processes progressing to dementia; seborrhea; diaphoresis; depression; autonomic dysfunction such as constipation, incontinence, impotence; infrequent blinking; blepharospasm; increased conjugate upward gaze; small, cramped handwriting; festinations; retropulsion and propulsion.

Diagnostic tests: Diagnosis is usually made based on signs and symptoms.

Tests	Result Indicating Disorder	CPT Code
Imaging: CT scan	Rules out brain stem or cerebellar atrophy, lacunar infarcts of basal ganglia, or those who do not respond to drug therapy	70450 without contrst 70460 with contrast
MRI	Rules out brain stem or cerebellar atrophy, lacunar infarcts of basal ganglia, or those who do not respond to drug therapy	70544 without contrast 70545 with contrast

CT, computed tomography; MRI, magnetic resonance imaging.

Differential diagnosis:
- Progressive supranuclear palsy (neck dystonia, rigidity, ocular changes)
- Wilson's disease (jaundice, ascites, peripheral edema, brown skin, decreased serum copper and ceruloplasmin, biopsy of liver)
- Lacunar infarctions (patient history)
- Side effects of medications that block striatal dopamine D_2 receptors, such as phenothiazines, or those that deplete striatal dopamine, such as reserpine (condition is reversible if the offending drug is withdrawn)
- Essential tremor
- Normal pressure hydrocephalus (lumbar puncture, CT or MRI imaging)
- Alzheimer's disease with extrapyramidal features (progressive mental deterioration with amnesia, aphasia and agnosia).

Treatment: No known treatment that will halt or reverse the underlying pathology and degeneration of the disease; treatment directed at relief of symptoms.

Pharmacologic
Early stages: use anticholinergics and amantadine. Later: gradually increase carbidopa or levodopa as tolerated. Late stage: when response to levodopa diminishes ("on/off" phenomenon), add anticholinergics or bromocriptine.
Carbidopa-levodopa (start with 1/2 of 100/25-mg tablet three times a day).

- Dopamine receptor agonists such as bromocriptine (start with 1.25 mg/day; increase 1.25 mg every 5 to 7 days to a maximum of 10 to 20 mg/day) or pergolide (0.125 mg/day; increase 0.125 mg every 5 to 7 days to a maximum of 3 to 4 mg/day).
- Monoamine oxidase (MAO) inhibitors such as selegiline (start with 2.5 mg twice a day at breakfast and lunch; can disturb sleep).
- Anticholinergics such as trihexyphenidyl hydrochloride (start with 1 mg/day; increase by 2 mg every 3 to 5 days to a maximum of 6 to 10 mg/day) or benztropine (start with 0.5 mg/day; increase by 0.5 mg every 5 to 6 days to a maximum of 6 mg/day).
- Amantadine (start with 100 mg/day; may increase to 100 mg twice a day).

Physical

Supportive care based on symptoms; may include physical therapy, occupational therapy, and speech therapy to assist with adaptation to decreasing functional ability.

Surgical

Deep brain stimulator insertion: pacemaker-like device that provides electrical stimulation of globus pallidus internus or subthalamic nucleus.

Thalamotomy, or modification of this procedure, may be appropriate late in disease progression when medications are no longer effective.

Fetal cell transplantation (midbrain dopaminergic cells) into putamen (under investigation).

Follow-up: Varies. See patient as needed depending on disease progression, response to treatment, presence of side effects from drug therapy, and ability to pursue activities of daily living.

Sequelae: Possible complications include disease progression to complete incapacity; death is usually caused by complications such as falls or aspiration pneumonia.

Prevention/prophylaxis: Prevention strategies include advising patient to avoid use of MPTP (for parkinsonism).

Referral: Refer to, or consult with, physician (neurologist) for definitive diagnosis and initial medication regimen; physical therapist, occupational therapist, and speech therapist as needed for assistance in maintaining activities of daily living.

Education: Explain disease process, signs and symptoms, and treatment (including side effects of medications). Discuss availability of local support groups, especially for significant others, and need for significant other to be involved in all aspects of patient care. Discuss methods of adapting home environment to meet patient's decreased functional abilities and to prevent falls. Advise patient's support persons to report depression.

SEIZURE DISORDER

SIGNAL SYMPTOMS▶ Loss of consciousness
Signs and symptoms vary with classification

| Seizure disorder (epilepsy) | ICD-9-CM: 780.3 |

Description: Seizure disorder, or epilepsy, is characterized by the episodic, abnormal electrochemical activity of the CNS, resulting in abnormal, uncontrollable behavior with or without an altered level of consciousness. There are numerous types of seizures, each with characteristic behavioral changes and electrophysiologic disturbances. Prognosis is difficult.

Etiology: The cause is idiopathic when onset is at age 20 or less. May also result from disruption in cerebral tissue or vasculature, such as from CNS trauma, infections, lesions, or cerebrovascular disorders; from metabolic disturbances, such as from electrolyte or metabolic imbalances; use of toxic agents such as heavy metals; hypoxia; uremia; eclampsia; or drug or alcohol use or withdrawal.

Occurrence: Approximately 5 per 1000 are diagnosed with seizure disorder (approximately 5% to 10% experience a single seizure).

Age: Occurs at any age; primary or idiopathic seizure disorder onset is usually at age 20 or under.

Ethnicity: No significant ethnic predisposition.

Gender: Occurs equally in men and in women.

Contributing factors: Drug or alcohol use, or withdrawal from drugs or alcohol; pregnancy (last trimester); fatigue; poor glycemic control in diabetes mellitus (individuals on insulin or oral hypoglycemic agents); emotional stress; external or exogenous stimuli (light, sound), hyperpyrexia such as fever or heat stroke.

Signs and symptoms: Signs and symptoms vary with classification. Refer to Figure 10-2 to determine seizure type.

Generalized seizures: Loss of consciousness. Absence (petit mal): altered awareness, blank stare, 5 to 30 seconds of eye blinking, onset in childhood. Myoclonic: brief, jerking contractions of one or both arms or legs, or trunk. Clonic: muscle contraction and relaxation. Tonic: abrupt muscle contraction and autonomic signs. Tonic-clonic (three phases): rigid extension of arms and legs (tonic), followed by sudden, quick jerking movements (clonic); receding gradually to flaccid muscles; and gradual returning to consciousness (postictal). Atonic: abrupt loss of muscle tone.

Partial seizures: Simple partial: awake, abnormal motor, somatosensory, autonomic, or psychic behavior. Complex partial: partial seizure progressing to loss of consciousness.

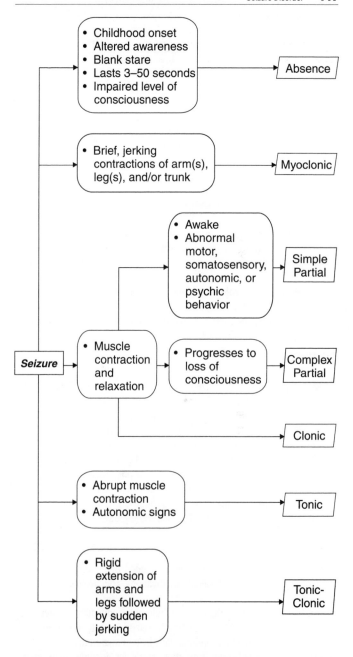

Figure 10–2. Determining seizure types.

Diagnostic Tests:

Test	Result Indicating disorder	CPT Code
CBC Basic chemistry panel (serum sodium, glucose, calcium, phosphorus, magnesium), and ammonia	Detects metabolic factors Specific to suspected or identified secondary causes, such as serum glucose for hypoglycemia, drug or toxicology screens	85025 80048 84140
EEG	May be nonspecific	95816
24-hour ambulatory EEG	Exacerbates seizures	95953
Video monitoring	Records seizure activity, progression, characteristics	96000 with computer read out
MRI (brain)	Rule out pathology such as tumor	70544 without contrast 70545 with contrast

Differential diagnosis: Seizures are associated with many diagnoses and conditions, and may be a symptom of many disorders; the type of seizure and underlying cause needs to be carefully differentiated by a neurologist.

Treatment: The neurologist should establish initial treatment, which should then be followed by practitioners with specialized knowledge in seizure disorders; the goal is to control seizures to enable patient to achieve optimal level of daily living functioning.

Pharmacologic

Begin with monotherapy; may need to change or add another agent.

Partial seizures: carbamazepine (Tegretol), 600 to 1200 mg/day, or phenytoin (Dilantin), 300 to 400 mg/day.

Generalized tonic-clonic seizures: valproic acid (Depakote), 750 to 2000 mg/day; lamotrigine (Lamictal), 150 to 500 mg/day; phenytoin (Dilantin), 300 to 400 mg/day (therapeutic range 10 to 20 mg/mL), or carbamazepine (Tegretol), 600 to 1800 mg/day (therapeutic range 4 to 12 mg/mL); add phenobarbital, 100 to 200 mg/day only as necessary (therapeutic range 10 to 30 mg/mL).

Absence seizures: ethosuximide (Zarontin), 250 to 1250 mg/day, or valproic acid (Depakene), 750 to 1500 mg/day.

Surgical

Ablation or resection of irritable foci.

Follow-up: Varies. See the patient as needed depending on type and control of seizures, overall health, medications, effectiveness, tolerance, and serum levels.

Sequelae: Possible complications include status epilepticus (emergency situation) and poor control resulting in seizure activity interfering with patient's ability to maintain optimal daily living functioning.

Prevention/prophylaxis: Prevention strategies include advising the patient to avoid known triggers, take medications as prescribed, and not to stop taking medications (if seizure-free for 2 years, the patient may consider a trial period without medication under care of a neurologist).

Referral: Refer to or consult with neurologist for evaluation and treatment.

Education: Explain disease process, signs and symptoms, and treatment (including side effects of medications). Discuss prevention strategies, methods to use to avoid trigger mechanisms, and importance of followup care. Encourage participation in local support groups. Teach family how to manage seizures. See Figure 10-2 for steps in determining seizure type.

TRANSIENT ISCHEMIC ATTACK

SIGNAL SYMPTOMS▶   Generalized deficits such as diplopia, vertigo, ataxia, facial paresis, Horner's syndrome, dysphagia, dysarthria, and visual blurring.

Transient Ischemic Attack	ICD-9-CM: 435.9

Description: TIA is a sudden onset of neurologic dysfunction caused by microemboli or decreased perfusion in either the carotid or vertebrobasilar circulations that resolves without residual deficit in less than 24 hours (usually within 1 to 2 hours from onset) or by platelet aggregates that form on atheromatous plaques and embolize to occlude a distal arteriole temporarily. A TIA is considered prognostic for CVA, or stroke.

Etiology: Most common causes include carotid artery occlusion and embolism from cardiac disease (mitral valve disease, anterior wall myocardial infarction, congestive cardiomyopathies, or atrial fibrillation). Other causes include hypercoagulable conditions (antiphospholipid antibody syndrome, oral contraceptives, presence of antithrombin 3, deficiency of protein S or C), and hypertension. It may also occur spontaneously or post trauma, such as from arterial dissection.

Occurrence: Incidence is 160/100,000; prevalence is 135/100,000.

Age: Usually occurs in patients older than 45 years of age; the highest risk is in persons older than 70 years of age.

Ethnicity: No significant ethnic predisposition; however, blacks have a greater incidence of CVAs.

Gender: Occurs in men three times more often than in women.

Contributing factors: Age, hypertension, cardiac disease, smoking, diabetes, antiphospholipid antibodies, family history.

Signs and symptoms: Vary with location of ischemia.

Carotid circulation involvement: Focal deficits such as hemiplegia, hemianesthesia, neglect, aphasia, visual field deficits (amaurosis fugax). TIA caused by carotid atherosclerosis is a predictor of MI.

Vertebrobasilar circulation involvement: Generalized deficits such as diplopia, vertigo, ataxia, facial paresis, Horner's syndrome, dysphagia, dysarthria, and visual blurring. TIAs may occur once or there may be multiple attacks.

Diagnostic tests:

Test	Results indicating disorder	CPT code
PT/PTT	Suggests hypercoagulopathies	85611 85732
Duplex carotid scan	Shows carotid stenosis	93880
CT scan	Detects "silent" ischemia or ischemic images	70450
Cerebral angiography	Detects stenosis and atheromatous ulcers	70496
EEG	Detects seizure activity	95816
ECG	Detects arrhythmias, valvular or structural abnormalities	93320
Transesophageal echo	Detects vascular tree abnormalities and stenosis	93318

CT, computed tomography; ECG, electrocardiography; EEG, electroencephalography; PT, prothrombin time; PTT, partial thromboplastin time.

Differential diagnosis:
- Migraine headache with aura (unilateral moderate to severe head pain, pulsating, photosensitivity, nausea, vomiting, phonophobia)
- Focal seizure (EEG)
- Hypoglycemia (blood glucose less than 50 mg/dL)

Treatment:

Pharmacologic
Anticoagulant medications can abolish TIAs. Enteric-coated aspirin (EC ASA), 325 mg daily, or clopidrogel (Plavix) 75 mg daily or ticlopidine (Ticlid) 250 mg twice a day—only if aspirin intolerant. Antihypertensive medications for patients with hypertension.

Physical
Measures to reduce risk factors such as smoking cessation; low-fat, low-salt diet; regular exercise; and measures to reduce blood pressure.

Surgical
Carotid endarterectomy (procedure of choice for patients with carotid TIAs and demonstrating >70% carotid bifurcation stenosis).

Follow-up: See the patient every 3 months for the first year, then at least yearly for neurologic and hypertension examination.

Sequelae: Approximately 33% have a CVA (completed stroke) within 5 years.

Prevention/prophylaxis: Prevention strategies include advising the patient to stop smoking; to control hypertension or diabetes; to maintain a regular exercise program; and to follow a low-fat, low-salt diet. For patient with a prior TIA, prevention strategies include the administration of aspirin or clopidrogel.

Referral: Refer to, or consult with, a neurologist and/or cardiologist for evaluation and diagnostic testing. Refer to Figure 10-3 for steps in the referral for suspected TIA.

Education: Explain the disease process, signs and symptoms, and treatment (including side effects of medications). Advise the patient of the potential for peptic ulcer disease and worsening of asthma symptoms from long-term ASA therapy. Discuss prevention strategies and risk factor reduction.

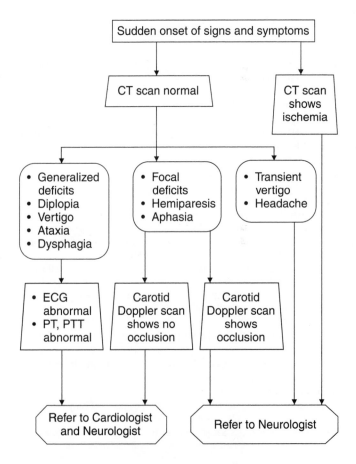

Figure 10–3. Referral for suspected TIA.

REFERENCES

General

Beers, MH, and Berkow, R (ed): The Merck Manual of Diagnosis and Therapy, ed. 17. Merck Research Laboratories, Whitehouse Station, NJ, 1999.

Braunwald, E, et al (ed): Harrison's Online. New York, McGraw-Hill, Harrison's Online.Com, 2001.

Cammermeyer, M, and Appledorn, C (ed): Core Curriculum for Neuroscience Nursing. American Association of Neuroscience Nurses, Chicago, 1993.

Cummins, RO (ed): ACLS Provider Manual. American Heart Association, Dallas, Tex, 2001.

Dambro, MR (ed): Griffith's 5 Minute Clinical Consult. Williams & Wilkins, Baltimore, 2002.

Dunphy, LM and Winland-Brown, JE (eds): Primary Care: The Art and Science of Advanced Practice Nursing. FA Davis, Philadelphia, 2001.

Greenberg, MS: Handbook of Neurosurgery, ed. 5.Thieme, New York, 2001.

Hurst, WJ: Medicine for the Practicing Physician, ed. 5. Appleton & Lange, Stamford, Conn, 2001.

Rowland, LP (ed): Merritt's Textbook of Neurology, ed 10. Williams & Wilkins, Baltimore, 2000.

Uphold, CR, and Graham, MV: Clinical Guidelines in Family Practice, ed. 3. Barmarrae Books, Gainesville, Fla, 1998.

Bell's Palsy

Grogan, PM, Gronseth,GS: Practice Parameters: Steroids, acyclovir, and surgery for Bell's palsy (an evidence-based review). Neurology 56:830, 2001.

Brain Cancer

Gutin, PH, and Posner, JB: NeuroOncology: Diagnosis and management of cerebral gliomas—past, present and future. Neurosurgery 47(1):1–8, 2000.

Cerebrovascular Accident

Brown, MM: Identification and management of difficult stroke and TIA syndromes. J Neurol Neurosurg Psychiatry 70(Suppl1):17–22, 2001.

Bryant-McKenny, H: Clinical management of the geriatric stroke patient. Advance for Nurse Practitioner 8(7):36–38, 43, 84, 2001.

Lewandowski,C, and Barsan,W: Treatment of acute ischemic stroke. Ann Emerg Med 37(2):202–216, 2001.

Llines, R, and Caplan, LR: Evidence based treatment of patients with ischemic cerebrovascular disease. Neurol Clin 15(1):79–105, 2001.

Encephalitis

Roos, KL: Encephalitis. Neurol Clin 17(4):813–833, 1999.

Meningitis

Davis, C, Schaad, LB, and Moeller, T (ed): Bacterial meningitis. Infect Dis Clin North Am 13(3):10–49, 1999.

Multiple Sclerosis

Fox, RJ, and Cohen, JA: Multiple Sclerosis: the importance of early recognition and treatment. Cleve Clin J Med 68(2):157–171, 2001.

National Multiple Sclerosis Society. Disease Management Consensus Statement. Available at: *http://www.nmss.org/include/newsclnclbulletin*. Accessed 2002.

Rolak, L: Multiple sclerosis treatment 2001. Neurol Clin 19(1):107–118, 2001.

Parkinson's Disease

Aminoff, MJ: Parkinson's disease. Neurol Clin 19(1):119–128, 2001.

The Deep Brain Stimulation for Parkinson's Disease Study Group: Deep brain stimulation of the subthalamic nucleus or the pars interna of the globus pallidus in Parkinson's disease. N Engl J Med 345(13):956–963, 2001.

Seizures

Marks, WJ Jr, and Garcia, PA: Management of seizures and epilepsy. Am Fam Physicians 57(7):1589–1600, 1603–1604, 1998.

Santilli, N, and Sierzant, TL: International classification of epileptic seizures. Clin Nursing Pract Epilepsy 1(1):8, 11, 1993.

Smith, D, and Chadwick, D: The Management of epilepsy. J Neurol Neurosurg Psychiatry 70(Suppl)2: 15–21, 2001.

Transient Ischemic Attack

Barnett, HJ, et al: Drugs and surgery in the prevention of ischemic stroke. N Engl J Med 332:238, 1995.

Bergman-Evans, B: Isolated hypertension in older adults. J Neurosci Nursing 4(9):23, 1996.

Chapter 11
ENDOCRINE AND METABOLIC DISORDERS

DIABETES MELLITUS, TYPE 1

SIGNAL SYMPTOMS ▶ Polydipsia; polyuria; polyphagia

Diabetes Mellitus, Type 1, uncontrolled	ICD-9-CM: 250.1

Description: Type 1 diabetes mellitus (formerly called insulin-dependent diabetes) is a chronic disorder of metabolic dysfunction; specifically, a derangement of carbohydrate, protein, and fat metabolism. It is accompanied by a profound predisposition to develop specific forms of renal, retinal, neurologic, and cardiovascular complications. The hallmark clinical feature is severe insulin deficiency, rendering the affected individuals prone to diabetic ketoacidosis (DKA)

Etiology: The condition results from a deficiency in insulin production caused by loss of pancreatic beta cells. An inherited chromosomal defect appears to cause an alteration in immunologic integrity, placing the beta cells at risk for inflammatory damage. The mechanism of this destruction is an autoimmune response. Most patients have circulating antibodies to islet cell components (islet cell antibodies) or to their own insulin (insulin antibodies).

Occurrence: The incidence is 12 to 14/100,000 per year.

Age: Occurs at any age. Most patients are diagnosed before age 30. There is a prevalence of 1/500 before age 16, with a decline in annual incidence after age 20. Latent autoimmune disease of the adult occurs at any age.

Ethnicity: There is a higher incidence in whites; the incidence is lower in blacks, Native Americans, and people of Hispanic and Asian heritage.

Gender: Occurs equally in men and women.

Contributing factors: Family history and environmental toxins such as viral infections (coxsackievirus B4 and congenital rubella) have been inconsistently implicated as triggers for the immunologic process. Emotional stress.

Signs and symptoms: Polydipsia, polyphagia, polyuria, anorexia, and weight loss (10% to 30%). Additional symptoms that may occur are increased fatigue, visual changes (blurriness), irritability, and emotional lability.

Diagnostic tests:

Test	Result Indicating Disorder	CPT Code
Fasting plasma glucose concentration	Greater than 126 mg/dL two times and/or random plasma glucose level exceeding 200 mg/dL with or without overt symptoms of diabetes	82962

Other tests that may be performed but are not needed to diagnose include an oral glucose tolerance test (OGTT) (fasting plasma glucose level is less than 126 mg/dL, plus sustained elevation of plasma glucose during at least two 75-g glucose load OGTTs in which the 2-hour level and one intervening level is greater than 200 mg/dL). Glycosylated hemoglobin (HgBA1c) is used for monitoring control of blood glucose.

Differential diagnosis:

- Type 2 diabetes mellitus (non-insulin-dependent)
- Impaired glucose tolerance (blood work results)
- Gestational diabetes (associated with pregnancy)
- Maturity-onset diabetes of the young (timed blood glucose)
- Pancreatic diseases such as chronic pancreatitis and cystic fibrosis (associated laboratory work)
- Endocrine diseases such as Cushing's syndrome, primary aldosteronism, and pheochromocytoma (check all associated blood work)
- Medications causing hyperglycemia such as thiazide diuretics, glucocorticoids, and estrogen preparations. (medication and medical history)

Treatment: Treatment goals are to restore and maintain near-normal glucose metabolism and to prevent or minimize complications. Goals for glycemic control are individualized and include: For pregnant women and women planning pregnancy: glucose 60 to 90 mg/dL before meals, less than 120 mg/dL 2 hours after meals, and HgBA1c within normal range. For the nonpregnant patient seeking average treatment: 80 to 160 mg/dL before meals, less than 200 mg/dL 2 hours post meals, and HgBA1c within 2% of normal range. For nonpregnant patient seeking intensive treatment: 90 to 130 mg/dL before meals, less than 180 mg/dL 2 hours post meals, and HgBA1c level within 1% of normal range.

 Clinical Pearl: for both Type 1 and Type 2 DM at every office visit examine patient's feet using monofilament to assess decreased sensation prior to ulceration development.

Refer the patient to an endocrinologist and a certified diabetic educator for initiation of therapy. Also, discuss the results of the Diabetes Control and Complications Trials with the patient and family, because treatment requires intensive therapy, including comprehensive education and lifestyle changes including daily injections of insulin, along with diet and exercise. Insulin pump (external) therapy is available for selected patients.

Pharmacologic

Insulin will be prescribed. Types, amounts, and dosage schedules will be adjusted according to the patient's glucose responses, metabolic needs, activities, and mode of administration (injection or insulin pump). Insulin preparations are categorized according to species (beef, pork, and human) and type (short-, intermediate-, and long-acting). Table 11–1 describes types of insulin and their actions.

Many insulin regimes may be used such as single-dose insulin (injection of Ultralente, NPH, or Lente with or without regular insulin once before breakfast or at bedtime, without regular), twice-daily insulin (injections before breakfast and dinner), three-shot regimen (injection of combined NPH and regular insulin before breakfast, regular insulin before dinner, and NPH insulin at bedtime), and CSII insulin pump (continuous delivery of buffered regular insulin through a syringe and needle into the subcutaneous tissue administered by a computerized pump). Usually, the patient is started on a twice-daily insulin injection regimen, beginning with a starting total dose of 0.2 units of insulin per pound of body weight or 0.4 to 0.6 units per kilogram of body weight.

Physical

Diet therapy: Because the food components that directly convert into glucose must be synchronized with the insulin that is needed to utilize it, refer the patient to a certified diabetes educator or dietitian to plan the patient's specific diet therapy. The American Diabetes Association diet is used as a guideline for calorie distribution and to promote realistic weight loss and overall

Table 11–1. Insulin Types

Type	Onset of Action	Peak	Duration	Route
Humalog	<15 min	0.55–2.5 h	3.55–4.5 h	SQ
Regular	0.5–1 h	15–5 h	35–10 h	SQ, IV, pump
NPH	15–4 h	45–14 h	105–24 h	SQ
Lente	15–4 h	45–14 h	125–24 h	SQ
Ultralente	35–4 h	85–30 h	185–36 h	SQ
Lantus	15–2 h	none	>24 h	SQ

cardiovascular fitness. Carbohydrate to insulin ratio is also being used in accordance to the patient's weight and response of the patient's blood sugar. A typical ratio is 1 unit of regular insulin to use 15 g of carbohydrate.

Exercise: Exercise has potent blood sugar–lowering effects; however, these effects are not predictable. Therefore, encourage the patient to exercise more for the improvement in cardiovascular fitness and overall sense of psychological well-being. Advise the patient of safeguards to take against hypoglycemia, hyperglycemia, and ketosis when exercising. General guidelines for exercise include: Check blood sugar before, and after exercise; eat a meal 1 to 3 hours before exercise. Take extra carbohydrates every 30 minutes for intense exercise. Reduce regular insulin prior to exercise. Delay exercise if glucose is greater than 250 and if ketoses are present. Inspect feet before and after exercise. Wear proper footwear to avoid injury.

Follow-up: See patient frequently until optimal glucose control is obtained and to monitor patient's adaptation to lifestyle changes and provide patient education. Telephone follow-up care may also be indicated. Once goals for education and glycemia control are met, see patient every 8 to 12 weeks for monitoring and evaluation. Use glycosylated hemoglobin (HgBA1c) every 3 months to monitor glucose control. Have patient perform daily home blood glucose monitoring and record results. Yearly measurement of serum lipids and thyroid function.

Sequelae: Possible complications include hypoglycemia, DKA, microvascular disease (retinopathy and peripheral neuropathy), macrovascular disease (arteriosclerotic heart disease [ASHD], peripheral arterial disease), hyperlipidemia, foot ulcers, and psychological problems related to living with a chronic disease. Cataracts.

Prevention/prophylaxis: Prevention strategies include advising the patient with a family history of diabetes to be closely monitored for the development of clinical diabetes. For the patient with diabetes, strategies for preventing complications include close adherence to and modification of the treatment plan and self-management strategies to meet the patient's metabolic needs, and sick day insulin management. Wear the Medic Alert bracelet at all times.

Referral: Refer to, or consult with, endocrinologist. Refer to an American Diabetes Association accredited diabetes program for comprehensive education and yearly podiatry and ophthalmology referral.

Education: Explain the disease process, signs and symptoms, and treatment (including side effects of medications). Discuss prevention strategies and when to seek medical care. Educational resource materials are available from the American Diabetes Association and the following web sites: *www.diabetes.org, www.diabetes-exercise.org, www.joslin. harvard.edu, and www.diabetes.org*

DIABETES MELLITUS, TYPE 2

SIGNAL SYMPTOMS Polydipsia; frequent infections

Diabetes mellitus, type 2, controlled	ICD-9-CM: 250.00
Diabetes mellitus, type 2, uncontrolled	ICD-9-CM: 250.02

Description: Type 2 diabetes mellitus (formerly known as adult-onset diabetes) is a chronic heterogeneous disorder characterized by hyperglycemia without predisposition to ketoacidosis. It is associated with chronic long-term complications related to macrovascular and microvascular diseases.

Etiology: Results from combination of insulin resistance and insulin secretory defect. Insulin resistance is a metabolic syndrome where the patient presents with central obesity, and where an increase in insulin is needed to transport glucose across cell membranes. The exact cause of beta cell dysfunction is not known. In the early stages of insulin resistance, glycemic control is normal because of hyperinsulinemia. However, when the beta cells can no longer compensate for the insulin resistance, hyperglycemia occurs.

Occurrence: Accounts for about 90% of all diabetes cases in the United States and affects about 7.4% of the entire population in 1995 and is expected to rise to approximately 9% by 2025. However, it is estimated that one third of all patients with diabetes may go undiagnosed. Prevalence increases with age and degree of obesity.

Age: Usually occurs after age 30 but is starting to be seen in obese children. Incidence increases with age.

Ethnicity: Occurs more often in blacks, Native Americans, and people of Hispanic heritage.

Gender: The condition is believed to be genetic. It occurs more in women in the white population, but equally in men and women in other ethnic groups.

Contributing factors: Obesity (more than 12% over ideal body weight), increased age, family history, race, and previous history of impaired glucose tolerance or gestational diabetes, hypertension, coronary artery disease (CAD), peripheral vascular disorders (PVD).

Signs and symptoms: Signal symptoms may be absent or classic symptoms such as polyuria, polydipsia, unexplained weight loss, blurred vision, fatigue, and frequent infections.

Diagnostic tests:

Test	Result Indicating Disorder	CPT Code
Random plasma glucose test level	Above 200 mg/dL with classic symptoms	82962
Fasting plasma glucose level	Above 126 on two occasions,	82962
Fasting plasma glucose level	Above 126 plus sustained elevation of glucose during at least two oral glucose tolerance tests (OGTTs) in which the 2-hour and one intervening level is above 200 mg/dL	82962 82591 OGTT

Differential diagnosis:
- Diabetes mellitus type 1 (anorexia, weight loss, fatigue)
- Diabetes insipidus (extreme polyuria and polydipsia)

Treatment: Treatment goals are to maintain near-normal blood glucose levels and to prevent or decrease macrovascular and microvascular complications. Therapies include a combination of diet therapy, exercise, medication, and blood glucose monitoring.

Physical

Diet therapy: Refer the patient to a certified diabetes educator or dietitian, because nutrition is the cornerstone of type 2 diabetes management. If the patient is overweight, weight reduction is indicated, because the loss of as little as 5% to 10% of body weight can dramatically improve blood glucose levels. Generally, a reduction of 500 to 1000 calories per day will result in a 1- to 2-lb weight loss per week. Customize the calorie distribution between protein, carbohydrate, and fat intake to meet the needs of the patient and any coexisting medical problems. In general, it is recommended that 10% to 20% of the total calories be from protein intake, 40% from carbohydrate, and 30% from fat, with 10% of that from saturated fat.

Exercise: Same as for type 1 diabetes. Additional benefits of exercise for the patient with type 2 diabetes include reduced cholesterol, blood pressure, and risk for peripheral arterial disease; improved glucose control; enhanced weight reduction, and an improved sense of well-being.

Pharmacologic

In many cases, the patient is able to discontinue oral agents or insulin when a consistent diet, exercise, and weight-maintenance regimen is established.

Oral hypoglycemic agents (sulfonylurea compounds, biguanides, alpha glucosidase inhibitors; and thiazolidinediones): Used as adjunctive therapy, medications are prescribed when diet and exercise are not sufficient to achieve near-normal blood glucose levels (usually when premeal glucose levels exceed 120). Individualize agent used and dosage to patient's blood glucose level and activities. Combination therapy may be used (Table 11-2).

Insulin: Insulin therapy is initiated when maximum dosage and/or combinations of oral hypoglycemic agents are not successful in meeting the goals for glucose control or temporarily in the newly diagnosed patient, during periods of major stress or infection, or during pregnancy. Type, amount, and dosage schedule are individualized to the patient's blood glucose level. Combination therapy with oral hypoglycemic agents may also be used.

Complementary Therapies

- Acupuncture has been shown to offer relief from diabetic neuropathy pain
- Chromium supplementation may improve diabetes control. Chromium is needed to make glucose tolerance factor, which helps insulin improve in action.
- Magnesium deficiency may worsen blood sugar control and may contribute to complications in type 2 diabetes.
- Vanadium, a compound found in plants and animals, has been shown to normalize blood glucose levels in animals with type 2 diabetes. A recent study found that when people with diabetes were given vanadium, they developed a modest increase in insulin sensitivity and were able to decrease their insulin requirements.
- Stress management techniques
- Yoga
- Exercise

Follow-up: Same as for type 1 diabetes.

Sequelae: Same as for type 1 diabetes. Patient may not be prone to develop DKA unless major stress or infection precipitates it; however, patient is usually more prone to develop hyperglycemic hyperosmolar nonketotic coma (HHNK).

Prevention/prophylaxis: Fasting blood glucose. Prevention strategies include advising the patient at risk to have yearly screening tests (patient with a family history of diabetes or history of impaired glucose hemostasis, ethnic predisposition, overweight or obese, woman with history of babies weighing greater than 9 pounds at birth, or woman with a previous history of gestational diabetes). Also advise the patient to decrease body fat, maintain a proper diet, and exercise regularly. Wear a Medic Alert bracelet at all times.

Referral: Same as for type 1 diabetes. Also refer patient to ophthalmologist and podiatrist for yearly screening examinations.

Education: Same as for type 1 diabetes.

Table 11–2. Oral Agents for Type 2 Diabetes

Class:	Generic Name	Mono-therapy	Combination with Sulfonylureas	Dosage
Amaryl	Glimepiride	Yes	Metformin, insulin	1, 2, 4 mg up to 8 mg /day
DiaBeta	Glyburide	Yes	Metformin, insulin	1.25–20g mg/day
Micronase	Glyburide	Yes	Metformin, insulin	1.25–20 mg/day
Diabinese	Chlorpropamide	Yes	Metformin, insulin	250–750 mg/day
Glucotrol	Glipizide	Yes	Metformin, insulin	5–10 mg Max 40 mg/day
Glucotrol XL	Glipizide	Yes	Metformin, insulin	5–10 mg Max 20 mg/day
Glynase prestab	Glyburide micronized	Yes	Metformin, insulin	0.75–12 mg/day
Class: Biguanides				
Glucophage	Metformin	Yes	Sulfonylurea, insulin thiazolidinediones	500 mg–2.55 g/day
Glucophage XR	Metformin	Yes	Sulfonylurea, insulin, thiazolidinediones	500 mg–2 g/day
Class: Combination				
Glucovance	Glyburide/ metformin	Yes	No	1.25/250 mg 2.5/500 mg 5/500 mg BID
Class: Alpha-Glucosidase Inhibitors				
Precose	Acarbose	Yes	No	25 mg/meal, up to100 mg /tid
Glyset	Miglitol	Yes	No	50 mg/tid max 100mg/tid
Class: Thiazolidinnedioes				
Actos	Pioglitazone	Yes	Metformin, sulfonylurea insulin	15, 30, 45 mg daily
Avandia	Rosiglitazone	Yes	Metformin, sulfonylurea	4–8 mg /24 h
Class: Amino Acid Derivatives				
Starlix	Nateglinide	Yes	No	120 mg before meals
Class: Meglitinides				
Prandin	Repaglinide	Yes	No	0.5–4 mg with each meal

HEAT-RELATED ILLNESSES (HEAT EDEMA, HEAT SYNCOPE, HEAT CRAMPS, HEAT EXHAUSTION, HEAT STROKE, MILIARIA)

Heat exhaustion	ICD-9-CM: 992.5
Heat stroke	ICD-9-CM: 992.0
Miliaria rubra	ICD-9-CM: 992.5 992.0 705.1

Heat Edema: Swelling of the feet and ankles associated with periods of prolonged sitting or standing.

Heat Syncope: Cool and moist skin, weak pulse, systolic blood pressure usually less than 100 mm Hg, and normal or mildly elevated core temperature.

Heat Cramps: Painful spasms of the voluntary muscles of the abdomen and extremities lasting 1 to 3 minutes; tender muscles; muscle twitching; moist or dry and cool or warm skin; normal or slightly elevated core temperature.

Heat Exhaustion: If a result of water depletion, signal symptoms may include weakness, intense thirst, decreased urine volume, marked central nervous system (CNS) symptoms, muscular incoordination, psychosis, delirium, coma, and hyperthermia. If a result of salt depletion, signal symptoms may include muscle cramps; nausea and vomiting; weakness; diarrhea; tachycardia; hypotension; thirst; pale, moist skin; rectal temperature above 37.8° C; and hyperventilation.

Heat Stroke: Cerebral dysfunction (with sudden onset in 80% of cases) with impaired consciousness, high fever, and absence of sweating.

Miliaria Rubra: Prickly (burning and itching) feeling on the skin; small papules surrounded by a red halo that begin to erupt and may develop into vesicles containing clear or milky fluid that are found mainly on the forearms in front of the elbows, shoulders and chest, waist, behind the knees, and intertriginous areas.

Description: There are a variety of heat-related illnesses. In *heat edema,* individuals who are suddenly exposed to hot climatic conditions without acclimatization develop swollen ankles and feet. In *heat syncope,* sudden unconsciousness occurs in unacclimatized individuals during the early stages of heat exposure. *Heat cramps* are cramps of heavily exercised muscles, often the calves, which occur during and after hard exertion in the heat. They usually occur in people doing hard exercise who sweat profusely and replace fluid losses with hypotonic solutions such as water. *Heat exhaustion* is a systemic reaction to prolonged heat exposure (hours to days), characterized by dehydration, sodium depletion, or isotonic fluid loss, or a combination of these factors, with an increased pulse rate, moist skin, and a rectal temperature over 37.8°C. *Heat stroke* is a life-threatening medical emergency resulting from failure of the thermoregulatory mechanism. It presents with altered mental status, elevated core body temperature in excess of 41°C (105.8°F), and variable sweating. *Miliaria rubra,* also known as prickly heat, heat rash, and lichen tropicus, is an acute inflammatory disorder of the skin caused by obstruction of the sweat ducts.

Etiology:

Heat edema: Caused by excessive vasodilation in the skin combined with venous stasis, increased antidiuretic hormone (ADH) secretion, and excessive intake of salt and water. Interstitial fluid then accumulates in the lower extremities.

Heat syncope: Results from cutaneous vasodilation, along with some decreased plasma volume caused by hypotension, peripheral venous pooling, and a decrease in vasomotor tone; does not represent a state of true dehydration.

Heat cramps: Results from the imbalance between the water and salt (sodium chloride) content in the extracellular and intracellular fluids.

Heat exhaustion: Results from water depletion (dehydration) or from salt depletion (when thermal sweating is replaced by an adequate intake of water but insufficient intake of salt).

Heat stroke: Caused by the inadequacy or failure of the body's heat loss mechanisms to regulate body temperature.

Miliaria rubra: Caused primarily by plugging of the ostia of sweat ducts with consequent ballooning and rupture of the sweat ducts (usually from continuous, prolonged sweating, especially in hot, humid environments).

Occurrence: Incidence of heat stroke in general population is unknown, but mortality increases threefold during heat waves; military recruits in basic training have an incidence of heat stroke of 180 in 100,000. Death rate in the United States due to heat related illness is approximately 175 to 200 persons per year.

Clinical Pearl: The incidence of heat-related illnesses is higher in areas with combined heat and humidity.

Age: Elderly persons are at an increased risk. Neonates are also at high risk owing to poorly developed thermoregulatory mechanism..

Ethnicity: No significant ethnic predisposition.

Contributing Factors: Living or working in non–air-conditioned environments in hot, humid weather; certain occupations such as workers in hot industries, those who must wear encapsulating protective clothing, people engaged in vigorous outdoor sports activities, and military recruits engaging in drill and training exercises; alcohol use; lack of sleep or proper diet; concurrent infection; immunization reaction; fatigue; excessive or constrictive clothing; lack of acclimatization; disorders such as skin diseases, obesity, dehydration, diminished cutaneous blood flow, hypotension, malnutrition, reduced cardiac output; medications such as antihistamines, anticholinergics, phenothiazines, tricyclic antidepressants, diuretics, monoamine oxidase (MAO) inhibitors, vasoconstrictors, beta-adrenergic blocking agents; illicit drugs such as lysergic acid diethylamide (LSD), amphetamines, cocaine, and phencyclidine; pre-existing fever; hyperactivity from psychosis, delirium tremens, drug withdrawal, and prolonged seizures; genetic factors.

Signs and symptoms:

Heat edema: Edema is not complicated by congestive heart failure (CHF) or lymphatic disease.

Heat syncope: Patient has a history of vigorous physical activity for 2 hours or more just preceding the episode.

Heat cramps: Patient has a history of vigorous activity just preceding the onset of symptoms.

Heat exhaustion: Heat exhaustion may progress to heat stroke if sweating ceases or if circulatory failure or seizures occur.

Heat stroke: In the early stage, patient has brilliantly red skin (from peripheral vasodilation). Premonitory findings include the following: visual disturbances; dizziness; headache; nausea; diarrhea; confusion; convulsions and possibly coma; dry, hot, flushed skin (cyanosis or sweating may be present); strong, rapid pulse followed possibly by cardiovascular collapse; elevated blood pressure that may fall with cardiac failure; rectal temperature above 41°C (105.8°F); hyperventilation; coagulopathy; loss of consciousness; and seizures.

Miliaria rubra: Patient has a history of constantly wet skin with salt concentration of the sweat layered over the skin for an extended period.

Diagnostic Tests:

Heat Edema, Heat Syncope, and Miliaria Rubra
Usually none indicated.

Heat Cramps
Rarely indicated; complete blood count (CBC) and electrolytes may reveal low serum sodium level, hemoconcentration, and occasionally hypokalemia.

Heat Exhaustion
Serum electrolytes (reveals markedly low sodium) and renal function (myoglobinuria indicates subclinical rhabdomyolysis).

Heat Stroke

Test	Results indicating disorder	CPT code
CBC	May reveal dehydration, leukocytosis, hemoconcentration	85022
Serum electrolytes/ chemistry Uric acid	May show hyperuricemia; decreased calcium, potassium, phosphorus	80054 84550 Uric acid
Coagulation studies	May show increased bleeding and clotting times, thrombocytopenia, fibrinolysis, consumption coagulopathy);	85610-85613
Creatine kinase, liver function tests, and blood urea nitrogen (BUN)	All elevated	82565 CK 80058 Liver function 84520 BUN
Urinalysis	Concentrated; may show anuria, proteinuria, hematuria; elevated myoglobinuria, protein, tubular casts	81007
Electrocardiogram (ECG)	May show ST-T changes, myocardial ischemia	93040

Differential diagnosis:

- Hypoglycemia (diaphoresis, blurred vision, headache, weakness, tachycardia, blood glucose-fingerstick)
- Dysrhythmias (EKG)
- Myocardial or cerebrovascular lesions (check EKG, imaging, lab work)
- Meningitis (fever, stiff neck)
- Encephalitis (fever, headache)
- Severe head trauma (head injury)
- Epilepsy (seizure)
- Thyroid storm (thyroid level)
- Neuroleptic malignant syndrome (diagnosis of cancer)
- Cerebrovascular accident (CVA)
- Diabetic ketoacidosis with infection (check blood work, inc CBC/diff)
- Drug rash (history of medication use)
- Folliculitis with miliaria (on physical examination)

Treatment:

Heat edema: Symptomatic treatment, such as use of support hose and elevation of lower limbs, because heat edema is self-limiting; diuretics are not indicated.

Heat syncope: Have patient rest in a recumbent position; provide cooling and oral rehydration.

Heat cramps: Place patient in cool environment. Provide oral saline solution (4 tsp of salt per gallon of water) to replace both salt and water. (Do not give salt tablets because of their slow absorption.) For intravenous (IV) treatment, give 1000 mL 0.9% NaCl over 1 to 3 hours.

Heat exhaustion: Place patient in shaded, cool environment. Hydrate with 1 to 2 liters of fluid over 2 to 4 hours. Give adequate cool water and salted fruit drinks, such as Gatorade. In severe cases, administer 0.9% NaCl or 5% dextrose in 0.45% NaCl based on patient's serum electrolyte levels; may require up to 4 liters of fluid over 6 to 8 hours. If sodium depletion is severe, administer IV 3% (hypertonic) saline.

Heat stroke: Rapidly reduce the core temperature within 1 hour. Remove clothing and spray body with water while passing air across the body with large fans. Alternatively, wrap patient in cold, wet sheets and blow air with a high-speed fan; continuously sprinkle sheets to keep them wet. Water should not be colder than 20°C (68 F) or patient will develop peripheral vasoconstriction. Continue treatment until rectal temperature drops to 38 C (100.4°F) because core temperature continues to fall after the cessation of cooling. Administer chlorpromazine 25 to 50 mg IV initially then every 4 hours to control shivering and other muscular activity. If hypovolemic shock is present, administer 500 to 1000 mL 5% dextrose in normal saline. Observe patient for renal failure; maintain urine output of 30 to 50 mL/h. Insert indwelling urinary catheter, and if myoglobinuria is present, alkalize urine with IV bicarbonate. Consider use of mannitol 0.25 g/kg IV to promote diuresis. If inotropic agents are required, administer dobutamine (does not have alpha-adrenergic renal effects).

Miliaria rubra: Wash off sweat and salt with antibacterial soap in a cool shower. Apply triamcinolone acetonide 0.1% or a mid-potency corticosteroid lotion or cream such as betamethasone (Valisone) bid for 3 days. Treat secondary infections with erythromycin or dicloxacillin, 250 mg orally four times a day. If sweating is related to fever, prescribe antipyretics and frequent, cool baths with Aveeno colloidal oatmeal. Provide dry and cool environment for 10 to 12 hours per day. Avoid sunlight.

Follow-up: See the patient as needed for further evaluation (especially if patient has chronic heat edema or if patient with heat exhaustion develops symptoms after discharge).

Sequelae: With early diagnosis and proper care, 80% to 90% of previously healthy patients will survive. Possible complications include potentially reversible neurological changes, permanent brain damage, cerebellar damage, reoccurrence (especially with heat stroke, heat exhaustion, or heat cramps), lower heat tolerance (with severe miliaria), rhabdomyolysis, cardiac disorders, acute renal failure, liver disorders, and disseminated intravascular coagulation (DIC).

Prevention/prophylaxis: Prevention strategies include teaching the patient signs and symptoms of heat-related illnesses and preventive measures such as decreasing extreme salt intake (for patient with heat edema); rest for 1 to 3 days with dietary salt supplementation (for patient with heat cramps); to take time for proper conditioning (such as exercising or working in graduated increases), acclimatization, and fluid replacement (cold water or weak electrolyte solutions for most people, 8 oz. for every 15 minutes of moderate exercise is recommended; salted fluids, such as Gatorade, for those who sweat heavily over extended period of time); removing clothing and maintaining skin exposure (with sunblock protection) in hot, humid conditions; to wear clean, lightweight, or cotton clothing and antibacterial preparations (for patient with miliaria); to take weight daily if exercising or working in hot, humid environments (3% weight loss indicates need for increased fluid intake; 5% weight loss indicates need to stop or cancel activity; 7% weight loss requires prompt fluid replacement).

Referral: Refer to, or consult with, physician if patient requires hospitalization (patient whose core temperature exceeds 41°C (105.8°F), is an older adult, has an underlying disease, or who shows little improvement after 2 to 3 hours).

Education: Explain the disease process, signs and symptoms, and treatment (including side effects of medications). Discuss prevention strategies and when to seek medical care.

HYPERLIPIDEMIA, HYPERCHOLESTEROLEMIA

SIGNAL SYMPTOMS▶   Elevated lipids, usually asymptomatic

Hyperlipidemia	ICD-9-CM 272.5
Pure Hypercholesterolemia	ICD-9-CM: 272.4 272.0
Carbohydrate-induced	ICD-9-CM: 272.1
Combined	ICD-9-CM: 272.4
Fat-induced	ICD-9f-CM: 272.3

Description: The hyperlipidemias, also referred to as hypercholesterolemias, are a group of disorders of lipid metabolism resulting in abnormally high circulating levels of lipids in the blood (high-density lipoprotein [HDL] fraction of cholesterol, low-density lipoprotein (LDL) fraction of cholesterol, very low-density lipoprotein [VLDL] fraction of cholesterol, and triglycerides). Hyperlipidemia is associated with atherosclerosis and pancreatitis and an increased risk of the development of CAD. The third report of the national cholesterol education program expert panel for detection, evaluation, and treatment of high blood cholesterol in adults (adult treatment panel III) identifies the LDL cholesterol as the primary target of lipid-lowering therapy. Research studies have shown that lowering LDL levels has decreased the risk of CAD.

Lipoproteins transport triglycerides and cholesterol in the plasma. Primary hyperlipidemia usually results from hereditary disorders involving deficiencies in various mechanisms of lipid metabolism. Secondary hyperlipidemia is associated with dietary intake of foods increased in lipids, and a variety of underlying disorders such as diabetes, Cushing's syndrome, acromegaly, hypothyroidism, alcohol, and liver diseases. Patients need their risk factors evaluated to assist with determining what treatment they need. Major risk factors include the presence or absence of CAD, Cigarette smoking, Hypertension > 140/90 mm Hg or on an antihypertensive drug, low HDL < 40 mg/dL, family history of CAD in male first-degree relative <55 or female <65, age men > 45, women >55. Each one of these risk factors alters the LDL cholesterol goal. A patient with known CAD or CAD risk equivalents (diabetes, peripheral vascular disease, 10-year risk assessment for CAD >20%) LDL goal is <100. Multiple risk factors >2 the LDL goal is <130, and zero to 1 risk factor the LDL goal is <160.

Occurrence: About 50% of the U.S. adult population has elevated blood lipid levels.

Age: The incidence increases with age.

Ethnicity: No significant ethnic predisposition.

Gender: Occurs more often in men than in women.

Contributing factors: Excessive alcohol intake, heredity, obesity, use of estrogen therapy and glucocorticoids, hypothyroidism, anorexia, liver and renal diseases, immunologic disorders, stress, sedentary lifestyle, cholestasis, and diabetes.

Signs and symptoms: There are no signal symptoms. The patient is often asymptomatic until signs and symptoms of advanced CAD appear, such as CVA, myocardial infarction (MI), angina, and claudication. Physical examination may reveal an arterial bruit, corneal arcus before age 50, or xanthoma.

Diagnostic Tests: A complete fasting lipid profile (total cholesterol, LDL, HDL, triglyceride levels) should be drawn at age 20 and repeated every 5 years. Thyroid function tests (may be performed as hypothyroidism may contribute to disorder). Hypothyroidism, nephrotic syndrome, and obstructive liver disease may alter laboratory results. Patients with a triglyceride level above 200 mg/dl need to have their triglycerides lowered before starting LDL lowering therapy.

Differential diagnosis: Primary versus secondary hyperlipidemia.

 Clinical Pearl: Anyone with an elevated LDL should undergo clinical or laboratory assessment to rule out secondary dyslipidemia before starting lipid lowering drug therapy.

Treatment: Treatment of hyperlipidemia is a lifelong endeavor and requires good knowledge of the patient and his or her motivation and risk profile. Begin treatment with diet and exercise, then re-evaluate the patient in 6to 12 weeks, depending on risk factors before beginning pharmacologic therapy. Table 11–3 lists Cholesterol goals based on risk factor assessment.

Physical

Diet: Dietary interventions remain a cornerstone of treatment. Medication alone will not lower the patient's LDL to acceptable levels without some adherence to healthful eating. Dietary therapy includes the following: Advise the patient to decrease all dietary fats, to use olive oil instead, and to increase the amount of fiber, fruits, vegetables, whole grains, and garlic in the diet. Encourage the patient to have vegetarian, meatless, eggless, and cheeseless meals; recommend meals with poultry, fish, and nonfat milk and yogurt. Also, advise the patient that even a minimal daily intake of alcohol may increase HDL levels.

Exercise: Aerobic exercise for at least 30 minutes three times a week helps increase HDL and decrease total cholesterol and body weight.

Pharmacologic

The decision as to which drug to use is often based on the patient's profile, cost of the medication, and working with the patient to determine which medication works best in regard to side effects and compliance with therapy. Overall, LDL cholesterol levels may decrease 30% to 40% on full-dose therapy. Start with the lowest dose and continue for 6 to 8 weeks to assess efficiency. Increase dosage only after rechecking cholesterol levels. Commonly prescribed medications include the following: Cholestyramine or colestipol, 2 scoops of bulk form twice or three times a day, begin with 1 scoop in the morning 30 minutes before eating, increase to twice a day, then 2 scoops twice a day; gemfibrozil, 600 mg

Table 11–3. LDL Cholesterol Goals Based on Risk Factors

Risk Category	LDL Goal	LDL level to start therapeutic lifestyle changes	LDL level to start drug therapy
CAD or CAD risk equivalents, 10 year risk >20%	<100 mg/dL	= 100 mg/dL	=130 mg/dL
2 + risk factors 10-year risk < 20%	<130 mg/dL	= 130 mg/dL	10-year risk 10% to 20% =130 mg/dL 10-year risk <10% = 160 mg/dl
0–1% Risk factor	<160 mg/dL	>160 mg/dL	>190 mg/dL

twice a day; fluvastatin, 20 to 40 mg/day, 30 minutes before meals; lovastatin (Mevacor), 20 to 80 mg/day; pravastatin sodium (Pravachol), 10 to 40 mg/day; simvastatin (Zocor), 5 to 80 mg/day, start with 5to 10 mg after evening meal, increase dosage every 6 weeks, and niacin, 500 to 1000 mg each day.

 Clinical Pearl: If patient is on statin therapy, a liver function test must be performed according to the drug manufacture recommendations.

Follow-up: See the patient two to four times a year or when indicated to monitor the cholesterol, HDL, LDL, and triglyceride levels; if cholesterol level is less than 200 mg/dL, repeat in 5 years.

Sequelae: Possible complications include CAD, CVA, pancreatitis, and atherosclerosis.

Prevention/prophylaxis: Prevention strategies include advising the patient to comply with treatment regimen, including diet and exercise, and to take measures to reduce risk of CAD.

Referral: Refer to, or consult with, nutritionist for dietary counseling if indicated; to cardiologist if the patient fails to respond to cholesterol-lowering diet, and monotherapy drug regimen for consideration of combination therapy.

Education: Explain disease process, signs and symptoms, and treatment (including side effects of medications). Discuss prevention and importance of compliance with diet, exercise, and drug therapy. Reinforce need to reduce CAD risk factors. *www.heartcenteronline.com*, *www.merckmedco.com*, *www.hivdent.org* are web sites available for patient education.

OBESITY

SIGNAL SYMPTOMS ▶ Body mass index (BMI) > 30; waist circumference >40 in for men and >35 in for women

Obesity	ICD-9-CM: 278.0

Description: Obesity is defined as weighing 20% above ideal body weight (IBW) and results from the accumulation of body fat in excess of that necessary for optimal body function. Obesity is one of the most common chronic disorders and is a risk factor for many other chronic diseases and psychological disabilities.

Etiology: Caused by multiple factors, including biologic, genetic, metabolic, psychological, environmental, and social factors, interacting simultaneously within the patient.

Occurrence: Occurs in about one third or more of the American population aged 20 and older.

Age: Incidence tends to increase with age but in recent years has been on the increase in school-age and adolescent children.

Ethnicity: Tends to occur more in black, Hispanic, American Indian, and Alaskan native women than in white or European-American women; more in white men than in black men; and more in lower socioeconomic groups.

Gender: Tends to occur more in women (30% to 40%) than in men (20% to 30%).

Contributing factors: Environmental factors such as lifestyle, including sedentary lifestyle and high-fat diets; various psychological factors; certain medications such as steroids and antidepressants; hypothyroidism; Cushing's syndrome; hypothalamic disorders; insulinoma.

Signs and symptoms: History may reveal a family history of obesity, recent weight changes, psychosocial factors, and past dieting experiences, as well as current motivation for weight loss. Ask about normal food intake and dietary habits; exercise habits; and alcohol, tobacco, and other drug use.

Patient may present with fatigue; inability to engage in physical activities; dyspnea on exertion; pain in weight-bearing joints or spine; or with signs and symptoms of hypertension, diabetes, cholecystitis, or cardiovascular disease.

Physical examination reveals an obese patient (classified as mild obesity, 20% t o 40% over IBW; moderate obesity, 41% to 100% over IBW; or over 100%, morbid obesity) and an android (apple) or gynoid (pear) body fat distribution.

Diagnostic Tests: Performed to determine metabolic alterations; may include

Test	Result Indicating Disorder	CPT Code
Random blood glucose	Assesses for hyperglycemia	82962
TSH, free and T_4	Free, decreased T_4 and elevated thyroid-stimulating hormone (TSH) levels indicates hypothyroidism	80091
Dexamethasone suppression testing	Rules out Cushing's syndrome	80420
Serum cholesterol level, triglycerides, and a lipoprotein panel	Assesses risk factors for cardiovascular disease	80061
Relative weights (RW) (used by insurance industry):	Weight of the patient divided by the IBW for a person of medium frame and the same height. RW for men equals 106 lb and 6 lb for each inch over 5 ft; RW for women equals 100 lb and 5 lb for each inch over 5 ft.	Physical examination

(Continued)

Test	Result Indicating Disorder	CPT Code
Body mass index (BMI) (measurement of choice):	Determined by dividing patient's weight in kilograms by patient's height in meters squared. Normal weight is defined as BMI of 18.5 to 24.9, overweight BMI 25 to 29.9, and obese is BMI of > 30.	Physical examination
Skin-fold thickness using a skin caliper on various parts of the body	Simple method for measuring body fat	Physical examination
"Pinch test" (estimated subcutaneous fat):	Skin folds measured in the midtriceps area, below the scapulae, lower part of the chest wall, buttocks, or thigh. Normal skin fold is less than 0.5 inch; excessive is more than 1 inch.	Physical examination

Differential diagnosis:

- Hypothyroidism (weight gain)
- Other metabolic derangements (check appropriate lab tests)

Treatment:

Physical

Diet: Encourage a healthy diet that meets all recommended daily allowances (RDAs) for nutrients; less than 30% total fat intake (10% only from saturated fat); 15% protein intake; and 55% carbohydrate intake (primarily complex carbohydrates). Many sources recommend a diet lower than 30% of daily calories from fat. Have patient submit a 3- to 5-day food diary and an exercise plan that can fit into his or her schedule. This information as well as information regarding outside stressors, emotional disorders, and substance abuse will provide an assessment of motivation as well as a basis for a treatment plan.

One pound of fat equals approximately 3500 calories. Therefore, to lose 1 to 2 pounds per week, a daily energy deficit of 500 to 1000 calories is required. The recommended caloric intake is obtained by multiplying the patient's IBW (in kg) by 30 then subtracting 500 to 1000 calories from it to obtain a 1- to 2-lb weight loss per week.

Exercise: Exercise increases energy expenditure, aiding in the energy deficit needed for weight loss and is essential for successful maintenance of weight loss. An exercise stress test may be needed for the patient with a sedentary lifestyle (especially for men over age 40 and women over age 50) or CAD risk factors. Have the patient select two aerobic exercises and perform either one of them four to five times per week for 20 to 25 minutes per day. Regular aerobic exercise also provides the patient with improved cardiovascular tone, decreased blood pressure, decreased appetite, improved glucose metabolism and insulin action, and improved lipid profile.

Lifestyle changes and behavior modification: Have the patient keep records of diet, exercise, and progress. Record keeping aids the patient in behavioral changes and assists the provider in assessing progress and making adjustments to the plan of care. Additional support may be obtained through involvement of family and peer support groups

Pharmacologic

Short-term use of appetite suppressants may be indicated in combination with lifestyle changes and may include the over-the-counter OTC medication phenylpropanolamine, 25 mg orally three times a day or 75-mg timed-release form once daily or prescription medications (Table 11–4).

Surgical

Usually used only as a last resort and for patient who has severe morbid obesity. Procedures include vertical-banded gastroplasty and gastric bypass.

Refer to Figure 11-1 for steps in the differential diagnosis of obesity.

Follow-up: See the patient on a regular basis to monitor progress and provide support. Close provider contact is a better predictor of success than the weight loss intervention. Long-term follow-up is also recommended to prevent further weight gain or weight regain after loss.

 Clinical Pearl: Monitor blood pressure closely (for elevation) when starting patients on prescription weight loss medications.

Sequelae: Android obesity (male pattern or abdominal obesity) is a greater risk factor for long-term health problems than is gynoid obesity (female pattern or gluteal obesity). Possible complications include death (primarily from coronary heart disease); the risk of developing type 2 diabetes, hypertension, hypercholesterolemia, surgical and obstetric complications; and tendency toward accidents, poor self-esteem, and job

Table 11–4. Prescription Medications for Obesity

Class	Generic Name	Brand Name	Dosage
C-4	Phentermine	Adipex, Ionamin	Adipex: 37.5 mg/day Ionamin: 15–30 mg/day
C-4	Sibutramine HCL monohydrate	Meridia	10–15 mg/day
C-4	Diethylpropion	Tenuate Tenuate Dospan	25 mg/tid 75 mg SR/daily
C-3	Phendimetrazine tartrate	Bontril Bontril SR	35 mg/tid 105 mg/daily
Not Controlled	Oristat	Xenical	120 mg/tid

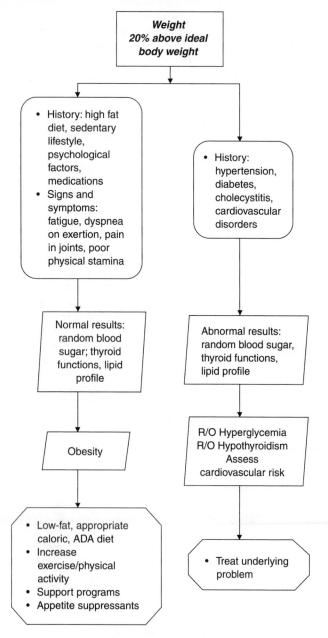

Figure 11–1. Steps in the differential diagnosis of obesity.

discrimination. Long-term obesity is associated with degenerative joint disease, gout, cholecystitis, esophageal reflux, thromboembolism, hypoventilation, and sleep apnea.

Prevention/prophylaxis: Prevention strategies include advising the patient to pay close attention to fluctuations in weight and providing the patient with guidelines for a healthy diet and adequate exercise.

Referral: Refer to dietitian, or consult with, physician as needed or a surgeon if surgical interventions are considered.

Education: Explain the disease process, signs and symptoms, and treatment (including side effects of medications). Discuss prevention strategies and need for life-long lifestyle changes (such as healthy diet and exercise). Also advise the patient about the potentially dangerous cardiovascular effects of weight fluctuations seen with cyclical weight gain and loss (so-called yo-yo dieting). See *www.shapeup.com www.weight.com* and *www.nhlbi.nih.gov* .

PANCREATITIS

SIGNAL SYMPTOMS Acute: Steady, dull or boring mid-epigastric pain radiating to back with associated nausea and vomiting. The pain lasts for hours and days rather than being transient.

Chronic: Intermittent or chronic, boring and dull midepigastric pain radiating to the back. Patients present with complaints of recurrent episodes of epigastric and upper left quadrant pain.

| Pancreatitis, acute | ICD-9-CM: 577.0 |
| Pancreatitis, chronic | ICD-9-CM: 577.1 |

Description: Pancreatitis is an inflammation of the pancreas that is generally classified as either acute or chronic. It is caused by the release of activated pancreatic enzymes into the surrounding parenchyma with the subsequent destruction of tissue, blood vessels, and supporting structures.

Etiology: Caused by excessive alcohol consumption and gallstones (90% of cases). Other causes include surgical injury from gastric and biliary operations, certain drugs (opiates, steroids, and thiazide diuretics), viral infections, and trauma (penetrating injuries to the upper abdomen.)

Occurrence: Approximately 15/100,000.

Age: Chronic pancreatitis occurs primarily in middle-aged adults (ages 35 to 45) unless it is a result of trauma or postoperative complications.

Ethnicity: No significant ethnic predisposition.

Gender: Occurs equally in women and men.

Contributing Factors: Alcohol abuse (at most risk), predisposition to formation of gallstones, hyperlipidemia, hyperparathyroidism, viral infections, nutritional and hereditary factors, metabolic hypercalcemia.

Signs and Symptoms:

Acute: Almost all patients present with abdominal pain, steadily growing worse in the epigastric area and eventually radiating straight through to the back. Other general complaints include nausea, vomiting, sweating, weakness, and pallor. Physical examination may reveal abdominal tenderness and distention and a low-grade fever.

Chronic: Other symptoms reported include anorexia, nausea, vomiting, constipation, flatulence, and weight loss. Physical examination may reveal tenderness over the pancreatic area, abdominal muscle guarding, paralytic ileus, dehydration, and occasionally mild jaundice.

 Clinical Pearl: Continual hiccups can be a sign of pancreatitis.

Diagnostic Tests:

Acute

Test	Result Indicating Disorder	CPT Code
Serum amylase and lipase	Elevated, increased on the first day of active symptoms then returns to normal in 3 to 7 days	82150 Serum amylase 83690 Lipase
Urinalysis	May reveal proteinuria, casts, glycosuria, and increased osmolality	81007
CBC	May show a marked leukocytosis; Hct will be as high as 50% to 55%	85022
Alanine aminotransferase (ALT)	Mildly elevated	84460
Alkaline phosphatase	Elevated	84075
Serum calcium	Decreased	82310
C-reactive protein	If elevated, suspect developing pancreatic necrosis	86140
Radiography-flat and upright of the abdomen	May show gallstones and intestinal air fluid levels	74241
CT scan	May show enlarged pancreas and extent of pancreatic swelling	78223

Chronic

Test	Result Indicating Disorder	CPT Code
Serum amylase, lipase, and bilirubin	All elevated	82150 Serum amylase 83690 Lipase 82251 BUN
Urinalysis	Shows glycosuria	81000
Stool sample	Shows high fecal fat content	Missing

(Continued)

Test	Result Indicating Disorder	CPT Code
Radiographic tests—imaging	May show presence of pancreatic calcification	78223
Radiographic tests—Ultrasound of abdomen	Pseudocyst formation/calcification	78223

Differential diagnosis:

- Perforated peptic ulcer (severe pain radiating to back)
- Biliary colic (right upper quadrant [RUQ] pain, imaging)
- Acute cholecystitis (RUQ pain, nausea and vomiting, ultrasound)
- Aortic aneurysm (acute onset of teary or nipping pain in chest, back and/or neck, pulse deficit, older age)
- Intestinal obstruction (decreased bowel sounds)
- Other malabsorption and/or malignant process.(diagnostic tests including imaging)

Treatment

Acute: Withhold food and fluids until symptoms subside. If ileus is present, apply nasogastric suction. Meperidine (Demerol) 50 to 100 mg intramuscularly (IM)/IV q 3–4 hours. Administer IV fluids to maintain intravascular volume; add calcium gluconate if severe hypocalcemia is present.

Treatment plan should include:

Pain control, Meperidine

Arrest, shock, IVF

Nasogastric tube/vomiting

Calcium monitoring

Renal evaluation

Ensure pulmonary function

Antibiotics

Surgery or special procedures in selected cases

Chronic: Absolute abstinence from alcohol is mandatory. Acetaminophen with or without oxycodone (Tylox) or hydrocodone (Vicodin) as needed for pain. Low-fat, low-cholesterol diet. Pancreatic enzyme supplements(Pancrease MT, Creon) should be included in patient's diet. Pharmacologic therapy includes histamine 2 (H_2) blockers (reducing gastric acid increases availability of pancreatic enzymes) and antacids. Pain: alcohol abstinence, avoid narcotics, celiac ganglionic block, surgery; maldigestion: pancreatic enzyme supplements; H_2 blockers, Diabetes mellitus: insulin.

Follow-up: See the patient immediately on discharge from hospital and at monthly intervals for collection of serum lipase and amylase, CBC to follow the white count, and urinalysis for glucose, bilirubin, and cast screening. For the patient with chronic pancreatitis, also perform ultrasound studies every 6 months to check for pancreatic pseudocysts. Continued elevation of amylase weeks after an attack of acute pancreatitis suggests a pseudocyst.

Sequelae: Acute pancreatitis resolves spontaneously 85% to 90% of the time. Monitor for addiction to pain medication. Possible complications include diabetes mellitus, pancreatic pseudocysts or abscesses, common bile duct stricture, and occasionally pancreatic cancer. Acute pancreatitis may become chronic.

Prevention/prophylaxis: Prevention strategies include advising the patient to limit alcohol consumption (single greatest preventive strategy) and to maintain a low-fat, low-cholesterol diet.

Referral: Refer to, or consult with, surgeon or gastrointestinal (GI) specialist once diagnosis is made; to nutritionist as appropriate; to psychologist, appropriate specialists, and programs for behavior modification, such as Alcoholics Anonymous or rehabilitation centers.

Education: Explain the disease process, signs and symptoms, and treatment (including side effects of medications). Discuss the importance of eliminating alcohol use, maintaining proper diet, and reporting symptoms.

See: *www.patient-education. com* and *www.gastromed.com*

THYROID CANCER

SIGNAL SYMPTOMS Hoarseness ; difficulty swallowing

Malignant neoplasm of thyroid gland	ICD-9-CM: 193

Description: Thyroid cancer is the unregulated, uncontrolled, disorganized cellular proliferation of the thyroid gland. There are four types of thyroid cancer: papillary, the most common and least malignant; follicular, less common and slightly more malignant; medullary, rare and moderately malignant; and anaplastic, very rare and highly malignant.

Etiology: Exact cause is unknown.

Occurrence: Approximately 16,000 new cases arise per year. Thyroid cancer accounts for 2% of all cancers but represents the most common cause of death from an endocrine cancer.

Age: Adult onset is most common

Ethnicity: Most common in whites; uncommon in blacks.

Gender: Papillary and follicular occur more often (70%) in women than in men; medullary and anaplastic occur equally in men and in women.

Contributing factors: History of head, neck, or upper thoracic low-dose radiation during childhood; iodine deficiency is a risk factor for follicular carcinoma; previous partial thyroidectomy for malignancy; positive family history for familial occurrence.

Signs and symptoms: A solitary painless thyroid nodule in an otherwise asymptomatic patient. Unexplained cervical adenopathy on routine examination may alert the clinician to underlying thyroid cancer.

Long-standing tumors may have hoarseness, stridor, or difficulty swallowing.

Diagnostic tests:

Test	Result Indicating Disorder	CPT Code
Thyroid hormone levels	Usually within normal limits	84439 80438-39 80418 80438-40 84443
Thyroid ultrasound	Helps distinguish between cystic and solid lesions; a solid lesion is more likely malignant	76536
Radionuclide testing	Helps distinguish between a "hot" functioning nodule versus a "cold" nonfunctioning nodule; "cold" nodules are more suspect for malignancy	78006 78000-78003
Fine-needle biopsy	Provides cytologic specimens from which a definitive diagnosis of Thyroid Cancer can be obtained	60100

Differential Diagnosis:

- Hashimoto's thyroiditis (affects men 8 times more than women, autoimmune thyroiditis, enlarged thyroid and hypothyroidism)
- Thyroid adenoma (biopsy)
- Benign thyroid cyst (biopsy)
- Multinodular goiter (review imaging, laboratory tests)
- Thyroglossal duct cyst (review imaging, laboratory tests)

Treatment:

Surgical

Thyroidectomy or partial thyroidectomy proved the best treatment of thyroid cancer and provides the best chance for survival. A small portion of the thyroid may be left adjacent to a parathyroid glands to protect its blood supply.

Pharmacologic

Post-thyroidectomy patients require thyroid hormone replacement. The goal of this treatment is to suppress thyroid hormone and maintain the TSH levels below 0.1 mU per liter.

Follow-up: Thyroid scan at 6 weeks, with administration of I_{131} (radioactive iodine) for any visible uptake. At 6 months the patient should have a thyroid scan and chest x-ray; then yearly. Thyroglobulin level should be checked yearly in cases of papillary and follicular thyroid cancer. Patient must be in hypothyroid state for scan and thyroglobulin level. This requires a 6-week withdrawal of levothyroxine or a 2- to 3-week withdrawal of liothyronine.

Sequelae: Possible complications include scarring, parathyroid involvement, reoccurrence, and difficulty maintaining euthyroid state. Papillary carcinoma has a 5-year survival rate of 90%; follicular carcinoma of approximately 80%. Patients with medullary carcinoma have a 5-year survival rate of 90% with negative nodes; 65% with positive nodes. Anaplastic carcinoma of the thyroid has a low survival rate. Recurrences are not uncommon.

Prevention/prophylaxis: Prevention strategies include advising the patient who has a history of radiation exposure in childhood or who has a family history to have an annual thyroid evaluation.

Referral: Refer to or consult with an endocrinologist if a patient has a solitary thyroid nodule.

Education: Explain disease process, signs and symptoms, and treatment including side effects of medications. Discuss prevention strategies and when to seek medical care. Monitor for recurrence.

See *www.endocrineweb.com/thyroidca.html, www.tsh.org/ptinfo/ guidecan.html, www.thyroidcancer.com*

THYROID IMBALANCE: GOITER

SIGNAL SYMPTOMS ▶ Palpable nodule in thyroid area; hoarseness; difficulty swallowing

Thyrotoxicosis with or without goiter	ICD-9-CM: 242.0
Toxic uninodular goiter	ICD-9-CM: 242.1
Toxic multinodular goiter	ICD-9-CM: 242.2

Description: Thyroid nodules, including goiter, are common. A palpable thyroid nodule can be detected in 4% to 7% of adults. Solitary thyroid nodules can be benign adenomas, carcinomas, or multinodular conditions in which only one nodule is palpable. Hashimoto's thyroiditis is an autoimmune condition that leads to multinodular goiters. Incidentalomas are nonpalpable thyroid lesions detected incidentally in the course of imaging the neck by ultrasound.

Etiology: Very little is known about the specific causes of thyroid nodules.

Occurrence: The prevalence of thyroid nodules on autopsy approaches 50%.

Age: The incidence of thyroid nodules increases with age.

Ethnicity: No significant ethnic predisposition.

Gender: Solitary or multiple nodules occur in 90% of women after age 60 and in 60% of men after age 80. Malignant potential is higher in men.

Contributing factors: Iodine deficiency; history of childhood neck irra-

Table 11–5 Signs and Symptoms of Thyroid Disease

Cause	Distinguishing Characteristics
Solitary Nodule	
Benign adenoma	Solid or mixed cystic and solid: most euthyroid and responsive to TSH: Those smaller than 3 cm may become autonomous and present as a hot nodule on scan.
Cancer	
Papillary or mixed	Single hard nodule: local adenopathy: cold on scan; slow growing; metastasizes very late.
Follicular	Metastasizes earlier, some cystic
Medullary	May be familial; multiple endocrine neoplasia; calcitonin elevated; cold nodule.
Lymphoma	Primary cancer arises in patients with chronic lymphocytic thyroiditis prominent regional nodes.
Multinodular	
Hashimoto's thyroiditis	Multinodular, rubbery gland, antithyroid antibodies, one-third hypothyroid, heterogeneous uptake, TSH responsive.
Multinodular goiter	Multiple nodules, enlarged gland, heterogeneous uptake on scan with some areas of decreased or absent uptake; clinically euthyroid although some with mild decrease in TSH; autonomous gland

diation (27% of all irradiated patients get nodules); exposure to excessive environmental radiation; history of thyroid cancer; use of goitrogenic substances such as lithium, turnips, beets, kelp, amiodarone, and iodides.
Signs and symptoms: See Table 11–5.
Diagnostic tests:
   The physical examination focuses on the gland and adjacent lymph

Test	Result Indicating Disorder	CPT code
Thyroid function tests	Usually within normal limits	84439 80438-39 80418 80438-40 84443
Thyroid ultrasound tests	Have good sensitivity in the detection of thyroid nodules and the ability to differentiate solid from cystic lesions. It is also excellent for determining multinodularity.	76536
Fine needle aspiration and biopsy (FNAB)	May be indicated to rule out malignancy. Malignancy is more associated with "cold" nodules.	60100

nodes. A solitary hard nodule that is irregular and fixed is suggestive of malignancy. A soft nodule could be cancerous but is likely to be benign.
Differential diagnosis:

- Thyroid cancer (imaging, biopsy)
- Hashimoto's thyroiditis (affects men 8x more than women,

autoimmune thyroiditis, enlarged thyroid and hypothyroidism)
- Parathyroid tumors (imaging, biopsy; surgical excision if necessary to differentiate)

Treatment:

Warm (Functional) Nodule: No treatment is needed unless hyperthyroidism is present. In that case, treat the hyperthyroidism. See also "Thyroid Imbalance: Hyperthyroidism," following.

Cold (nonfunctional) nodule: Fine-needle aspiration and biopsy is suggested. Higher association with malignancy.

Progressively enlarging goiter: Surgical interventions, such as a thyroidectomy, may be necessary if the goiter makes it difficulty to swallow, talk or breath.

Nodule associated with a hyperthyroid or hypothyroid state: Treat underlying thyroid imbalance. Suppressive L-T$_4$ therapy may be used; however, the success rate of this therapy is variable. Stop all substances that may be goitrogens.

Follow-up: See patient with an asymptomatic nodule as needed for re-evaluation and diagnostic testing ("watchful waiting").

Sequelae: Possible complications include the potential for suffocation related to upper airway obstruction and the potential for a "cold" nodule to progress to a "hot" one.

Prevention/prophylaxis: Prevention strategies include advising the patient to maintain a diet that includes the intake of iodized salt.

Referral: Refer to endocrinologist for multinodular goiter and/or evaluation to confirm diagnosis. Refer to or consult with surgeon if malignancy is suspected.

Education: Explain disease process, signs and symptoms, and treatment (including side effects of medications). Discuss signs and symptoms of upper airway obstruction, need for regular follow-up, and when to seek medical attention.

See *www.endocrineweb.com/goiter.html*

THYROID IMBALANCE: HYPERTHYROIDISM (THYROTOXICOSIS)

SIGNAL SYMPTOMS Weight loss despite increased appetite; tremor; nervous palpitations

Thyrotoxicosis	ICD-9-CM: 242.0 242.9

Description: Hyperthyroidism or thyrotoxicosis is a condition in which excessive amounts of free thyroxine (T_4) and triiodothyronine (T_3) are found in the blood.

Etiology: Most common cause is Graves' disease (an autoimmune phenomenon in which antibodies are produced that attack various components of the thyroid gland). Goiter and ophthalmopathy are common characteristics of Graves' disease. Other causes include toxic adenomas of the thyroid, subacute thyroiditis (inflammation thought to be caused by a viral infection), thyrotoxicosis factitia (results from ingestion of excessive amounts of thyroid hormones), struma ovarii (thyroid-secreting tissue found in ovarian teratomas), and TSH-secreting tumor of the pituitary glan.

Occurrence: Hyperthyroidism is common in the population with a prevalence of 1.9% in women and 0.16% in men.

Age: Fifteen percent of cases in persons older than 60 years; Graves; disease is more common in persons younger than 40 years.

Ethnicity: No significant ethnic predisposition.

Gender: Occurs more often in women than in men.

Contributing factors: Other autoimmune disorders, positive family history, female gender, iodine repletion after iodine depletion.

Signs and symptoms: Patients often complain of many symptoms, including nervousness (85%); dyspnea on exertion (75%); heat intolerance (70%); palpitations (75%); weight loss (52%); tremor (65%); warm, moist skin (72%); fatigue (60%); and increased appetite (40%).

Physical examination may reveal a goiter (may be smooth and diffuse or nodular in texture; tender or nontender and firm (87%), exophthalmos (34%), tremor (65%), hyperkinesis, and lid lag.

Diagnostic tests:

Test	Result Indicating Disorder	CPT Code
Tests include T_3, T_4, and free thyroxin index (FTI)	All will be elevated	84439 80438–39 80418 80438–40 84443
TSH	Will be depressed	80418 80438–40 84443
Ultrasound of thyroid	Diffuse in Graves' disease; focal in toxic nodule	76536
Radionuclide studies	Shows increased uptake of radioactive iodine in Graves' disease and multinodular goiter	78006 78000–78003

Differential diagnosis:
- Thyroid neoplasm (check ultrasound, biopsy)
- Tumors, and goiters (check ultrasound, biopsy)
- Atrial fibrillation (EKG, Holter monitor)
- CHF (echocardiogram, chest x-ray study)

Table 11–6. Drugs for Hyperthyroidism

Drug	Mechanism of Action	Dose
Propylithiouracil	Inhibits T_4 to T_3 conversion peripherally as well as thyroid hormone formation and release	150 - 600 mg in divided doses given twice or three times daily.
Methimazole	Decreases the release of thyroid hormone. Does not inhibit conversion of T_4 to T_3 peripherally	15–30 mg in divided doses given twice daily
Iodine	Used only when preparing a patient for surgery	5–10 mg/day
Beta-blocker	Inhibits T_4 to T_3 conversion, blocks catecholamine effect and controls tachycardia	10–360 mg divided doses

- Panic or anxiety/depression disorder (resolve with treatment)
- Menopause (check hormone levels)
- Pregnancy (positive pregnancy test, history)
- Diabetes (elevated blood glucose)
- Pheochromocytoma (check epinephrine/norepinephrine, imaging for tumor)

Treatment:

Pharmacologic

See Table 11–6 for drugs used in hyperthyroidism.

Surgical:

Subtotal thyroidectomy (rare; preferred for pregnant women who do not respond to antithyroid medications and patients with large goiters).

Physical

Sufficient calories to prevent weight loss.

Follow-up: See the patient using radioactive iodine monthly until patient reaches euthyroid state; then see the patient every 6 months to check for hypothyroidism. See patient taking propylthiouracil at the end of treatment then every 3 months to check T_4 levels; every 6 months for 1 year, check liver enzymes; CBC (propylthiouracil may cause dermatitis, agranulocytosis, or hepatotoxicity). Patient undergoing surgical treatment will be followed by surgeon for routine postoperative care.

Sequelae: Possible complications include hypothyroidism from treatment. Most patients return to the euthyroid state. In general, excellent prognosis with appropriate diagnosis and treatment.

Prevention/prophylaxis: Prevention strategies include advising the patient to avoid excessive intake of iodine and abuse of exogenous thyroid hormones and to minimize physical and emotional stress.

Referral: Refer to, or consult with, ophthalmologist for exophthalmic complications; surgeon for surgical intervention, or endocrinologist for radioactive iodine therapy and evaluation.

Education: Explain disease process, signs and symptoms, and treatment (including side effects of medications). Stress importance of compliance with drug therapy. Diet must be sufficient in calories to maintain weight until treatment re-establishes euthyroid state. Discuss need for follow-up care.

THYROID IMBALANCE: HYPOTHYROIDISM

SIGNAL SYMPTOMS▶   Fatigue; lethargy

Acquired hypothyroidism	ICD-9-CM: 240.9 242.0 244.2
Iodine hypothyroidism	ICD-9-CM: 244; 244.2

Description: Hypothyroidism is a decrease in function of the thyroid gland causing reduced thyroid activity with concomitant decrease in the amounts of thyroid hormones secreted. Hypothyroidism may be classified as primary or secondary.

Etiology:

Primary

In developed countries, commonly caused by primary thyroid gland failure such as from autoimmune thyroiditis (Hashimoto's), congenital hypothyroidism, and radioactive iodine therapy for hyperthyroidism or thyroid surgery. Other, less common causes include drug-induced hypothyroidism (lithium, methimazole, excessive iodine ingestion) and postpartum thyroiditis (usually transient). Worldwide, the most common cause is an iodine-deficient diet.

Secondary

Caused from failure of the hypothalamic-pituitary axis from either a deficient secretion of thyroid-releasing hormone from the hypothalamus (TSHRF) or the lack of secretion of TSH from the pituitary.

Occurrence: The occurrence of hypothyroidism in the general population is 0.8%.

Age: Commonly occurs in three age groups: newborns (cretinism), people age 30 to 50 years (Hashimoto's), and people age 60 years and older (adult-onset).

Ethnicity: No significant ethnic predisposition.

Gender: More common in women than in men (10:1).

Contributing factors: Environmental factors, such as iodine-deficient diets, radioactive iodine exposure, and certain medications (propylthiouracil, amiodarone, and lithium); surgery (total or partial thyroidectomy; increased age; genetic predisposition; postpartum period.

Signs and symptoms: Onset may be insidious and subtle. Symptoms include lethargy, cold intolerance, constipation, depression, mental confusion, high cholesterol levels, menorrhagia, weight gain or loss, hoarseness, decreased sweating, muscle cramps, arthralgia, and paresthesia.

Physical examination may reveal dull facial expression; cool, coarse, dry skin; periorbital puffiness; swelling of hands and feet; hypothermia; bradycardia; decreased body and scalp hair including scanty eyebrows; coarse hair; slow speech; and delayed return of deep tendon reflexes.

Diagnostic testing:

Test	Results indicating disorder	CPT code
TSH, serum T_4 and free T_4	High levels of TSH with low levels of serum T_4 and free T_4 are diagnostic. In subclinical hypothyroidism, levels of TSH are low but serum T_4 levels are normal. Both overt hypothyroidism and subclinical hypothyroidism should be treated.	84439 80438-39 80418 80438-40 84443

Differential Diagnosis:

- Other thyroid dysfunction such as thyroid cancer and hyperthyroidism (check appropriate laboratory tests)
- Liver, adrenal, and pituitary diseases (check appropriate laboratory tests)
- Nephrotic syndrome (check BUN, creatinine; urine output)
- Depression (depression screen, normal laboratory tests)
- CHF (echocardiogram, EKG)
- Dementia (decreased score on mini-mental status examination [MMSE]; not reversible with treatment of thyroid dysfunction)

Treatment:

Primary Hypothyroidism

Treatment of choice is thyroid hormone replacement, most commonly with levothyroxine (Synthroid, Levothroid), starting with 50 to 100 µg/day with increases of 25 µg/day every 4–6 weeks to a maximum dosage of 300 µg; dosage depends on clinical condition, laboratory results, and varies with age. Increase dosage until BH is within normal range. Elderly patients may require lower dosages. Contraindicated in thyrotoxic heart disease. Dosages of anticoagulant and hypoglycemic drugs may need to be modified. Monitor for drug interactions (e.g., insulin, corticosteroids, estrogens).

Hypothyroidism from Dietary Deficiency

Supplementation with iodine.

Postpartum (Transient) Hypothyroidism

Usually self-limiting; no treatment needed unless patient is bothered by signs and symptoms.

Follow-up: See patient monthly to monitor response to hormone replacement therapy. Once TSH serum concentrations have stabilized, see patient every 6 months to 1 year for clinical and laboratory (TSH and T_4 levels) evaluation.

Sequelae: Most patients return to a euthyroid state with treatment. Possible complications include myxedema coma (life-threatening), treatment-induced CHF in patient with CAD, increased susceptibility to infection, megacolon, infertility, and sensitivity to opiates.

Prevention/prophylaxis: Prevention strategies include advising the patient to maintain an adequate dietary intake of iodine.

Referral: Refer to, or consult with, endocrinologist if patient is unresponsive to treatment.

Education: Explain the disease process, signs and symptoms, and treatment (including side effects of medications). Discuss prevention strategies, importance of compliance with therapy, and when to seek medical care.

See *www.endocrineweb.com/hypo1.html;www.hsc.missouri.edu/~daveg/thyroid/thy_dis.html*

REFERENCES

General

Dambro, M: Griffiths 5-minute Clinical Consult, ed. 1. Lippincott, Williams & Wilkins, Philadelphia 2001.

Dunphy, LM, and Winland-Brown, JE: Primary Care: The Art and Science of Advanced Practice Nursing. FA Davis, Philadelphia, 2001.

McCann, J.S. Rapid Differential Diagnosis. Lippincott, Williams & Wilkins, Philadelphia 2002.

Rakel, R: Textbook of Family Practice, ed. 6. WB Saunders, Philadelphia, 2001.

Diabetes

Cefalu,W: Practical Guide to Diabetes Management, ed. 2. Medical Information Press, New York, 2001.

Cincinnati, R, and Veliko, S: Diabetes update oral medications. RN 64(8):30–36, 2001.

PDR: Diabetes Disease Management Guide, ed. 2. Medical Economics Company, New Jersey, 2002.

Heat-Related Illnesses

Kunihiro, A: Heat exhaustion and heat stroke. eMedicine Journal 3(4):1–13, 2002.

McGeehin, Ma, and Mirabelli, M: The potential impacts of climate variability and change on temperature-related morbidity and mortality in the United States. Environmental Health Perspectives 109:185–190, 2001.

Hyperlipidemias

Gotto, A: Contemporary Diagnosis and Management of Lipid Disorders, ed. 2. Handbooks in Health Care Co, Newton, PA, 2001.

National Cholesterol Education Program: Third report of the expert panel on detection, evaluation, and treatment of high blood cholesterol in adults (Adult treatment panel III). National Heart, Lung, and Blood Institute, Bethesda, MD. NIH Publ No 01-3670, 2001.

Obesity

Kearns, P: Are there benefits from long term pharmacotherapy of obesity. Arch Intern Med 162(9):1070, May 2002.

Leslie, M: Weighing in on clinical guidelines for obesity. Advance for Nurse Practitioners: 78-81. March 2000.

McLeelan, F: Obesity rising to alarming levels around the world. Lancet 359(9315):1412, 2002.

Pancreatitis

Proca, DM, et al: Major pancreatic resections for chronic pancreatitis. Arch Pathol Lab Med 125(8):1051-1054, 2001.

Thyroid

Canaris, G, et al: The Colorado thyroid disease prevalence study. Arch Int Med 160(4):526–432, 2000.

Caraccio, N et al:) Subclinical Hypothyroidism: Response to levothyroxine replacment. J Clin Endocrinol Metab 87(4):1533–1538, 2002.

Cecil, R, et al: Cecil's Textbook of Medicine. WB Saunders, New York, 2000.

Goroll, A, et al: Primary Care Medicine Office Evaluation and Management of the Adult Patient. Lippincott, Williams & Wilkins, Philadelphia, 2000.

Chapter 12

HEMATOLOGIC AND IMMUNOLOGIC DISORDERS

ANAPHYLAXIS

SIGNAL SYMPTOMS▶ Shortness of breath; rash; dizziness; lightheadedness

Anaphylactic shock	ICD-9-CM 995.60
Secondary to medicine	ICD-9-CM: 995.0
Immunization	ICD-9-CM: 999.4
Overdose or wrong substance given	ICD-9-CM: 977.9

Description: Anaphylaxis is an acute, systemic, immunoglobulin E (IgE)–mediated, antigen-antibody reaction. An anaphylactic reaction occurs when sensitized persons are exposed to an antigen to which they have an allergy. The manifestation of anaphylaxis varies according to the route of administration, dose, release of and sensitivity to vasoactive substances and the sensitivity of the organs affected by these substances. Anaphylactic shock is a potentially fatal acute shock state caused by an allergic reaction, occurring within 5 to 10 minutes of antigen exposure.

Etiology: The anaphylactic response occurs when IgE antibodies release mast cells, histamine, prostaglandins, leukotrienes, and cytokines, which cause an acute inflammatory reaction.

Occurrence: Injected penicillin and sulfa drugs are the most common cause of fatal anaphylaxis in the United States today. Between 100 and 500 deaths or 75% of all anaphylactic deaths each year have been attributed to penicillin. Stinging insects, such as bees and fire ants, account for 40 to 50 anaphylactic deaths per year. Nonsteroidal anti-inflammatory agents have triggered anaphylactic reactions due to the inhibition of the enzyme cyclo-oxygenase. Blood transfusions have caused anaphylactic reactions in persons with IgA deficiencies. IgA deficiency prevalence is 1:500 to 1:700 individuals. Latex allergy and exercise in persons with severe physical allergies have caused anaphylaxis. Severe food allergies, such as allergy to peanuts, has caused anaphylaxis.

Age: Occurs in all age groups.

Ethnicity: No significant ethnic predisposition.

Gender: Occurs equally in men and in women.

Contributing factors: Previous anaphylaxis, exposure to allergen, history of asthma.

Signs and symptoms:

History: Quickly obtain a history of events (including time of exposure and location) to determine the allergan involved. Signs and symptoms can occur independently or concomitantly in each involved organ system.

Early Signs and Symptoms: Initial manifestations of anaphylaxis include skin erythema, pruritus, and generalized feelings of warmth, anxiety, lightheadedness, shortness of breath, nausea and vomiting.

 Clinical Pearl: Signs and symptoms of bronchospasm and impending respiratory failure include hoarseness, dyspnea and high-pitched breath sounds (stridor).

Cutaneous signs and symptoms: The most common manifestation of anaphylaxis is urticaria. The rash is well circumscribed; erythematous, intensely pruritic, exhibiting raised wheals with blanched centers. Angioedema may occur with swelling of the face, eyes, lips, tongue, and pharynx or extremities.

Respiratory symptoms: These include upper-airway compromise secondary to soft tissue edema and angioedema of the epiglottis. Early symptoms of this include hoarseness, cough, dysphasia, or a "lump" in the throat. Laryngeal edema and laryngospasm result in stridor, choking, hoarseness, and loss of voice. Lower airway obstruction produced by bronchoconstriction and bronchospasm result in dyspnea, wheezing, and chest tightness. Complete airway obstruction can also result.

Cardiovascular symptoms: These include hypotension, tachycardia, and vascular collapse secondary to vasodilatation and increased vascular permeability. Diaphoresis, lightheadedness, and syncope also occur. Cardiac dysrhythmias occur secondary to hypoxia, acidosis, and myocardial hypoperfusion.

Gastrointestinal and urinary symptoms: These include nausea, vomiting, diarrhea (may be bloody), abdominal cramps, dysphasia, urinary incontinence, and vaginal bleeding.

Central nervous system: Symptoms include delirium, and seizures that are due to hypoxemia or hypotension.

Diagnostic tests:

Test	Result Indicating Disorder	CPT Code
Serum/urine histamine	Elevated levels of histamine	83088
Serum tryptase level	Initial elevation with return to normal range confirms anaphylaxis	82570
Electrocardiogram (ECG)	Dysrhythmias/heart blocks and conduction delays	93270
Arterial Blood Gases	Acidosis	36600/82805/82810

Differential diagnosis:

- Pseudoanaphylactic reaction (no triggering substance)
- Pulmonary embolus (very short of breath with pink frothy sputum)
- Foreign-body aspiration (evidence of choking—grasping neck, unable to speak)
- Arrhythmia (syncope, evidence of arrhythmia on electrocardiogram [ECG])
- Carcinoid syndrome (symptoms are prolonged)
- Scombroid fish poisoning (person must have consumed raw fish)
- Vasovagal reactions (syncope)
- Viral or bacterial infections of the upper airway (fever, dark colored sputum, malaise)

Treatment:

Clinical Pearl: Call for emergency assistance (911) immediately if patient experiences signs of respiratory distress, especially if this occurs after taking a drug, eating, or being bitten or stung by an insect. Check airway, breathing, and circulation, and initiate CPR if necessary until assistance arrives.

Begin treatment as soon as anaphylaxis is suspected. Place conscious patient in comfortable position, ensuring unimpeded ventilation; place hypotensive patient supine in level or Trendelenburg's position if respiratory status allows (Table 12–1).

Discharge therapies: When stable, the patient may be discharged with an antihistamine such as diphenhydramine, 25 to 50 mg orally every 6 to 8 hours as needed and possibly several days of a corticosteroid such as prednisone, 60 mg orally daily.

Follow-up: Observe patient for at least 3 hours after stabilization before being discharged home. Late phase reactions such as edema of the airway may require rapid treatment and the patient may need hospitalization. Schedule a follow-up appointment. If the patient is discharged, advise the patient of sedative effects of antihistamines.

Table 12–1. Treatment for Anaphylaxis

System	Symptom	Treatment	Dose
Airway Support	Oxygenation	Oxygen by nasal cannula at 2 LPM or mask at 6 to 10 LPM	5 to 10 L/min
	Laryngeal and posterior pharyngeal angioedema	Inhaled racemic epinephrine	2.25% (0.5 mL in 2 mL normal saline) nebulized
	Inadequate oxygenation, or profound shock	Prepare for endotracheal intubation or cricothyrotomy if severe angioedema precludes intubation	Epinephrine
	Isolated cutaneous anaphylactic responses—mild bronchospasm	Epinephrine	0.2 to 0.5 mg of 1:1000 dilution SQ or IM every 15 to 20 minutes
	Insect sting or allergen injection site	Inject epinephrine directly into the affected site	0.1 to 0.2 mg
	Vasodilatory anaphylactic responses—hypotension, laryngeal edema, bronchospasm	Epinephrine Slow IV push over 5 minutes	0.1 mg (1 mL of 1:10,000 solution) in 10-mL NS
	Antihistamines: second line therapy—usually given in combination	Diphenhydramine	1–2mg per kg up to 50 mg IV over 5 to 10 minutes or IM every 6 to 8 hours as needed.
		Hydroxyzine	25 to 50 mg IM every 6 to 8 hours
		Cimetidine	300 mg IV every 6 hours
		Ranitidine	50 mg IV every 6 to 8 hours
	Beta$_2$ agonists	Aminophylline	5.6 mg per kg (up to 500 mg) administered IV
Breathing and Pulmonary Support:	Bronchospasm	Albuterol	2.5 to 5 mg nebulized every 20 minutes as needed
		Aminophylline	6 mg/kg IV loading dose (if patient not on aminophylline) Followed by a continuous IV infusion

(Continued)

Table 12–1. Treatment for Anaphylaxis (Continued)

System	Symptom	Treatment	Dose
Circulatory Support	Hypotension	Normal saline or lactated Ringer's	0.5 to 1 liters every 20–30 minutes based on blood pressure, cardiac status, and urine output
Prolonged reactions	Corticosteroids	Methylprednisolone	125 mg IV, repeat dose every 6–8 hours
		Hydrocortisone	250 mg IV, repeat dose every 6–8 hours

Sequelae: Possible short-term complications include full cardiovascular collapse and death. Possible long-term complications include increased sensitivity to antigen and possibility of future anaphylactic reactions.

Prevention/prophylaxis: Prevention strategies include advising the patient with a serious anaphylactic reaction to carry an Epi-Pen or Ana-Kit, and instruct the patient and family in its use; to wear medical identification such as a Medic-Alert bracelet indicating allergies. The patient should remain in practitioner's office for at least 30 minutes after administration of any medications; and advise practitioner of medication use and reactions. For the patient allergic to insects, advise the patient to avoid areas where insect exposure is likely to occur; to always wear shoes when outdoors; and to avoid perfumes, after shave lotions, and brightly colored clothing. For the patient allergic to foods, advise the patient to avoid those foods and to read food labels carefully and to advise food preparers of allergy.

Referral: Immediate referral to physician or clinical emergency department if patient has an acute attack. Refer to or consult with allergist if the cause of the anaphylaxis is unclear or if desensitization immunotherapy to the antigen is considered.

Education: Explain disease process, signs and symptoms, and treatment (including side effects of medications). Discuss prevention strategies.

Web Site: *www.doctorpage.com*

ANEMIAS

SIGNAL SYMPTOMS▶ *Iron deficiency:* fatigue, tachycardia; *Aplastic:* bleeding, fatigue; *Hemolytic:* fever, jaundice; *Pernicious:* tingling of extremities, beefy red tongue

Unspecified	ICD-9-CM: 285.9
Iron deficiency anemia	ICD-9-CM: 280.9 285.1 280.0
Aplastic anemia	ICD-9-CM: 284.9
Hemolytic anemias	ICD-9-CM: 282.9
Pernicious anemia	ICD-9-CM: 284 283.0 281.0 281.9
Thalassemia	ICD-9-CM: 282. 4
Sideroblastic anemia	ICD-9-CM: 282.0

Description: *Anemia* means "lack of blood" or an insufficient number of red blood cells (RBCs) to carry oxygen. Specifically, a hemoglobin level below 13 g/dL in men and 12 g/dL in women is considered diagnostic for anemia. Abnormally low hemoglobin concentration or inadequate red blood cell population can be the result of blood loss, deficient erythropoietin, or excessive red blood cell hemolysis. The type of anemia can be diagnosed from the complete blood count based on RBC shape (morphology), which is evident in the mean corpuscular volume (MCV) and RBC color, which is evident in the mean corpuscular hemoglobin concentration (MCHC). In normocytic anemia, the RBCs are normal size and the MCV is within normal limits; normochromic anemias exhibit a normal hemoglobin concentration and therefore color as noted by an MCHC within normal limits. In microcytic anemia, the MCV is low, indicating that the RBCs are smaller than normal; a hypochromic anemia is evident when the MCHC is low, indicating that the hemoglobin concentration is reduced. In macrocytic anemia, the RBCs are oversized because of a defective nuclear maturation; the MCV is also elevated (Tables 12–2 and 12–3).

Table 12–2. Signs and Symptoms of Anemia

Type of Anemia	Cause	Laboratory Results Indicating disorder	Physical Signs and Symptoms
Iron Deficiency	Blood loss Inadequate dietary intake Inadequate absorption	↓ Hgb/Hct ↓MCV/MCHC ↓ Serum Ferritin ↓ Serum Iron ↑ RDW ↑ TIBC Anisocytosis	Fatigue, headache, paresthesias, irritability, dysphasia, pica, atrophic glossitis, spooning of nails
Anemia of Chronic Disease	Inflammation Malignancy HIV infection	↓ HCT/HgB Normocytic Hypochromic Normal Ferritin ↓ Serum Iron ↑ ESR	Fatigue, headache Weakness
Thalassemia	Genetic disorder Among persons of Mediterranean ancestry and in rare cases African Americans	↓Hgb/Hct ↑RBC count ↓MCV ↓MCHC ↑Hemoglobin A Target cells, poikilocytosis, anisocytosis are present	None in early stages Fatigue, weight loss, weakness

(Continued)

Table 12–2. Signs and Symptoms of Anemia (Continued)

Type of Anemia	Cause	Laboratory Results Indicating disorder	Physical Signs and Symptoms
Vitamin B$_{12}$ Deficiency	Pernicious anemia	↓ Hct/Hgb ↑ MCV ↑ MCHC	Anorexia, diarrhea, peripheral numbness and tingling, atrophic glossitis, disturbances of position and vibration, lack of coordination, spasticity, depression and irritability
Folate deficiency	Inadequate dietary intake Alcohol intake pregnancy, hemolysis, malignancy, severe psoriasis, phenytoin, methotrexate, Bactrim	↓Hgb, Hct ↑ MCV, MCHC	Increased risk for thrombosis In pregnant women—increased risk of neural tube deficit in newborns Anorexia, diarrhea, depression
Hemolytic anemia	Intrinsic red cell defects. Immunologic and mechanical injury	↑ Reticulocyte Normochromic Normocytic Nucleated red cells Schistocytes Polychromatophilia + Coombs' test	Chills, fever, abdominal and back pain, shock, splenomegaly, hepatomegaly, melena, epistaxis, hemoglobinuria and hemosiderinuria as well as jaundice.
Sickle cell anemia	Genetic disease	>50% of hemoglobin is hemoglobin S, which decreases the ability to carry oxygen	Joint pain, shortness of breath, leg ulcers, hepatomegaly, hematuria, jaundice, fever, leukocytosis
Aplastic Anemia	Idiopathic, toxin, drugs, and viral infections	↓Hct, Hgb Normochromic, normocytic Diminished platelets ↓Reticulocyte Count Pancytopenia	Onset gradual Fatigue, bleeding, infection No organomegaly seen
Glucose-6-phosphate Dehydrogenase Deficiency (G6PD)	Sex-linked red blood cell defect seen more in African Americans or in persons of Mediterranean ancestry	Unoxidized Hemoglobin	Hemolysis after exposure to sulfonamides or antimalarials or infection

(Continued)

Table 12–2. Signs and Symptoms of Anemia *(Continued)*

Type of Anemia	Cause	Laboratory Results Indicating disorder	Physical Signs and Symptoms
Sideroblastic Anemia	Associated with Rheumatoid arthritis, chronic alcoholism, cancer, lead poisoning and pyridoxine deficiency	↓Hgb/Hct ↓ MCV/MCHC ↑Serum Iron ↑ Transferrin Marrow stains show ringed cells Anisocytosis and poikilocytosis	

Etiology: The most common form of anemia encountered in primary care is iron deficiency anemia. The most frequent cause of this type of anemia is blood loss. Anemia may also develop as a secondary consequence of defects in other body systems.

Occurrence: Iron deficiency anemia occurs in 10% to 30% of the population in the United States. About 500 to 600 million people worldwide are estimated to have iron deficiency anemia. Blood loss is the most common cause of iron deficiency anemia. After iron deficiency anemia, the anemia of chronic disease, caused by underlying infection, inflam-

Table 12–3. Types of Anemia

Type of Anemia	Special Diagnostic Tests Beyond the Anemia Profile	Treatments
Iron deficiency anemia	Serum ferritin Total iron-binding capacity	Iron replacement, transfusion, Diagnose reason for blood loss and treat
Thalassemia	History of Mediterranean heritage Hemoglobin electrophoresis to look for hemoglobin A	Avoid drugs that induce oxidative stress, blood transfusions splenectomy in severe cases, avoid iron over treatment
Sideroblastic anemia	Serum Iron Level, Total Iron Binding Capacity, Transferrin saturation. Bone marrow aspirate to look for ringed sideroblasts	
B_{12} deficiency	History of gastric or bowel inflammation, Hashimoto's thyroiditis, or vitiligo Neuropsychiatric symptoms Serum B $_{12}$ level Shilling Test	Replacement of B_{12} usually by injection
Folate deficiency	Folate level	Replacement of folate at 1 mg per day by mouth
Hemolytic anemia		Red blood cell transfusion, hydration, provide oxygen control hemorrhage diuresis, treat underlying cause

mation, and malignancy is the second most common cause of anemia worldwide. Incidence of aplastic anemia is about 4/1 million.

Age: Occurs primarily in adults older than age 60 and women of child-bearing years.

Ethnicity: Thalassemia and glucose-6-phosphate dehydrogenase (G6PD) deficiency occurs more often in people of Mediterranean and African descent. Vitamin B_{12} deficiency occurs more often in people of northern European descent, particularly Scandinavians, and black women.

Gender: Occurs more commonly in women than in men.

Contributing factors: Certain medications, including nonsteroidal anti-inflammatory (NSAIDs) and sulfa drugs; chronic use of alcohol, and caffeinated coffee. Pregnancy. Malignancies. Viral infections. Excessively heavy menstrual periods.

Diagnostic tests: Anemia is identified and classified by laboratory evaluation. Complete blood count with differential, electrophoresis, and other laboratory studies are needed for complete diagnosis.

Test	Results indicating disorder	CPT code
Bone marrow studies	Diagnoses aplastic anemia, leukemia, myelodysplasia, or neoplastic infiltration of bone marrow	78102–78104
Bone marrow aspiration and biopsy	Diagnoses iron deficiency anemia, anemia of chronic disease, or the macrocytic anemias	85095–85102
Upper GI series, barium enema, sigmoidoscopy, esophagoscopy, gastroscopy, and a gastric analysis	Rules out intestinal problems as a cause for anemia	74246 UGI 74270 BA enema 45330 Sigmoidoscopy 74220 Esophagoscopy 43234–43235 Gastroscopy

BA, barium; GI, gastrointestinal.

Differential Diagnosis:

- Malignancy (weight loss)
- Intestinal or gastric disorders (nausea, weight loss)
- Hypothyroidism (cold intolerance, constipation, weight gain)
- Chronic diseases such as HIV (rule out with laboratory studies)
- Renal Failure (oliguria, anuria, uremic frost)
- Chronic liver disease (clotting disorders, altered glucose metabolism)
- Myelodysplastic syndromes (pain)

Treatment: The main treatment goal is to correct the cause and ensure adequate tissue oxygenation. Moderate to severe anemia may require a blood transfusion. Depending on the type of anemia, treatment includes providing supplements of the deficient component, correcting the cause of the blood loss, or alleviating the hemolytic component (see Table 12–3)

Follow-up: See patient every few months or as needed to monitor the response to treatment and to obtain appropriate diagnostic tests.

Sequelae: Possible complications include cardiopulmonary problems such as angina pectoris, myocardial infarction (MI), congestive heart failure (CHF), cardiomegaly, pulmonary and systemic congestion, ascites, and peripheral edema; excessively enlarged spleen with resultant RBC destruction and hemolysis resulting in pain, renal failure, shock, serious illness, and gallstones (with hemolytic anemia); infertility and increased susceptibility to infection (with folic acid deficiency); and neurologic complications such as paresthesias, altered gait, difficulty with coordination, and mental deterioration (with vitamin B_{12} deficiency anemia).

Prevention/prophylaxis: Prevention strategies include advising the patient to eat a diet rich in all nutrients, including iron, vitamin B_{12}, and folic acid; to take medications that cause gastric irritation such as non steroidal antiinflammatory drugs (NSAIDs) with food to prevent bleeding; to avoid injuries; to maintain effective gas exchange, adequate cardiac output, and tissue perfusion; to reduce stress; to obtain adequate sleep; to watch for signs and symptoms of bleeding; to avoid or modify activities that may result in bleeding; and to avoid excessive use of alcohol, over-cooking food, use of oral contraceptives and anticonvulsants, and smoking (increases need for folic acid). Genetic testing may alert couples to the possibility of certain hemolytic anemias such as thalassemia and G6PD deficiency.

Referral: Refer to, or consult with, physician/hematologist as needed.

Education: Explain disease process, signs and symptoms, and treatment (including side effects of medications). Discuss prevention strategies. Educational resource materials are available from the National Heart, Lung and Blood Institute, Communications and Public Information Branch, National Institutes of Health, Building 31, Room 4121, 9000 Rockville Pike, Bethesda, MD 20892.

Web Sites:
American Sickle Cell Anemia Association – *www.ascaa.org*
Aplastic anemia – *www.aplastic.org*
Thalassemia – *www.thalassemia.org*

CHRONIC FATIGUE SYNDROME

SIGNAL SYMPTOMS▶   Fatigue; insomnia

Fatigue/lethargy/malaise	ICD-9-DM: 780.79
Chronic fatigue	ICD-9-DM: 780.71

Description: Chronic fatigue syndrome (CFS), also known as chronic fatigue immune dysfunction syndrome (CFIDS), is a disease characterized by debilitating fatigue, exhaustion, fibromyalgia (joint and muscle pain), sore throat, headaches, lymph node pain, sleep disturbance, flu-like symptoms, and a deficit in information-processing efficiency and cognitive performance. Other symptoms may include anxiety, depression, and decreased sexual drive. The illness lasts at least 6 months and often lasts years. The typical patient is a person who was previously physically active, often an overachiever, who describes sudden flulike symptoms that never go away. The patient may be devastated by this disease; unable to work, or even unable to get out of bed (Box 12–1).

Etiology: Chronic fatigue is diagnosed based on patient history and the exclusion of other illnesses that can cause fatigue such as hypothyroidism, depression, chronic active hepatitis, schizophrenia, dementia, bipolar disorder, anorexia, bulimia, substance abuse, and obesity. Recurrent viral (such as Epstein Barr), fungal, and bacterial infections, the reaction of the immune system to vaccination and immunizations, hormonal imbalance, hyperventilation, alcohol abuse, mercury toxicity from dental amalgams, and increased muscle tension can cause CFS. These immunologic abnormalities that cause chronic fatigue are often preceded by a stressor, which may be environmental, physical, or emotional. Many researchers believe that the condition is latent and only exacerbates as a result of stress.

Occurrence: Incidence is 10/100,000 adults in the United States.

Age: Tends to occur in the middle of an individual's most productive years (commonly around age 35 to 45); rarely seen in older adults; may be seen in adolescents.

Ethnicity: Primarily seen in whites.

Gender: Occurs primarily in women.

Contributing factors: Infectious illness (seen at the onset); trauma; allergies; surgery; recent life event changes such as a new job, marriage,

---

Box 12–1
Definition of Chronic Fatigue

Classify as chronic fatigue syndrome (CFS) if both of the following criteria are met. Unexplained persistent or relapsing fatigue of new or definite onset that is not due to ongoing exertion, is not relieved by rest, and results in a substantial reduction in previous levels of activity

Four or more of the following symptoms are concurrently present for 6 months or longer

- Impaired memory or concentration that impairs everyday activities
- Sore throat
- Tender cervical or axillary lymph nodes
- Muscle pain
- Multijoint pain
- New headaches lasting more than 24 hours
- Unrefreshing sleep
- Postexertion malaise

moving, and problems with a relationship; borderline anemia; hypothyroidism; mental fatigue; anxiety; depression; fibromyalgias; multiple low-grade viral infections.

Diagnostic Tests

Test	Results indicating disorder	CPT code
CBC, SMA21, thyroid profile, urinalysis, HIV, and antinuclear antibody	To rule out other causes for symptoms	85022/81000/ 84295/84132/ 84520/86038
Flow cytometry	Evaluate the immune system	88180
Immune globulins, including subclasses	Decreased immunoglobulins, especially IgG, indicate chronic fatigue	86332
Rheumatoid factor	Increases indicate possible connective tissue cause of fatigue	86430-86431
Erythrocyte sedimentation rate (ESR)	Increased ESR indicates inflammation	85652
Epstein-Barr viral titer	Increases often seen in chronic fatigue	86663-86665
Cytomegalovirus titers	Increases often seen in chronic fatigue	86645

CBC, complete blood count; HIV, human immunodeficiency virus; IgG, immunoglobulin G; SMA21, complete metabolic panel.

Differential diagnosis:

- Malignancies (weight loss, imaging, biopsy, associated laboratory studies)
- Autoimmune disease (increased ESR, associated laboratory studies)
- Localized infection such as occult abscess (lymph nodes, fever, check, white blood cell [WBC] count)
- Lyme disease (rash, fever)
- Fungal or parasitic disease (rash, diarrhea)
- Toxic agent exposure (rash)
- Drug abuse (altered mentation, drug seeking behavior)
- Menopause (cessation of menses, hot flashes)
- Allergic fatigue (increased sputum production)
- Hypothyroidism (weight gain, cold intolerance)
- Depression (often concomitant with chronic fatigue)
- Multiple sclerosis (decreased strength)
- HIV disease (night sweats, opportunistic infections)
- Uncontrolled diabetes mellitus (polyuria, polydipsia, polyphagia)

Treatment: Treatment goals are to establish a diagnosis, alleviate symptoms, and preservation of strength to enable the body to break the cycle of fatigue and sleeplessness, and treatment of any underlying condition, such as infection, hypothyroidism, or anemia. One of the most important aspects of the initial visit with the patient is to verify that CFS does exist and may be the reason for the fatigue and pain. Verification by a healthcare provider can be a first step in helping the patient recover. Providing reassurance and emotional support, referrals to support groups and counseling, lifestyle management, and the prevention of further disabilities are the hallmarks of CFS management.

Physical

A balanced diet, adequate rest, and as much physical conditioning as the fatigue will allow is the initial recommended regimen. A diet of high nutrient, high protein, and complex carbohydrate foods are helpful in boosting immune function. Neuromuscular massage, heat, and myofascial trigger point release techniques (at least two treatments a week for 6 weeks) for treatment of fibromyalgia.

Pharmacologic

Tricyclic antidepressants (to break the wake-sleep cycle and allow the patient to sleep for at least 6 uninterrupted hours) such as trazodone, 50 to 75 mg at bedtime, or serotonin reuptake inhibitors such as sertraline, 50 mg once a day, or fluoxetine, 20 mg a day. Selective serotonin reuptake inhibitor (SSRI) antidepressants paroxetine (Paxil) 10 to 20 mg/daily, fluoxetine (Prozac) 20 mg daily, sertraline (Zoloft) 50 to 100 mg daily. The atypical SSRI nefazodone (Serzone), starting at 50 mg at hs increasing to a maximum of 300 mg daily in divided doses, is indicated.

Complementary Therapy

- Vitamin supplements, especially vitamin C, magnesium, zinc, and B vitamins.
- Herbal therapies that have demonstrated effectiveness for chronic fatigue include:
- Short courses of Echinacea, goldenseal, and ginseng—during acute exacerbations
- Ginseng, and Ginkgo biloba for chronic management
- Herbal therapies are not without risk and side effects must be considered before recommending these methods to any patient with chronic fatigue.

Follow-up: Individual follow-up needed for support, symptom relief, continued assessment, for underlying medical problems. Condition tends to wax and wane with very slow improvement over months or years.

Sequelae: Possible complications include depression, isolation, and socioeconomic hardship.

Prevention/prophylaxis: Prevention strategies include advising patients to maintain a diet high in carbohydrates, moderate in protein, and low in fat; to obtain adequate sleep (at least 6 hours a night); to continue therapy to help prevent a relapse; and to contact their health-care provider if signs of exacerbation occur. Encourage patients to reduce the stressors in their lives and provide information on support groups.

Referral: Refer to, or consult with, physician specializing in CFS if patient requires gamma globulin therapy or psychiatrist as needed. Refer patient to support groups, including those on the Internet.

Education: Explain the disease process, signs and symptoms, and treatment (including side effects of medications). Discuss prevention strategies and when to seek medical care, such as with fatigue, sleep interruptions, and fibromyalgia (signs of exacerbation). Support groups are available. Contact the CFS Association, 3521 Broadway, Suite 222, Kansas City, MO 64111 (816-931-4777); CFIDS Association, P.O. Box 220398, Charlotte, NC 28222-0398; International Chronic Fatigue Syndrome Society, P.O. Box 230108, Portland, OR 97223. See *www.chronicillnet. org/cfs; www.cfs-recovery.org*

HIV DISEASE

SIGNAL SYMPTOMS▶   Generalized lymphadenopathy; night sweats

HIV Disease	ICD-9-CM: 042 079.53
HIV, asymptomatic	ICD-9-CM: V08

Description: HIV disease encompasses the clinical spectrum seen with HIV infection. It ranges from asymptomatic HIV infection to infection that culminates in a group of symptoms known as acquired immunodeficiency syndrome (AIDS).

Etiology: The human immunodeficiency virus is a retrovirus infecting cells with CD4 receptors. Caused by infection by HIV type 1 (associated with non-African HIV infection) or type 2 (associated with African HIV infection). HIV type 1 infects and nearly destroys CD4+ T lymphocytes. All HIV-infected persons with less than 200 CD4 cells are categorized as AIDS patients. HIV is transmitted through sexual contact (through the exchange of body fluids), exposure to blood and blood products (such as through the use of contaminated needles by IV drug users), and maternal to fetus or infant (vertical) transfer.

Occurrence: AIDS is the primary killer of persons between the ages of 25 and 44 worldwide. The World Health Organization estimates that there are 17 million people infected with HIV, over six million people have died of AIDS, and five million children have been orphaned by AIDS. The incidence of AIDS has shifted from gay and bisexual men to IV drug users and their sex partners. The incidence is increasing in women and children (Table 12–4).

Age: Occurs in all ages. Children progress from primary HIV infection to AIDS more quickly than adults.

Ethnicity: Incidence of new cases of AIDS is greater in blacks and Hispanics than in whites.

Gender: HIV infection occurs more in men than in women; however, incidence of women with HIV infection is rising. At present, there is no demonstrable difference between men and women with respect to progression to AIDS.

Table 12–4. Percentage of Cases of HIV Infection Accounted for by Risk Factor

Exposure Category	Percentage of Cases World Wide
Vaginal intercourse	70–85%
Anal intercourse	10–15%
Intravenous drug abuse	5–10%
Blood transfusion	2–8 %
Perinatal	5–10%
Working as a health-care worker	< 0.01%

From Phair, JP, and King, E: Medscape HIV/AIDS Annual Update 2000. Northwestern University Medical School Comprehensive AIDS Center, New York, 2000. www.medscape.com/hivdisease/html

Contributing factors: The three known routes for transmission of HIV are (1) directly from person to person by sexual contact; (2) contact with contaminated blood products, or needles; (3) infected mothers transmitting HIV to the fetus or newborn child.

Signs and symptoms: The clinical manifestations of HIV infection include chills, fever, night sweats, dry productive cough, lethargy, confusion, stiff neck, seizures, headache, malaise, fatigue, oral lesions, skin rash, abdominal discomfort, diarrhea, weight loss, and lymphadenopathy. Many of these symptoms, however, can be related to other illnesses, and people infected with HIV may not have any symptoms for many years. The only way to determine HIV infection is by testing.

Diagnostic tests:

Test	Result Indicating Disorder	CPT Code
Rapid HIV test	Negative—Repeat in 6 months Positive—Evidence of HIV	86701
Enzyme immunoassay (EIA)	Negative—Repeat in 6 months Positive—Evidence of HIV	86701
Western blot	Confirm EIA test that is positive	86689
Radioimmunoprecipitation assay (RIPA)	Confirms HIV when antibody levels are very low or difficult to detect.	86701
Rapid latex agglutination assay	Inexpensive test in areas with high rate of HIV infection	86701
Dot-blot immunobinding assay	Inexpensive rapid screening for HIV	86701
VDRL	Positive VDRL indicates secondary syphilis	86592
PPD testing with controls	To evaluate the current state of the immune system No reaction to PPD or controls indicates a failing immune system. No reaction to PPD but positive control indicates functional immune system but no exposure to TB. Positive PPD and Control indicates functional immune system and exposure to TB	86280

(Continued)

Test	Result Indicating Disorder	CPT Code
Complete blood count	Decreases in white blood cells or platelets may be evident in HIV	85022
CD4/CD8 cell count (also called T4/T8 or T-helper/T-suppressor cells):	Marker of progression of HIV Decreased levels indicate progressive HIV disease If CD4 is less than 500, start PCP prophylaxis; if less than 50 consider MAC /CMV prophylaxis	87390/87391
RT-PCR viral load	Increases in viral load indicate progression of disease or that current therapy is not affective	87534/87536/ 87537/87539

CMV, cytomegalovirus; MAC, *Mycobacterium avium* complex; PCP, *Pneumocytis carinii* pneumonia; PPD, purified protein derivative; RT-PCR; reverse transcriptase–polymerase chain reaction.

Differential diagnosis:

 Clinical Pearl: According to the Centers for Disease Control and Prevention (CDC), AIDS is an illness characterized by one or more indicator diseases with coexisting laboratory evidence of HIV infection. Many conditions can mimic HIV infection; however when there is an unexpectedly prolonged illness, HIV testing is indicated.

Treatment: Treatment depends on the stage of the infection and the patient's CD4 cell count. Refer to the diagnostic test table for timetables in testing for initial diagnosis and evaluation of HIV disease.

Physical

Treatment includes encouraging proper nutrition, a well-balanced diet, and adequate fluid intake, and maintaining adequate rest, sleep, physical activity, and exercise. Support, reassurance, and psychosocial, financial, and health-care counseling are also a part of care. If the patient asks about alternative/complementary therapies, provide the patient with current information or refer as appropriate.

Pharmacologic

Antiretroviral Therapy: As we have progressed in our ability to measure plasma viral burdens, impressive gains in HIV/AIDS treatment have been achieved. Unprecedented benefits have resulted from highly active antiretroviral therapy (HAART). Antiretroviral therapy is the cornerstone of HAART. Nucleoside reverse transcriptase inhibitors were the first major classification of antiretroviral drug developed. They work by substituting nucleoside analogues for natural substrates necessary for the formation of viral DNA. These drugs inhibit the formation of viral DNA and prevent viral replication. Examples of nucleoside reverse transcriptase inhibitors are zidovudine (AZT), didanosine (Ddl), lamivudine (3TC), and stavudine (d4T). Common side effects of these drugs are anemia, pancreatitis, peripheral neuropathy, and stomatitis

Non-nucleoside reverse transcriptase inhibitors combine directly with reverse transcriptase, causing this enzyme to be inactivated. This blocks the process by which the HIV RNA becomes HIV DNA. Examples of non-nucleoside reverse transcriptase inhibitors are delavirdine and abacavir. These drugs have fewer side effects than the other classifications of anti-retroviral drugs.

The third classification of drug used to reduce viral load and prevent the progression of HIV are the protease inhibitors. These drugs inhibit protease enzymes from splitting immature larger proteins within the CD4+ cell so that they can become smaller, structurally essential proteins that are necessary to manufacture HIV cells. Examples of protease inhibitors are saquinavir, ritonavir, indinavir and nelfinavir. Side effects of these drugs include hyperglycemia, elevated liver enzymes, hyperbilirubinemia, and nephrolithiasis.

Some complementary therapies have been shown to benefit those with HIV/AIDS. Self-help measures such as relaxation, meditation, and guided imagery can increase resiliency and foster a sense of control in persons with HIV infection. Healthy dietary habits not only promote physical health but also allow the HIV-infected person to assume some control over the therapeutic process. These and other complementary therapies can foster an increased adherence to treatment regimens, one of the greatest challenges to caring for individuals who are infected with HIV/AIDS.

Failure to consistently take medications leads to resistance in the virus that not only harms the individual but also increases the possibility of drug resistant strains of HIV within the general population. A recent study demonstrated that 63% of perinatally infected children treated early in life with an antiviral drug, had adequate virologic responses and unde-tectable viral loads. The best predictor of the success in these children was adherence to the medication regimen

Complementary Therapy:

- Glutathione is a natural antioxidant that may help HIV patients live longer. *N*-acetylcysteine (NAC) is a natural substance that raises glutathione levels in the body.
- Dehydro-3-epiandrosterone (DHEA), an adrenal steroid present in decreased amounts in persons with HIV, has been reported to have antiretroviral and immunomodulatory effects in vitro. Therefore, DHEA supplementation has been shown to be effective for HIV-infected individuals.

Follow-up: The best indicator of the effectiveness of antiretroviral therapy is the viral load. Viral load increases as the CD4+ cell count decreases and as the disease progresses. PCR is used to measure viral load and is sensitive enough to measure viral loads < 50 copies/mL. A decrease in viral load of 0.5 log10 indicates that the therapy is effective. If the viral load remains the same or does not drop 0.5 log 10 after instituting a new therapy, the treatment regimen should be re-evaluated and modified, if necessary. Antiretroviral therapy is usually begun when the CD4+ cell count is < 500 cells/mm or when blood tests show a rapid decline in CD4+ cell counts even though the total remains > 500 cells/mm. A significant reduction in CD4+ cells indicates that the treatment plan needs to be re-evaluated and possibly changed.

The diagnosis of opportunistic infections or opportunistic malignancies is often the first indicator of HIV infection and the point at which HIV becomes AIDS. Table 12–5 lists all classifications of opportunistic infections and malignancies, the most common site involved, and signs and symptoms.

Table 12–5. Opportunistic Infections and Malignancies Seen in HIV Disease

Classification	Organism	Common Site	Signs and Symptoms
Fungi	Pneumocystis carinii	Lungs	Dyspnea, tachypnea, cough, fever
	Candida albicans	Oropharyngeal	Dry mouth, altered taste
		Esophageal	Dysphagia, fever, odynophagia, weight loss
		Vaginal	Purulent discharge, pruritus, frequent urination
	Cryptococcus neoformans	Central nervous system	Headache, fever, malaise, stiff neck
	Coccidioides immitis	Lungs	Fever, chills, weight loss, cough, dyspnea
	Histoplasma capsulatum	Lungs Lymphatic system	Fever, weight loss, lymphadenopathy, hepatomegaly
Viral infections	Herpes simplex	Mouth, lips, or genital area	Headache, pain, fever, red painful pustules
	Varicella-zoster (shingles)	Along any dermatome or cranial nerve	Painful macular-papular rash with crusty papules
	Cytomegalovirus	Retina of the eye, brain, lung, liver, GI tract	Decreased visual acuity, hemorrhages on the retina, colitis, esophagitis, pneumonia
Bacterial infections	Mycobacterium tuberculosis	Lung, CNS, pericardium, GI tract	Productive cough, malaise, chest pain, fever, night sweats, hemoptysis
	Mycobacterium-avium complex	Systemic infection	Septicemia, fever, fatigue, weight loss, anorexia, nausea and vomiting, night sweats, diarrhea, abdominal pain, lymphadenopathy

(Continued)

Table 12–5. Opportunistic Infections and Malignancies Seen in HIV Disease (Continued)

Classification	Organism	Common Site	Signs and Symptoms
Protozoa	Cryptosporidium	GI tract	Profuse watery diarrhea, weight loss, abdominal pain, nausea, vomiting.
	Microsporidia	GI tract	Same as cryptosporidium but not as severe
	Isospora belli	GI tract	Diarrhea, abdominal cramping, dehydration.
	Giardia lamblia	GI tract	Flatulence, abdominal cramping, dyspepsia, diarrhea, dehydration
Malignancies	Kaposi's sarcoma	Multi nodular, red macular patches on torso, arms, head, neck, or mucous membranes	Plaqueike eruptions on skin or mucous membranes
	Hodgkin's and non-Hodgkin's lymphoma	Lymph nodes	Fever, night sweats, weight loss, diarrhea, lymphadenopathy
	CNS Lymphoma	Cerebellum, basal ganglia, brainstem	Decreased level of consciousness, weakness, confusion, lethargy, aphasia, and memory loss.
	Cervical cancer	Cervix	

Prevention/prophylaxis: HIV infection is a reportable disease. Check with your local and state health department concerning reporting requirements. Ensure that the patient is aware of the extent and limits of confidentiality and disclosure of HIV test results. Provide appropriate counseling when disclosing HIV status to the patient and when discussing whether or not the patient will disclose status to others. Prevention strategies for primary HIV infection include advising the patient to avoid behaviors that transmit the virus and to follow safe sex practices, avoid IV drug use, and use standard (universal) precautions when in contact with body fluids.

Referral: Refer to or consult with infectious disease specialist for co-management of opportunistic infections. Refer patient with HIV infection and a CD4 cell count $<$ 50 to an ophthalmologist for funduscopic examinations every 6 months.

Education: Explain the disease process, signs and symptoms, and treatment (including side effects of medications). Discuss prevention strategies and the need for compliance with therapy and follow-up care. Provide counseling regarding travel, immunizations, and self-care regimens for maintaining wellness and preventing disease, and information on local support groups. Financial, home care, and emotional and spiritual counseling may also be indicated. National AIDS Hotline (800-342-2437 [Spanish, 800-342-7432]); National Institute of Health AIDS Clinical Trials Group (800-874-2572); American Foundation for AIDS Research (212-719-0033). See *www.hivatis.org; http://hivinsite. ucsf.edu*

INFECTIOUS MONONUCLEOSIS

SIGNAL SYMPTOMS▶ Lymphadenopathy; fatigue

| Mononucleosis, infectious | ICD-9-CM: 075 |

Description: Infectious mononucleosis is an acute viral syndrome with a classic triad of fever, pharyngitis, and lymphadenopathy.

Etiology: Most often caused by Epstein-Barr virus (EBV). Other causes include cytomegalovirus, HIV, and toxoplasmosis. A contagious virus, EBV transmission is fecal-oral and occurs through intimate contact and exchange of saliva, such as by kissing. The incubation period is 20 to 50 days.

Occurrence: Most people become infected with EBV by adulthood; about 50% of the population seroconverts by age 5 years. EBV is excreted from oropharyngeal secretions for up to 18 months after a primary infection resolves and intermittently throughout life.

Age: Occurs at any age; most frequently seen in people ages 15 to 24 years.

Gender: Occurs equally in men and in women.

Ethnicity: No significant ethnic predisposition.

Contributing factors: Prior contraction of EBV; disease manifestation delayed until adolescence or adulthood.

Signs and symptoms: The Patient may complain of fever, malaise, headache, pharyngitis, myalgias, and arthralgias.

Physical examination may reveal tired-looking patient with flushed or jaundiced skin, possibly with rash; red, irritated pharynx, possibly with exudate; lymphadenopathy; and splenomegaly or hepatomegaly.

Diagnostic tests:

Test	Result Indicating Disorder	CPT Code
Heterophil antibody test (HAT) or a "spot" test	HAT titer at least 1:56 diagnostic for Mononucleosis	86308
WBC with differential	Increased mononuclear leukocytes and lymphocytosis with an increased percentage of atypical lymphocytes indicates disease	85540
Throat culture	If positive, treat for strep bacteria	87060

WBC, white blood cell.

Differential diagnosis:

- Pharyngitis (less lymphadenopathy)
- Herpes virus (rash, burning and itch)
- HIV/AIDS (night sweats, opportunistic infections)

Treatment:

Physical

Supportive care including rest and adequate fluid intake (at least 8 glasses of water or juice per day during periods of high fever). Convalescence may take several weeks. Avoid stress. No contact sports (possibility of splenic rupture).

Pharmacologic

Antipyretics and analgesics such as ibuprofen or acetaminophen asindicated (for fever, headaches, and myalgias). Avoid aspirin because of suspected association with Reye's syndrome. In most cases, antiviral therapy is not indicated. Antibiotics are necessary for only secondary infection. Avoid use of ampicillin because 90% of patients develop a rash following administration. For the patient with oropharyngeal lymphoid tissue swelling, a short course of IV corticosteroids, such as methylprednisolone 1 mg/kg per day given in divided doses is helpful.

Follow-up: See the patient in 1 to 2 weeks after initial assessment unless complications develop. The acute phase usually lasts from 7 days to several weeks; fatigue may continue for several months.

Sequelae: Possible complications include splenic rupture, laryngotonsillar obstruction, encephalitis, Bell's palsy, Guillain-Barré syndrome, autoimmune hemolytic anemia, granulocytopenia, thrombocytopenia, and hepatitis or massive hepatic necrosis. Fever subsides in about 10 days, adenopathy and splenomegaly in about 4 weeks.

Prevention/prophylaxis: Prevention strategies include advising the patient to use proper hand-washing techniques and to not share eating utensils or drinking cups. Advise the patient that a healthy diet, exercise, and adequate sleep help increase immune resistance. Avoid contact sports for 3 months.

Referral: Refer to, or consult with, immunologist or specialist if complications develop. Usually referral is not necessary.

Education: Explain the disease process, signs and symptoms, and treatment (including side effects of medications). Discuss contagious status of disease, prevention strategies, and when to seek medical care (temperature above 102°F, upper abdominal pain, yellowing of skin, or difficulty swallowing or breathing). Advise the patient to avoid strenuous activities, including sports, for 1 to 2 months to avoid splenic rupture.

See *http://blunix.hl.ut.us/els/epidemiology*

LYME DISEASE

SIGNAL SYMPTOMS Erythematous rash; malaise

| Lyme disease | ICD-9-CM: 088.81 |

Description: Lyme disease is a multisystem infection and is the most common vector-borne illness in the United States

Etiology: Caused by the spirochete *B. burgdorferi*. It is usually transmitted to humans by the bite of an infected *Ixodes* tick. Once introduced into the skin, spirochetes may remain localized or disseminate hematogenously to any organ.

Occurrence: Varies by region of the country, with highest incidences (about 6.1/100,000) in the mid-Atlantic and New England (3.7/100, 000) areas of the United States, specifically Connecticut, Rhode Island, New York, New Jersey, Pennsylvania, and Maryland.

Age: Occurs at any age; most common in children younger than 15 years of age and adults age 25 to 44 years.

Ethnicity: No significant ethnic predisposition.

Gender: No significant gender differentiation.

Contributing factors: Exposure to tick-infested area, especially during the months of May to September when infected ticks pass the organism to humans during the nymph stage.

Signs and symptoms:

Stage 1

History may or may not reveal history of tick bite. Only about 30% of patients remember a tick bite. Patient may be asymptomatic. Classic local lesion is seen: erythema migrans (EM), a painless annular lesion up to 15 cm or greater in diameter; may be erythematous with a clearing center and may be hot to the touch. The initial EM lesion may be followed within days by other similar lesions in other locations, which usually fade after 3–4 weeks. Other signs and symptoms include fever, chills, aching, headache, and local lymphadenopathy.

Stage 2

This stage usually begins several weeks after the initial infection if antibiotic therapy has not been initiated and may involve one or more organ systems. Signs and symptoms may include multiple EM lesions, including a lupus-like macular rash and urticaria; conjunctivitis (occasionally); cardiac problems (seen in about 10% of patients), commonly atrioventricular (AV) block; migratory arthralgia, and myalgias (about 80% of untreated patients); neurologic symptoms such as acute facial nerve palsy and meningitis-like illnesses (about 15% of untreated patients); malaise; and fatigue. By the end of stage 2 at 1 year or more, there may be evidence of frank arthritis.

Table 12–6. Treatment for Lyme Disease Dependent on Stage Diagnosed

Stage	Treatment
Stage One	Doxycycline 100 mg orally every 12 hours for 14 for 21 days OR amoxicillin 500 mg orally every 8 hours for 14 to 21 days.
Stage Two	Doxycycline 100 mg orally each 12 hours or amoxicillin 500 mg orally every 8 hours for 28 days. CNS is involved—Medrol Dose Pack over 6 days ceftriaxone 2 g IV each day or cefotaxime 2 g IV every 8 hours

Stage 3

This stage begins after 1 year in about 50% of untreated patients. Signs and symptoms are varied and include neuropsychiatric symptoms, such as memory loss, sleep disorders, depression; peripheral neuropathic symptoms, such as carpal tunnel syndrome or neuropathies; and there are often recurrent synovitis, tendonitis, or bursitis (Table 12–6)

Diagnostic tests:

Test	Result Indicating Disorder	CPT Code
ELISA tests (IgM and/or IgG) for antibody to *B. burgdorferi*.	Positive antibodies indicate disease	82239
Skin, blood, cerebrospinal fluid, and/or synovial fluid cultures	Culture for *B. burgdorferi*	CPT code assigned by pathology after specimen analyzed

Differential diagnosis:

- Viral syndromes (no rash)
- Rocky Mountain spotted fever (geographical area of infection)

Follow-up: See the patient with stage 2 and 3 disease closely for a period of months to years for careful monitoring; if refractory to treatment, see patient for re-evaluation.

Sequelae: Possible complications (especially without proper diagnosis and treatment) include recurrent synovitis, tendonitis, bursitis, chronic neurologic symptoms, and peripheral neuropathy.

Prevention/Prophylaxis: The U.S. Food and Drug Administration (FDA) approved the first vaccine against Lyme disease for human use in 1998. LYMErix has shown a 50% effective rate if vaccinations were given as two injections 2 months apart. The vaccine is designed to be part of a total plan to reduce the risk of getting Lyme disease in the event of an exposure, not a guarantee against the disease. Prevention strategies include advising the patient about the disease and increasing awareness of tick activity in the area (ticks are most active from April through September). Advise the patient to wear protective clothing, such as long-sleeved shirt and pants tucked into socks, when in wooded areas (light-colored clothing makes ticks easier to spot); to wear an insect repellent containing up to 30% DEET; and to check entire body for ticks after spending time in high-risk areas. If a tick is found, advise the patient to grasp it with a pair of tweezers, as close to the head of the tick as possible. Pull straight out, gently but firmly.

Referral: Refer to, or consult with, physician, especially patients with stage 2 and 3 disease.

Education: Explain the disease process, signs and symptoms, and treatment (including side effects of medications). Discuss preventive strategies. Educational resources are available from the Lyme Borreliosis Foundation, P.O. Box 462, Tolland, CT (203-871-2900).
See www.lymenet.org; www.lymealliance.org

RHEUMATOID ARTHRITIS

SIGNAL SYMPTOMS▶ Swollen joints, especially proximal interphalangeal joints, and metatarsal joints; Pain/heat in joint areas

Arthritis, rheumatoid	ICD-9-CM: 714.0

Description: Rheumatoid arthritis (RA) is an autoimmune disease that causes chronic inflammation of connective tissue, primarily in the joints. The first joint tissue to be affected is the synovial membrane, which lines the joint cavity. Eventually, inflammation may spread to other related structures, such as the ligaments and tendons. RA is divided into four stages: disease is present but not causing disability; disease is beginning to interfere with daily activity; major compromise in function affects life and work; and incapacitation, where the patient is mostly confined to bed or chair.

Etiology: Genetic predisposition is implicated.

Occurrence: Affects 1% of adults worldwide. RA increases morbidity including increased medical expenditures, lost income and a decreased quality of life.

Age: Occurs at any age; peak onset in the fourth decade

Ethnicity: More common in Native Americans.

Gender: Occurs three times more in women than in men.

Contributing factors: Family history, genetic factors.

Signs and symptoms: Key symptoms are morning stiffness that persists for at least 1 hour along with painful, swollen joints. There is symmetric joint involvement, typically of the wrists, knees, elbows, ankles, shoulders, metatarsal-phalangeal and subtalar joints. Stiffness tends to abate with activity. Other symptoms may include malaise, muscle weakness, fatigability, weight loss, and low-grade fever. Patients with RA and a single joint inflamed out of proportion to the rest of the joints must be evaluated for coexistent septic arthritis.

Key signs include the symmetric joint findings described above with associated tenderness, warmth, and a typically "boggy" feel to the affected joints. Later, there may be joint effusion or joint destruction, including subluxation, dislocations, and ankylosis. At least four of these features must be present for at least six weeks for diagnosis

- Morning stiffness
- Arthritis of three or more joint areas
- Arthritis of hand joints
- Symmetrical arthritis
- Rheumatoid nodules
- Serum rheumatoid factor
- Radiographic changes

Diagnostic tests:

Test	Result Indicating Disorder	CPT Code
Rheumatoid factor (RF)	Titer greater than 1:80 is detectable in 70 to 90% of patients does not establish diagnosis unless coupled with associated clinical findings	86430
ESR	Elevated indicating inflammatory process	85652
Antinuclear antibodies (ANA)	Levels are elevated in about 30% of patients	86038
Synovial fluid	Yellowish white and turbid increased WBC protein levels decreased viscosity and decreased glucose levels	CPT code assigned by the pathologist after specimen analyzed

Differential diagnosis:

- Osteoarthritis (Heberden's nodes, pain later in the day, no warmth)
- Ankylosing spondylitis (Back pain and stiffness)
- Systemic Lupus Erythematosus (Butterfly rash on face)
- Gout, pseudogout (Only in one asymmetrical joint)
- Lyme disease (Rash)
- Sjögren's syndrome (dry eyes and mouth)

Treatment:

Physical

Emphasize exercise and mobility, including reduction of joint stress, and physical and occupational therapy. Encourage full activity but avoidance of vigorous exercise and heavy work during acute phase as these can increase joint inflammation. Hydrotherapy or water therapy is effective. Use hot and cold packs.

Pharmacologic

NSAIDS improve symptoms and result in a significant decrease in pain and swelling. Disease-modifying antirheumatic drugs (DMARDS) are the cornerstone of treatment for RA. Methotrexate 7.5 to 20mg per week is generally well tolerated. Hydroxychloroquine (Plaquenil) is the second most commonly used DMARD at a usual dose of 6.5 mg per kg per day in two divided doses. These drugs have many side effects and require close monitoring. Corticosteroids are potent anti-inflammatory drugs and are used often with RA. Systemic corticosteroids should be used for treatment of exacerbations of RA but avoided for long periods of time due to GI toxicity, increased osteoporosis, and infection. Doses of < 10 mg daily are usually sufficient. Tumor necrosis factor (TNF) agents are the newest class of drug to combat RA. Tumor necrosis factor stimulates the release of proinflammatory agents responsible for the joint destruction in RA. The inhibition of TNF reduces the amount of proinflammatory agents in the blood stream of patients with RA.

Surgical

May be used to help relieve symptoms, improve function, and correct deformities. Common procedures include tendon transfers, osteotomy, synovectomy, arthroplasty, and total joint replacement.

Complementary Therapy:

- Blueberries, cherries, and hawthorn berries are rich sources of flavonoid molecules, particularly proanthocyanidins, which exhibit membrane and collagen stabilizing, antioxidant anti-inflammatory properties.
- Ginger (eaten or in a tea) has demonstrated the ability to decrease joint pain and swelling in patients with RA. Ginger compresses have also been shown to benefit those with RA-inflamed joints.

Follow-up: See patient frequently to assess efficiency of treatment.

Sequelae: Possible complications include erosive joint destruction, arthritis, skin vasculitis, intracardiac rheumatoid nodules, pericarditis, renal involvement, and side effects of prolonged drug therapies, decreased functional abilities, and depression.

Prevention/prophylaxis: Prevention strategies include advising the patient to splint affected joint to help relieve pain and prevent deformities and contractures; to avoid physical or emotional stress that may exacerbate the illness; to seek supportive care; to exercise to maintain joint function and flexibility; to use warm compresses to relax muscle spasm and facilitate joint movement; to obtain adequate rest (8 to10 hours of sleep nightly, 1 to 2 hours during the day); to eat a well-balanced diet; and to lose weight if overweight.

Referral: Refer to, or consult with, physician for further diagnosis and treatment; to physical therapist, occupational therapist, social services, and support groups as indicated.

Education: Explain the disease process, signs and symptoms, and treatment (including side effects of medications). Discuss prevention strategies and when to seek medical care. Advise patient about various types of assistive devices as indicated. American Rheumatism Association (800-282-7023). See *www.help4rheumatoid.com; www.allaboutarthritis.com; www.rheumatology.org/patient/factshee*

ROCKY MOUNTAIN SPOTTED FEVER

SIGNAL SYMPTOMS▶ Fever; rash

| Rocky mountain spotted fever | ICD-9-CM: 082.0 |

Description: Rocky Mountain spotted fever (RMSF) is the most virulent form of a group of tick- and mite-borne zoonotic infections known as spotted fevers and caused by various *Rickettsia* species. The *Rickettsia* invades and destroys blood vessels in all systems of the body. Most patients suffer a moderate to severe illness, but the disease can be life threatening.

Etiology: Caused by *R. rickettsii*, a small, gram-negative, obligate an intracellular bacterium that is capable of invading the nucleus of host cells. It is transmitted by the bite of ticks (*Dermacentor andersoni* and *D. variabilis*). The American dog tick is the prevalent vector in the eastern United States; the Rocky Mountain wood tick in the western United States, and the lone-star tick in the southwestern United States and in Central and South America.

Occurrence: Only the adult tick feeds on humans, so infections usually occur in late spring to end of summer.

Age: Occurs in all ages; more likely in children and young adults.

Gender: Occurs more in men than in women.

Contributing factors: Exposure to vectors, outdoor activities in tick-infested areas, contact with dogs.

Signs and symptoms: Classic presentation includes the triad of fever, rash, and a history of tick exposure (however, such a history is lacking in 10% to 40% of patients). Initial symptoms are nonspecific and can be abrupt or gradual. Early symptoms include fever; malaise; headache that is often severe, with associated myalgias; nausea; vomiting; anorexia; abdominal pain; and photophobia.

Physical examination may reveal a rash that presents in 85% to 90% of patients. The rash usually appears 3 to 5 days after the onset of fever. Early in the disease it is maculopapular, and as it evolves, it becomes more defined and petechial. It usually begins on the extremities and spreads to the trunk.

Diagnostic tests: Diagnosis is often presumptive, based on symptoms and history of exposure in an endemic area.

Tests	Result Indicating Disorder	CPT Code
Serum proteus OX-19	Fourfold increase in acute and convalescent or solitary titer greater than 1:320 (relatively specific).	82905
Serum complement fixation (CF) antibody	Fourfold increase or solitary titer greater than 1:16.	86171
Punch skin antibody biopsy direct immunofluorescence testing	Early confirmation of RMSF rickettsia appears as early as 3 days after onset of the illness in the skin lesions).	CPT code assigned by pathology after specimen analyzed
CBC with differential	Thrombocytopenia/Anemia suggestive of RMSF	85022/86025
Chemistry	Hyponatremia	84295

CBC, complete blood count, RMSF, Rocky Mountain spotted fever.

Differential diagnosis:

- Measles (maculopapular eruption over entire body, general rash, extremely rare; check immunization status)
- Rubella (Forchheimer's spots, small rose-colored to reddish spots located on soft palate that appear before general rash)
- Koplik's spots (on buccae mucosa preceding rash, highly communicable characterized by fever, general malaise, sneezy, nasal congestion, cough)
- Meningoencephalitis (intense headache, light and sound sensitivity, delirium, irregular fever)
- Idiopathic thrombocytopenia (profoundly decreased WBC, RBC, platelets; weight loss, pale, weak)
- Purpura (characterized by hemorrhage into skin, mucous membrane, internal organs)
- Rheumatoid arthritis (symmetric joint involvement, pain, swelling, erythema, warmth, positive RA factor)
- Rheumatic fever (systemic, febrile illness, pericardia discomfort, murmur, migratory polyarthritis)
- Toxic shock syndrome (severe hypotension, fever, rash, cardiopulmonary collapse)
- Salmonellas (diarrhea)
- Lyme disease (rash, history of tick exposure)
- Allergic drug reactions (history of drug ingestion)

Treatment:

 RF 12–1 Red Flag: Cases of RMSF must be reported to the CDC and local and/or state health departments.

Doxycycline 100 mg orally or intravenously every 12 hours, tetracycline 25 to 50 mg/kg orally divided into four doses daily, or chloramphenicol 50 to 75 mg/kg/day orally or intravenously divided into four daily doses with a maximum dose of 4 g daily are all effective against this organism. Chloramphenicol IV is preferred if central nervous system (CNS) manifestations are prominent. Symptoms resolve within 72 hours, and therapy can be discontinued after 7 days. .

Follow-up: If patient is not hospitalized, see every 2 to 3 days until symptoms subside.

Sequelae: Poor prognosis and increased mortality are associated with a delay in starting appropriate antibiotic treatment, increasing age, and absence of the history of tick exposure.

Prevention/prophylaxis: Prevention strategies include advising the patient to avoid contact with ticks; to have pets undergo appropriate treatment for tick infestations; and to wear protective clothing (such as long pants and long-sleeved shirts), use insect repellent, and inspect skin daily for tick bites when in tick-infested areas or areas endemic for RMSF. If a tick is found, carefully remove tick and dispose of it in a container of alcohol or flush down the toilet.

Referral: Refer to, or consult with, physician; report case to CDC.

Education: Explain the disease process, signs and symptoms, and treatment (including side effects of medications). Discuss prevention strategies. See *http://blunix.hl.state.ut.sus/els/epidemiology; www.lyme.org/otherdis/rmsf*

SJÖGREN'S SYNDROME

SIGNAL SYMPTOMS▶   Dry eyes and mouth; decreased saliva and tear production; dryness of bronchus, skin, and vagina

Collagen disease: ICD-9-CM: 710.9

Description: Sjögren's syndrome is a common autoimmune disorder that often occurs secondarily to an inflammatory connective tissue disease such as RA or systemic lupus erythematosus (SLE). It is characterized by decreased lacrimal and salivary gland secretions caused by a chronic dysfunction of the exocrine glands.

Etiology: The cause is poorly understood. Genetic, immunologic, hormonal, and environmental factors may contribute to its development. It is thought that an insult to the immune system, such as a viral syndrome or bacterial infection, may trigger the disorder in a genetically susceptible person, which results in the deposition of auto antibodies to two protein RNA complexes, termed SS-A/RO and SS/B/LA, which cause the tissue damage.

Occurrence: It is the most common connective tissue disorder; approximately 4 million Americans affected; about 50% of all persons with rheumatoid arthritis develop Sjögren's syndrome.

Age: Occurs between ages 30 and 60 years, with a mean age of approximately 50.

Ethnicity: No significant ethnic predisposition.

Gender: Occurs in women nine times more than in men.

Contributing factors: Connective tissue disorders, RA, scleroderma, SLE, primary biliary cirrhosis, Hashimoto's thyroiditis, polyarteritis, pulmonary fibrosis, Raynaud's phenomenon, vasculitis, family history of autoimmune disorders.

Signs and symptoms: There is usually a slowly developing siccant complex (dry eyes, mouth, and nasal mucosa). The patient might complain of a "gritty" sensation in the eye along with redness, burning, and photophobia. A classic complaint is a "film" across the eye. There may also be abnormal sensations of taste or smell. Other signs and symptoms may include dry nasal and respiratory passages, cough, vaginal dryness and dyspareunia, fatigue, arthralgia, low-grade fever, and occasionally, hair loss and generalized itching.

Physical examination may reveal mouth ulcers, dental caries, "chipmunk faces," and enlarged parotid glands and lymph nodes.

Diagnostic tests:

Test	Result Indicating Disorder	CPT Code
ESR	Elevated in more than 90% of patients	85652
Rheumatoid factor	Present in 75% to 90% of patients	86430
Serum protein electrophoresis	Hypergammaglobulinemia in 50% of patients	86320
Schirmer test	Measures quantity of tears produced in 5 minutes	86235
Lacrimal or salivary gland biopsy	Confirms diagnosis; shows infiltration of the tissue by lymphocytes, plasma cells, and macrophages	68510

Diagnostic criteria are keratoconjunctivitis, diminished salivary flow, and a positive salivary gland biopsy showing mononuclear cell infiltration, and presence of autoimmune antibodies in a serum sample.

Differential diagnosis:
- Xerostomia (occurs in conjunction with Sjögren's disease)
- Salivary duct stones (pain and swelling in salivary duct area)
- Mumps (pain and swelling general malaise)
- Chronic thyroiditis (thyroid gland enlargement, signs of hyper/hypo thyroidism)
- Chronic active hepatitis (jaundice)
- Gastric achlorhydria (stomach pain, lower abdominal discomfort)
- Acute pancreatitis (abdominal pain)
- Polymyositis (muscle pain)

Treatment:

Pharmacologic

Symptomatic treatment may include artificial tears (for eye dryness), methylcellulose swab or spray (for mouth dryness), nystatin (for fungal infection of the mouth), corticosteroids (may be prescribed), K-Y jelly (for vaginal lubrication), and normal saline solution drops or aerosol spray (for respiratory dryness).

Physical
Symptomatic treatment such as soft contact lenses or special chamber moisture glasses (to protect the cornea), a cool mist ultrasonic humidifier (to help add moisture), warm compresses or heating pad (for relief of joint pain or swollen gland discomfort), and adequate oral fluid intake.

Follow-up: See the patient as needed depending on symptoms and periods of exacerbation.

Sequelae: Possible complications include respiratory infections, increasing disability and, occasionally, renal failure and extra glandular proliferation may become malignant, for example, lymphoma.

Prevention/prophylaxis: Prevention strategies include advising the patient to have meticulous oral hygiene and regular dental visits, to ingest adequate fluids, to use sugarless gum or candies to moisten mouth, and to avoid foods such as sugar (which contributes to dental caries), spicy foods, tobacco, and alcohol (which may contribute to mouth irritation). If mouth lesions become painful and interfere with nutritional status, protein-rich liquid supplements should be provided. Also advise the patient to wear sunglasses when outside, not to rub eyes, and to use eye drops and ointment as instructed. Also advise the patient to use a humidifier at home, to avoid hot showers or baths, and to avoid saliva-decreasing medications.

Referral: Refer to, or consult with, rheumatologist if systemic disease is suspected, to other specialist depending on organ involvement.

Education: Explain the disease process, signs and symptoms, and treatment (including side effects of medications). Discuss prevention strategies and signs and symptoms of ear, nose, mouth, respiratory, and vaginal infections. Educational resources are available from Sjögren's syndrome Foundation, 382 Main Street, Port Washington, NY 11050 (516-767-2866). See *www.sjogren's.com; http://members.tripod.com*

REFERENCES

General

Dambro, M: Griffith's 5-Minute Clinical Consult. Williams & Wilkins, Baltimore, 2001.

Dunphy, LM and Winland-Brown, E: Primary Care: The Art & Science of Advanced Practice Nursing. FA Davis, Philadelphia, 2001.

Goldman L, and Bennet C: Cecil Textbook of Medicine. WB Saunders, Philadelphia, 2000.

Goroll, A. and Mulley, A: Primary Care Medicine: Office Evaluation and

Management of the Adult Patient, ed. 4. Lippincott, Williams & Wilkins, Philadelphia, 2000.

Noble, J (ed): Primary Care Medicine, ed. 3. Mosby, St Louis, 2001.

Rakel, R, and Bope, E: Current Therapy. WB Saunders, Philadelphia, 2002.

Sellers, R: Differential Diagnosis of Common Complaints, ed. 3. WB Saunders, Philadelphia, 2000.

Uphold, C, and Graham, MV: Clinical Guidelines in Family Practice, ed. 3. Barmarrae Books, Gainesville, Fla, 2000.

Anaphylaxis

Genasi, F: Anaphylaxis management. Professional Nurse 16(9):1331, 2001.

Anemia

Brill, JR, and Baumgardner, DJ: Normocytic anemia. Am Fam Physician 62(10):2255-2264, 2000.

Call-Schmidt, T: Interpreting lab results: A primer. Medsurg Nursing 10(4):179–184, 2000.

Ludwig, H, and Strasser K: Symptomatology of anemia. Semin Oncol 28(2), 2001.

Chronic Fatigue Syndrome

Millea, PJand Holloway RL: Treating chronic fatigue. Am Fam Physician 62(7):1575–1582, 2000.

Robertson, TJ: Comical notebook. Misunderstood illnesses: Fibromyalgia and chronic fatigue syndrome. Alberta RN 55(3):6–15, 1999.

Wright, JB, and Beverley, DW: Current topic. Chronic fatigue syndrome, Arch Intern Med 79(4):368-374, 1999.

HIV

Boyle, B: HAART and adherence. The AIDS Reader 10(7):392–396, 2000.

Boyle, B: Issues in Antiretroviral Therapy: When to Start? The AIDS Reader 11(2):66–70, 2000.

Ferri, et al. AIDS Update. Clinician Review 8(7):114–115, 2001

Florida Department of Health. HIV/AIDS Update. Tallahassee, Fla, 2000

Groer, M: Advanced Pathophysiology: Application to Clinical Practice. Lippincott, Philadelphia; 2001.

Northwestern University Medical School Comprehensive AIDS center. Medscape, New York, 2000.

Phair JP, and King E: HIV/AIDS Annual Update 2000. Medscape, New York, 2000.

Riley, S: Legal and Legislative Issues in HIV/AIDS. Bureau of HIV/AIDS, Tallahassee, Fla., 2000.

Mononucleosis

Godshall, SE, and Kirchner, JT: Infectious mononucleosis; complexities of a common syndrome. Postgrad Med 107(7):175–179, 2000.

Lyme Disease

Lapp, T: Practice guidelines. AAP issues recommendations on prevention and treatment of Lyme disease. Am Fam Physician 61(11): 3453–3454, 2000.

Sigal, LH: Lyme disease: A clinical update Hosp Pract 36(7):31–32, 2001.

Rheumatoid Arthritis

Blumberg, SN, and Fox, DA: Rheumatoid arthritis: Guidelines for emerging therapies. American Journal of Managed Care 7(6):617–626, 2001.

Ignatavicius, DD: Rheumatoid arthritis and the older adult. Geriatric Nursing 22(3):120, 2001.

Rocky Mountain Spotted Fever

Goudeau, J, and Roberts, GH: Rocky Mountain spotted fever. Journal of Continuing Education Topics and Issues 2(1):37–40, 2000.

Sjögren's Disease

Anaya, J, and Talal, N: Sjögren's syndrome comes of age. Semin Arthritis Rheum 28(6):355-359, 1999.

Chapter *13*
PSYCHOSOCIAL PROBLEMS

ABUSE, ALCOHOL, UNSPECIFIED DRINKING BEHAVIOR

SIGNAL SYMPTOMS▶ Behavioral manifestations in a variety of areas
Need for a drink in early A.M.

Alcohol dependence	ICD-9-CM: 303.90
Alcohol abuse	ICD-9-CM: 305.00
Acute alcoholic intoxication	ICD-9-CM: 303.0
Alcohol withdrawal	ICD-9-CM: 291.81

Description: According to the *Diagnostic and Statistical Manual of Mental Disorders, Fourth Edition (DSM-IV)* **alcohol abuse** is a maladaptive pattern of excessive alcohol use leading to impairment or distress. The person continues the drinking behavior despite significant alcohol-related problems. **Alcohol dependence** is a maladaptive pattern of alcohol use characterized by the need to use alcohol more frequently in greater amounts with greater tolerance and by the inability to reduce use despite efforts and knowledge of the harmful effects.

Etiology: Complex etiology that includes biological, psychological, and sociocultural factors. The physiologic cause is thought to be genetic flaw in metabolizing alcohol. The psychodynamic view relates alcohol abuse to an expression of intrapsychic conflict with the repetitive use of alcohol to alleviate anxiety or emotional stress. Learning theorists view alcoholism as a learned behavior, and sociocultural schools of thought attribute the abuse to social and cultural influences.

Occurrence: Lifetime prevalence is of alcohol disorder is between 11% and 15%, with a high of 15.9% seen in ages 18 to 29, and a low of 7.4% during middle adulthood. It is thought to increase with aging, but statistics on this are unclear. Frequently coexists with other mental disorders, especially depression. Twenty percent of all primary care encounters may be alcohol related.

Age: Occurs in all ages; high prevalence in people age 18 to 29 and 65 and 74.

Ethnicity: People of some cultures, such as Native Americans, appear to be affected more than others. Many Japanese people have a deficiency in aldehyde dehydrogenase, which impairs metabolism and makes the person more susceptible to the effects of alcohol.

Gender: Occurs more in men (10%) than in women (3.5%).

Contributing factors: Easy accessibility of alcohol, family history of alcohol abuse, alcoholic spouse or family member of the spouse, use of other psychoactive substances, poor self-esteem, peer group pressure, adolescence, social nonconformity, stressful life events, loss, depression, other psychiatric disturbances all may contribute to abuse. Being the last child born into a large family, being of Irish, Scandinavian, or Native American descent, history of maternal depression for more than one generation, and upbringing in a broken home have all been identified as contributing factors. Some associated conditions are nicotine addiction, prescription drug abuse, depression, bipolar disorder and antisocial personality. Women may have associated reproductive tract disorders, as well as histories of sexual abuse or incest. Being single or divorced has been identified as a risk factor, unemployment, and occupation as a bartender, house painter, or traveling salesperson.

Signs and symptoms: The patient rarely presents with a chief complaint of alcohol abuse or dependence. Rather, common problems include psychological issues such as irritability, mood changes, anxiety, depression, insomnia, and impotence; or somatic symptoms such as gastric upset, headaches, fatigue, palpitations, and neuropathies. Alcoholics' desire to deny or conceal their problem makes it challenging to detect.

 Clinical Pearl: In the primary care setting 50% to 90% of patients who abuse alcohol or drugs are not recognized as abusers and only about 10% are referred for treatment.

History

Obtain information about recent stressors such as job loss, divorce, and legal problems. Suicide and domestic abuse often involve alcohol and alcohol is also a major factor in assaults and rapes. Consider a history of alcohol abuse with medical problems such as gastritis and other gastrointestinal (GI) complaints, hepatitis, or liver dysfunction. Because the patient often denies or minimizes alcohol use, it may be necessary to interview family members.

 Clinical Pearl: Alcoholism may present as a history of trauma. Even an old finding of thoracic vertebral or rib fracture on chest x-ray may prompt suspicion of potential alcohol dependence or abuse. These injuries occur 22 more times in alcoholics than nonalcoholics. Patient rarely present with reports of alcohol abuse.

Physical Examination

Because there are medical complications associated with alcoholism, a complete physical examination including laboratory tests is necessary. Physical examination may reveal weight loss or gain, labile or refractory hypertension, skin vascularization, tongue or hand tremors, epigastric tenderness, hepatomegaly, cognitive deficits, and signs of previous or current trauma. Special attention needs to be focused on the liver and central nervous system.

Diagnostic tests:

The CAGE questionnaire that may be used to screen or help diagnosis. Two or more yes responses to the following questions may signify a problem with alcohol:

> **C**ut down—Have you ever felt should cut down drinking?
>
> **A**nnoyed—Are you annoyed when others criticize your drinking or suggest you have a problem?
>
> **G**uilty—Do you feel guilty about your drinking?
>
> **E**ye opener—Have you ever had an eye opener in the morning to steady your nerves or to get rid of a hangover?
>
> Score > 2 is 79% to 95% specific for alcohol disorder (74% to 89% sensitive); less sensitive (43% to 73%) for early problem drinking or heavy drinking.

Two other psychological questionnaires are the MAST (Michigan Alcohol Screening Test) with a sensitivity of 90% and specificity of 74% and the AUDIT (Alcohol Use Disorders Identification Test), which is 70% to 92% sensitive and 73% to 94% specific.

A score of 2 or higher on the five-item Trauma Scale of the Addiction Research Foundation is another indicator of alcohol abuse/dependence. Ask in the following order:

1. Have you had any fractures or dislocations since you were 18?
2. Have you been injured in a traffic accident?
3. Have you had a head injury?
4. Have you been injured in an assault or fight?
5. Have you been injured after drinking?

Test	Result Indicating Disorder	CPT Code
Blood alcohol level (provides level of intoxication).	The following are all considered diagnostic for abuse: 300 mg/100mL at any time; 100 mg/100mL during a routine physical examination; and 150/100mL without evidence of intoxication	82055

Diagnostic tests that may be performed include liver enzymes and erythrocyte mean corpuscular volume (MCV) (may show increase) and gamma glutamyl transferase level (GGT) (is the most sensitive indicator of alcohol-induced liver damage. If levels are more than 30 units/L, it is suggestive of heavy drinking). If both MCV and GGT are elevated, it is likely that there is a significant drinking problem. Serum amylase and ammonia level (elevated in an acute episode), nutritional and vitamin profiles (shows nutritional deficiencies), and liver biopsy (helps diagnose alcoholic hepatitis or cirrhosis) all help in the diagnosis of alcohol problems.

Differential diagnosis:
- Nonpathologic alcohol use (no physical or emotional disturbances related to alcohol)
- Alcoholic withdrawal syndrome (tremors or shaking of hands; increased pulse, respiration, temperature; anxiety, panic, hallucinations)
- Chronic alcoholic brain syndrome (pathologic, irreversible changes to brain from alcohol)
- Alcoholic hallucinosis (serious mental disorder caused by alcoholism marked by fear or anxiety and visual and auditory hallucinations)
- Wernicke-Korsakoff syndrome (Severe mental disorder caused by alcoholism characterizes by psychosis and hallucinations; may be irreversible)
- Viral hepatitis (absence of behavioral disorders)
- Other cerebellar ataxia (can be distinguished during neurologic workup)
- Benign essential tremor (may be a separate benign disorder)
- Affective disorders
- Other forms of substance abuse, and major depressive disorders

The high incidence of physical and psychological co-morbidities may make the diagnosis difficult.

Treatment: Management of alcoholism may run the gamut from inpatient treatment to a brief, educational intervention. It may be necessary to confront the patient with the diagnosis of alcohol abuse or dependence and present alcoholism as a treatable disease. Do not tell the patient to stop drinking because it may induce withdrawal, which is a medical problem with significant morbidity and mortality. Referral or consultation with a specialist in alcohol abuse are usually necessary.

The goal of treatment is for the patient to maintain sobriety and complete abstinence from alcohol. The severity of the disease and the ability of the patient to cooperate with treatment will be considered when deciding on in-patient or outpatient treatment. If there is a risk of a major alcohol withdrawal (delirium tremens), concurrent and severe medical or psychiatric problems, inadequate social supports, or failure to complete an outpatient, an in-patient program is warranted. Short-term counseling intervention may include discussion of the risks, of the physical and psychological consequences, comparison of the patient's alcohol intake with deteriorating physiologic markers and a recommendation for abstinence. It may be necessary to assist the patient in identifying high-risk situations for drinking, providing advice and referral, identifying motives to reduce drinking, monitoring intake with a self-report diary, use of self-help books, and negotiating a treatment goal.

General Therapy for Outpatient Treatment

Strongly encourage the patient to seek counseling and provide positive support. Various community resources are available for the patient and family, the most common being Alcoholics Anonymous (AA) for the patient and Al-Anon for family. Concurrent management includes encouraging proper nutrition with vitamin supplements, adequate physical exercise and rest. Other therapies such as stress management, relaxation techniques, and biofeedback may also be used. Once the patient is sober, advise the patient to avoid all alcohol, including products containing alcohol such as cough syrups.

Pharmacologic

Disulfiram, 125 to 500 mg/day, is an aversive drug used to discourage alcohol abuse once the patient is sober. It may be a helpful adjunct in short-term management but is contraindicated if the patient cannot maintain sobriety because of the severity of the side effects. Disulfiram is contraindicated in the elderly population. The patient should ingest no alcohol 24 hours before the start of treatment. Naltrexone (ReVia) 50 mg orally each day, is sometimes effective as a short-term management tool to reduce cravings. Neither of these drugs should be used in the potentially suicidal patient. Thiamin and Folic Acid are supplemental to all.

For inpatient detoxification and management of alcohol withdrawal: chlordiazepoxide, diazepam, or lorazepam is used for patients with severe liver disease; phenobarbital is less frequently used. Beta blockers are used for persistent sinus tachycardia, and clonidine for autonomic hyperactivity (tremor, tachycardia, and hypertension).

Follow-up: Inpatient treatment and detoxification will include necessary medical care. Outpatient treatment necessitates regular and close medical monitoring of symptoms, especially if the patient has associated medical problems or comorbid psychiatric problems. The patient also need social support or outpatient referral.

Sequelae: Possible complications include alcoholic dementia, alcoholic hallucinosis, hypertension, neuropathy, Wernicke-Korsakoff syndrome, central and peripheral nervous system complications such as chronic brain syndrome, and peripheral neuropathies, hypertension, cardiomyopathy, cirrhosis, and esophageal varices, as well as, relapses, trauma, malignancies. If the patient is pregnant, fetal alcohol syndrome in the infant must be considered. Alcoholism is a progressive disease; it eventually causes death, usually related to cirrhosis and liver failure.

Prevention/prophylaxis: Prevention strategies include advising the patient to seek prevention counseling if the patient has a family history of alcoholism and get support during times of life changes and stressors. Teach and encourage use of relaxation and stress reduction techniques.

For the patient who is pregnant or considering pregnancy, advise her to avoid drinking during the pregnancy. Encourage and support public health and education and "no drinking while driving" measures.

Referral: Refer to, or consult with, psychiatrist or addiction specialist. If indicated, refer for inpatient treatment care. For outpatient care, refer to addiction support groups such as AA; Al-Anon; employee assistance programs; or appropriate individual, family, or group therapy.

Education: Explain the disease process, signs and symptoms, and treatment (including side effects of medications). Discuss prevention strategies. Encourage patient and family participation in support groups. Educational resource materials available from local AA programs (*http://www.alcoholics-anonymous.org*) and the National Clearinghouse for Alcohol and Drug Information (800-729-6686 or *http://www.health.org*). Encourage the patient and family to read "Alcohol: What to Do If It's a Problem for You," available from the American Academy of Family Physicians, 8880 Ward Parkway, Kansas City, MO 64114-2797 (800-944-0000).

SUBSTANCE USE DISORDERS

SIGNAL SYMPTOMS▶ Weight loss, Perforation of nasal septum (cocaine use), Pupillary dilation (opioids)

Drug dependence	ICD-9-CM: 304
Opioid dependence	ICD-9-CM: 304.00
Sedative, hypnotic, or anxiolytic dependence	ICD-9-CM: 304.10
Cocaine dependence	ICD-9-CM: 304.20
Cannabis abuse	ICD-9-CM: 305.20
Sedative, hypnotic, or anxiolytic abuse	ICD-9-CM: 305.40
Opioid abuse	ICD-9-CM: 305.50
Cocaine abuse	ICD-9-CM: 305.60

Description: Substance abuse, as defined by the *Diagnostic and Statistical Manual of Mental Disorders, Fourth Edition (DSM-IV)* is a maladaptive pattern of substance use leading to clinically significant impairment or distress. It is manifested by one or more of the following with-in a 12-month period: recurrent substance use resulting in a failure to fulfill major role obligations at work, school, or home. Recurrent substance use in situations in which it is physically hazardous; recurrent substance-related legal problems; or continued substance use despite having persistent or recurrent social or interpersonal problems. **Substance dependence** is a maladaptive pattern of substance use leading to significant impairment and/or distress as manifested by three (or more) of the following items occurring at any time in the same 12-month period:

- Tolerance, as defined as a need for markedly increased amounts of the substance to achieve the desired effect, or markedly diminished effect with the continued use of the same amount of the substance; substance is taken in larger amounts or over a longer period of time than intended

- Withdrawal
- Persistent desire or unsuccessful efforts to cut down on use of the substance
- A great deal of time is spent procuring the substance
- Other activities are given up in favor of the substance

All of the above continue despite the patients awareness of the sequelae

Etiology: Cause is not clear. Many factors contribute including genetic, psychodynamic, behavioral, and socio-cultural factors. Transgenerational drug abuse is becoming more common and some patients become addicted to substances as a way to self medicate their undiagnosed psychiatric disorders.

Occurrence: It is estimated that 10% to 16% of all primary care patients suffer from problems relating to substance abuse. Only about 10% of patients who meet diagnostic criteria are actually diagnosed with the disorder. (Numbers are approximate because of the illegal nature of many substances.) 36% have used an illicit substance at least once. 13.9 million or 6% (11.4% for ages 12 to 17) have used in past month.

Age: Predominate age is 18 to 25, although may occur in all ages.

Clinical Pearl: Maintain a high level of suspicion in elderly patients whose substance dependence and abuse problems are often overlooked.

Ethnicity: Incidence higher in blacks and people of Hispanic heritage. However, more white middle-class individuals are using these substances.

Gender: Usage in men is greater than in women.

Contributing factors: Being a young man is a risk factor for substance abuse, as are unemployment and low socioeconomic factors. Likewise, social difficulties, low self-esteem, criminal activities, family or peer-use approval and accessibility of substances puts an individual at risk. Family history of substance abuse, use of other psychoactive substances, peer group pressure, social nonconformity, stressful life events, loss, depression, other psychiatric disturbances, and chronic pain syndromes.

Signs and symptoms: The patient rarely presents with chief problem of substance abuse. Signs and symptoms vary with the substance abused. Generally, they are subtle, but they tend to become more apparent as the substance abuse increases. Common signs and symptoms include personality changes, irritability, decline in schoolwork or work activities, isolation, decreased ability to concentrate, depression, and weight loss or gain.

Cocaine abuse may lead to irritability, changes in mood, nasal bleeding, headache, fatigue, insomnia, chronic hoarseness, anxiety, and depression. Moderate use of stimulants such as cocaine produces hyperactivity, irritability, and labile mood. Moderate use of opioids produce apathy, pupillary constriction, impaired judgment, and impaired social functioning. Some chronic users of either substance may have symptoms of paranoia.

If the patient presents with signs and symptoms of overdose, immediately transport patient to clinical emergency department.

History

History is often unreliable. Obtain information about recent stressors such as job loss, divorce, and legal problems. Obtain a history of substance abuse including family substance abuse history. Inquire about social and behavioral problems such as job problems, unstable relationships, and criminal incarceration. Ask about blackouts, mood swings, repetitive injuries, and infections such as sexually transmitted diseases (STDs) or human immunodeficiency virus (HIV) status, as well as frequency of emergency room visits. It may be necessary to interview other family members if substance abuse is strongly suspected, because the patient will often deny or minimize the problem.

Physical Examination

The physical examination may be nonspecific, and findings will depend on the substance abused. The examination may reveal findings such as needle marks, dilated or constricted pupils, and perforation of the nasal septum (cocaine abuse). Refer to Table 13–1 for symptoms of and treatment for abuse of commonly abused substances.

Diagnostic tests:

- Diagnosed by the following *DSM-IV* criteria for opioid abuse:
    Vital sign changes
    Pupillary constriction
    Drowsiness
    Inattentiveness
    Perspiration or chills
    Sclerosed veins in IV users.
- Diagnosed by the following DSM-IV criteria for Cocaine Abuse:
    Weight loss
    Increased energy
    Rambling speech
    Impaired judgment
    Changes in vital signs
    Pupillary dilatation
    Perforated nasal septum

Test	Results indication disorder	CPT code
Urine or blood toxicologies or screens	Will determine substance and level of intoxication for both substances).	

Table 13–1. Symptoms and Treatment of Selected Commonly Abused Substances

Type	Substance	Symptoms	Treatment
CNS Depressants	Barbiturates and benzodiazapines.	*Marked:* Reduced insight and judgment. *Moderate:* Euphoria, depression. *Mild:* Anxiety	Phenobarbital in divided doses that are decreased daily, or diazepam in decreasing doses; for benzodiazepines, gradually reduce dose over 10 to 14 days or more.
Opioids	Codeine, meperidine, morphine, hydromorphone, heroin.	*Marked:* Euphoria, reduced insight and judgment. *Mild:* Depression, anxiety.	Naloxone for overdose; methadone in decreasing doses over 10 or more days for withdrawal. Clonidine 0.1 mg for increased B/P.
CNS Stimulants	Cocaine and amphetamines.	*Marked:* Euphoria, delusions, hallucinations, hyperactivity, tremors, pupil dilation, hypertension, tachycardia, hyperthermia, reduced insight and judgment. *Mild:* Depression, anxiety	Diazepam for agitation; propranolol for tachycardia.
Hallucinogens	Phencyclidine (PCP), lysergic acid diethylamide (LSD), mescaline.	*Marked:* Hallucinations, hyperactivity, reduced insight and judgment. *Moderate:* Euphoria, depression, anxiety, delusions, tremors, pupil dilation, hypertension, tachycardia, hyperthermia.	Diazepam for mild agitation and anxiety; haloperidol for severe episodes; use phenothiazines only with LSD, can be fatal if used with other hallucinogens.

- Urine tests usually identify the use of specific drugs during the 1 to 3 days before the submission of the sample; blood tests usually identify drug use within 4 to 12 hours before testing.
- Other diagnostic tests performed depend on the substance abused and the patient's condition. Obtain a serum sample for complete blood count (CBC), blood chemistry panel, and liver enzymes (LFT).

Differential Diagnosis: Organic dysfunction versus functional illness. Consider polysubstance abuse, depressed mood, and generalized anxiety disorders, which are clarified by blood toxicology results. Diagnosis may be difficult because of co-morbidities, drug interactions, and underlying medical conditions such as malnutrition, fluid and electrolyte imbalance, and respiratory disorders.

Treatment:

Emergency Treatment

Emergency treatment of the patient who has overdosed or is unconscious includes immediate transport to clinical emergency department through emergency medical services. The major priorities are to establish an adequate airway, support circulation, control hemorrhaging, and then deal with any destructive behavior.

General Measures

Confront the patient with the diagnosis of substance abuse or dependence, and present it as a treatable disease. Merely telling the patient to stop taking the drug may be futile and dangerous. Referral or consultation with a specialist in substance abuse. The goal of treatment is for the patient to have complete abstinence from the substance. Whether treatment is conducted in an inpatient or outpatient setting depends upon the severity of the disease, the presence of comorbid conditions, history of seizure disorders, threat of harm to self and others, and abilities of the patient. The risk of major substance withdrawal, concurrent and severe medical and/or psychiatric problems, inadequate social supports, and failure to complete an outpatient program may all warrant hospital admission.

General Therapy for Outpatient Treatment

The chemically dependent patient usually benefits from a multiple-treatment approach that includes psychologic and physiologic treatment and support, as well as sociocultural and spiritual counseling. If recovery is to be successful, a total change in lifestyle is usually required. Strongly encourage the patient to seek counseling and provide positive support. Various resources are available for the patient and family and include individual, group, and/or family therapy; half-way houses; and employee assistance programs. Twelve-step programs such as Alcoholics Anonymous or Narcotics Anonymous are extremely important for both the patient and the family. Other support groups include Rational Recovery and secular organizations for sobriety. Medical management includes treatment of any concurrent medical problem. Common medical problems associated with substance abuse include malnutrition with vitamin deficiencies, fluid and electrolyte imbalances, respiratory infections, skin abscesses, cellulitis, dental caries and loss of teeth, hepatic dysfunction, bacterial endocarditis, thrombophlebitis, pulmonary embolism, seizures, amenorrhea, and impotence.

Follow-up: Monitor the patient closely during the initial treatment phase; may initially require daily follow-up, then weekly following treatment, then less frequently.

Sequelae: HIV, hepatitis, malnutrition, abscesses, social and legal problems. Marital and family difficulties often occur. Overdoses resulting in seizures, arrhythmias, cardiac and respiratory arrest, coma, death. May require inpatient treatment and detoxification. Patients who stay in treatment for at least a year have a higher success rate.

Prevention/prophylaxis: Prevention strategies include advising the patient to seek prevention counseling if the patient has a family history of drug abuse and support during times of life changes and stressors. Reduce risks through education, especially of young adults. Early detection and treatment are crucial.

Referral: Refer to psychiatric provider or addictions specialist. If indicated, refer for inpatient treatment care. For outpatient care, refer to addiction support groups, employee assistance programs, or appropriate individual, family, or group therapy.

Education: Explain the disease process, signs and symptoms, and treatment (including side effects of medications). Teach proper nutrition and need for physical activities and rest. Discuss prevention strategies. Encourage patient and family participation in support groups. Educational resource materials are available from local support programs and the National Clearinghouse for Alcohol and Drug Information (800-729-6686 or *http://www.health.org*). Groups such as Cocaine Anonymous and Narcotic Anonymous use approaches from Alcoholic Anonymous (*http://www.alcoholics-anonymous.org*). Alternative approaches such as Rational Recovery and Secular Organizations for Sobriety are also available.

ANOREXIA NERVOSA

SIGNAL SYMPTOMS▶ Significant weight loss, absence of menses for 3 months, bradycardia, dehydration,

Anorexia nervosa   ICD-9-CM: 307.1

Description: Anorexia nervosa is diagnosed according to the DSM-IV by three criteria: weight loss leading to a weight at least 15% below ideal body weight, absences of three consecutive menses, and intense fear of weight gain. Most patients with anorexia have a disturbed body image as well. There are two types or anorexia. The first is the restricting type characterized by diet, fasting, or exercise. The second type is the binge/purge type characterized by self-starvation alternating with episodes of bingeing and purging with the use of self-induced vomiting of the use of laxatives, diuretics, enemas to prevent weight gain.

Etiology: No organic cause is known; it is a complex psychiatric illness. No psychiatric hypothesis explains anorexia. However, a psychological thesis is that anorexia is an attempt to regain a sense of control through the refusal to eat. Many anorexic patients exhibit obsessive-compulsive personality characteristics and rigid perfectionistic thinking. Many also exhibit symptoms of depressive disorders.

Occurrence: In the United States, about 0.5% to 1% of the female population meets the *DSM-IV* criteria; about 5% of those age 16 to 25 are estimated to have subclinical anorexia. Anorexia is more prevalent in industrialized societies. Anorexia is rarely found in men.

Age: The onset is usually between ages 12 and 22 years for anorexia for women; later for men. Onset is rare after 40 years of age.

Ethnicity: Occurs predominately in whites and Japanese.

Gender: Occurs more (90%) in girls and women than in boys and men; however, the incidence in boys and men is increasing.

Contributing factors: Sociocultural stressors and pressures, such as, multiple school or social activities, and acceptance of culturally condoned ideas of beauty related to thinness. The person often exhibits rigid perfectionist thinking and has an anxious, self-critical, overachieving personality. Physical stressors include early puberty, unstable body image, perceptual distortions. At high risk are ballet dancers, gymnasts, models, cheerleaders, runners, other athletes in whom low weight is desirable.

Signs and symptoms:

History

Obtain information on any patterns of bingeing and purging, other self-destructive behavior, and previous psychiatric history. Patients may switch back and forth between anorexia and bulimia.

Signs and Symptoms

Common complaints include cold intolerance, emaciation, lanugo, constipation, amenorrhea, bradycardia, loss of body fat, dry skin and hair, dehydration, swelling of the hands and feet, abdominal bloating and parotid enlargement with purging.

Physical Examination

Often presents as emaciated (less than 85% of desired weight) and amenorrheic (usually for longer than 3 months). Physical examination may reveal impaired renal function, dental problems, and osteoporosis. Physical examination may reveal the following: hair (dull, dry, brittle, sparse), eyes (xerophthalmia, increased vascularity, keratomalacia), lips and buccal cavity (cheilosis; angular fissures; red, swollen lesions), tongue (smooth, swollen, beefy red, atrophic papillae), gums (spongy, recessed, bleed easily), skin (rough, dry, pale petechiae, lacking subcutaneous fat, lack of turgor), muscles (wasted, flaccid, tenderness, weakness, loss of tone), nervous system (decreased or absent knee and ankle reflexes, lethargy), cardiovascular (cardiomegaly, bradycardia at rest, tachycardia with exercise, hypotension), skeletal (prominent ribs, scapula, bowed legs or knock-knees), and abdomen (enlarged, hepatomegaly). Evaluate for suicidal intent.

Diagnostic Tests: Diagnosed by the *DSM-IV* criteria described earlier. Most laboratory findings are related to dehydration and starvation; no findings are specific for anorexia and all tests may be within normal limits.

Vital signs may reveal orthostatic hypotension and EKG may reveal bradycardia or cardiac irregularities such as prolonged QT interval if weight loss or purging is significant. There may be abnormal liver enzymes, diminished serum BUN and creatinine, low CD4/CD8 ratio, low serum zinc level, neutropenia with relative lymphocytosis, diminished plasma, LH, FSH, T_3 and elevated growth hormone, cortisol, cholesterol, vasopressin. Osteoporosis may be present (order a bone density examination).

Differential Diagnosis: Other psychiatric disorders include:

- Major depressive disorder (may cause significant weight loss; however, weight control is not a focus in major depression)
- Schizophrenia (may also cause weight loss. These patients do not fear gaining weight but may not eat because of delusion that food is poisoned or so impaired by psychoses that self-care neglected or non-existent.)
- Social phobia (similar in that patients may avoid eating in public places. Dissimilar in that with social phobia, the focus is general public scrutiny)
- Obsessive-compulsive disorder (similar in that patients exhibit compulsions and obsessions related to food. It should be diagnosed only if the patient exhibits additional obsessions and compulsions in addition to food and body image.)
- Bulimia nervosa, and eating disorder NOS (recurrent episode of binge eating to maintain at or above 85% of body weight)
- Other medical conditions to consider include the following: gastrointestinal disorders, brain tumors, acquired immunodeficiency syndrome (AIDS), hypothyroidism, superior mesenteric artery syndrome. Also consider metabolic disorders such as celiac, Crohn's disease, panhypopituitarism, as well as tuberculosis, lymphoma, and hypothalamic disorders.

Treatment: If the patient's physical condition is life-threatening, factors that justify involuntary hospitalization include starvation resulting in cognitive impairment and patient expressing psychotic beliefs about his or her weight and shape. The goal of treatment is to restore normal body weight and restoration of menses. Two to six percent develop complications of the disorder, and there is a 10% mortality rate associated with anorexia. Death usually results from starvation, suicide, or electrolyte imbalance.

Physical

- Therapy: Individual, family, or group therapy, including cognitive psychotherapy. Common topics include body image and factors that led to eating disordered behavior.
- Nutritional therapy and education: Teaching about basic nutrition, discussing ritual and forbidden foods, and maintaining a regular meal plan. Involve the patient in establishing target weight with gradual weight gain. Weigh weekly at first, then monthly. Challenge fear of uncontrollable weight gain.

Pharmacologic

The antidepressant fluoxetine, along with a short-acting benzodiazepine such as lorazepam or oxazepam, in low doses, 30 minutes before meals, may be helpful for short-term treatment. Other selective serotonin reuptake inhibitors (SSRIs) may be used to treat the obsessive-compulsive symptoms.

Follow-up: See the patient as indicated by the condition. Long-term therapy and follow-up is usually required.

Sequelae: Prognosis is poor, especially for the patient who has had the disorder for more than 10 years; mortality is estimated to be about 10% to 15%, with no more than 50% of patients recovering completely. Relapses are common, especially when stressful situations occur. Possible complications include depression and suicide attempts. There may be potassium depletion, cardiac arrhythmias, cardiomyopathy, congestive heart failure (CHF), delayed gastric emptying, convulsions, peripheral neuropathy, nitrogen depletion, exhaustion, collapse.

Prevention/prophylaxis: Prevention strategies include helping the patient and parents focus on the psychosocial development of the adolescent. Raising children in an environment with an emphasis on caring and good communication rather than appearance is important. Encourage a rational attitude about weight and involvement in a team or competitive sport where there are built-in constraints to the amount of exercise and where the activity is nonisolating and includes a social component. Adolescents need help with social, schoolwork, and leisure skills to mature.

Referral: Refer to or consult with, psychiatric health professional specializing in eating disorders. Consultations with other members of the multidisciplinary team managing the patient care, such as nutritionist, and physical or occupational therapists is also necessary.

Education: Explain disease process, signs and symptoms, and treatment (including side effects of medications). Discuss prevention strategies. Advise patient and family when to seek medical attention and when to seek emergency medical care (life-threatening symptoms such as rapid, irregular heartbeat; chest pain, or loss of consciousness). Encourage patient and family participation in support groups. Provide reassurance and support. Educational resources are available from the Anorexia Nervosa and Related Eating Disorders Association, PO Box 5102, Eugene, OR 97405 (503-344-1144); and the National Association of Anorexia Nervosa and Associated Disorders, PO Box 7, Highland Park, IL 60035 (708-831-3438).

BULIMIA NERVOSA

SIGNAL SYMPTOMS ▶   **Parotid gland enlargement, dental enamel loss**

Bulimia nervosa   ICD-9-CM: 307.51

Description: The *DSM-IV* describes bulimia nervosa as binge eating and the inappropriate use of compensatory methods to prevent weight gain. Recurrent episodes of binge eating are followed by purging by self-induced vomiting, use of diuretics, laxatives, or enemas. Bingeing may also be followed by self-imposed starvation, which leads to hunger, which precipitates another binge and subsequent self-loathing over loss of control. Bulimia often represents an unsuccessful attempt at dieting or weight loss. Hunger from dieting leads to binge eating, later followed by remorse, intense exercise, or purging. Bulimia continues to be a very private disorder; there is much secrecy about the bingeing on high-carbohydrate foods, so it is difficult to detect. Patients may switch back and forth between anorexia and bulimia.

There are two types of bulimia nervosa. The first is the purging type. In this type, the patient regularly engages in self-induced vomiting or misuse of laxatives, diuretics, or enemas.

In the nonpurging type, the patient uses other inappropriate compensatory behaviors, such as fasting or excessive exercise.

Etiology: No organic cause; it is a complex psychiatric illness. There is often a hereditary predisposition for mood disorders, an inability to discriminate between hunger and satiety, neuroendocrine dysfunction affecting metabolism, and psychological and sociocultural factors.

Occurrence: In the United States, 2% to 5% of female adolescents are estimated to meet the *DSM-IV* criteria, with an estimated 5% to 15% experiencing dimensions of the disorder. Prevalence in college age women may be as high as 19%. Bulimia generally occurs in young middle-to-upper class women.

The true incidence is not known because this is a secretive disorder.

Age: Onset is usually between age 15 to 25 years for bulimia for women; later for men. May occur at any age.

Ethnicity: Occurs predominately in whites.

Gender: Occurs more (90%) in girls and women than in boys and men.

Contributing factors: Sociocultural pressures, stressful life events, multiple responsibilities, tight scheduling, competition. Mood disorders such as depression, use of alcohol or drugs, behavior and personality that include emotional reactivity, elements of impulsivity, histrionics, and a general disgust or intense loathing of the body followed by severe caloric restriction. Ambivalence about dependency vs. independence. Often part of a "dual-diagnosis."

Signs and symptoms:

History

Obtain information on bingeing and purging, self-destructive behavior, previous psychiatric history, and weight pattern (frequent fluctuations of weight of 10 pounds or more is common; patient is often of normal or higher-than-normal weight for height).

Signs and Symptoms

Common complaints include parotid gland enlargement, swelling of the hands and feet, abdominal bloating, depression, headaches, fatigue, and muscle cramps or weakness. Evidence of self-mutilation inflicted by cutting or burning on arms, legs, or abdomen. Menses is usually preserved with bulimia.

Physical Examination

May reveal skin changes ranging from abrasions to scarring in the dorsum of the hand (from trauma associated with using the hand to stimulate the gag reflex), hypertrophy of parotid glands (from repeated vomiting), and dental erosion (associated with an acid bath to the back of the throat). Evaluate for suicidal intent.

Diagnostic tests: Serum blood tests include complete blood count (CBC) and a chemistry panel including electrolyte levels. Frequent purging may lead to hypokalemia, hyponatremia, and hypochloremia with elevated serum bicarbonate levels. Some patients have increase levels of serum amylase due to excessive vomiting and elevated BUN, along with a positive dexamethasone suppression test.

Differential diagnosis: Psychiatric disorders such as

- Anorexia nervosa (eating disorder marked by excessive fasting)
- Binge/purge type (repetitive behavioral cycle around eating)
- Mood disorders (alteration in affect)
- Substance abuse or dependence especially stimulant abuse (maladaptive pattern of substance abuse)

Physical considerations include

- Gastrointestinal disorders (associated disturbances)
- Psychogenic vomiting (vomiting induced by patient)
- P pharyngitis (sore throat from repeated vomiting)
- G asteric dilation (from intermittent bingeing)
- Pancreatitis (inability to digest fat)

- Esophagitis (from wear and tear on esophagus from repeated vomiting)
- Electrolyte disturbances (second to decreased food/oral intake)
- Dehydration (second to decreased food/oral intake)
- Constipation (second to decreased food/oral intake)
- Hemorrhoids (frequent straining to move bowels)

Treatment:

Physical

Therapy: Individual, family, or group therapy, including cognitive behavioral techniques.

Nutritional therapy and education: Teaching about basic nutrition, discussing ritual and forbidden foods, and maintaining a regular meal plan. Identify precipitants to binging or purging, as well as alternatives; address ruminations

Pharmacologic

Fluoxetine may be given at a higher dose (60 to 80 mg) than the recommended antidepressant dose. Other SSRI such as fluvoxamine (Luvox) 50 to 300 mg/day (higher doses often needed) are also seeking indication for treatment of bulimia. Occasionally augmented with buspirone (BuSpar). Tricyclics, such as imipramine (Tofranil) 10 mg with gradual increase to 250 mg if needed (monitor with EKGs) may also be tried. If there is an underlying bipolar disorder, patients may benefit from lithium (Eskalith) 300 mg. twice a day, increase gradually to therapeutic blood level of 0.6 to 1.2 mmol/L). Ondansetron (Zofran) 4 to 8 mg three times a day between meals may help with prevent vomiting. Psyllium (Metamucil) preparations may help prevent constipation during laxative withdrawal.

 Clinical Pearl: Lithium and tricyclic medication can be lethal when administered to hypokalemic patients. Additionally, dishonesty and noncompliance are common.

Follow-up: See the patient as indicated by condition. Long-term therapy and follow-up is usually required. Monitor binge-purge activity, repeat any laboratory tests that had abnormal values weekly or until stable. Monitor ruminations and depression, exercise, comfort with body, self and others.

Sequelae: Prognosis is highly variable, especially for the patient who has had the disorder for more than 10 years. A relapse rate of 30% to 50% per year for several years is not uncommon. Patients with personality disorders have a generally poor prognosis. Death is rare from this disorder unless there is co-morbid depression and suicide attempts. May spontaneously remit. Those who stay in therapy tend to improve. Impulsive patients may engage in stealing, suicide gesture, substance abuse, and promiscuity.

Prevention/prophylaxis: Prevention strategies include helping the patient and parents focus on the psychosocial development of the adolescent. Raising children in an environment with an emphasis on caring and good communication rather than appearance is important. Encourage a rational attitude about weight and involvement in a team or competitive sport where there are built-in constraints to the amount of exercise and where the activity is nonisolating and includes a social component. Adolescents need help with social, schoolwork, and leisure skills to mature. Goal is a balanced diet with adequate calories and resumption of a normal eating pattern.

Referral: Refer to a psychiatric health professional specializing in eating disorders. Consultations with other members of the multidisciplinary team managing the patient care, such as nutritionist, and physical or occupational therapists is also necessary.

Education: Explain the disease process, signs and symptoms, and treatment (including side effects of medications). Discuss prevention strategies. Advise the patient and family when to seek medical attention and when to seek emergency medical care (life-threatening symptoms such as rapid, irregular heartbeat; chest pain; or loss of consciousness). Encourage patient and family participation in support groups. Provide reassurance and support. Educational resources available from the Anorexia Nervosa and Related Eating Disorders Association, PO Box 5102, Eugene, OR 97405 (503-344-1144); and the National Association of Anorexia Nervosa and Associated Disorders, PO Box 7, Highland Park, IL 60035 (708-831-3438).

DEPRESSION

SIGNAL SYMPTOMS▶ Sad or depressed mood for a 2-week period
Feelings of hopelessness

Depressive disorder, not elsewhere classified	ICD-9-CM: 311
Major depressive disorder, single episode	ICD-9-CM: 262.2
Major depressive disorder, recurrent	ICD-9-CM: 296.3

Description: According to the *DSM-IV,* the essential feature of major depression is a two-week period with a depressed mood or loss of pleasure (anhedonia) or interest in the usual activities of life. Neurotransmitter systems are disrupted with mood disorders. Unipolar relates to mood disorders in which only depressive episodes occur. Bipolar relates to mood instability in which episodes of depression and mania or hypomania occur.

 Clinical Pearl: May be a life-threatening disorder. Always assess for suicidal intent.

Etiology: Mood disorders occur as a result of genetic tendencies, psychosocial stressors, general medical illnesses, and/or grief reaction. Metabolic changes and substance abuse may contribute to the occurrence of a mood disorder. The primary neurotransmitters involved in mood disorders are serotonin and norepinephrine. Learned behavior and environmental factors may effect neurotransmitters or have an independent influence on depression. Lack of these neurotransmitters cause certain types of depression e.g., depressed norepinephrine causes dullness and lethargy, while decreased serotonin causes irritability, hostility and suicidal ideation. Various theories, biologically and psychodynamically based, abound.

Occurrence: It is estimated that 15% of the population will experience a major depression at least one time during their lives. Approximately 10% to 15% or more of major depressive conditions are caused by general medical illness. Five to twelve percent of patients seen in the primary care offices have major depressive disorder. Depression is the fourth most common reason people visit their primary care provider. Ten to fifteen percent of postpartum women will experience a mood disorder within 2 weeks to 6 months of delivery. Thirty to fifty percent of patients with medical disorders such as cancer, cardiac disease, or cerebrovascular accident develop depression.

Age: Major depressive disorder may occur at any time in life, whereas bipolar disorder usually begins in late adolescence or early adult life. Mean age for unipolar depression is in the 40s and peaks again in older adults.

Ethnicity: No significant ethnic predisposition.

Gender: Occurs more in women than in men.

Contributing factors: Family history of depression, prior episodes of depression, prior suicide attempt, lack of social supports, stressful life events, current substance, or alcohol abuse. Certain medications may contribute to depression such as reserpine, digitalis, benzodiazepines, oral contraceptives, glucocorticoids, levodopa, beta blockers, and other hypertensive agents. Illnesses such as rheumatoid arthritis, multiple sclerosis, chronic heart disease are associated with depression too. Hormone fluctuations are also implicated in mood disorders. Chronic pain, insomnia, and advancing age may also contribute to depression. Situational changes and crises, such as loss of a loved one or loss of a job, may precipitate a depressive episode. Female gender and advancing age are both risk factors.

Signs and symptoms:

History

Obtain information about any prior depression or suicide attempt, family history of unipolar or bipolar disorder or family history of suicide attempt, concurrent medical or psychologic illnesses, substance or alcohol abuse, stressful life events, and lack of social support. If there is a history of prior episodes of depression, ascertain the type of treatment, level of recovery. Ascertain if there is a history of manic or hypomanic episodes.

Clinical Pearl: Depression in primary care may present as fatigue, somatic complaints (backache, chest pain, dyspepsia, limb pain), anxiety symptoms, depressed mood, weight loss or gain, or insomnia.

Signs and Symptoms

DSM-IV criteria for major depression state that at least five symptoms must be present for longer than a 2-week period. One of the symptoms **must** be either depressed mood or loss of interest in pleasure. Other symptoms include significant weight loss unrelated to dieting; insomnia; fatigue or low energy; psychomotor agitation or retardation, feelings of worthlessness, or excessive guilt; decreased concentration; indecisiveness; or recurrent thoughts of death and suicide with or without a plan. Common somatic complaints may include pain, headache, body aches, apathy, anxiety, malaise, sadness, and or sexual complaints.

Bipolar disorder with manic symptoms includes labile mood, elevation of mood, hyperactivity, easily distracted, hyperverbal, pressured speech, irritability, and decreased need for sleep. Hypomania is a less intense mood instability. The mood changes may occur suddenly and may last from a day to several months.

Clinical Pearl: No screening tool for serious suicidal ideation has high sensitivity; ask about intent, plan, access to means, and ability to contract for safety.

Diagnostic Tests:

- Diagnosed by *DSM-IV* criteria. See Table 13–2. A quick assessment of depression is facilitated by the following mnemonic SIGECAPSS:

Table 13–2. DSM-IV Diagnostic Criteria: Major Depressive Episode

Must include at least five of the following symptoms; at least one of the symptoms must be either depressed mood or loss of interest or pleasure. These symptoms must represent a change from previous level of functioning and be present for more than 2 weeks.

To be defined as a major depressive episode, the symptoms must not be attributable to the effects of substance use, bereavement, or a general medical condition; must cause clinically significant distress or impairment in function.

- Depressed mood, most of day, on a daily basis, by subjective report or observation by others (e.g., feels sad, empty)
- Diminished interest or pleasure in most activities
- Increase or decrease in appetite with associated weight loss or gain (5% of body weight in a month)
- Insomnia or hypersomnia nearly every day
- Psychomotor Retardation or agitation as observed by others
- Fatigue, decreased energy nearly every day
- Inappropriate guilt (may be delusional); feelings of worthlessness
- Indecisiveness; poor concentration
- Recurrent thoughts of death or suicide

American Psychiatric Association: Diagnostic and Statistical Manual of Mental Disorders, ed. 4. American Psychiatric Association, Washington D.C., 1994.

S	Sleep pattern changes
I	Interest in normal activities diminished
G	Guilty feelings
E	Energy decrease
C	Concentration decreased
A	Appetite changes
P	Psychomotor retardation or excitation
S	exual desire diminished
S	Suicidal thoughts

- Psychological testing that may be performed includes self-report scales such as the Beck Depression Inventory (BDS), Zung Self-Rating Depression Scale (ZSRDS), and The Hamilton Rating Scale for Depression (HRD-S) is a clinician generated rating scale used in psychiatry. Children's Depressive Inventory (CDI) is a depressive inventory for use with children; Yesavage's Geriatric Depression Scale is for use with older adults.
- Laboratory tests may be performed to rule out physiologic causes. Serum blood should be drawn for complete blood count (CBC), thyroid-stimulating hormone (TSH), and chemistry profile. Estrogen levels are also important to evaluate in perimenopausal women.
- Mental status examination, including level of alertness, orientation, mood, affect, thought content (hallucinations, delusions, suicidal/homicidal ideation, if present), thought processes, psychomotor activity, speech, insight, and judgment. Flostein's Mini-Mental Status Examination may help identify a delirium or dementia.
- Depression is primarily a clinical diagnosis that depends on skillfully eliciting family, social and psychosocial data.

Differential Diagnosis: Grief reaction and concurrent medication use or polypharmacy may lead to depression. In some cases, the disturbed mood is a result of a physiologic condition. The following conditions must be considered: hypothyroidism, renal or liver disease, cardiac disease, seizure disorder, infection, or cancer; organic brain syndrome; chronic fatigue syndrome, and vitamin deficiencies. Psychiatric disorders such as panic and other anxiety disorders, alcohol abuse and/or substance abuse, and schizophrenia must be ruled out. May be a dual-diagnosis.

Treatment: If the depression is caused by physical illness, treat the condition. Then, if the depression continues, treatment should be initiated. The plan should be developed with the patient and include pharmacology and psychotherapy for maximal results. Initial intervention is for 6 to 12 weeks to bring about a response and decrease in symptoms. Continued treatment for 9 to12 months is necessary to prevent a relapse. Provide patient education prior to the treatment; monitor for side effects of medication; monitor regularly for signs of worsening depression; adjust the plan as necessary.

Red Flag: Hospitalization is indicated if serious suicidal deation is present, if patient is a danger to self or others, if there is a significant medical co-morbidity, or lack of support system as home.

Physical
Encourage proper nutrition and adequate physical exercise and rest. Treat any underlying nutritional deficiencies.

Psychotherapeutic
Individual, group, or family therapies may be used. Support groups are also helpful.

Pharmacologic
The severity and persistence of the symptoms, recurrent episodes, presence of psychotic features, family history, prior response to treatment, incomplete response to psychotherapy, and patient preference may influence the decision to use medication. Most patients experience marked improvement or complete remission of symptoms. If the patient has severe depression, combination therapy may be needed along with referral. Electroshock therapy (ECT) be indicated in resistant cases of depression and hospitalization is required initially for this treatment.

- The antidepressant drugs are classified as tricyclics (TCAs), selective serotonin reuptake inhibitors (SSRIs), atypicals, and monoamine oxidase inhibitors (MAOIs). See Table 13–3 for dosage, and possible adverse effects. Each patient initiating antidepressant therapy needs to know that 2 to 3 weeks may pass before any response occurs.

 Clinical Pearl: Monitor for increasing suicidal ideation during this period.

- Full effects of the antidepressants take 4 to 6 weeks to achieve.

Table 13–3. Selected Antidepressants

Name	Dosage (range/day)	Possible Adverse Effects
Selective Serotonin Reuptake Inhibitors (SSRIs)		
Best given in A.M.; all may cause anxiety, insomnia, appetite suppression, sexual dysfunction [main reason for patients discontinuing use]; overdose less likely to be fatal; abrupt discontinuation may result in withdrawal symptoms; decrease beginning doses by half for children and elderly		
Fluoxetine	10–80 mg every A.M.	Insomnia, nausea
Paroxetine	10–50 mg every A.M.	Insomnia, nausea
Nefazodone	300–600mg	Insomnia, nausea. Start at 100 mg twice a day
Citalopram	10–60 mg every A.M.	Insomnia, nausea
Sertraline	25–200 mg every A.M	Insomnia, nausea

(Continued)

Table 13–3. Selected Antidepressants (Continued)

Name	Dosage (range/day)	Possible Adverse Effects
Polycyclic (Mostly Tricyclic [TCAs]) Antidepressants		
All have the potential for fatal overdose; prescribe in small amounts initially to prevent overdose		
TCAs may produce arrhythmias and lower seizure threshold		
Decrease beginning dose by half in children and elderly		
Amitriptyline	75–300 mg	Sedation, anticholinergic effects, orthostatic hypotension Take at HS
Amoxapine	100–300 mg	Sedation, anticholinergic effects, orthostatic hypotension, insomnia Give in divided doses
Desipramine	75–300 mg	May have activating properties, insomnia, anticholinergic effects, insomnia, anxiety
Doxepin	75–300 mg	Sedation, anticholinergic effects, orthostatic hypotension, take at HS
Imipramine	75–300 mg	May have activating properties; anticholinergic effects, insomnia, anxiety
Maprotiline	75–200 mg	Sedation, anticholinergic effects, orthostatic hypotension, take at HS
Nortriptyline	75–150 mg	Sedation, anticholinergic effects, orthostatic hypotension, take at HS
Trazodone	150–300 mg	Sedation, anticholinergic effects, orthostatic hypotension, take at HS
Trimipramine	75–250 mg	Sedation, anticholinergic effects, orthostatic hypotension, take HS
Protriptyline	10–30 mg	May have activating properties, anticholinergic effects, insomnia
Monoamine Oxidase (MAO) Inhibitors		
Significant drug and food interactions limit their use, but may be helpful in refractory cases		
Phenelzine	30–90 mg	Sedation, orthostatic hypotension, insomnia
Tranylcypromine	10–60 mg	Orthostatic hypotension, insomnia, nausea
Others		
Bupropion	75–450 mg	Seizure risk in higher doses; minimal risk of sexual dysfunction Give in divided doses
Mirtazapine	15–45 mg	Somnolence, appetite increase, risk of agranulocytosis
Venlafaxine	50–375 mg	Anxiety, insomnia, anorexia - allow approximately 2 week "wash out" of other medications before instituting therapy - Give in divided doses.

If the patient is pregnant, use caution in prescribing psychotropics; fluoxetine has been used safely in patients with severe depression who are in the second trimester. Dosage may need careful titration.

Follow-up: See patient 2 weeks after starting medication and at least every 2 weeks until symptoms improve, then every 3 months. If depression does not improve, referral may be necessary. Plan to treat the patient for 12 months to 2 years after initial response occurs. During follow-up visits, evaluate side effects, dosage, and effectiveness of medications. The nature of the relationship between the patient and nurse practitioner is important to treatment success. Each plan must be individualized to the patient. Anticipate recurrences. Provide continued support.

Sequelae: Possible complications include suicide (70% of patients who commit suicide have depressive illness) and recurrence (over 50% of patients). However, in general, this is a treatable, reversible, and temporary illness with an excellent prognosis.

Prevention/prophylaxis: Prevention strategies include providing close and careful monitoring of the patient with a family history or prior episodes. Work on treatment of any underlying physical, chronic conditions.

Referral: Refer to, or consult with, psychiatric specialist if the patient has potential for suicide, recalcitrant symptoms, or frequent recurrence; is very young, very old, or pregnant; or as indicated.

Education: Explain the disease process, signs and symptoms, and treatment (including side effects of medications). Discuss prevention strategies. Advise the patient when to seek medical attention. Encourage participation in support groups. Suggest that the patient or family read, "How to Cope with Depression" by Depaulo and Avlow. Educational resource material available from the National Depression/Manic-Depression Association (800-82M-DMDA).

DOMESTIC VIOLENCE

SIGNAL SYMPTOMS Numerous injuries at multiple sites in various stages of healing, recurrent fractures

Domestic violence	
Sexual abuse of an adult	ICD-9-CM: 995.81
Physical abuse of an adult	ICD-9-CM: 995.81

Description: Domestic violence, often referred to as spousal or partner abuse, involves physical, emotional, or sexual abuse. Domestic violence may extend to children and relatives, and may involve destruction of personal property and pets. Domestic violence is the single major cause of injury to women. It is estimated that nearly 25% of women in the United States are abused by a current or former partner, and 50% of all women killed in the United States are killed by their partners.

Etiology: Domestic violence is an issue of power and control. A cycle of violence (physical and sexual) characterizes the relationship. Power and control are at the center, with the abuser using intimidation, emotional abuse, isolation, minimizing, denying, blaming, threatening the children, male privilege, economic abuse, coercion, and treats to maintain dominance. Abusers are often not violent toward anyone except the people they love. Fear usually motivates the victim to stay in the abusive environment.

Occurrence: Common; acts of domestic violence occur every 18 seconds in the United States. A woman's lifetime risk for abuse is 22%. Between 17% and 31% of women and up to 30% of men in same-sex partnerships experience violence in relationships. The prevalence of abuse during pregnancy is estimated between 2% to 17%.

Age: Occurs at any age.

Ethnicity: No significant ethnic predisposition; occurs in all socioeconomic, racial, ethnic, and religious groups.

Gender: Most acts of domestic violence occur against women; 95% are committed by men.

Contributing factors: Past history of abuse, personality with a need for power, poor self-image, sees violence as natural, poor communication skills, or intense jealously; history of or current alcohol or substance abuse; pregnancy.

Signs and symptoms:

History

History is most important. The patient may present with nonspecific symptoms such as abdominal or chest pain, headaches, insomnia, pelvic pain, fatigue, back pain, or a choking sensation. In the case of injury, ask directly, "Did someone hurt you? Were you hit?" If domestic violence is suspected, the most important step is to ask the patient directly if he or she is or has been abused. Asking this question may help break the silence often imposed by victims. The information gathered helps determine the nature of the injuries and helps establish a trusting relationship. If domestic violence is suspected, try to question the patient alone. If this is not possible, observe the behavior between the patient and the partner. Ask when and how the injuries occurred; a delay in seeking treatment may occur. Often, the victim will take responsibility for the injury or take blame for the partner's behavior. If the patient states that abuse has occurred, question about the abuse and plans the patient may have for dealing with the abuse.

Signs and Symptoms

There may be clear evidence of trauma from unclear or suspicious etiology or there may be more subtle cues. Common injuries include contusions; abrasions; sprains; lacerations; fractures; injuries to head, neck, chest, breasts, abdomen, and/or genitals. Frequently, these are not "fresh" injuries, but injuries in various stages of healing. There may be numerous injuries at multiple sites, at various stages of healing, or repeated or chronic injuries. Subtle cues may include chronic pain; sleep or appetite disturbances; fatigue; or chronic headaches. Other symptoms may include abdominal or GI complaints; palpitations; dizziness; atypical chest pain. Women may have frequent urinary tract infections (UTIs), sexually transmitted diseases (STDs), or vaginal infections; dyspareunia; or sexual dysfunction. Psychological disturbances such as anxiety, depression, isolation, and panic attacks may occur. Victims may use or abuse of drugs or alcohol.

Clinical Pearl: Suspect domestic violence if unexplained injuries are present, if the patient's explanation seems unlikely. Victims often avoid eye contact and seem overly agitated or wary. Cancellation of appointments is common. An abuser may attempt to stay close to monitor what patient is saying.

Physical Examination

Physical examination may reveal a "bathing-suit pattern" of injuries, where injuries, such as contusions and bruises, are located in areas that are not normally seen. Multiple anatomic sites of injury often indicate abuse as contrasted with single-limb injury from true accidents.

Diagnostic tests: Diagnosed primarily by history and physical examination. Diagnostic tests, such as x-ray studies, help confirm or rule out specific injuries. Pattern of old, healed fractures on x-ray studies.

Differential diagnosis:

- Trauma of soft tissue (bruises, red areas, black and blue, discoloration of tissue)
- Bone fractures (x-ray study)
- Numerous other medical disorders (review diagnostic tests)

Also consider psychiatric disorders such as

- Anxiety (excessive worries may be in response to situation)
- Depression (due to loss of self esteem, change is social situation, occupational functioning)
- Alcohol or substance abuse (abuse to decrease anxiety, decrease insomnia, stop distressing thoughts or recollections)

Treatment: In most states, abuse must be reported. Check with your local and state laws. Photographic and other evidence may need to be obtained. Use nonjudgmental, factual language in charting; chart is a legal document.

- Treatment of the specific injury as indicated
- If patient is in immediate danger, intervene as is appropriate and safe. Do not question the patient's sense of danger. If the patient senses danger, it exists. Establish a safety plan with the patient. Victims are at increased risk when attempting to leave the abuser; most murders happen then. Remain with patient until domestic violence counselor or specialist trained in domestic violence counseling or appropriate support person is with patient.

- Provide unconditional positive regard. Recognizing and naming the abuse is an essential intervention. Be explicit that in all cases physical or sexual assault is unacceptable.
- Provide appropriate support and reassurance. Reinforce the fact that domestic violence is a crime; it is not the victim's fault. Advise patient of local resources and provide appropriate telephone numbers. Follow-up closely. Assess psychological and childcare needs.
- Resist the desire to "fix" the problem. Respect the abused person's ability to make appropriate choices. It is up to the patient to decide when and if they will leave the relationship. This time frame may be long. Take care of self. You may need to "de-brief" when working with these patients.
- Provide an office milieu of safety. For example, posters that say something like "It is okay to talk about family violence here" may be helpful. Provide patient information materials.

Follow-up: See patient as indicated by situation. Close follow-up helps build trusting relationship and allows for early intervention if needed.

Sequelae: Possible complications depend on the type and extent of injury; may also include emotional disorders, risk of future injuries to patient or other family members, and financial stresses.

Prevention/prophylaxis: Prevention strategies include advising the patient on community resources and options available (including shelters, hotline numbers, and legal and financial services), how to access those services, and helping the patient develop a safety plan. Refer to Table 13–4 for steps in the screening of domestic violence.

Referral: Refer to, or consult with, local domestic violence counselors or psychologist or social worker trained in domestic violence counseling.

Education: Explain disease process, signs and symptoms, and treatment (including side effects of medications). Discuss prevention strategies. Provide patient with the National Domestic Violence Hotline telephone number, 800-333-SAFE (7233), and other resource telephone numbers. Educational resources available from the National Resource Center on

Table 13–4. Screening for Domestic Violence

When to Screen:
- Initial and annual examinations; premarital, OB, pre-employment examinations.
- Screen patient in private; ask direct questions; assure confidentiality; if pre-employment physical, do not note on employer's form.

What to Screen for:
- Angry, jealous domineering partner; patient will not speak in front of partner; partner accompanies patient to examination room or shows anger or aggressive behavior.
- Signs and symptoms: Suspicious injury, "bathing suit" pattern of injuries (those appearing in concealed areas), mechanism of injury inconsistent with findings, multiple injuries in various stages of healing, cigarette or friction burns (especially symmetric injury of wrists, forearms, and neck), injury during pregnancy, multiple sites of injury, delay in seeking care, stress-related illness, frequent vague complaints, sexual dysfunction, drug or alcohol abuse by partner, suicide attempt, history of sexually transmitted diseases.

Table 13–4. Screening for Domestic Violence

What Specific Questions to Ask:
- Does (s)he control most of your daily activities?
- Has (s)he ever threatened to kill you? Do you believe (s)he is capable of it?
- Is (s)he violent toward you, your children, or your pets?
- Has (s)he ever threatened or attempted suicide?
- Is (s)he constantly jealous?
- Has (s)he ever forced you to have sex?
- Is physical violence increasing in frequency?

What to Do:
- Help patient assess danger; plan for safety, support, and a safe place to go; provide patient with domestic violence hot line number and legal resources; refer to domestic violence counselor or social services.
- Document all injuries, behavior objectively and nonjudgmentally; quote patient when possible; obtain photographs, drawings, and/or other evidence as indicated; report as indicated by local, state, federal laws.
- Follow up with patient and counselor.

Domestic Violence (800-537-2238); National Coalition Against Domestic Violence (202-638-6388); National Council on Child Abuse and Family Violence (508-793-6166); and Center for the Prevention of Sexual and Domestic Violence (206-634-1903).

GENERALIZED ANXIETY DISORDER (GAD)

SIGNAL SYMPTOMS▶   Excessive worry, nervousness, hyperarousal

Anxiety disorder	ICD-9-CM: 300.0
Simple phobia	ICD-9-CM: 300.29
Agoraphobia	ICD-9-CD: 300.22
Social phobia	ICD-9-CM: 300.23
Obsessive-compulsive disorders	ICD-9-CM: 300.3

Description: Generalized anxiety disorder (GAD) is characterized by the *DSM-IV* as a chronic state of anxiety (more than six months) manifested by worry, nervousness, being easily fatigued, irritable, restless or on-edge, along with muscle tension.

DSM-IV criteria for a panic attack, an exacerbation of GAD, include a discrete period of intense fear or discomfort developed abruptly and accompanied by at least four somatic symptoms listed: pounding heart or increased heart rate; chest pain or pressure; sweating, chills, or hot flashes; shaking or trembling; shortness of breath; shocking; feeling dizzy or faint; paresthesias; nausea; fear of dying or feeling trapped; derealization (feelings of unreality); or depersonalization (detached from oneself). These symptoms peak within 10 minutes, and are not related to the direct physiologic effects of a substance or medication such as caffeine or cocaine, or general medical condition such as hyperthyroidism. Panic disorder develops with recurrent attacks and worry about having future attacks. Panic may lead to avoidance behavior and isolation, leading to the development of agoraphobia. Panic disorder is defined as at least two unexpected panic attacks and at least 1 month of concern over more attacks, worry about implications of the attack, or a significant change in behavioral pattern.

 Clinical Pearl: Almost 70% of patients with panic disorder have either past or present history of depression. Half of the time, a depressive episode will precede the onset of panic attacks, and half of the time it will follow. Panic attacks are seen in 30% of depressed patients.

Phobias are defined as persistent, irrational fears about an object, a situation, or an activity that arouses an intense desire to avoid the perceived fear and thus whatever causes it. Simple phobias tend to focus on a discrete stimulus such as animals, insects, or heights. Agoraphobia is defined as fear of being trapped in a situation where escape is impossible. It may center on (1) fear of being alone, (2) fear of being away from home. Most often seen in association with panic disorder. Social phobias are fear of humiliation or embarrassment in social situations when under scrutiny. Fear of public speaking is a good example.

Obsessive disorders classified as an anxiety disorder that manifests itself recurrent, obtrusive thoughts (obsessions) and ritualistic behaviors (compulsions). Thought to be defensive measures in warding off more generalized anxiety.

Etiology: Variety of theories including a genetic or familial link (biorelations of patients have a four to seven times greater chance of developing panic attacks or generalized anxiety. Psychosocial stressors may trigger the onset of panic and the dysfunction of several neurotransmitters (norepinephrine, serotonin, gamma-aminobutyric acid, dopamine, and cholecystokinin) may be involved. Stressors also may lead to the chronicity of GAD.

Occurrence: Anxiety disorders are the most common psychiatric disorders in the United States. 40 million adults may suffer from one form or another of GAD. May be present in up to 20% of all primary care patients; 3.5% of people experience a panic attack in their lifetime. Lifetime prevalence of phobias is thought to be approximately 12.5%. Obsessive-compulsive disorders have a lifetime prevalence of 2.5%. The incidence of comorbid conditions are high, especially depression.

Age: Occurs at any age. Many with GAD report having been anxious all their lives. The onset of panic disorders varies. Most panic attacks occur by the mid-thirties, and onset after 45 is unusual. Panic Disorder usually develops within the first year of developing panic attacks. Up to 50% of patients diagnosed with panic disorder develop agoraphobia.

Ethnicity: No significant ethnic predisposition.

Gender: GAD is more common in women (4.3%) than in men (2.0%).

Contributing factors: Depression (seen in 40% of patients with GAD), agoraphobia (33% of patients), alcohol abuse (26%), psychosocial

stressors such as loss or financial stress, family history, underlying medical conditions. Traumatic experience also may precipitate panic attacks.
Signs and symptoms: Patients presenting to primary care settings with anxiety usually have somatic complaints such as chest pain, palpitations, and breathlessness in the absence of cardiac disease, GI symptoms, nervousness, dizziness, headache, chronic fatigue. The patient is also likely to reveal a recent period of stress and may be a frequent user of medical services.

Diagnostic Tests:

- Interview may reveal a history of anxiety leading to impairment of social and occupational functioning.
- Psychological tests such as the Zung anxiety self-assessment, and Hamilton's Anxiety Scale are often used.
- Laboratory tests such as drug screens or toxicologies rule out substance abuse while CBC, chemistry panel, and TSH rule out physiologic causes.

Differential diagnosis: Physiologic disorders such as cardiovascular disease, respiratory disorders, CNS disorders such as transient ischemic attack (TIA) or seizure disorder, and metabolic disorders such as hyperthyroidism; alcohol or substance abuse, or withdrawal. Panic disorders must be distinguished from a cardiac event.

Treatment:

Pharmacologic

SSRIs are the drugs of choice and include fluoxetine, begin with 10 mg, increase by 10 mg every 7days to a maximum daily dose of 40 mg; sertraline, begin with 25 mg, increase by 25 mg every 7 days to a maximum dose of 200 mg; and paroxetine, begin with 10 mg, increase by 10 mg every 7 days to a maximum dose of 60 mg; citalopram begin with 10 mg, increase by 10 mg every 7 days. Because SSRIs have a slow onset (4 to 6 weeks), short-acting benzodiazepines may be needed for the initial control of symptoms. Full therapeutic response usually takes 6 weeks. A 3-month trial period, followed by 9 to 12 months or longer of maintenance therapy is usually indicated. See Table 13–3 for additional information on antidepressants.

Physical

Therapies including cognitive behavioral training, where the patient learns to recognize and re-evaluate prodromal symptoms of an attack and learns that there is nothing reality-based occurring and nothing to fear, and exposure therapy (desensitization), where the patient gradually increases exposure to the feared situation, may be used. Relaxation, distraction, and controlled breathing techniques may be taught to help the patient avoid attacks. Advise patient to keep a diary of attacks, learn stress management techniques, and maintain regular physical exercise. Provide reassurance and support.

Follow-up: See patient as indicated for close evaluation of effectiveness and side effects or dependence of medications and for support, education, and reassurance.

Sequelae: Possible complications include impaired social and occupational functioning, isolation, depression, agoraphobia, drug dependence (benzodiazepines), cardiac arrhythmias, and increased risk of suicidal thoughts and attempts.

Prevention/prophylaxis: Prevention strategies include advising the patient on the importance of regular exercise, balanced diet, decreased caffeine intake, and stress management. Encourage patient to recognize situations that trigger the attack and implement strategies to minimize the attack. Teach patient techniques to minimize hyperventilation such as rebreathing with a paper bag and slow deep breathing. Yoga exercises are beneficial for all forms of anxiety.

Referral: Refer to psychiatric specialist as indicated. Concurrent management with the specialist planning the care and the primary care provider implementing the plan may occur as a result of the trusting relationship developed with the patient.

Education: Explain the disease process, signs and symptoms, and treatment (including side effects of medications). Discuss prevention strategies. Advise patient when to seek medical attention. Educational resource materials available from the National Institute of Mental Health, National Anxiety Awareness Program, 9000 Rockville Pike, Bethesda, MD 20892 (800-64-PANIC).

POSTTRAUMATIC STRESS DISORDER

SIGNAL SYMPTOMS Recurrent intrusive recollection of event(s), emotional numbing, diminished responsiveness to social relationships, sleep difficulties

Posttraumatic stress disorder, specify if acute or chronic with delayed onset	ICD-9-CM: 293.9

Description: Posttraumatic stress disorder (PTSD) is a disabling anxiety disorder that has a high rate of comorbidity with depression. PTSD is characterized by three diverse clusters of symptoms: re-experiencing or flashback, avoidance of stimuli, and hyperarousal. PTSD is caused by exposure to a major external stressor such as, rape, sexual abuse, severe burns, military combat, disasters, or any event that is a significant threat to one's physiologic and/or psychological integrity. Witnessing a violent event or disaster that involves death, massive destruction, injury or death of family members or close associates may also lead to PTSD.

Etiology: The person experiences or witnesses a traumatic events. The person's response to the traumatic event(s) involves intense fear, help-lessness, and horror.

Occurrence: Approximately 30% of all victims of disaster or severe trauma develop PTSD. Lifetime prevalence rates reported in the community range from 1% to 14%. One of 12 adults in the general population may experience PTSD at some time in their lifetime.

Age: Occurs in all ages; young children and older adults are more vulnerable.

Ethnicity: No significant ethnic predisposition.

Gender: Occurrence varies with the type of stressor: men are more likely to experience combat situations or job trauma, young men are more vulnerable to trauma in general, and women are more vulnerable to trauma from rape and/or assault. A ratio of 2:1 female to male lifetime prevalence of PTSD is reported.

Contributing factors: Severity of the stressor, history of childhood neglect, abuse, or dysfunctional family. Children of alcoholic parents.

Signs and symptoms: The symptoms may be precipitated or exacerbated by distant events that are a reminder of the original stressor. Symptoms may begin soon after the traumatic event, within 3 to 6 months, or be delayed to six months or more. Some experience a long latency period before symptoms appear. Three clusters of symptoms coexist with this disorder. The patient has flashbacks or re-experiences the traumatic event, avoidance or decreased responsiveness to current events with the trauma and physiologic hyperarousal leading to psychosomatic difficulties. The three clusters:

- The re-experiencing cluster includes symptoms including recurrent intrusive distressing memory of the event, recurrent distressing dreams, flashbacks or acting as if the event were occurring again. Patient experience intense psychological or physiologic distress at exposure to internal or external cues that symbolize or resemble an aspect of the event.
- The avoidant cluster includes emotional numbing as well as symptoms that may superficially resemble agoraphobia. Symptoms may include efforts to avoid thoughts, feelings, or conversations associated with the event; efforts to avoid activities, places, or people that arouse recollections of the event; inability to recall an important aspect of the event; markedly diminished interest or participation in significant activities; feeling of detachment or estrangement from others; restricted range of affect; or a sense of a shortened future.
- The hyperarousal cluster may manifest with insomnia, irritability, anger, and difficulty concentrating and hypervigilance and exaggerated startle response.

If the symptoms persist for longer than 3 months the patient has chronic or delayed PTSD.

Diagnostic Tests:

- Psychometric and psychophysiologic assessment and testing administered by a psychologistand/or hypnosis may be helpful in determining etiology.
- Neuropsychologic testing may be helpful to rule out dementia and subtle cognitive dysfunction.
- Diagnostic tests such as sleep studies or EEG (rules out sleep disorders, brain damage) may be indicated.

Differential Diagnosis:

- Cognitive disorders (age-related reduction in working memory, may or may not interfere with activities of daily living)
- Sleep disorders (inability to fall asleep or stay asleep; interferes with functioning)
- Dementia (memory and cognitive disorder that impairs an individual's ability to function or have social relationships)
- Adjustment disorders (alterations in behavior/personality)
- Affective disorders (alterations in mood)
- Panic disorder (primary fear of having a panic attack in public setting)
- Personality disorders (antisocial and borderline personality)
- Acute stress disorder (symptoms last less than one month)

Treatment: Primarily treated on an outpatient basis unless there is gross dysfunction in activities of daily living or suicidal intent, in which case, referral to a psychiatric health professional is made for evaluation of need for possible hospitalization.

Physical

A variety of psychotherapeutic approaches may be used. Therapeutic modalities include behavioral interventions to achieve anxiety reduction. Cognitive and psychodynamic therapy also are used. Management also includes treating concurrent problems, such as sleep disorders, and encouraging a healthy diet (consisting of complex carbohydrates, proteins, vitamins, and minerals along with avoidance of fatty foods) and adequate balance of physical exercise and rest.

Pharmacologic

SSRIs such as fluoxetine, 20 to 80 mg; sertraline, 50 to 200 mg; paroxetine, 20 to 60 mg; or citalopram, 20 to 60 mg per day may improve symptoms of intrusion and avoidance as well as the coexisting depression often seen in these patients. Venlafaxine 75 to 300 mg and low doses of Risperidone, 0.5 to 1 mg, have proved helpful in the treatment of some patients with PTSD. Trazodone, 25 to 300 mg/day given at bedtime or nefazodone, which improves REM sleep, 100 to 600 mg/day, may be prescribed for sleep problems. Because of the high potential for abuse, use benzodiazepines very selectively and with caution. If the patient has psychophysiologic hyperactivity during intense flashbacks, propranolol and clonidine may be used to control the hyperactivity. Mood stabilizers such as Neurontin, 100 to 400 mg three times a day or oxcarbazepine (Trileptal) 300 to 600 mg per day may decrease irritability and improve impulse control.

Follow-up: See patient very closely and intensely after the traumatic event. If condition is a delayed or chronic reaction, see patient as indicated; long-term therapy is usually required. Assess for suicidal ideation.

Sequelae: If the patient meets the diagnostic criteria, there is a high incidence of a severe comorbidity such as major affective disorders, substance or alcohol abuse, and anxiety or personality disorders. Possible complications include suicide, self-inflicted violence, occupational and interpersonal impairments, and in some cases, severe, persistent, and debilitating psychiatric disorders.

Prevention/prophylaxis: Prevention strategies include advising the patient to undergo crisis intervention immediately after the traumatic event and to continue ongoing individual or group therapy to help prevent delayed or chronic PTSD. Also, advise the patient to maintain good mental hygiene (diet, activity, interpersonal support, leisure activities, avoidance of drugs and alcohol, meaningful work, involvement with others), seek treatment for any co-morbidity.

Referral: Refer to psychiatric health professional specializing in PTSD.

Education: Explain disease process, signs and symptoms, and treatment (including side effects of medications). Discuss prevention strategies, avoidance of triggering events and experiences, and when to seek medical attention. Encourage participation in support groups. Suggest patient and family read *Too Scared to Cry* by L. Terr (Harper & Row, 1990).

REFERENCES

General

American Psychiatric Association: Diagnostic and Statistical Manual of Mental Disorders, ed. 4. American Psychiatric Association, Washington, DC, 1994.

Dambro, M: Griffith's 5-Minute Clinical Consult. Williams & Wilkins, Baltimore, 2002.

Dunphy, LM & Winland-Brown, J: Primary Care: The Art and Science of Advanced Practice Nursing, FA Davis, Philadelphia, 2001.

Graber, M, and Lanternier, M: University of Iowa Family Practice Handbook, ed. 4.St. Louis, MO: Mosby, 2001.

Lucas, B.D: Coping with psychiatric emergencies in the office. Patient Care for the Nurse Practitioner, Feb, 1999.

Nemeroff, CB, and Schatzberg, AF: Recognition and treatment of psychiatric disorders: A psychopharmacology handbook for primary care. Am Psychiatric Press, Washington, DC, 1999.

Taylor, R: Manual of Family Practice, ed 2. Lippincott Williams & Wilkins, Philadelphia, 2002.

Uphold, C, and Graham, MV: Clinical Guidelines in Family Practice, Barmarrae Books, Gainesville, Fla, 2003.

US Preventive Service Task Force: Guide to Clinical Prevention Services, ed. 2. Williams & Wilkins, Baltimore, 1998.

Abuse, Alcohol and Abuse, Substance

Anton, R. F: Pharmacologic approaches to the management of alcoholism. J Clin Psychiatry. 62(Suppl 20):444, 2001.

Ewing, JA: Detecting alcoholism: the CAGE questionnaire. JAMA 252:323, 1984.

Graham, J.D: Rock bottom: Recognizing alcoholism in your patients. Advance for Nurse Practitioners 30, 2000.

Martin, AC, et al: Managing alcohol-related problems in the primary setting. The Nurse Practitioner 24(8):14–39,1999.

National Institute on Alcohol Abuse and Alcoholism, National Institutes of Health. Alcoholism. Getting the Facts. NIH Publication No. 96-4153, 1996.

Anorexia Nervosa and Bulimia Nervosa

Garner, DS, and Garfinkel, PE: Handbook of Treatment for Eating Disorders, ed. 2. Guildford Press, New York, 1997.

Orbanic, S: Understanding bulimia: Signs, symptoms & the human experience. AJN 101:3, 2001.

General Anxiety Disorder

Culpepper, L: Generalized anxiety disorder in primary care: emerging issues in management and treatment. J Clin Psychiatry. 63(Suppl 8):24, 2002.

Gorman, J. M: Treatment of generalized anxiety disorder. J Clin Psychiatry. 63(Suppl 9):56, 2002.

Greco, N, and Zajecka, , JM: Evaluating and treating comorbid depression and anxiety in women. 3:5, 2000.

Lecrubier, Y: The burden of depression on anxiety in general medicine. J Clin Psychiatry 62(Suppl 8):4, 2001.

Pollack, F H: Therapeutic spotlight: Comorbid anxiety disorders in primary care. A self-study. Supplement to Clinical Reviews 6:16, 2001.

Schatzberg, A: New indications for antidepressants. J Clin Psychiatry. 61(Suppl 11):9, 2001.

Zal, HM: Social Anxiety disorders: How to help. Consultant 8:89, 2000.

Domestic Violence

Barton, P, and Carbone, C: Domestic violence. Bert Rodgers Schools of Continuing Education, Sarasota, FL, 2000.

Jensen, LA: The cycle of domestic violence and the barriers to treatment. The Nurse Practitioner 25:5, 2000.

Pollack, MH, et al: Trauma & stress: Diagnosis & treatment. J Clin Psychiatry Audiograph Series 5:3, 2002.

Stewart, J: Becoming advocates for battered women. Clinil Rev 10:6, 2000.

Veenema, TG: Children's exposure to community violence. J Nursing Scholarship 33:2, 2001.

Major Depression

Antai-Otong, D: Dark days: Treating major depression. Advance for Nurse Practitioners 9:3, 2001.

Compton, M. T: The evaluation and treatment of depression in primary care.http://primarycare.medscape.com/ExerptalMed/ClinCornerstne/200.../pnt-clc303.04.comp.htm Accessed 7, 2001.

Craighead, WE, and Miklowitz, DJ: Psychosocial interventions for bipolar disorder. J Clin Psychiatry 61(13): 58–64, 2000.

Culpepper, L: Early onset of antidepressant action: Impact on primary care. J Clin Psychiatry. 62(suppl 4):4, 2001.

D'epiro, N. W: Chronic depression: Now, a treatable condition. Patient Care for the Nurse Practitioner 1:32, 2000.

Glaser, V: Effective approaches to depression in older patients. Patient Care for the Nurse Practitioner 9:24, 2000.

Goldberg, JF: Treatment guidelines: Current and future management of bipolar disorder. J Clin Psychiatry. 61:13, 2000.

Greco, N, and Zajecka, , J. M: Evaluating and treating comorbid depression and anxiety in women. Women's Health in Primary Care 3:5, 2000.

Kornstein, SG, and Schneider, RK: Clinical features of treatment resistant depression. J Clin Psychiatry, 62(Suppl 16):18, 2001.

Manji, HK, and Lenox, RH: The nature of bipolar disorder. J Clin Psychiatry 61(Suppl 13):42, 2000.

Shell, RC: Antidepressant prescribing practices of nurse practitioners. Nurse Practitioner 26:7, 2001.

Stahl, SM: Essential psychopharmacology of depression and bipolar disorder. Cambridge University Press, 2001, Cambridge, Mass.

Trivedi, MH, and Kleiber, BA: Algorithm for the treatment of chronic depression. J Clin Psychiatry 62(Suppl 6):22, 2001.

Weitzel, C, and Jiwanlal, S: The darker side of SSRIs. RN 64:8, 2001.

Posttraumatic Stress Disorder

Davidson, JRT: Pharmacotheraphy of PTSD: Treatment options, long-term follow-up and predictors of out come. J Clin Psychiatry 61 (Suppl 5):52, 2000.

Foa, EB, and Davidson, J RT(eds): The expert consensus guideline series: Treatment of posttraumatic stress disorder. J Clin Psychiatry, 60(Suppl 16), 1999.

McConlay, TE, Sole, ML, and Holcomb, L: Assessing the female sexual assault survivor. Nurse Practitioner 22:44, 2001.

Shalev, AY: What is PTSD? J Clin Psychiatry 62(Suppl 17):4, 2001.

INDEX

Page references followed by f reference a figure
Page references followed by t reference a table

A

Abdomen
  bloating
    in anorexia nervosa, 533
    in bulimia nervosa, 537
  chest pain and, 24–30
  disorders of, 277–348
  heat cramps and, 462
  hernias, 318–320
  lactose intolerance and, 328–329
  pain, 330
    abdominal disorders and, 279, 286,
      289, 293, 297, 303, 317, 321,
      324, 344
    differential diagnosis, 283f
    psychological problems and, 546
    symptom-based problems and,
      31, 64
ABGs. *See* Arterial blood gases (ABGs)
ABPI. *See* Ankle-Brachial Pressure Index
  (ABPI)
Abuse
  alcohol, 522–527
  irritable bowel syndrome (IBS) and,
    324
  physical, 545–549
  sexual, 545–549
  substance, 527–532
ACE inhibitors
  acute renal failure (ARF) and, 339
  for congestive heart failure (CHF), 240
  for hypertension, 248t
Acetaminophen
  chest disorders and, 227

head and neck disorders and, 148,
  186, 193, 196, 203
hematologic and immunologic
  disorders and, 509
musculoskeletal disorders and, 395,
  406
skin disorders and, 120, 172
symptom-based problems and, 50, 53
Acetazolamide (Diamox), for angle-
  closure glaucoma, 168
Acetic acid, in Condyloma acuminata, 352
Acne, 91–95
Acne rosacea, 91–95
Acne vulgaris, 91–95
Acquired hypothyroidism, 485–487
Acquired immunodeficiency syndrome
  (AIDS), 502
Actinomyces, 184
Active range of motion, in fibromyalgia,
  387
Acute alcoholic intoxication, 522–527
Acute otitis media, 188–194
Acute renal failure (ARF), 338–341
Acyclovir
  for Bell's Palsy, 426
  for encephalitis, 435
  (Zovirax), for Herpes Zoster infection,
    120
Aerobic and anaerobic cultures, in
  animal/human bites, 97
AF. *See* Atrial Fibrillation (AF)
AFP. *See* Alpha-fetoprotein (AFP)
African-Americans, prostate cancer and,
  362
Agencies Websites, 10t

3